CONCEPTS BASIC TO NURSING

LIST OF CONTRIBUTORS

Miss Margaret E. Auld, R.N., M.N.
Assistant Professor, University of Washington School of Nursing, Seattle

Mrs. Doris Carnevali, R.N., M.N.
Associate Professor, University of Washington School of Nursing, Seattle

Miss Susanna Lee Garner, R.N., M.A.
Former Instructor, University of Washington School of Nursing, Seattle

Miss Barbara Innes, R.N., M.S.
Instructor, University of Washington School of Nursing, Seattle

Dr. Madeleine Leininger, PhD.
Professor and Dean, School of Nursing; Professor and Lecturer in
Anthropology, University of Washington, Seattle

Mrs. Pamela Holsclaw Mitchell, R.N., M.S.
Assistant Professor, University of Washington School of Nursing, Seattle

Mrs. Jurate Abromaitis Sakalys, R.N., M.S.
Assistant Professor, University of Colorado School of Nursing, Denver

Miss Judith West, R.N., M.N.
Instructor, University of California, San Francisco Medical Center

Miss Rosemary Witt, R.N., M.N.
Assistant Professor, University of Nevada School of Nursing, Las Vegas

CONCEPTS BASIC TO NURSING

PAMELA HOLSCLAW MITCHELL

Assistant Professor of Physiological Nursing
University of Washington
School of Nursing

McGRAW-HILL BOOK COMPANY
A BLAKISTON PUBLICATION

New York   St. Louis   San Francisco   Düsseldorf   Johannesburg
Kuala Lumpur   London   Mexico   Montreal   New Delhi
Panama   Rio de Janeiro   Singapore   Sydney   Toronto

Library of Congress Cataloging in Publication Data

Mitchell, Pamela, 1940–
Concepts basic to nursing.

Includes bibliographies.
1. Nurses and nursing. I. Title. [DNLM: 1. Nursing care. WY 100 M681c 1973]
RT69.M55   610.73   72-10080
ISBN 0-07-042580-9

 2 3 4 5 6 7 8 9 0 MURM 7 9 8 7 6 5 4 3

This book was set in Times Roman by Rocappi, Inc. The editors were Cathy Dilworth and Barry Benjamin; the designer was Rita Naughton; and the production supervisor was Ted Agrillo. The drawings were done by Textart Service, Inc.
The printer was The Murray Printing Company; the binder, Rand McNally & Company.

CONTENTS

Preface   *vii*

PART 1   NURSING AND HEALTH CARE

Introduction   *1*
Chapter 1   The Meaning of Health and Illness / *Jurate Sakalys*   *3*
Chapter 2   Nursing in the Context of Health Care / *Pamela Mitchell*   24
Chapter 3   Nursing in the Context of Social and Cultural
                   Systems / *Madeleine Leininger*   *34*

**PART 2   THE PROCESS OF DIAGNOSIS AND
                   INTERVENTION IN NURSING PROBLEMS /** *Pamela Mitchell*

Introduction   *47*
Chapter 4   Interpersonal Relationships in Nursing   *49*
Chapter 5   The Scientific Method in Nursing   *69*
Chapter 6   The Process of Diagnosis   *74*
Chapter 7   Intervention: Planning Nursing Care   *107*

PART 3   CONCEPTS BASIC TO NURSING PRACTICE

Introduction   *131*
Chapter 8   Conceptualizing, A Nursing Skill / *Doris Carnevali*   *133*

v

Chapter 9   Psychosocial and Mental-Emotional Status / *Rosemary Witt
              and Pamela Mitchell*   *139*
              Basic needs, sociocultural influences on behavior, the family,
              developmental levels, stress and anxiety, learning, consciousness

Chapter 10   Environmental Status / *Barbara Innes*   *177*
              Safety, infection control, environmental effects on illness

Chapter 11   Sensory Status / *Pamela Mitchell*   *194*
              Sensation, sensory-perceptual restriction and overload

Chapter 12   Motor Status / *Pamela Mitchell*   *220*
              Mobility, immobility, rehabilitation

Chapter 13   Nutritional Status / *Pamela Mitchell*   *270*
              Regulation of food intake, food habits

Chapter 14   Elimination Status / *Margaret E. Auld*   *295*
              Bladder and bowel function

Chapter 15   Circulatory and Fluid-Electrolyte Status / *Pamela
              Mitchell*   *320*
              Measurement of function, fluid homeostasis—distribution, volume,
              concentration; thirst, edema, shock

Chapter 16   Respiratory Status / *Pamela Mitchell, Judith West,
              and Margaret E. Auld*   *363*
              Respiration—ventilation, circulation, cell utilization; problems
              related to dysfunction

Chapter 17   Body Temperature Status / *Margaret E. Auld*   *390*
              Temperature regulation, temperature measurement, hyperthermia,
              hypothermia

Chapter 18   Integumentary Status / *Barbara Innes*   *410*
              Skin integrity, skin breakdown

Chapter 19   Comfort and Sleep Status / *Susanna Lee Garner and
              Pamela Mitchell*   *437*
              Sleep, pain

Index   *463*

PREFACE

This textbook is prepared for the student of professional nursing—the person preparing to be the primary agent of nursing care for the various consumers of nursing services. It is based upon the premise that the professional nurse is the practitioner who determines the need for nursing care, plans the care, gives or directs its implementation, and evaluates the efficacy of the care. Nursing is a means to help people whose actual or potential deviations from health have impaired their ability to cope with some aspects of daily living. Nursing care may be aimed at preventing the initial or further deviations from health, at restoring or enhancing the ability to cope with daily activity, and at maintaining or sustaining the person's capacities through a health problem. These services may be provided independently of other health professions or in collaboration with them.

The book was conceived to meet the needs of beginning students for depth in the basic concepts upon which their practice of nursing will rest. Most textbooks in the "fundamentals" of nursing are oriented to the care of the hospitalized sick person, with passing reference to his extrainstitutional needs. This textbook is meant to provide explicitly the basis for determining the need for nursing care of well or ill people in whatever area they may be—home, institution, work.

As the book evolved, talks with registered nurses seeking the baccalaureate degree and with some of their instructors led me to believe that the text will also meet the needs of these students for a systematic approach to the nursing process, and for a conceptual approach to practice.

Beginning students deal primarily with individuals, rather than with groups of people. Consequently, the focus of this book is upon the application of basic concepts to the nursing care of individuals. The family members or others in the immediate social environment are considered as they represent, relate to, interpret for, or impinge upon the individual. Nursing service to the family group as an entity, to groups of patients or staff, or to community groups is not within the scope of the book.

The textbook is organized into three major sections. The first deals with professional nursing in the context of modern health-care systems, the second with a systematic use of the scientific method in determining the client's need for help and in planning care, and the third with the basic concepts needed to make the diagnosis and plan intervention.

A discussion of health and illness initiates Part 1 to help place health care in perspective with society's values regarding health. Health and illness are described as socially and culturally defined phenomena, with illness being a change from the culturally accepted state of health. Definitions of health vary within subsystems of our culture, and these variations should affect the manner and type of service offered by health professions to a particular subculture.

The discussion of the delivery of health care describes nursing care in relation to the care provided by other professions. Inherent in this approach is consideration of the changing roles of nursing and of its various kinds of practitioners. In addition, social systems in which nurses practice are described. Students of professional nursing must learn early to observe and evaluate the systems in which they practice in order that they may eventually make changes in those systems.

Part 2 presents in detail a framework of diagnosis and intervention in the health and illness problems of people. Frequent reference is made to the expanding literature related to systematic assessment of the status of the patient and to planning of nursing care. Little of this literature has appeared to date in textbooks for beginning practitioners. The framework presented in this text may be used in any setting in which nursing services are given. It is a paradigm which may be used by students and practitioners, from the beginning student to the clinical specialist; their own knowledge and experience determine the depth to which they may go.

The major focus of Part 3 is upon the concepts basic to determining daily living problems and interventions. All textbooks emphasize the use of scientific principles in nursing care, but these principles often appear as statements of fact which the student is expected to accept at face value. The presentation of principle and theory in the context of their underlying concepts in this book is designed to enable both student and teacher to evaluate their validity. This approach also provides a model to lead the student into critical analysis of concepts as he learns to apply principles and theories on his own. The presentation of concepts is based on the assumption that the student already has an introductory background in both the natural and social sciences.

The concepts are organized in the same categories as those in the assessment outline presented in Part 2. This will enable the student to see what kinds of information are needed and the use to which the data will be put in determining nursing care. The concepts included are ones which pertain to all nursing specialties and to people in many age groups. Technical procedures related to these concepts are not presented here. The numerous audiovisual aids and textbooks currently available may be used to enable the student to apply the concepts presented to the technical procedures that he may be called upon to perform.

Acknowledgments

I cannot begin to acknowledge the help of the many students and colleagues who have influenced the philosophy of nursing and nursing education that shaped this textbook. Students and faculty involved in first-level clinical courses at the University of California San Francisco Medical Center, Emory University, and the University of Washington all contributed, knowingly and unknowingly, to the work.

More specifically, I should like to thank the following people for their review of specific chapters and their suggestions:

Judy Atwood, University of Washington, for review of the section on problem-oriented records, Part 2, Chapter 7

Doris Carnevali, for many hours spent in considering ideas and giving her reactions to them

Dorothy Crowley, University of Washington, for review of the section on pain, Part 3, Chapter 19

Johanna Horton Flynn, Emory University, for review of relationships with children, Part 2, Chapter 4

Joleen Klocke Heath, University of Washington, for review of the fluid and electrolyte concepts in Part 3, Chapter 15

Donald W. Mitchell, M.D., Seattle, for review of respiratory concepts, Part 3, Chapter 16

Jurate Sakalys, University of Colorado, for review of all of Part 2

Carol Smith, Seattle, for many of the drawings

Barbara Walike, University of Washington, for review of nutrition concepts, Part 3, Chapter 13

Margeret A. Williams, University of Colorado, for review of Part 2, Chapter 1

Finally, my appreciation to my husband for his patience and his answers to many questions about medical science, and to my children, whose antics enlivened the whole affair.

Pamela Holsclaw Mitchell

Part One

Nursing and Health Care

What is a nurse? Is a nurse someone who takes care of sick people, gives pills, helps the doctor, and gives "shots"? Yes—but a nurse is also someone who helps people stay well, helps disabled people learn how to take care of themselves, and represents the ill or well person to the health-care system. Most people can define some things which nurses do to help ill people; fewer can articulate a nurse's role with well people; and fewer still are aware of the complex relationships that exist among nurses, people who need nursing help, and the systems of health care in which they seek help.

Nursing and nurses exist because people who have actual or potential health problems need help in coping with difficulties in their daily living which are posed by these problems. Because nursing help does not exist independent from the total system of health care or cultural definitions of health and illness, the introductory portion of this book is intended to present some ideas about health and illness, nursing in the context of health care, and health care as a social system. These concepts may help the beginning practitioner view his own practice as one involving not only himself and his client but also the social and cultural framework in which his work occurs.

The Meaning of Health and Illness

Jurate A. Sakalys

This book is based on the premise that contacts between nurses and their clients, or patients, include prevention of illness, help with the problems of illness, and promotion of wellness. But just what is meant by wellness and by the deviation from wellness that is variously known as illness, disease, or sickness?

It seems logical that in order to intervene in states of wellness and illness, the nurse must be able to distinguish between these states in a variety of situations. Though it is virtually impossible to explore every variation in health and illness, it *is* possible to identify and to categorize many of the known and significant factors which differentiate these phenomena. The effort to categorize a variety of events having common features, such as states of health and illness, is part of the process of conceptualization. Conceptualization—identifying similarities from separate parts of our experience and subsequently defining a class of phenomena having similar characteristics—is a way of reducing the complexity of our experience and making it unified and manageable. With an understanding of the concepts of health and illness, the student of nursing can progress to an identification of these states in a variety of situations from a variety of perspectives.

Differentiation between concepts of health and illness, therefore, is not purely a question of semantics or an attempt to keep intellectual discourse logical. Rather, definitions of these

3

concepts help the nurse clarify his thinking, which, in turn, gives direction to his professional attitudes and behavior.

It is the purpose of this chapter to explore the concepts of health and illness from clinical and behavioral frames of reference; to identify behavioral aspects of wellness and illness; and to delineate some appropriate nursing interventions.

ORIENTATIONS TO HEALTH AND ILLNESS

Although health and illness are universal phenomena, these concepts are variable, relative, and do not have absolute or universal definitions. What is health for one person at one time may be illness for another, or even for the same person at another point in time. The sickle-cell trait, for example, was an adaptive condition for African Negroes and some Mediterranean residents, providing them with a higher resistance to malaria. For people living in nonmalarial regions, however, the possession of sickle-cell genes was dysfunctional and defined as illness. Therefore, some concept of what is normal for a given person within a given environment is implicit in all definitions of health and illness. The conceptualization of normal physiological and behavioral function, in turn, depends on needs imposed by the environment, on the nature of health-care institutions in a society, and on the cultural context within which health problems are defined. These definitions have evolved together with the evolutions of societies and technologies and differ from one social group to another. What is considered health varies widely between a highly industrial, technological society such as ours and nonindustrialized, underdeveloped societies.

Scientific and Nonscientific Orientations

Since time immemorial, men have searched for causes of illness. Their beliefs and attitudes regarding causes of illness, in turn, have determined definitions of illness, the role of the ill person, the role of the healer, and the system of care. Scientific and nonscientific orientations to health and illness are similar in their goals: they share a search for causes of illness; they diagnose; prescribe treatment; and evaluate treatment. Differences in these orientations derive largely from the ways in which these goals are achieved.

In underdeveloped societies, or in insulated segments of modern, industrial society, men often construct theories of life that are based on cosmic elements they cannot perceive. That is, when observable causes of illness are not present in man's environment, he attributes illness to nonscientific or supernatural causes, such as divine retribution, sin, or unbalanced phlegms. Treatment of illness, consequently, is based on religious or magical techniques, and the healer is likely to be a religious person who intercedes for the sick. The belief that the cause and treatment of illness are supernatural is characteristic of primitive medicine, a prime example of nonscientific orientations to health and illness.

Folk medicine may also be founded on nonscientific or on quasiscientific beliefs. This health-illness orientation is based on definitions of diseases according to physical or natural causes which may be similar to scientifically defined causes. Adherents of folk medicine will identify illnesses such as colds, heart disease, arthritis, but will treat illnesses with home-originated remedies, which result from ancestral trial-and-error methods. These curative regimens frequently derive from natural resources (such as minerals or herbs) or from physical treatments (such as massage, application of heat and cold, or manipulation). Successful therapeutic procedures are then relayed through generations within a social group and become traditions that are uncritically accepted by group members.

Scientific orientations to health and illness, in contrast, are predicated upon beliefs and practices requiring the systematic and controlled establishment of objectively verifiable laws of etiology and treatment. These laws, moreover, are expected to be constantly and critically reexamined in search for more effective health practices. In scientifically oriented health-care systems, care is entrusted only to persons who are highly qualified academically.

While nonscientific orientations to health and illness are common in underdeveloped societies and scientific orientations are common in modern, industrialized societies, the two are not mutually exclusive. That is, scientific and nonscientific orientations may coexist within the same social group. Moreover, even in scientifically oriented health-care systems, there is acknowledgment of the presence of undefined aspects of health and illness that are important even if they are not subject to scientific categorization, measurement, and experimentation.

Although scientific and nonscientific orientations to health and illness share similarities and may coexist, their differences serve to point out that concepts of health and illness are highly variable and complex. In addition, their definitions are largely dependent on the nature of the sociocultural group defining these phenomena and upon the degree of technological development in that social group.

Development of Scientific Orientations

Single-agent Theories Illness has traditionally been easier to define than health. Until the early twentieth century, common views of health and illness focused upon illness, which was defined as an "intrusion" upon an otherwise perfect state of being. The cause of this "intrusion" was viewed as a single agent and was variously identified as mythological, spiritual, or bacteriological in character. As such, the "intrusion" was ascribed to mythical figures or to gods wishing to punish the afflicted person. As science progressed, this belief eventually evolved into a highly sophisticated "germ theory," which ascribed all illness to bacteriological "intrusion." Health, on the other hand, was defined only as an absence of illness.

Throughout its evolution from primitive times to the present, this theoretical perspective had in common what Engel (1962) describes as the tendency to focus upon a single etiological factor in illness. Furthermore, this etiological factor was identified as bad and undesirable, qualifying for attack and eradication. Contemporary theories of illness which describe causes only in terms of anatomical lesions or of biochemical defects are concepts of the same order. That is, they also represent an attempt to identify a single defect to explain illness and represent a linear, cause-and-effect relationship: a specific etiological agent affecting a specific organ or organ system, thereby producing disease.

There is no doubt that such theorizing was a most constructive force. The doctrine of specific etiology has been a crucial element in the development of scientific orientations to health and illness, as is poignantly demonstrated in the present degree of control of many communicable diseases. Single-agent theories, however, have proved inadequate to explain many kinds of illnesses, most notably those that have psychosomatic components and chronic illnesses. Moreover, single-agent theories have been found lacking in that they are based on a view of man as distinct and separate from his environment. The linear, cause-and-effect relationships of single-agent theories have a way of obscuring the fact that it is virtually impossible to separate environmental factors (i.e., agents of illness) from the central figure (i.e., man). A conceptualization of illness premised on a view of man not in interaction with his environment leads to a division of man into his component parts and maintains that man who is only biological is affected by an environment that is only biological. Such a conceptualization denies that man is a biopsychosocial being who relates to his environment holistically.

Single-agent theories were also limiting in their definitions of wellness. Definition of health only as the absence of illness relegated health to a secondary position, meriting little exploration and conceptualization. Consequently, single-agent theories taught much about illness but little about health, as evidenced by the fact that health professionals have a tendency to focus more on episodes of illness and less on a continuum of health care.

Multiple-causation Theories As understanding of man grew, it became apparent that man himself, as well as the etiological agent, was a factor in the causation of disease. Increasingly refined theories regarding man's functioning took into account all levels of human function, including biochemical, cellular, organic, psychological, interpersonal, and sociocultural aspects. Consideration of the interaction of these functional aspects necessitated a departure from single-agent theories and from the idea of health and illness as things in themselves, unrelated to the individual and his internal and external environments. Accordingly, the definitional focus of health professionals shifted toward a delineation of other factors which influence health and illness, such as genetic endowment. Multiple-causation theories emerged, maintaining that illness rarely, if ever, results from a single, discrete, disease-causing agent acting upon an otherwise normal and healthy man. Man's relationships to his internal and external environments were emphasized, and the effects of these relationships on health-illness statuses were elucidated. As a result, a frame of reference was formed which maintained that health and illness cannot be rigorously defined in a manner appropriate to all persons, places, and times. Rather, health and illness came to be perceived as dynamic states or processes (instead of as static entities) which change with times and circumstances.

Attempts to define health similarly took into account man as a biopsychosocial being who relates to the biopsychosocial components of his environment. In 1946, the World Health Organization, in the preamble to its constitution, made a beginning attempt to broaden the definition of health by stating that it is "a state of complete physical, mental, and social well-being, not merely the absence of disease or infirmity." Dunn (1959) approached the problem more vigorously, contending that there is a difference between good health and wellness. He defined the former as a passive state of adaptability to one's environment. Wellness, in contrast, represents a dynamic growth toward fulfillment of one's potential. Dunn's is an open-ended concept of wellness, depicting a goal which is constantly changing as the person matures and his environment changes. It may be that there is no state of optimum wellness, Dunn stated, "but rather [that] wellness is a direction in progress toward an ever higher potential of functioning." [1] In similar vein, Dubos (1959) stated that "perfect health . . . is an illusion . . . to be alive means to struggle for existence in the interplay between man and his environment . . . complete freedom from disease and from struggle is almost incompatible with the process of living . . . health is a state constantly to be modified and strived toward as society and environment change." [2] Engel (1962) also presented a definition of health similar to that of Dubos. Health exists, he maintained,

when the organism is successfully adjusting in its environment and is able to maintain this state free of undue excitation, capable of growth, develop-

[1] H. L. Dunn, What High Level Wellness Means, *Canadian Journal of Public Health,* **50**:447–457 (1959).
[2] R. Dubos, "Mirage of Health," Harper and Row Publishers, Inc., New York, 1959.

ment, and activity in an integrated and effective sense. . . . This is an active, dynamic process taking place in the face of ever-changing environment. There is continued need for adjustment and adaptation to maintain this state in face of tasks imposed from the outside or from within the organism itself.[3]

Therefore, as multiple-causation theories emerged, health and illness were no longer defined as the linear, cause-and-effect phenomena described in the past. Rather, these states came to be defined as multivariate in causation and complex in composition. Furthermore, in being viewed as expressions of man's relationship to his internal and external environments, health and illness came to be conceptualized as aspects of human ecology.

Ecological Systems Theory Conceptualization of man's health-illness status as resulting from his interaction with his environment led to the development of an ecological theoretical perspective. Integral to this perspective is a broadened understanding of man, who is perceived as part, product, and determiner of his environment. Moreover, man is perceived as a system (a set of interrelated parts which mutually react and maintain themselves by exchanging energy) which transacts with other systems within the environment. That is, the health status of an individual is seen as being determined by the interaction and integration of two ecological universes: the internal environment of man himself and the external environment in which he lives and to which he relates. Because these environments are interrelated, a change in one part of a system will necessarily produce change in other parts of the system. Therefore, all man's interactions with his environment have an effect on his health status.

[3] G. Engel, "Psychological Development in Health and Disease," W. B. Saunders Company, Philadelphia, 1962.

Central to the ecological systems theoretical approach is the concept of adaptation. According to this view, man's health status is viewed as a function of current and accumulated effects of his environment upon his mind and body. That is, healthy man is able to adapt to his environment in a meaningful and successful manner. In illness, on the other hand, either adaptive mechanisms fail or adaptive capacity is limited in some way; illness is viewed as an expression of a basic imbalance in man's adaptation to the multiple physical and emotional stresses in the environment. The concept of adaptation originated in the works of Claude Bernard and Walter B. Cannon, who stated that health and survival depend on the ability of an organism appropriately to use regulatory systems which would enable it to maintain its internal environment in an approximately stable state, despite unceasing changes in the external environment. This successful stable state is commonly known as *homeostasis,* a state of dynamic equilibrium which occurs in health.

Rogers (1960) states that two basic types of environment can affect a person's health status: (1) the material environment, which is composed of (*a*) intrinsic, somatic factors, such as age, sex, hereditary characteristics, and of (*b*) extrinsic factors such as the physical environment, the biological environment, and the social environment, and (2) the nonmaterial environment, which also contains intrinsic and extrinsic factors such as inherent mentality, temperament, those factors affecting man's conscious and/or unconscious, his beliefs, values, goals, ideologies, social norms, and life experiences, such as socialization, education, trauma, stress, satisfactions, and rewards. Although he does not schematically relate these factors to health and illness, Rogers sees health as a spectrum ranging from perfect health to complete absence of health, or death. Man may move up or down on this scale,

Health Status Scale Showing Focus of Major Forms of Health Service

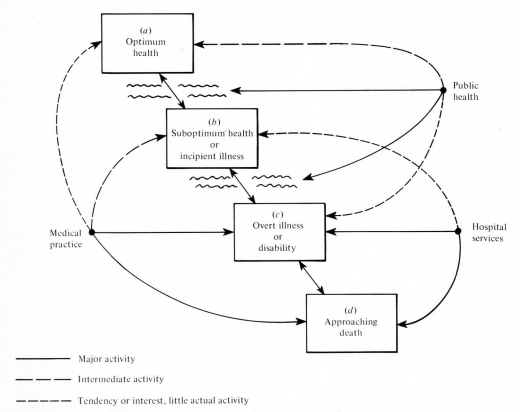

Figure 1-1 Rogers's health-status scale, depicting health and illness as part of a single continuum, ranging from perfect health to death. *(Reprinted with permission of The Macmillan Company, New York, from "Human Ecology and Health," copyright by Edward S. Rogers, 1960.)*

and between the two extremes are all degrees of health.

Some theorists postulate that another environmental factor, the rate of change in a person's life, could be one of the most important environmental factors of all. Researchers have attempted to devise ways of measuring impact of life changes characteristic of the American way of life. These include changes in family constellation, occupation, economics, group relationships, residence, and education. Holmes and Masuda (1970) postulate that such life changes evoke adaptive efforts on the part of the involved

persons which tax health and, therefore, increase susceptibility to disease. The mechanisms by which stress or change predispose to illness are still being researched and are not well understood. It is apparent, however, that stress plays a role in causing or contributing to the occurrence of illness, and work in psychosomatic medicine is based upon an awareness that all psychological and social experience is associated with changing physiological states.

Dunn (1961) also perceives health and illness as being influenced by one's environment. He views health and illness as dynamic processes

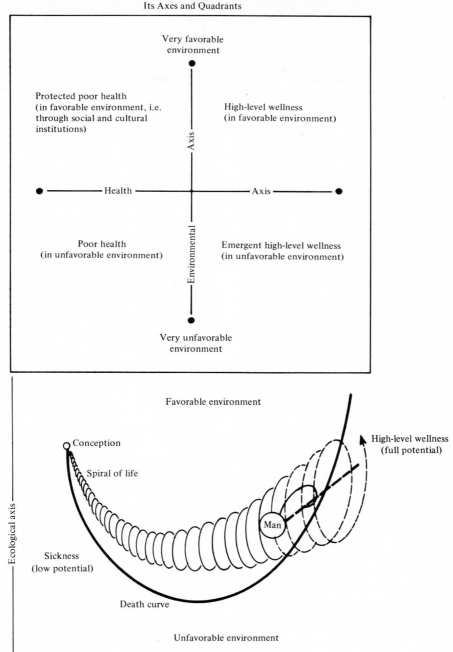

Figure 1-2 Dunn's ecological conceptualization of health and illness, depicting the interaction between a person's health status and his environment. *(From H. L. Dunn, "High Level Wellness," R. W. Beatty Company, Arlington, Va., 1961. By permission of the publisher.)*

and defines health in terms of high-level well-ness:

> High level wellness for the individual is defined as an integrated method of functioning which is oriented toward maximizing the potential of which the individual is capable. It requires that the individual maintain a continuum of balance and purposeful direction within the environment within which he is functioning.[4]

Dunn's definition of high-level wellness therefore embodies three assumptions: (1) a direction in progress to a consistently higher level of function; (2) an open-ended and always expanding future which challenges the person to pursue his potential; and (3) the integration of the whole being of a person—body, mind, and spirit.

Like Rogers, Dunn also theorizes about health and illness in terms of a graduated scale, a scale which he schematizes as a "health grid." This grid is composed of two axes: (1) the environmental axis, which is made up of the physical, socioeconomic components of the environment, and (2) the health axis, which ranges from death to peak wellness. The area between these two points represents various and relative states of wellness or illness. Consequently, Dunn's grid is divided into four quadrants: (1) poor health in an unfavorable environment; (2) protected poor health in a favorable environment; (3) emergent high-level wellness in an unfavorable environment; and (4) high-level wellness in a favorable environment (Fig. 1-2). Another schematic representation of health-illness theory developed by Dunn characterizes the dynamic state of illness and wellness, depicting man "as a whirling globe moving in a spiral course through time and through environment (favorable and unfavorable) from conception to death."[4] High-level wellness is represented by the ever-changing, emergent side of the spiral traveled by man. Sickness, or low potential, lies to the rear of the spiral (Fig. 1-2).

Health and Illness as Separate Entities In both of the previous theoretical perspectives, health and illness are defined as parts of the same entity, or as parts of one continuum. There is, however, another way to view the interrelationship between health and illness by representing health and illness not as poles of a graduated scale, but as two distinct, parallel entities. Although this perspective does not focus on multiple causation or ecological theories of illness, it implicitly acknowledges these theories. In describing this double continuum, Jahoda (1958) states: "Assuming that health is qualitatively different from disease, the extreme pole of sickness would be absence of disease; of health, absence of health"[5] (Fig. 1-3).

[4] H. L. Dunn, "High Level Wellness," R. W. Beatty Company, Arlington, Va., 1961.

[5] Excerpted from "Current Concepts of Positive Mental Health" by Marie Jahoda (Joint Commission on Mental Illness and Health, Monograph Series, No. 1), Basic Books, Inc., Publishers, New York, 1958.

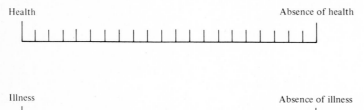

Figure 1-3 A schematic representation of health and illness as separate but parallel entities.

Jahoda proceeds to state: "The advantage of having established pure types [of health and illness] and of conceiving them as qualitatively different consists in drawing attention to the health potential in patients and the sickness potential in healthy persons." [5] The hope embodied in such a perspective is valuable to health professionals, and the alertness to healthy aspects in a person who is ill renders the health worker more truly a "health" professional, not a person who deals only in illness.

Thus far, some scientific and nonscientific perspectives regarding health and illness have been explored. The significance of exploring these perspectives lies in that each will influence a different goal of health care and a different pattern of health-care delivery. When, for example, it was believed that illness was caused by a specific agent which could be predicted to pursue a specific course, the processes of diagnosis, treatment, and prevention became the three basic elements in all medical-care systems.

Today, with the evolution of new concepts of health and illness embodied in multiple-causation theories and in ecological perspectives, the goals and the nature of health-care delivery are changing. From a predominantly individual-oriented clinical science, medicine is progressing to a community science, with goals surpassing the relief of symptoms and the cure of disease. The concept of comprehensive care, for example, focuses the attention of health professionals on the entire continuum of a person's health, with the goals of maintaining adaptation and promoting wellness, rather than on an isolated episode of illness. Moreover, since the individual lives within a community, health care must focus upon the community as well as upon the patient-client, and health services must be located within the community. The incorporation of multiprofessional personnel to deal with the complex etiologies of illness is resulting in drift from the doctor-patient dyadic relationship toward a team approach to the patient-client. Conceptual-

ization of man as a biopsychosocial being has led to increased utilization of the behavioral sciences and the growth of psychosomatic medicine. And, lastly, because ecological systems imply a mutual reciprocity, the ill person is becoming known more frequently not as a patient, but as a client with a more active, decision-making role in his health care.

Nursing must follow suit. If the nurse believes that man's health status is influenced by the nature of his interaction with his environment, then he must take the environment into account in planning care for the patient. The "rehabilitated" cardiac patient, for example, who returns to the same stressful environment which caused him to channel his stresses into his cardiovascular system, and who has not been helped to cope with or to change his environment in a qualitatively different way, will not be rehabilitated or cured for long.

Application of Definitions How do we know when someone is ill or well? That is, how do we operationalize the definitions of health and illness heretofore presented? This is a difficult task in relation to health, for, although a definition is available, health professionals know very little about optimum health. We do not yet know how to measure it, study it, maintain, or obtain it. Consequently, few professional functions can be directed specifically toward that goal (Rogers, 1960). However, definition may be perceived as the first step in measurement and operationalization.

Again, operationalization of a definition of illness presents less of a problem than application and utilization of definitions of health. This is particularly true when illness is consciously experienced, expressed by the patient, and objectively observable in signs and symptoms. Such a composite picture of illness generally exists and is used to evaluate a person's relative state of wellness or illness. The sources of evaluation forming this composite picture are the individual himself, health professionals, and lay observers who influence the person's definition of illness or wellness.

Traditionally, physicians have tended to rely predominantly upon a clinical definition of illness based on the presence of a clearly identifiable pathological condition. But there are a vast number of conditions that do not lend themselves to such facile clinical definitions, and Engel cautions that lack of a clinically observable syndrome or lack of presenting complaints does not necessarily mean that there is no illness. The person who feels well but is found during routine medical examination to have some pathological condition is a case in point. Is he ill or well? We might ask the same question about the person who seeks medical assistance because he feels ill but has no demonstrable, definable pathologic condition. When a pathologic condition cannot be detected, even definitions of illness become obscure. Part of the difficulty in defining illness in such cases arises because traditionally, definitions of illness were closely related to what physicians do in society. That is, illness was defined as something that is treated by a physician. If an illness is undefinable, it is untreatable; therefore, there is no illness.

It may be seen that professional definitions of illness have heretofore been more influential than lay definitions. Definitions of illness result, however, from a series of social actions based on subjective judgments (self-perceptions of the individual) and objective observations (observations of significant other persons, including health professionals). Moreover, viewing illness as a holistic response of the individual necessitates consideration of the social dimensions of illness. Organic illness and social patterns of illness do not necessarily coincide. Thus, if we are to understand fully the processes of illness and wellness, it is necessary to examine social definitions of illness, i.e., to explore ways in which individuals have decided whether they are well or ill and whether they will seek care.

PSYCHOSOCIAL AND CULTURAL PROCESSES IN HEALTH AND ILLNESS

Norms of health and illness are socially and culturally as well as clinically determined. As indicated previously, what is considered illness in one social group at a given time may be considered health in another group. The ancient practice of binding the feet of Oriental women, for example, was viewed as indicating high status, for women who participated in this practice did so not only to preserve the beauty of their feet but also to show that they did not have to perform the menial task of independent locomotion. Instead, they were carried from place to place. In Western cultures, the results of such a practice were perceived as a deviation from health and normal functioning. Indeed, they were perceived as gross disability. More currently, in North American social groups, values in relation to health and illness likewise reflect sociocultural influence. Myocardial infarctions and peptic ulcers, for example, though serious pathological processes, frequently are thought to bestow status because they are seen as related to the stress of achievement. Each society (and social groups within societies) influences the development of behavioral and biological norms, which are rules of conduct, or social expectations that arise from consensually held values within the group. Concepts of illness derive from these norms in that illness represents a deviation from expected standards of performance. Because these norms are variable among and within societies, deviations (illnesses) are also variably defined, rendering sociocultural definitions and expressions of illness extremely relativistic.

Social norms affect not only definitions of health and illness but also the processes by which illness is defined. The behavior of persons who think themselves ill is significantly governed, often regardless of the effects of the disease, by the social groups to which they belong. Differences among sociocultural groups often create different health and social problems and may require different modalities of care. For instance, health professionals who work in cultures other than the North American find that it is difficult to persuade native people to follow therapeutic regimens without first interpreting these regimens into the common cultural context.

Thus, recognition of health or illness depends on implicit ideas regarding which physical, mental, and social states are "normal" and which are not. These ideas are based upon personal experience, cultural orientations, and knowledge regarding health and illness.

Lay Definitions of Health and Illness

Freidson (1970) describes several sociocultural elements involved in lay definitions of illness and responses to illness. These elements may derive from social class, ethnic orientation, or religious affiliation and include the person's view of the body, his knowledge of illness, his interpretation of pain and of various symptoms, and his attitudes toward modern medicine. Knowledge about health and illness will particularly influence the recognition of symptoms and the significance attached to them, and seems to vary with socioeconomic and educational achievement. Generally, in our society, education and affluence tend to encourage stricter definitions of health and decreased tolerance for the discomforts of illness. Freidson attributes this to the fact that persons of higher socioeconomic status and education tend to have more scientific notions of health and illness and tend to have life styles and values closer to those of health professionals than persons from other strata. Lower-class persons, on the other hand, tend to have limited knowledge regarding causes and treatments of illness and may be more likely to subscribe to nonscientific theories. Their definitions of possible illness tend to arise directly from concrete observations or experiences, such as pain and

incapacity, and they appear to seek health care when sickness is experienced, not before. Freidson describes lower-class persons as subscribing to a parochial structure, characterized by limited knowledge of bodily functions, lack of information about the range and nature of health services available, and timidity in consulting physicians.

How different these attitudes are in segments of our society is poignantly revealed in the outlook of a lower-class person quoted by Koos (1954):

> I wish I really knew what you mean by being sick. Sometimes I've felt so bad I could curl up and die, but had to go on because the kids had to be taken care of, and besides, we didn't have the money to spend for a doctor—how could I be sick?—how do you know when you're sick anyway? Some people can go to bed most any time with anything but most of us can't be sick—even when we need to be.[6]

This example illustrates that in addition to knowledge about health and illness, several other factors influence lay definitions of illness. One of these is the degree to which signs and symptoms interfere with "normal" functioning. Lay definitions of illness are intimately influenced by perceptions of wellness and well behavior. Baumann (1961), in her analysis of lay definitions of health, states that these definitions are distinguished by three criteria: (1) a subjective feeling of well-being; (2) an absence of symptoms; and (3) a state of being able to perform those activities that a person in good health should be able to perform. Freidson reinforces this perspective, stating that if one defines illness as that which interferes with ordinary activities, then what an individual selects as a symptom of illness is influenced by what his ordinary daily activities are. Therefore, if an individual's "well role," for example, does

[6] E. L. Koos, "The Health of Regionville," Columbia University Press, New York, 1954.

not include the need for visual acuity, beginning visual disturbances may be unnoticed. On the other hand, a seamstress not only would recognize more quickly that such symptoms indicate deviations from health but also would attach more significance to them.

A second important variable in laymen's definitions of illness is also demonstrated in the Koos quote, that of situational factors which make it more or less difficult to obtain medical attention (Ludwig and Gibson, 1969). Though finances was the specific situational factor mentioned in the example, this variable can be broadened to include the costs of seeking medical help in terms of time, peer-group sanctions, availability, and physical proximity of health-care resources. It seems logical that the less available the resources are, the less they will be utilized except in cases of extreme need. Also, if the use of health-care resources is likely to be met with peer-group disapproval or rejection (as sometimes occurs in mental illness), these resources are less likely to be utilized.

A third major factor influencing lay definitions of illness consists of attitudes toward health-care delivery systems and their personnel—i.e., faith and trust in health professionals may serve as motivation for heeding signs and symptoms and for defining them as illness (Ludwig and Gibson). Conversely, persons who mistrust health-care professionals are less likely to define symptoms as illness and to approach scientifically oriented health workers.

In summary, then, the layman's definition of illness is culturally and socially variable and is importantly influenced by definitions of "normal" functioning, situational factors that help or hinder him in getting medical attention, and attitudes toward the health-care delivery system, as well as by the structure of the lay system in which he participates.

Social Processes in Illness

In the preceding exploration of factors that influence an individual's definition of illness, we can see that his definition depends upon the meaning and interpretations learned in his social life. Consequently, it may be said that the behavior in which an individual engages when he feels ill is largely socially determined.

The transitional phase between health and illness is often vague and ambiguous. The individual who thinks himself ill may feel some literal *dis*-ease, some discomfort, or merely something indefinably different and discomforting in his functioning. The beginning phases of most illnesses are extremely nonspecific, and laymen generally have difficulty in defining illness at this time. This process of transition is rarely defined as part of the illness process, even though it is accompanied by various significant behaviors. Mechanic (1968) terms the social actions engaged in during this phase "illness behavior," which he defines as "the way in which symptoms are perceived, evaluated, and acted upon by a person who recognizes some pain, discomfort, or other signs of organic (we may add emotional) malfunction."[7] Illness behavior may be viewed as part of a broader sociological analysis of the illness process. In discussing illness behavior, Freidson (1970) identifies the social course of illness for laymen as beginning with the experience of discomfort, progressing to a search for the meaning of the discomfort and then to a search for ways of coping with it, and culminating in the person's entrance into medical consultation. At any stage of illness behavior, Freidson states, people may withdraw and progress no further. Lederer (1952) and Suchman (1965) have defined stages of social adaptation to illness, of which illness behavior is only the beginning. Lederer defines three stages in the social experience of illness: (1) transition from health to illness; (2) stage of accepted illness; and (3) convalescence. Suchman's delineation of these phases is somewhat more detailed, and he categorizes the process in the following way: (1) symptom experience; (2) assumption of the sick

[7] Reprinted by permission of The Macmillan Company, New York, from "Medical Sociology," copyright by The Free Press, New York, 1968.

role; (3) medical-care contact; (4) dependent-patient role; and (5) recovery or rehabilitation. These stages are generally experienced in some form by all persons who become ill, regardless of the nature, duration, and intensity of their illness.

Transition from Health to Illness Illness behavior, however, characterizes the beginning of the social experience of illness and may be said to correspond to the first stages defined by Lederer and Suchman. When a person experiences unusual, unpleasant emotional or bodily changes, he undergoes stress, which he may handle in some way that is characteristic, or normal, for him. His stress is often manifested as anxiety; he may try to handle his anxiety by plunging into healthy activities in an attempt to deny the symptoms, or by trying self-treatment in an attempt to convince himself that the symptoms are not serious. Whatever his behavior, it is affected by a number of factors, some of which have been mentioned. However, continuing discomfort and increasing symptoms often pressure him into seeking help of some kind. Generally, he first consults his reference group, the group with which he most identifies and the values and norms of which he shares. Freidson (1970) terms this group the "lay referral system." The lay referral system functions to reflect norms of health to the ambivalent individual and to help him arrive at some decision as to whether his symptoms represent illness and what he should do about them. The nature of illness behavior at this point is crucial in determining whether medical diagnosis and treatment will begin. According to Freidson, help-seeking and advice-giving behavior among laymen organizes illness behavior. The person may independently become aware that something is wrong with him; nevertheless he generally needs some agreement by his social group that his symptoms do indeed represent illness. A large part of the significance of social structure lies in its role in encouraging or discouraging the individual's movement toward medical consultation. Hadley

(1966) points out that interaction between the individual and his reference group at this point may result in any one of four possible outcomes:

1 The individual claims illness, but his reference group denies its presence.
2 The individual claims illness, and his reference group affirms its presence.
3 The individual does not claim illness, and his reference group does not affirm its presence.
4 The individual does not claim illness, but his reference group affirms its presence.

In this transitional phase of illness, the nurse may be called upon to perform significant professional functions. (1) He is in a unique position to reflect a highly discriminating norm of health to the person seeking advice and to direct him to appropriate resources. (2) He has a responsibility to disseminate accurate information regarding health and illness to public audiences, thereby helping to make this transitional phase less ambiguous. (3) The nurse has a significant responsibility in this phase of illness to allay the fears and anxieties that inevitably accompany recognition of illness and to help the patient cope with feelings of shame, guilt, or disgust which may also mark the transition. (4) The nurse can encourage the patient to trust in health professionals.

Stage of Accepted Illness Given that the individual and his reference group agree on the presence of a deviation from health, a number of other social processes transpire. As stated previously, implicit in defining deviance from health is the sociological definition of illness as an incapacity for normal role and/or task performance (Parsons, 1958). That is, illness is an incapacity of a person to perform within his expected social framework, in terms of either interpersonal relations or the physical tasks that accompany these relations, or both. The ill person, therefore, ceases to be a useful, productive member of the social group and is generally excluded from the group until his deviance or the disruptive effect of his illness is rectified. He is therefore subject to a set of expectations that modern, industrial society places before him. These expectations, which constitute the "sick role," include the following:

1 The person is not held responsible for his incapacities.
2 He is released, to varying degrees, from normal role obligations.
3 He must recognize that illness is undesirable and have an expressed desire to "get well."
4 He must seek competent help, cooperate with treatment, and relinquish the right to make decisions to the physician and to other health-care professionals (Parsons, 1958).

In assuming the sick role, the person exchanges freedom and autonomy for control, but simultaneously gains care, protection, and freedom from responsibility (Folta and Deck, 1966). The sick-role mechanism is part of the process of social control, assuring that the ill are insulated from the well and are obligated to obtain health care. Though the Parsonian typology is a valuable conceptual tool, it gives no information regarding the context in which sick-role behavior may occur. That is, enactment of the sick role is dependent upon a number of factors such as sociocultural patterns, socioeconomic status, and specific attributes of the illness.

Whether a person assumes the sick role, with its rights and obligations, depends upon a balance of forces between perceived sanctions for disregarding his symptoms (i.e., what will happen if he neglects treatment) and the sanctions for acknowledging illness (expense, disruption in family life, rejection).

However, when his deviant position is legitimized by his conformity to these expectations, the person generally abandons any pretense of being healthy and begins to seeks medical care. The person's interaction with his physician is, again, socioculturally determined. The physician, in this stage of illness, has the mandate of arriving at a diagnosis. Primary sources of information for this process include the person himself and direct and technological observation of the person's health status. Since symptoms are highly subjective and influenced by the person's knowledge, the significance he attaches to them, his anxiety, and his perception of health professionals, their presentation will necessarily be selective. Moreover, cultural differences will determine what information is to be presented and what information may be considered shameful and consequently concealed.

Thus, the physician is largely dependent on how the patient reports his experiences. However, as Mechanic (1968) states,

> physicians and patients come together holding somewhat different conceptions of illness. The physician's views are largely molded by his professional training and clinical experience, [while the] patient's views are influenced by a need to cope with a particular problem and his social and cultural understanding of the nature of the problem.[8]

One of the greater problems in the delivery of health care stems from such differences in perception of illness and the resulting lack of communication. The health professional has the responsibility not only of helping the patient, but also of striving to understand clearly what he is expressing. Because the physician's energies are frequently focused upon treating the patient, the nurse may function as a valuable facilitator of the patient's expression of illness. By spending time with the patient, allaying his anxiety, and attempting to comprehend his presentation, the nurse can help the patient to define his health-illness position. In the course of such a relationship, the nurse may derive a great deal of information, much of which may not lend itself to categorization. Yet, as Engel (1962) states, this

[8] Reprinted by permission of The Macmillan Company, New York, from "Medical Sociology," copyright by The Free Press, New York, 1968.

unclassifiable information may also be essential for the physician's understanding of how, and perhaps why, the person is ill. In these and other ways, nurses are increasingly assuming the role of the patient's advocate in all areas of health care, and promoting a climate in which the patient-client can act optimally in his own interests.

Often, we assume that when a person seeks verification of his illness, it is readily accorded. However, such is not always the case. The two most notable variations in this process occur when (1) the person seeks verification of illness and the physician does not accord it; and (2) the person does not seek verification of illness, but the physician identifies him as ill. Perhaps the most striking example of the first kind of situation occurs when complaints of illness seem to have no distinguishable cause. Health professionals often term the person with this kind of complaint "crocky" and consider him deviant from both well-role and sick-role expectations. The result is that the individual attempts to enact a role for which there is no satisfactory counter-role. That is, he attempts to enact the sick role, but health professionals refuse to adopt a therapeutic role. Severe frustration often results, sometimes with the ultimate result that when the person does have a legitimate illness, his complaints are discredited. Perhaps for this reason, health professionals have been said to be biased toward illness and have maintained that it is better to impute illness rather than deny it and risk overlooking its presence (Freidson, 1970).

The other notable variation in the process of verifying illness is exemplified by refusal to accept the sick role. This might occur when a person feels well, is active, and is not incapacitated in any way, but is found during a routine physical examination to have a pathological condition. Because of his subjective feelings of wellness, the individual may refuse to enact the sick role. Variations in role transitions of this nature, which may have roots in psychological

denial of the threat of illness, are often dangerous to the patient's well-being. In either case, failures in consensual validation serve to divert individuals from medical care, and it is often the nurse's responsibility to act as a patient's advocate in such situations.

Assuming, however, that verification of illness is accorded, some form of treatment begins and the individual becomes a patient-client, dependent upon health professionals for curing him and caring for him—i.e., for performing those functions which he is unable to perform for himself. Within the stage of accepted illness, therefore, the patient or the client becomes dependent to some degree. In addition, the patient may also exhibit a number of other constrictive and regressive personality characteristics, such as egocentricity, constriction of interests, and hypochondriasis. This process of divesting energy from the environment and investing it in one's self, Lederer points out, may be essential to the process of healing. Other reactions that the patient in the accepted stage of illness manifests may derive largely from the symbolic meanings his illness holds for him. As Dubos (1965) states, "Man's responses to his physical illness are often less affected by the direct stimulus on his body than by the symbolic interpretation he attaches to the stimulus."[9] The fear of symbolic or real loss seems to be a major component of reactions to illness. Engel states that this fear can relate to loss of body function and image, social roles, goals, persons, ideals—all those things which constitute the basis of one's self-concept and are necessary for effective ego function. Moreover, the threat of injury is no small one; mutilation and pain are also commonly feared.

A patient's perception of his illness plays an important part in his acceptance of it, his relationships with health professionals, his acceptance of therapy, and his progress toward health.

---

[9] R. Dubos, "Man Adapting," Yale University Press, New Haven, Conn., 1965.

It has been demonstrated that perceptions of illness and adaptations to illness not only are significant for success in treating the present illness, but also determine the nature of future health-oriented experiences. Health professionals cannot know how a person is experiencing his illness until they explore the meanings that a patient attaches to his condition. Assuming that nursing is largely concerned with situational aspects of a patient's illness—i.e., those aspects which derive from the patient's reaction to being ill, to his diagnosis, to his treatment, rather than those aspects deriving directly from his disease (Wooldridge et al., 1968)—it behooves the nurse to obtain some information from the patient about his experience of illness. A nurse's effectiveness is influenced by his understanding of the patient's perception of the situation, and nursing care planning cannot begin until the nurse has some information regarding the extrinsic and intrinsic processes affecting the patient. The nurse's own perceptions of health and illness, which are partly influenced by his sociocultural background, will also influence his effectiveness. For example, some nurses find it easier to work with patients who have sociocultural backgrounds similar to their own. Some knowledge, some perception of the way in which the patient is experiencing his illness is crucial; the nurse needs to gather data about the patient's experience. The tools and processes of such data collection are described in Part 2 of this book. However, the following are some guiding thoughts particularly appropriate to gathering data about the patient's experience:

1 When does the patient consider himself ill? (When he feels pain? When he cannot work?)

2 Does the patient think he is presently ill?

3 What is the patient's interpretation of his health-illness problem? How does he define and describe his illness? What does he think caused his illness?

4 Did the patient notice signs and symptoms of illness, or was he labeled ill by someone else?

5 If the patient noticed signs and symptoms, what did he experience (physically and emotionally) when he began feeling ill? What did he think was occurring? Did he attempt home remedies? If so, what kind?

6 Did the patient consult anyone about his feelings? If so, whom? How did his consultants respond?

7 How much time elapsed before the patient discussed his feelings with anyone?

8 What precipitated the patient's decision to seek medical advice?

9 What does the patient know about treatment of his illness? What does he expect treatment to accomplish? (Complete cure? Relief of symptoms? Nothing?)

10 Has the patient experienced previous illness? If so, how was he sick before? What was his illness? How did he feel? What does he remember best about previous experiences with illness?

11 How is being ill affecting the patient's everyday life? How is his life changed as a result of his illness? Does the patient feel disabled in any way as a result of his illness? How does he feel about these changes? How is he attempting to cope with them?

12 What aspects of the illness experience does the patient perceive as pleasant and favorable, as unpleasant and unfavorable?

13 How did the patient come into contact with the health-care agent or agency? (Through his physician? Through referral? Through the telephone directory?)

14 What factors facilitated or hindered the patient's arrival at the health-care delivery system?

15 How does the patient feel about health professionals? What expectations does he have of them?

In your clinical experiences, you will undoubtedly discover other questions which can help you to appreciate the patient's experience of illness and to empathize. Presented in an appropriate and nonthreatening manner, such questions can yield a great deal of information regarding the factors which influence definitions of illness, such as knowledge about health and illness, the significance attached to symptoms and the symbolic meaning of the illness, attitudes toward the health-care system, and the costs and rewards of being ill. In other words, answers to these and related questions can give the nurse insights about the patient's perceptions of his internal and external environments which are not readily observable. Subsequent chapters will deal with how to establish relationships with patients that will facilitate gathering such information. Once this information is obtained, some assessment of the patient's experience of illness is possible, and the nurse can then pursue planning for highly individualistic needs of the patient.

In the stage of accepted illness, then, primary nursing functions derive from gathering information regarding the patient's internal and external environments; modifying the external environment until the patient is able to adapt to it; helping the patient to accept the fact that he is ill and understand his illness; allowing the patient the necessary degree of dependency; assessing the patient's coping abilities, with the support of effective mechanisms and the teaching of new ones, if necessary; and reinforcing motivations to get well.

Ideally, the period of accepted illness ends after the patient has been allowed the degree of dependence he needs in order to cope with his illness and when medical treatment has reversed or controlled the pathogenic process.

Transition from Illness to Wellness The stage of convalescence or recovery and rehabilitation is a transition from illness to a state of optimal wellness for a given person, involving a change from sick role to well role. Again, there are four options in this phase. According to Hadley (1966), the person may:

1 Continue to enact the sick role and have his behavior validated by his reference group
2 Continue to enact the sick role and not have his behavior validated by his reference group

3 Attempt to relinquish the sick role and have his performance validated by others
4 Attempt to relinquish the sick role and not have his behavior validated by others

Some of the essential prerequisites to the stage of convalescence are (1) physical *and* emotional readiness to resume well roles (sometimes physical improvement may progress more rapidly than emotional coping capacities); (2) environmental and interpersonal incentives to leaving the sick role; and (3) validation of readiness by one's reference group. However, role changes in convalescence may be just as complicated as role changes in the transition from health to illness. Patients who wish to resume their well roles earlier than is medically advisable are not uncommon, possibly because of an essential discomfort with dependency. On the other hand, patients who do not wish to resume their well roles when they are judged to be capable of doing so are probably overcomfortable with the dependency legitimized by illness and are receiving secondary gains from the sick role. In the latter situation, the privileges and exemptions of the sick role become satisfying to the patient, who is then, often unconsciously, motivated to remain ill.

Assuming, however, that the patient-client and his reference group, including health professionals, agree that return to a well role is indicated, this phase of illness is marked by a return to optimal function, an emotional reintegration, and the beginning of any necessary changes in life style effected by the experience of illness. It may be a turbulent stage for the person, who must experiment with renewed strengths and adapt to remaining incapacities while working through his feelings about his illness. Nursing functions in this stage may derive largely from Jahoda's conceptualization of both ill and well aspects within the same person; i.e., the nurse may focus upon well aspects in his goal of moving the patient to a maximally independent level of functioning. The nurse may direct his efforts toward reinforcing the patient's incentives to get well and toward decreasing secondary gains from the illness. Other nursing functions in this stage include helping the patient to resolve his feelings about his illness and to integrate the experience into his self-concept. What does this illness mean in this person's life? Examination of this question may lead to expression of feelings of discouragement or failure which need to be resolved. If these feelings are unresolved, residual disturbances in psychosocial adjustment may occur. The nurse needs to be alert to signs of such residual disturbances, for, as Engel states (1962), they constitute no less an illness and may prove to be even more disabling or incapacitating. It is only after such disturbances are resolved that the patient can integrate the meaning of his illness into his self-concept and arrive at an intrapsychic equilibrium. [Other examples of how nurses may function in this stage of illness are included in discussion of the concept of rehabilitation, which is explored in Part 3, Chapter 12.]

Variations in the Social Processes of Illness

What has been discussed thus far is a prototype of the social aspects of the process of illness, a pattern which is largely similar for all persons who experience illness in our society. This is not to say, however, that all persons everywhere, or even within our society, will experience illness in exactly the same way. Not all patients will progress through the stages of illness in a consecutive, regimented fashion, nor will they all fulfill sick-role expectations. The nurse must be cognizant of factors that will influence variations in illness behavior and sick-role enactment.

Variations in the social process of illness may stem from many sources and may result in qualitatively different needs of the patient and needs for nursing interventions. Previously identified factors which influence illness behavior and the nature of the sick role include socioeconomic status, education, and sociocultural orientation. Other factors that will create differences in the social experience of illness include (1) variations in the process of role change; (2) the nature of the illness; (3) the context of health-care delivery; and (4) the goals of health care.

Variations in the Role Change   Earlier in the discussion, it was pointed out that two role transfers occur in illness, the transition from well role to sick role and the transition from sick role back to well role. These are dependent, to a large degree, upon validation from the person's social and medical reference groups. In either transition, complications are common, as has been described. Some of the most common types of deviation from acceptable sick-role behavior include the preference of well persons for the sick role and the refusal of ill persons to enact the sick role. When patients deviate from role expectations, the nurse's empathic ability and problem-solving skills are particularly challenged. It is often easier not to deal with perceptions and experiences which cause a patient to behave in unusual ways but rather to judge and categorize the patient as deviant from sick-role expectations—a "problem patient." Labeling behavior as abnormal often has the effect of absolving one's self of any responsibility in relation to such behavior. However, the nurse's responsibility to such patients does not end with a diagnosis of their social status vis-à-vis sick-role expectations. Indeed, an assessment of the problem is often only the beginning of a potentially complex problem-solving process. As an initial step in this process, the nurse should validate his assessment, because assessments of deviance from the sick role frequently carry judgmental and negative overtones. Judgmental and categorical labels such as "malingerer" or "crock" tend to cloud an objective and thorough diagnosis of the problem at hand. Objective exploration of factors precipitating the situation yields data which, in turn, may lead to an understanding of the person's attempts to adapt to his environment and to the development of nursing interventions designed to foster satisfactory adaptations.

Variations in the Nature of the Illness   A second major way in which the social process of illness may vary derives from the nature of the illness. Illnesses are generally classified as acute or chronic, short-term or long-term. In the chronic, long-term category a variety of illnesses are found which are complex and difficult to categorize, understand, and treat. Illnesses with the greatest number of causes are frequently placed in this category, illnesses about which medical science has not yet satisfactorily crystallized its knowledge. It is in this category also that many variations in the social process of illness occur, stages of illness are distorted, and sick-role expectations are unfulfilled.

For our purposes, let us classify illnesses as temporary, progressive, and permanent. Temporary illness may be viewed as an impermanent deviance from a norm of health which has a definite time limit, the duration being relatively short, with rapid improvement and ultimate removal of etiological factors. In temporary illness, signs and symptoms are frequently familiar, making the transition from health to illness readily verifiable. The apparent progress toward a higher level of wellness also makes the change from sick role to well role relatively facile. Progressive and permanent illnesses, however, by their very nature, cannot legitimately be called illnesses; they become disabilities which do not provide conditions for fulfillment of sick-role expectations. Progressive disability, such as multiple sclerosis, is characterized by an incapacity that advances in stages and subjects the person to constant changes in all spheres of life, making role transition difficult. The onset of illness may be insidious, with vague signs and symptoms; periods of ability may vary with periods of disability; and the stage of transition from health to illness may be markedly ambigu-

ous. The person is frequently described as neither ill nor well and is therefore unable to fulfill the expectations of either role with any consistency. Moreover, because progressive disabilities are often accompanied by emotional disturbances, other questions arise, concerning the person's responsibility for his condition and his motivation to get well. There is no stage of convalescence, no transition from illness to wellness for the person who has a progressive disability; his condition is usually irreversible and ends in either permanent disability or death.

In permanent disability, such as paralysis or amputation, the sick role may become a major, primary life role, but it must be defined in a qualitatively different manner. Depending upon the nature of the disability, the individual may be released from some well-role obligations. Moreover, in order to express a desire to "get well," the individual is expected to cooperate with rehabilitation programs directed toward maximizing his ability to perform well roles. It is in permanent disability that Jahoda's conceptualization of health and illness as double, parallel continua becomes particularly meaningful, for it helps health professionals to see the patient and the patient to see himself as "abled" as well as disabled.[10] Moreover, the person who is disabled cannot totally relinquish decision making to health professionals. His disability is lifelong, and he must be a comanager in his rehabilitation. Stages of illness in permanent disability are also different. Because the disability is permanent, the last stage of illness, that of rehabilitation, is the one in which the patient invests his life's energies.

Variations in the Context of Health-care Delivery   A third major factor affecting variations in the social aspects of illness relates to the social context in which health care is delivered. Health

[10] For much more complete discussion of psychosocial aspects of physical disability, the student is encouraged to refer to the works of Beatrice Wright (1960) and Constantina Safilios-Rothschild (1970).

care may be administered in a variety of settings: the community health center, the outpatient clinic, a physician's office, a hospital—each setting differentially influencing certain aspects of illness and sick-role behavior. Every health-care delivery agency has its own social structure, its own pattern of organization or relationships, and its own normative expectations of the patient's role. In some cultures and in some illnesses it is possible for an individual to experience all stages of illness outside the hospital. In our society, however, and for more serious illnesses, a hospital stay for various lengths of time is often necessary, for the hospital contains the most concentrated gathering of the personnel and equipment necessary to diagnose and treat disease. It is in the hospital that all the characteristics of the sick role are most strictly enforced, perhaps because of the hospital's predominant orientation to treatment of acute, temporary illness and because the patient is expected to be in the dependent-patient role throughout the major portion of his hospitalization. Everything about the hospital reinforces such expectations, and deviations are generally poorly tolerated by health professionals. Because the patient loses physical and social mobility, he is isolated from information he would need in order to assume an active role in managing his illness. His behavior is, as a result, more amenable to organization by health professionals.

Other health-care delivery settings are more tolerant of deviations from the sick role, and, indeed, encourage them, because such deviations are necessary for the patient-client to function effectively within these settings. To administer care in outpatient clinics, for example, requires that the patient not be released from his role obligations to such a degree that he cannot transport himself from home to clinic. Moreover, in such a situation, more than in a hospital (which has, in effect, a captive audience), pressure is brought to bear on the patient to seek competent help and cooperate with treatment,

because the patient who receives health care in such an institution is often totally responsible for implementing treatment (there is no nurse around at home to see that he takes his medications) and is severely sanctioned when he fails to fulfill this particular expectation. Freidson states that when an ill person remains in the community, his behavior is organized more by the life of the lay community than by health professionals and the sick role may not be adopted at all.

Variations in the Goals of Health Care A fourth major factor influencing variation in the social aspects of illness relates to the goals of health care. If health care is segmented and we address ourselves to incidents of acute illness, then the aforementioned social processes apply. If, however, we address ourselves to the goal of promotion and maintenance of health in an already healthy person, we find ourselves at a loss in defining the social processes which accompany this aspect. We have also seen that social processes differ when the goals of health care are oriented to care and rehabilitation, as with permanent and progressive disability, rather than to total cure. Social processes in disability are also disparate, a fact which has been elucidated by theorists such as Safilios-Rothschild and Wright.

SUMMARY

There is much current emphasis in health-care delivery systems on prevention, early diagnosis, and early treatment of health problems. As our perspective of illness has incorporated the theory of an ecological balance between man and his environment, and our perspective of health has enlarged to include the idea of constant striving to fulfill individual potentials, we have emerged with an unlimited mandate for health professionals.

In order to participate in fulfilling this mandate, the nurse needs a frame of reference from which to view the physiological and behavioral phenomena of health and illness. Awareness of professional definitions of health and illness and awareness of the sociocultural dynamics accompanying these states should enable the nurse to maximize his professional potential in the delivery of health care.

REFERENCES

Books

Coe, R., "Sociology of Medicine," McGraw-Hill Book Company, New York, 1970.

Dubos, R., "Man Adapting," Yale University Press, New Haven, Conn., 1965.

———, "Mirage of Health," Harper and Row, Publishers, Inc., New York, 1959.

Dunn, H. L., "High Level Wellness," R. W. Beatty Company, Arlington, Va., 1961.

Engel, G., "Psychological Development in Health and Disease," W. B. Saunders Company, Philadelphia, 1962.

Folta, J., and E. Deck, "A Sociological Framework for Patient Care," John Wiley & Sons, Inc., New York, 1966.

Freidson, E., "Profession of Medicine," Dodd, Mead, & Company, Inc., New York, 1970.

Jahoda, M., "Current Concepts of Positive Mental Health," Joint Commission on Mental Illness and Health, Monograph Series, No. 1, Basic Books, Inc., Publishers, New York, 1958.

Koos, E. L., "The Health of Regionville," Columbia University Press, New York, 1954.

Mechanic, D., "Medical Sociology," The Free Press, New York, 1968.

Parsons, T., Definitions of Health and Illness in Light of American Values and Social Structure, in E. G. Jaco (ed.), "Patients, Physicians and Illness," The Free Press, New York, 1958.

Rogers, E. S., "Human Ecology and Health," The Macmillan Company, New York, 1960.

Safilios-Rothschild, C., "The Sociology and Social Psychology of Disability and Rehabilitation," Random House, Inc., New York, 1970.

Sakalys, J., Adaptation to Illness and Disability: A Psychosocial View, in M. Duffey et al., "Current Concepts in Clinical Nursing," vol. 3, The C. V. Mosby Company, St. Louis, 1971.

Wilson, R. N., "The Sociology of Health: An Introduction," Random House, Inc., New York, 1970.

Wooldridge, P., et al., "Behavioral Science, Social Practice, and the Nursing Profession," The Press of Case Western Reserve University, Cleveland, 1968.

Wright, Beatrice, "Physical Disability: A Psychological Approach," Harper & Row, Publishers, Incorporated, New York, 1960.

Periodicals

Apple, D.: How Laymen Define Illness, *Journal of Health and Human Behavior,* **2**(1):39–46 (1961).

Baumann, B.: Diversities in Conceptions of Health and Physical Fitness, *Journal of Health and Human Behavior,* **2**(1):40–45 (1961).

Dunn, H. L.: High Level Wellness for Man and Society, *American Journal of Public Health,* **49**:786–792 (1959).

———: What High Level Wellness Means, *Canadian Journal of Public Health,* **50**:447–457 (1959).

Kasl, S. and S. Cobb: Health Behavior, Illness Behavior, and Sick-role Behavior, *Archives of Environmental Health,* **12**:531–541 (1966).

Lederer, H.: How the Sick View Their World, *Journal of Social Issues,* **8**(4):4–15 (1952).

Ludwig, E. G., and G. Gibson: Self-perception of Sickness and the Seeking of Medical Care, *Journal of Health and Social Behavior,* **10**(2):125–133 (1969).

Suchman, E.: Stages of Illness and Medical Care, *Journal of Health and Social Behavior,* **6**:114–128 (1965).

Wylie, C. M.: The Definitions and Measurements of Health and Disease, *Public Health Reports,* **85**:100–104 (1970).

ADDITIONAL READINGS

Hadley, B. J.: "Becoming Well: A Study in Role Change," unpublished doctoral dissertation, Department of Sociology, University of California, Los Angeles, January 1966.

Holmes, T., and M. Masuda: "Life Change and Illness Susceptibility," presented as part of a "Symposium on Separation and Depression: Clinical Research Aspects," at the Annual Meeting of the American Association for the Advancement of Science, Chicago, Ill., Dec. 26–30, 1970.

Nursing in the Context of Health Care

Pamela Mitchell

MODELS OF HEALTH CARE

When people need help in maintaining their health, in dealing with illness, or in coping with problems related to health and illness, they turn to "experts" or "professionals" in the fields of health and the care of the ill. In cultures and groups which see religion, health, and the environment as inseparable, people turn to the shaman, the curandero, the witch doctor, or other religious practitioners (such as the Christian Science practitioner). These practitioners are persons who perform whatever rituals are culturally prescribed in relation to health. In technological or scientific societies persons in need of health help turn to the physician, in some groups to the chiropractor or naturopath, to the dentist, and to medically allied practitioners. Although

these professional groups consider themselves purely scientific, they, too, go through certain intellectual and ritual processes (the physical examination, the laying on of hands) related to health. Although the practices and premises of the medical and nonmedical ("primitive") practitioners differ markedly, both have evolved as specialized groups or systems for meeting the health needs which individual members of a culture cannot meet themselves. Midway between the "primitive" and "scientific" systems is the "folk-medicine" system—the folklore and ways of laymen which are used before consulting the professionals. The mustard plaster, herb concoctions, and over-the-counter remedies familiar to all are examples of the folk system. The lay referral system described by Sakalys in Chapter 1 is another example.

No one set out to design any of these systems; they simply evolved in response to each culture's needs and values regarding health and illness. As noted in Chapter 1, the scientific medical system has grown around discoveries about the causes and cures of illnesses. Only recently has the promotion of *wellness* become a focus. Conversely, primitive or aboriginal systems tend to focus on the harmony or disharmony of man with his environment, and thus upon maintaining wellness.

Folk systems are used both in maintaining wellness and combatting illness. Witness the advertisements for vitamin and mineral preparations to keep fit, and the current stress among some young people on "natural" nutrition as the key to a full life. Many Americans, particularly among the low-income and lower working class, rely extensively upon folk and lay referral systems before seeking help from professionals. Even then, they are more likely to seek help from a chiropractor or naturopath than from a physician or osteopath.[1]

People from groups in which nonmedical practitioners predominate often use both the healers from their own culture and physicians as we know them. If the illness or disability is judged to be purely physical in nature (e.g., a broken arm, sprained ankle), outside help may be readily sought. However, most psychological distress and unobservable diseases (such as some forms of cancer and tuberculosis) are often considered to be resulting from imbalance and disharmony between the person and his physical and spiritual environment, and therefore are thought to be inaccessible to the scientific practitioner. The beliefs of Christian Scientists about the relationship between harmony with God and health are similar to those of many aboriginal cultures.

Nursing and Health-Care Models

Nursing as a caring, comforting, and nurturing art is not specific to any one of these systems. Assistance in meeting daily physical needs of the ill has always been associated with nursing care, whatever the culture or technology. Ill people needed assistance with their bodily functions long before nursing became a profession or organized occupation. Family members or servants have always been called upon to bathe, feed, and otherwise comfort the ill. Until relatively modern times, these activities occurred in the home, and hospitals were reserved for the poor, who had no place else to die. In many countries throughout the world, the comforting and the physical ministrations associated with nursing are performed in hospital settings by the patient's family, rather than by "trained nurses." Only more recently has nursing been associated with helping persons cope with daily life in nonphysical functions, for example, in relationships with others, or in preventing injury and ill health. In many areas of the world, these aspects of daily life are still not considered a proper area for nursing concern.

As modern medicine evolved its scientific base, nursing became more allied with the profession of medicine, and implementation of many of the curative therapies was delegated to nurses. Thus, nursing has become associated in the public mind with physicians and medical care. Consequently, many nurses and most laymen do not appreciate the role which nurses can play in bridging cultural gaps between medical and nonmedical modes of health care. Because nurses seek to help persons cope with difficulties in daily living, they can offer this help in any

[1] A *chiropractor* is a member of a pseudomedical group which believes that all disease is the result of physical derangement of the nervous system and is amenable to cure by manipulation of the spine. A *naturopath* is also a pseudomedical practitioner, who believes that natural remedies such as diet, rest, and fresh air will cure all disease. An *osteopath* is a member of a medical group which utilizes physical measures somewhat more extensively than medical physicians (M.D.'s). The osteopath (D.O.) may also be licensed as an M.D. in many states. Chiropractic and naturopathy are considered dangerous by scientific health professions because such therapies often cause delay in the treatment of disorders for which there are efficacious medical remedies (Cohen, 1968; A.P.H.A., 1969). Many problems of psychosocial origin respond well to the ministrations of chiropractors and naturopaths.

context in which a person lives and can serve as "translator" between the systems, provided the nurse understands the culture and health beliefs of the person to be helped. The increasing interest in cross-cultural knowledge and practice promises to expand the roles of nurses among the existing health-care systems. References pertinent to understanding health beliefs of cultural and subcultural groups are given in Part 2, Chapter 7, and Part 3, Chapter 9.

The Recipients of Health Care

Before turning to the providers of health care, we need first to look at the ways in which we speak of the recipients of care—the patients and the clients.

Within the scientific or medical model, people who seek help are usually called *patients.* The word patient is derived from the Latin verb *pati,* "to suffer," and is traditionally used to designate sick people. However, the use of the word has expanded to include all those who are under medical care, whether they are ill or not. Because nursing has become so allied with the medical system of care, the term patient is the one most commonly used to describe recipients of nursing care as well.

As health care (in the scientific model) has increased the focus on health as well as illness, the term "patient" has become increasingly restrictive and inaccurate to classify recipients or "consumers" of care, particularly of nursing care. The connotations of "patient" center exclusively around dependence, infirmity, and disease, whereas many of those who seek and use medical and nursing help are predominately independent and are not ill.

The term *client* is being used increasingly by nurses and by some groups of physicians (notably psychiatrists). Client is derived from the Latin *cliens,* a "follower" or "retainer." This word also connotes dependence, in the sense of needing to lean upon another and to give the

other the authority to act in his behalf. Client connotes collaboration, active seeking of help, and interdependence with the helper. Social workers and lawyers have always regarded the persons seeking their help as clients; only recently have members of the health professions done so. Table 2-1 shows the marked differences in connotations of the two terms.

Table 2-1   Comparison of the Denotations and Connotations of *Patient* and *Client*

Patient	Client
Under medical care	Follower
Sufferer	Retainer
Dependent	Dependent (of one engaged
Ill	to act in his behalf)
Ailing	Customer
Not well	Patron
Laid up	
Diseased	
Out of health	

Sources: "American Heritage Dictionary," 1969; "New World Dictionary," 2d College Edition, G. C. Merriam and Company, New York, 1971; "Roget's Pocket Thesaurus," Pocket Books, Inc., New York, 1959.

Nurses attempt to help those who may be in either or both of these roles—that of patient or that of client. The common picture of a nurse is of one who is comforting an acutely ill person, and assisting the physician in cure; e.g., the nurse with a patient. Less commonly do lay persons think of a nurse as one who might counsel a mother in maintaining the health of her family—e.g., a nurse with a client. In this book, we will frequently use the term *patient-client,* to help remind the reader of the collaborative, or active, as well as the passive roles of the persons we help. The term is purposefully clumsy, in the hope that no one will add it to the lexicon of stereotypes about the recipients of our care. As Travelbee (1966) so aptly noted, the terms patient and nurse are both shorthand words which classify the persons so named into certain stereotypes. One of the goals of the interpersonal relationships which are basic to nursing is to move from seeing each other as patient-client and nurse to being people (see Part 2, Chapter 4, for expansion of this theme).

THE FOCUS OF NURSING

Nursing is just one of the many services available to people who need help with health or illness problems. Physicians, nurses, social workers, physical therapists, and dentists are among the many occupational groups so involved. The patient or client has one primary goal—to become more healthy or to relieve his suffering, illness, or disability. Each of the health-care groups has a particular focus on helping him to do this. These focuses overlap to some extent, as they must if the person seeking help is not to be "picked apart" by highly specialized attentions. However, there are certain identifiable differences among the focuses.

Ways of Looking at Nursing

Nurses and sociologists for years have debated among themselves just what the "unique" focus of nursing is—just what nurses contribute to the well-being of patient and client that no one else does. Some have looked at nursing *functions*— what nurses do. For example, the American Nurses' Association defined nursing as having three functions: care, cure, and coordination (A.N.A., 1965). Certain activities were defined within these categories, but the distinction did not really indicate what nursing could offer which was different from the help of other fields. For example, the physician cares for and about his patients, certainly tries to cure them, and considers himself as the coordinator of all other health workers (including the nurse).

Sociologists turned to the *roles* which nurses assume. Role refers to the behaviors associated with a particular position and status and modified by interactions with others in the situation. Johnson and Martin (1958), Schulman (1958),

Skipper (1965), and others have been primary in defining nursing roles as mothering, expressive ones, as opposed to the physician's instrumental or action-oriented roles. These roles would appear to have evolved from the origins of nursing in the comfort of the sick at home, and from the predominance of women in the growth of nursing as a profession. Expressive, nurturing roles are obviously the ones that we equate with women in our society. Many have discussed the conflicts and problems surrounding the increasing delegation of instrumental or curative tasks to nurses (e.g., the medical therapies) and the corresponding diminution in status of the expressive or psychosocial functions. The problems appear to stem both from concern by nurses lest their help to people be "swallowed up" in delegated medical procedures, and from the reluctance of women in our culture to be independent and assertive in those areas which they deem important.

The emphasis on role and function tended to define nursing solely in terms of care of the ill, rather than in the broader context of *health* care. In the late 1950s and early 1960s, nursing leaders began to discuss their contributions in terms of the effects of illness *and* wellness on daily living. Henderson (1960) described nursing as helping persons do those things which they would do for themselves if they were able. Johnson (1959) wrote somewhat more broadly of helping to support the person physically and emotionally until his own resources enable him to deal with the illness or health-threatening situation—providing a "steady state." Rogers (1961) felt that nursing's goal was to help man achieve the optimum health possible. Orlando (1961) and Weidenbach (1964) emphasized looking at the patient's needs from *his* point of view. These approaches recognize more explicitly nursing help in both psychological and physiological functioning, in wellness as well as illness, and emphasize the supporting, sustaining character of nursing.

A Definition of Nursing Focus

Health and illness problems actually or potentially affect a person's ability to cope with or carry on his daily living—for example, his eating, his movement, his relationships with others. Therefore, we may define the focus of nursing as *helping people cope with those difficulties in daily living which are associated with their actual or potential health/illness problems or the treatment thereof.* Orem calls this ability to cope with daily living, "self-care" (1971).

This focus of nursing differs from that of medicine in that the physician is concerned primarily with determining and removing the cause or in treating the health/illness problem, and only secondarily with the person's daily functioning during the course of it. Nurses have an interdependent role with physicians in the therapy of a disability or illness, but they have a primary role in helping the person live with or avoid further disability, and in promoting wellness—living to one's fullest capacities. The model in Fig. 2-1 shows the differing and overlapping focuses of physician and nurse in helping the client.

Changes in Nursing Focus   In its beginnings, nursing functioned quite independently from medicine; the religious nursing orders ran their own hospitals for the sick poor and consulted physicians and surgeons only when they thought necessary. Medicine at that time had little to offer in the cure of disease, and tended to dissociate itself from hospitals, which were places to die in. Gradually, as the science of medicine emerged, physicians began to exert more control over hospitals and over the activities of the nurses who cared for the patients. As medicine developed the tools to fight disease, physicians began to delegate more and more of the actual administration of the therapy to the nurses, who by now were "trained" ladies rather than unprepared pauper women off the street.

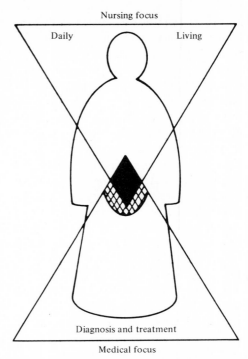

Figure 2-1   Differing and overlapping focuses of nursing and medicine. The *triangles* represent the primary focus of the nurse and the physician in helping a person with his health or illness problem. The *shaded area* is the area of overlap. Nurses are involved in observation and care of the patient as related to diagnostic and therapeutic procedures; physicians are concerned with how their therapy affects the person's daily functional ability. The *cross-hatched* area represents expansion of the nursing focus into responsibility for diagnosis and treatment of some illness. Bates (1970) conceptualizes the expanded role of the nurse as encompassing the nursing focus plus the added medical role (cross-hatched area above). The physician's assistant, in contrast, is seen as functioning only within the medical triangle.

Nurses prior to World War II practiced in hospitals only as students or nursing administrators; graduate nurses were relatively independent as private-duty nurses or public health nurses. As nursing schools gradually changed emphasis from apprenticeship and institutional service to clinical work as selected laboratory experiences, the majority of graduate nurses became hospital employees. Consequently, the average nurse has moved from the relatively independent position of a private practitioner, to the dependent status of an employee. This change, plus the generally dependent position assumed by women in our culture, has led to an unbalanced view, with emphasis more on the assisting roles of nurses and less on the independent contributions to client care. During the major feminist movement in the early 1900s, nursing gained in status as a respectable potential career for women. Some members of the current women's liberation movement downgrade nursing as the prime example of the dependent role of women in society. It is to be hoped that the same movement will provide impetus for recognition of the important independent contributions which nurses can make in health care.[2]

If your own conception of nursing is still that of a lay person, you may see the nurse as assisting the physician in the treatment of disease, and as following his "orders." You may have a mental image of the comforting "angel of mercy," or you may have joined a large part of the population in seeing the registered nurse as one who gives the medicines, and the nurse's aide as the one who takes care of people. By the time you finish your nursing program, perhaps you will see that the professional nurse can have both an independent role and a collaborative role with other health workers, including the physician. In coping with problems of daily living, the nurse may be the expert, but in other areas, or even in selected areas of daily living, other workers may have more expertise. For example, the physical and occupational therapists may focus on selected aspects of daily living—mobility and retraining in physical activity; the dietitian may focus on diet therapy.

New Roles for Nurses One of the current trends in health care is the movement away from institutional care (in hospitals) to community-based care. Along with this trend has come increasing use of the expertise of the nurse and physician to give the client the best help, regardless of the traditional function of nurse and physician. Community health nurses have long provided a great deal of "well" care in guidance, counseling, and support, in addition to traditional home care of the ill. To these skills are being added the ongoing medical management of persons with stable medical problems. Nurses functioning in such roles are given the titles "nurse practitioners," "pediatric associates," "Primex," among others. Such positions are often collectively called the "expanded" or "extended" roles of the nurse. This simply means that in addition to the traditional roles of helping people to cope with problems of daily living, nurses are sharing with physicians some of the responsibility in the treatment of disease and disability. References regarding both the pros and cons of such roles are included at the end of this chapter.

The role of clinical specialist or nurse-clinician has been developed over the past eight to ten years. This type of nurse works with patients and clients in a specialized medical or nursing setting, either having direct patient-care responsibility or functioning as a consultant to the nursing team caring for the patient-client. Nurse-specialists function primarily within the nursing focus, and assist in devising new technologies and approaches in collaboration with medical therapy. Coronary care, hemodialysis and renal transplantation, and psychotherapy are examples of the areas in which nurse-specialists function. The bibliography contains several readings for more information about this role.

The Health Team

When several groups of workers are involved with the care of one client, a health team may be

---

[2] A fascinating account of nursing history and its relationship to the status of women is found in Bullough and Bullough (1969).

formed, in order to coordinate their efforts. Traditionally, physicians have been at the head of such teams. More and more, nurses and other members of the team are assuming leadership for those clients whose major problems are in the area of daily living. In the community, the nurse who visits in the home often takes the initiative for coordinating efforts of other health and community groups. For example, in helping a mother cope with the behavior of a retarded child, the nurse may serve as liaison and interpreter between the parents and such persons as the special education teacher, the diagnostic clinic physician, and the health department consultant in mental retardation.

Basically, all members of the health team utilize their skills in four main ways to aid the patient or client. They help him to *maintain function* (which includes preventing dysfunction), to *sustain him during dysfunction,* to *restore function,* or to *rehabilitate function* if restoration is not possible. Nurses tend to focus primarily on maintaining and sustaining function, and to work with others to restore and rehabilitate. The emphasis in beginning courses in clinical nursing is often on maintaining function and preventing dysfunction.

The Nursing Team

Within health teams, the various professional groups may have their own teams of workers. Up to this point we have spoken of nursing as if it were one entity. However, although nursing may be defined as having one focus, various kinds of persons, with differing educational and training backgrounds, actually provide nursing service to patients and clients. When persons with several levels of training and background provide service to a group of patients or clients, these persons form a nursing team. The leader of the team is usually the person with the greatest amount of education or experience. This nurse generally works with the group in planning to meet the needs of the client or patient (or group) and works through the team to accomplish care. The amount of direct patient-client contact by this leader depends upon the numbers of clients served and the level of expertise of the team members.

The team may be composed of nurses—professional, technical, and vocational; and non-nurses—aides, orderlies, community health workers. The non-nurse members of the team are usually trained on the job, either through formal classes or by simply plunging into the work. In community health agencies, many of the homemakers and clinic workers are recruited from the community served in order to increase communication between the health professionals and those whom they seek to help.

The designations within the category "nurse" are based primarily upon type of licensure and type of nursing education. The registered nurse (R.N.) may be a graduate of a baccalaureate, an associate degree, or a diploma (hospital) program. The initials "R.N." signify simply that the nurse has passed a basic licensing examination. The licensed practical (or vocational) nurse (L.P.N., L.V.N.) has passed a licensing examination allowing him or her to practice under the supervision of a registered nurse or a physician.

Practical or vocational nurses are educated in one- to two-year vocational programs, usually at community colleges or technical schools. They are prepared to assist nurses and physicians in therapy of illness, and to provide for the basic bodily needs of patient-clients. In some settings, such as nursing homes or other stable groups, such a nurse may act as the leader of the care team, under the general supervision of a registered nurse.

Registered nurses have completed two-, three-, or four- and five-year programs leading to a diploma, an associate degree, or a baccalaureate degree. In 1965 the American Nurses' Association issued a position paper on nursing education which stated that the minimum level for professional nursing was the baccalaureate degree; the minimum for technical nurses, the associate degree. Further, the paper stated that all educational preparation for registered nurses should be within institutions of higher learning—e.g., junior and senior colleges. Since that time, there has been a gradual but by no means complete phasing-out of hospital-based diploma programs. Currently, diploma programs continue to graduate the largest number of nurses prepared for licensure as registered nurses.

Although it was hoped that the professionally educated nurse would lead the nursing team (in both hospital and community), the number of nurses so prepared is far below the number of leadership positions already existing; therefore, nurses with other educational backgrounds willingly and unwillingly fill them. The comprehensiveness of planning by registered nurses in leadership roles depends on both their educational background and their clinical experience.

The use of the terms *professional* and *technical* in categorizing registered nurses has prompted many emotional and heated discussions. "Technical" suggests to many people second-best and mechanical, particularly if contrasted with "professional," which connotes higher status. Consequently, the real differences in functions and contributions to the care of patients by nurses prepared in the educational programs so labeled have become blurred.

Nurses in baccalaureate programs are educated to work with individuals and groups in both institution and community, to determine the needs for care, to plan care needed, and to work both independently and through teams of nursing personnel in providing that care. They are prepared to apply this process in a variety of institutional and community settings. In addition, they have the foundation to apply research findings of nurses and other health professionals in designing new approaches to care and to begin to formulate new knowledge in the field.

Nurses educated in the associate degree and diploma programs are prepared primarily for institutional nursing. They, too, have been educated to see the need for and to plan nursing care, but on the basis of more immediate needs related to illness. They have been prepared to use established nursing approaches to common problems, and to function under the general prescriptions of nurses with more advanced education (Waters, 1972; Dechow, 1970; Chater, 1969; Johnson, 1966).

The California Nurses' Association, in attempting recently to redefine the functions of the registered nurse members of the team, omitted the emotionally charged professional and technical designations. They defined practice as *implemental* and *supplemental*. Implemental practice is aimed toward implementing and using established or new technologies in illness care, and focuses on immediate needs; supplemental care attempts to develop the client's abilities to cope for himself, has long-term as well as immediate objectives, and tests new or innovative approaches. The commission does not attempt to define levels of education basic to each approach (Waters, 1972).

The National Commission for the Study of Nursing and Nursing Education recently proposed that nursing follow two career patterns. One pattern they call *episodic*—directed primarily toward persons with diagnosed disease, and concerned with restoration and curative function. The *distributive* pattern is concerned with noninstitutionalized persons and the maintenance of their health (Lysaught, 1970). The report and its recommendations have been criticized for artificially separating aspects of nursing care which are not separate in the persons for whom we care, and in defining nursing primarily on the basis of where the nurse is employed (institution or community) (Christy et al., 1971; Rogers, 1972).

The controversy regarding levels of nursing preparation, functions of varying categories of nurses, the need for career ladders (for easy movement from one level to another), and the intellectual and technical focus of each group of nursing personnel is far from resolved. Those of you who are beginning your nursing education will certainly be touched by these debates, and some of you will be among those who will help define the new roles of nursing.

REFERENCES

American Nurses' Association: First Position on Education for Nursing, 1965, *American Journal of Nursing*, **65**:106–111 (Dec., 1965).

American Public Health Association: Policy Statement, Nov. 19, 1969, quoted in H. T. Ballantine, Will the Delivery of Health Care Be Improved by the Use of Chiropractic Services? *New England Journal of Medicine*, **286**:241 (Feb. 3, 1972).

Chater, Shirley (ed.), "Toward Differentiation of Associate and Baccalaureate Nursing Education and Practice," University of California Press, San Francisco, 1969.

Christy, Teresa, Muriel Poulin, and Julie Hover: An Appraisal of An Abstract for Action, *American Journal of Nursing*, **71**:1574–1579 (1971).

Cohen, Wilbur J.: Independent Practitioners under Medicine: A Report to Congress, U.S. Dept. of Health, Education, and Welfare, 1968.

DeChow, Georgeen: Preparing the Technical Nurse Practitioner, *The Journal of Nursing Education*, **9**:2–4 (Aug., 1970).

Henderson, Virginia, "Basic Principles of Nursing Care," International Council of Nurses, London, 1960.

———: The Nature of Nursing, *American Journal of Nursing*, **64**:62 (Aug., 1964).

Johnson, Dorothy: A Philosophy of Nursing, *Nursing Outlook*, **7**:198–200 (Apr., 1959).

———: The Significance of Nursing Care, *American Journal of Nursing*, **61**:63 (Nov., 1961).

———: Competence in Practice: Technical and Professional, *Nursing Outlook*, **14**:30–33 (Oct., 1966).

Johnson, Miriam, and Harry W. Martin: A Sociological Analysis of the Nurse Role, *American Journal of Nursing*, **58**:373–377 (Mar., 1958); also in J. Skipper and R. Leonard (eds.), "Social Interaction and

Patient Care," J. B. Lippincott Company, Philadelphia, 1965.

Lysaught, Jerome P., et al., "An Abstract for Action: Report of the National Commission for the Study of Nursing and Nursing Education," McGraw-Hill Book Company, 1970. [Summarized in the *American Journal of Nursing*, **70**:279–294 (Feb., 1970).]

Orem, Dorothea E., "Nursing: Concepts of Practice," McGraw-Hill Book Company, New York, 1971.

Orlando, Ida Jean, "The Dynamic Nurse-Patient Relationship," G. P. Putnam's Sons, New York, 1961.

Rogers, Martha, "Educational Revolution in Nursing," The Macmillan Company, New York, 1961.

———: Nursing: To Be or Not to Be? *Nursing Outlook*, **20**:42–46 (Jan., 1972).

Schulman, Sam: Basic Functional Roles in Nursing: Mother Surrogate and Healer, in E. G. Jaco, (ed.), "Patients, Physicians, and Illness," The Free Press, Glencoe, Ill., 1958.

Skipper, James: The Role of the Hospital Nurse: Is It Instrumental or Expressive? in J. Skipper and R. Leonard (eds.), "Social Interaction and Patient Care," J. B. Lippincott Company, Philadelphia, 1965.

Travelbee, Joyce, "Interpersonal Aspects of Nursing," 1st ed., F. A. Davis Company, New York, 1966.

Waters, Verle H.: Nursing Practice—Implemental and Supplemental, *American Journal of Nursing*, **72**:88–92 (Jan., 1972).

———, Shirley S. Chater, Mary L. Vivier, Judithe H. Urrea, and Holly S. Wilson: Technical and Professional Nursing: An Exploratory Study, *Nursing Research*, **21**:124–131 (Mar.-Apr., 1972).

Weidenbach, Ernestine, "Clinical Nursing: A Helping Art," Springer Publishing Company, New York, 1964.

ADDITIONAL READINGS

General

Bullough, Bonnie, and Vern L. Bullough, "New Directions in Nursing," Springer Publishing Company, New York, 1971. (A book of readings which represents both sides of the controversies about changing roles and directions of the profession.)

——— and Bonnie Bullough, "The Emergence of Modern Nursing," The Macmillan Company, New York, 1969.

Cleland, Virginia: Sex Discrimination: Nursing's Most Pervasive Problem, *American Journal of Nursing,* **71**:1542–1547 (1971).

King, Stanley, Systems of Beliefs and Attitudes about Disease, in "Perceptions of Illness and Medical Practice," Russell Sage Foundation, New York, 1962, pp. 91–131.

Nursing Forum, **9**(4) (1970). (Entire issue devoted to the effects of a changing world on nursing.)

New Roles for Nurses

Expanded and Extended Roles

Andrews, Priscilla, and Alfred Yankauer: The Pediatric Nurse Practitioner, *American Journal of Nursing,* **71**:504–515 (1971).

Bates, Barbara: Doctor and Nurse: Changing Roles and Relationships, *New England Journal of Medicine,* **283**:129–134 (July 16, 1970).

Bergman, Abraham: Physician's Assistants Belong in the Nursing Profession, *American Journal of Nursing,* **71**:975–977 (1971).

DeTornyay, Rheba: Expanding the Nurse's Role Does Not Make Her a Physician's Assistant, *American Journal of Nursing,* **71**:974–976 (1971).

Leininger, Madeleine, Delores Little, and Doris Carnevali: Primex, *American Journal of Nursing,* **72**:1274–1277 (July, 1972).

Lewis, Charles, and Barbara Resnik: Nurse Clinics and Progressive Ambulatory Care, *New England Journal of Medicine,* **277**:1236–1241 (1967).

Nursing at the Crossroads, *Nursing Outlook,* **20**: (1972). (Entire issue; includes report of the Secretary of HEW's Committee to Study Extended Roles for Nurses.)

Clinical Specialist

Lewis, Edith P. (ed.), "The Clinical Nurse Specialist," American Journal of Nursing Company, Educational Services Division, New York, 1970.

Little, Dolores E., and Doris Carnevali: Nursing Specialist: Effect on Tuberculosis, *Nursing Research,* **16**:321–326 (1967).

Reiter, Frances: The Nurse Clinician, *American Journal of Nursing,* **66**:274–280 (1966).

Nursing in the Context of Social and Cultural Systems

Madeleine Leininger

Since nursing practices take place within a designated social and cultural system, it is essential for nurses to acquire an understanding of some of the basic ideas about the characteristics of system behavior. To understand and apply knowledge of social and cultural systems is a relatively new trend in nursing, but one of major significance if one hopes to help people effectively and successfully. Without an understanding of system behavior, the nurse might readily become frustrated and baffled about the "why" of human behavior. In addition, system behavior may indirectly and directly affect the patient-client in his working relationships with staff in an agency or hospital. Moreover, an awareness of system behavior enables the nurse to design effective nursing plans and to utilize appropriate strategies for care of the patient. With such

knowledge and its application, the nurse will be able to grow considerably in his professional skills and be stimulated to cope with complex individual and staff behavior that is influenced by social and cultural system behaviors.

Although system behavior is complex, it can be observed, understood, and evaluated (Taylor, 1970). Both cultural and social systems are people-centered and people-oriented. As one thinks about system behavior it is important first to clarify one's ideas of a system, a social system, and a cultural system.

DEFINITIONS: SYSTEM, SOCIAL SYSTEM, CULTURAL SYSTEM

In a general sense, *a system may be viewed as an organization of persons who are linked together and who show signs of being interrelated and interdependent upon one another to achieve certain functions or goals.* A system reflects that each person is important in contributing to the work of all the persons in the structure. Furthermore, each person is dependent upon the others in some way, whether it is a close or very loose form of dependency. Thus, each phrase in this definition has meaning and should be given careful thought for an understanding of the essence of a system. Let us next consider the definitions of social and cultural systems.

A social system may be viewed as a network of persons who regularly interact with one another and manifest signs of being interdependent and interrelated in order to achieve common institutional goals. A social system is primarily *group-oriented* and *group-directed.* One may also view a social system as an identifiable pattern of social interaction with a number of persons communicating with one another and sharing common interests and concerns about activities in a designated setting. Indeed, it is almost impossible to conceive of a social system having socially isolated or alienated individuals, as all individuals are expected to function with other persons in the system. Furthermore, one might conceive of the hospital, the community, a public health agency, or a family as a social system. Each of these large or small kinds of social system has identifiable patterns of behavior that make it a somewhat unique or distinct type of social system. Social systems are functional systems in that persons interact in a regular way with one another and are interdependent and interrelated (Leininger, 1970).

A cultural system refers to the norms, values, and action patterns of a designated group of people who are interdependent upon one another to maintain their life ways. The key terms related to a cultural system are the words norms, values, and actions of being interdependent. Every cultural system has rules of behavior (norms) which guide the group's thinking, actions, and ways of living.

Cultural norms of a designated group of people in a social system may be slightly or markedly different from those of another group. Thus it is important for the nurse to understand the norms of a social system in order to interact appropriately with the group and determine courses of action with patients and staff that will be acceptable to those in the system. Knowledge of the cultural norms of any system is essential to the nurse's functioning, especially if he is attempting to change patterns of health care with a family or in a designated community. Today, he must understand the norms of behavior that influence or determine social and cultural system behaviors. To change health practices of a family, a community, or a hospital system without an awareness of its cultural norms would be like trying to change the life style of one's parents without a logical reason.

Individual and group behavior reflects the norms and values of a particular cultural system. Some persons adhere to the cultural norms of the system, others tend to be more flexible and try to accommodate a range of variation in the behavior norms. Sometimes subgroups in a system diverge considerably from the norms of the system (Leininger, 1970). The extent to which a group supports or rejects the specific cultural norms of a system is generally related to the group's desire to retain or relinquish traditional norms. Hospitals, too, adhere to certain norms and then in time drop or change them (Taylor, 1970). For example, in one hospital, a nurse was not expected to visit with or do any health counseling with parents when they brought their child to the hospital. However, five years later in the same hospital these norms or cultural rules were reversed.

In most hospitals there are both *implicit* and *explicit* norms; the nurse should identify and study both kinds, as both are important. Implicit norms are the informal, subtle, and covert rules of behavior; explicit norms are the formal, overt, and usually written rules of behavior. Implicit norms are the most difficult to identify and are often more significant than the explicit ones. For example, an explicit norm of behavior in a hospital is the written statement in the ward handbook that nurses meet at 3 P.M. for a so-called "change-of-shift" ward conference. An implicit norm of behavior is the unwritten statement, and an informal rule, that certain nurses meet together in a coffee shop about 2:30 P.M. to identify ward problems and gossip about the latest hospital events.

SYSTEMS WITHIN AND OUTSIDE THE HOSPITAL SETTING

Although the hospital may be perceived and recognized as having a social and cultural system, the nurse needs to know that other kinds of institutions in a community also have these systems. For example, public health departments, day-care centers, mental health clinics, rehabilitation centers, nursing homes, and a variety of other community agencies also have cultural and social systems. Each agency has its *own* pattern of social interaction (the social system) and its own peculiar rules of behavior (the cultural system). It is the responsibility of the nurse of tomorrow to study and identify the essential attributes of these systems to determine his mode of operating and ways of working successfully in these settings. Usually the greater the number of employees in an agency, the more complex are its social and cultural systems and the more difficult it is to identify the essential components of the systems. Thus, it is often wise for the nurse to start with a small system, such as a small clinic or a family, before trying to identify the complex system of the hospital. Because hospitals are complex, it is becoming common practice to have an anthropologist or sociologist employed in the hospital to identify social and cultural system behavior at different periods of time. If the hospital has such an employee, the nurse can draw upon his knowl-

edge. There are also a few nurse-anthropologists and nurse-sociologists who can be most helpful to nurses in understanding such system behavior.

Hospitals in urban areas are usually stratified (or layered), with persons working in subordinate and superordinate positions to one another. The hospital functions as an organization to serve people, mainly sick ones, in contrast to some nonhospital agencies, which may serve to prevent people from becoming ill through health counseling and education. Within a hospital system there are subsystems, such as ward units. These subunits constitute the total hospital system, but each unit may have rules and patterns of social interaction that differ slightly from those prescribed by the hospital administrators.

As a general system principle, the total hospital environment must be in relative harmony with the outside environment and with its constituent agencies in the community. The hospital must also be in relative harmony with the culture in which it functions. Traditional values and norms within and outside the hospital must be considered if the hospital hopes to achieve its goals effectively (Taylor, 1970). In summary, there are systems within and outside the hospital, and all are important to health care and to nurse practitioners.

WHAT TO OBSERVE, STUDY, AND EVALUATE ABOUT SYSTEM BEHAVIOR

In any system, there are essential components which the nurse needs to observe, study, and evaluate in order to understand *what* to do, *why* to do the activity in a certain way, and *how* to give nursing care in what appears to be the best way. The nurse's interpersonal strategies are also contingent upon understanding system behavior. In the remainder of this chapter, some of the key components of system behavior will be identified and briefly discussed. The nurse who desires a more comprehensive understanding of these components will find additional information and research findings in social science helpful. In addition, nursing conferences and seminars with nurse-anthropologists and nurse-sociologists would be helpful in applying the theory and research findings to nurse-patient-staff situations and in the general assessment of health systems. The following components of system behavior have been selected as important in understanding system structure and behavior and will be discussed below: (1) social organization and role behavior, (2) interactional and communication patterns, (3) social status, rank, and prestige, (4) authority, power, and politics, (5) cultural norms and values, and (6) cultural and social changes.

Social Organization and Role Behavior

In social or cultural system behavior, individuals and groups are organized to achieve the goals or purposes of the institution. The way in which the people are organized and assume different roles to get the work accomplished in the institution is the *social organization.*

Social organization is concerned with the interactional behavior of subgroups of people within an institution and the way they function to fulfill the purposes of the institution. Health institutions have goals and a philosophy which guides behavior (King, 1962). Some institutions are highly organized in an efficient and democratic way; others may be rigidly organized with norms which are impersonal and autocratic (Taylor, 1970).

Within any social organization, there are persons who occupy and perform certain roles so that they can get the work done in the setting. In the simplest sense, *role behavior refers to the cluster of functions and activities which persons are expected to perform in an institution or in a given society.* For example, the nurse is expected to help clients with their health concerns. He performs caring functions to relieve clients of undue discomforts, stresses, and illness problems and to help them retain their health status. In his

nursing role, the nurse is expected to perform a number of role activities, such as health counseling, health teaching, coordination of health services, curing, monitoring of machines, and other activities. The nurse may fully endorse all role activities as highly essential to the nursing role, or he may question or reject a number of role activities which do not seem to be in accord with the expected nursing role. For example, the nurse may fully accept health counseling and reject the monitoring of a machine. If the system role expectations do not *fit* the nurse's perceptions and those of the nursing profession, role conflict and ambiguities occur, with the nurse trying to clarify the nurse's role in the institution (King, 1962).

In most social organizations, the roles of different staff members tend to overlap with another professional group. For example, the role of the physician and the role of the nurse commonly overlap in the area of health assessment and diagnosis of the patient-client's problems and needs. Such *role overlaps* are common and exist when health services are perceived to be an integral part of the duties of several persons giving health care. These role overlaps can be used in a positive way to validate and reinforce interprofessional skills and knowledge. Sometimes they come in direct conflict with role-performance expectations and are a source of interprofessional tension. For example, the nurse's role activities in providing continuity of care as the patient-client moves from the hospital back to his home may be a source of role conflict with the social worker as he makes arrangements for the patient to go home. However, since both the nurse and social worker are involved in home-care plans, they should use their combined knowledge and skills in a collaborative way to help the patient get the best kind of health service possible when he goes home. Sometimes role conflicts between professional staff become sources of hostility and the patient gets caught in the conflict. Thus it is important for the nurse to be aware of the likelihood of the problem and to try and resolve it through interprofessional communication, rather than having the patient experience the conflict along with his other illness stresses.

Occasionally, one can also find *role gaps* in that no professional group is performing important functions to meet the needs of a patient or of an institution. When this occurs, it is often the patient who reveals the role gap. He may say, for example, "I couldn't find anyone to help me with this problem." Professional staff need to remain alert to such comments and to look for role gaps. For example, a critical role gap was revealed a few years ago when parents were asking professional staff for help with children who had fears associated with surgery. This need was recognized, and nurses were prepared to fulfill the role functions related to health counseling of parents and children prior to and after surgery. Frequently, the invention of new machines and the discovery of new kinds of illness lead to the need for new role functions.

Role behaviors of different professional groups generally *complement* one another and are essential to provide the full complement of health services. It is, therefore, important that the nurse have an understanding of the general role activities of *each* health professional group, so that he will know the contributions of each to health care. Since interdependency exists among health professionals, no professional group can function in an isolated manner from another group. Knowledge of one another's roles is essential to effective interdisciplinary work and interprofessional communication. In addition, a knowledge of the various professional roles helps one to understand role changes, role conflicts, role gaps, and areas of role satisfactions and dissatisfactions of persons within a health organization. In summary, the social organization and the roles of persons within the organization constitute the key structural ingredients to understanding social and cultural systems.

Interactional and Communication Patterns

Because interactional and communication patterns are dynamically interrelated to one another, they are discussed together in this section. Whom people in an institution communicate with in the day-to-day work situation largely determines the patterns of interaction and the way in which the goals of an institution are achieved. Generally the pattern of communication follows the pattern of professional interaction. Or the reverse of this statement probably holds, in that the patterns of interaction determine the patterns of communication in social and cultural systems. Thus it is difficult to separate communication and interaction modes in a social system. It is, however, possible; we know that communication can exist without direct contact between persons and that symbolic interaction can occur without direct physical interaction between two or more persons in the setting.

The important question is *what* should the nurse observe about interactions and communication. Most important, he should observe *who* communicates with *whom* and about *what* in the health setting. The nurse observes *patterns of interaction* among various persons in the social system. Whom do the nurse, physician, social worker, and others interact with, and about which matters? The key questions which the nurse needs to consider in observing and studying interactional and communication patterns are the following: (1) Who interacts and communicates with whom and for what purposes? (2) Where and how do they usually communicate with each other? (3) What is the predominant way they communicate with each other? (4) Are there problems or areas of stress concerning the communication or the interaction? (5) What appears to be the consequence of the interaction, i.e., was it helpful? agreeable? satisfying? argumentative? informative? sharing? or what? (6) Was the interaction more oriented to problems of patients, to institutional concerns, or what? (7) Was the interaction a recurrent or typical kind of encounter? (8) How did persons involved use the communication to help people in the hospital or agency? (9) What problems or barriers could you identify as you observed the interaction or communication encounter? (10) What do you believe would facilitate more effective patterns of communication, and why?

As the nurse observes interaction and communication modes, he may find the following models of communication helpful to him (the arrow in these models indicates the direction of the communication or interaction):

A. Linear Model. This is a two-way flow of communication going in a straight direction between two individuals (*a* and *b*).

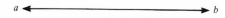

B. Inverted-Y Model. The flow of communication goes from the person in a top-level position (superordinate role) to others below him in the social system (subordinate roles). It is a stratified model of communication.

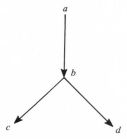

C. Circular Model. The communication starts with *a* and flows around to *b, c, d,* and back to *a,* in a one-directional pattern.

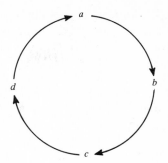

D. Wheel Model. One key person sends and receives all communication from the center of the wheel to other persons in subunits of the system. Thus the flow of communication is essentially back and forth from the "executive communicator" to others in between *a* and *b, a* and *d,* etc.

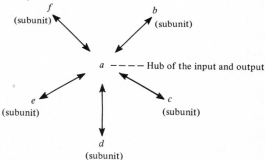

E. Star Model. The goal is to have the communication or interactions occur between all persons in the social system. The flow of communication is multidirectional, with all modes possible between individuals and subsystems.

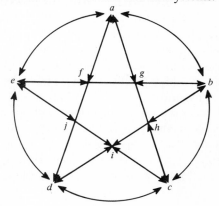

As one considers these samples of communication models, one can identify the strengths and limitations of each pattern. This exercise will be left to the reader and his interested colleagues to discuss and apply to hospital and nonhospital settings. Interestingly, the inverted-Y model is one of the most common models of communication used in hospitals. If one can identify the model used in an institution or agency, it helps him to explain, predict, and refer to behavior patterns more precisely than by using a long descriptive account.

Social Status, Rank, and Prestige

It is well established today that in every social and cultural system, persons who occupy certain roles in the system have an identifiable social status and prestige associated with the role. *Social status* refers to the particular position which a person has who occupies a particular role in the system. *Prestige* refers to the importance of and the recognition accorded to a person who occupies a particular position in a system or society. *Rank* refers to the ordered position above and below persons in the system. It is usually viewed in relation to persons in a higher or lower position in the system who are designated with a particular title to refer to their rank. For example, we speak of the rank of a nursing director, assistant director, and staff nurse. Certain positions in a system tend to offer more status and prestige than others. Accordingly, some positions are of lesser significance and do not offer much prestige or honor. The role of the physician in the hospital setting and in our society almost automatically accords the physician a high prestige, high social status, and high rank in the system. This high status, prestige, and rank of the physician can be visibly identified in most hospital systems today by such signs as: "Only for Physicians," "Physicians' Lounge," "Physicians' Conference Room," "Silence—Physicians' Room." Such status and prestige signs become clearly evident when one attempts to find similar signs of deference, recognition, and special privileges for the nursing staff in the hospital. Thus one notes frequently less status, less prestige, and lower ranks for nurses in the hospital system. Differences in status and rank between the nurse and physician can be noted in relation to salary differences, special privileges, annual honors, deferential behavior toward the physician, signs of respect to the physician, and availability to the physician of many services in the hospital.

Differences in status and prestige may also be related to long-term sex-discrimination practices. Nurses are becoming more aware that the profession is largely female, and that nurses have less status, fewer top institutional positions, and less prestige by virtue of the sex factor alone. It is to be hoped that with the current liberation movement for women this obvious inequity will be changed soon.

Status may be either ascribed or achieved. An *achieved status* is acquired through hard work, years of education and experience, and solid efforts based upon one's knowledge and experience background. For example, a nurse faculty member may have an achieved status by virtue of her years of teaching students. In contrast, an *ascribed status* may be acquired by virtue of one's birth, sudden rise to fame (i.e., luck), or acquaintance or association with certain persons in social and work situations. For example, the son of a well-known physician may receive an ascribed status by virtue of being the physician's son. He did not receive his recognition through achieved-status means. Or a woman who suddenly becomes a millionaire by winning money may acquire an ascribed status almost overnight.

Status and prestige differences can have both positive and negative effects upon persons in the system. Of course, those with higher status tend to be content, as high status offers power, special privileges, and many other benefits not given to people of low status or rank. In our culture, persons with low status often struggle "up the social and occupational ladder" in order to gain equal status, prestige, and rights which are supposed to be an ideal norm for all Americans and not just a few.

Most research findings today show that patients or clients in our health system are given generally low status and prestige, especially in the hospital setting. Patients often change their social rank and status considerably when they enter the hospital, and this is of much concern to some patients. They may find themselves with less power, less responsibility, and less authority, and they may be shown less respect. All these factors greatly reduce the patient's social status and prestige. A reduction in social status can seriously affect the emotional, social, and cultural health problems of the patient. Thus differences in status and respect provide valuable clues about how people behave and how they are perceived, valued, and respected in the system. Knowledge of social status, rank, and prestige can help the nurse predict which persons will probably communicate and interact with one another, and possible changes in health behavior.

Authority, Power, and Politics in Health Systems

Anyone working in a hospital or other type of health system will soon discover that authority, power, and politics exist in different forms and different degrees of influence. Like any other social or cultural system which hopes to survive in our society, the system needs to have persons in authority roles who will be ultimately responsible for the institution—its people, practices, and services. These authority persons carry heavy responsibilities in most of our complex and stratified hospital systems. In general, persons in an *authority role* are designated to have rightful legal power and to command others under them to perform certain acts in order to maintain the operation of the system.

Currently in our society, persons in authority roles tend to be viewed with contempt; the feeling seems to be that they are trying to take away one's own power and rights. Many Americans do not like to have any restraints upon their freedom and rights. Complete freedom in thoughts and actions is often considered one's due, and this freedom is sometimes coupled with limited responsibility to others in society. Values related to self-interests, high emphasis upon individual needs, and the desire for autonomy in thinking and action challenge persons in authority roles today and are a source of interpersonal tension between leaders and followers. This autonomy-authority conflict is apparent between nursing service directors and nursing staff in nonauthority roles in hospitals. It is, therefore, important for the nurse to observe and evaluate the role of persons in authority and to understand leader-follower problems stemming from conflicts with our values.

Observing behaviors and measures employed by effective leaders in authority roles is valuable in helping nurses become respected, helpful leaders in a social system. Some leaders are positively democratic in their mode of operation. They actively seek and encourage group and individual participation in decision making, opinion giving, communication, and implementing plans bearing upon group decisions. Other leaders in authority are autocratic and operate in a manner that is the opposite of democratic. And finally, there are leaders who tend to ride the "middle-of-the-road" position (neutral leaders) and never seem to exert any direction, advice, or group leadership in one way or another. These leaders seem to be afraid to be either democratic or autocratic; they maintain a truly neutral attitude and are generally ineffective as leaders in a large social system such as the hospital.

Indeed, leadership behavior is extremely important and fascinating to observe, study, and evaluate, as it offers guidelines to nursing success in a social system. The effectiveness of the nurse's leadership in the hospital, agency, and community is largely determined by the role models the nurse emulates in handling complex problems related to care of the patient and to interdisciplinary leadership in health settings.

Power and politics are intrinsically interwoven into the concept of authority. Power often is possessed by persons other than the officially designated leaders. It is always of interest to discover *who* exerts the most power in a system and *why*. Essentially, *power is concerned with the capacity for action or with producing an effect upon someone or something.* Persons with power possess a controlling influence over others, such as an individual, group, social system, government, etc. Often persons with power are invested with authority, but again an individual who is not officially vested with authority may still greatly influence others. Political power and politics might be viewed as a means by which an individual (or more than one) exerts a *weighty influence* (intellectually or by sheer group-experience tactics) upon others, whether within or outside a social system, in order to achieve individual interests or for a variety of other reasons.

Politics as the art and science of managing the affairs of groups and political parties exists within and outside a hospital environment and consequently affects the quality of nursing care to patients. The modern nurse must be knowledgeable about politics, power, political affairs, and authority behavior. The author contends that these factors are some of the most important that are influencing professional nursing practices and health-care services today. We are in an era in which nurses must deal directly with political, cultural, and social issues and problems. Such issues cannot be glossed over as nonprofessional interests of nurses. Our interests in quality of health care and in the management of nursing care are vitally related to authority controls, politics, and power within and outside health agencies and in schools of nursing.

Cultural Norms and Values

As indicated earlier, the nurse must observe and study the cultural norms (rules of behavior) and the values that direct and guide the behavior of patients and staff in any system. The cultural values of the patient-client, the staff, and the hospital may differ, one from another, and may produce areas of great conflict and tension (Leininger, 1970).

Indeed, the hospital has identifiable cultural norms to which the patient is generally expected to conform; if he fails to conform to these norms it may seriously affect his recovery (Taylor, 1970). Each hospital has fairly unique cultural norms which may be very strange to the patient-client (King, 1962).

In order to develop meaningful nursing-care plans and implement them, the nurse must be knowledgeable about the values of different **cultural and subcultural groups such as the Mexican-Americans, Japanese-Americans, Afro-Americans, North American Indians, Appalachian peoples,** and many other cultural groups in our society. With our rapid modes of transportation and communication, he will also be providing health care to peoples in other countries and should have some beginning knowledge of them and their cultures. Without such knowledge of the values of different cultural groups, the nurse often unintentionally or intentionally imposes his own ethnocentric health values and norms upon the patient. This is a highly questionable practice and may have unfavorable consequences and nontherapeutic long-range effects. Thus, in order to make valid and reliable judgments about cultural values, the nurse must first understand the values of the patient, group, or family he is trying to help. While this remains largely a new area of focus in nursing, the nurse may have to seek culture information through independent study and reflective experiences. Anthropological courses and literature regarding different culture groups will be helpful in increasing the nurse's knowledge. Examples of the use of such knowledge in nursing care are given throughout this book.

Cultural and Social Changes

Cultural and social systems are not static. They change through time and from place to place in the world. Some systems tend to change very slowly; others change fairly rapidly and over a short span of time. It is the people living and working in any system that are primarily the change agents. The nurse is an important change agent within the hospital and in other kinds of community-based agencies.

Currently, there is a prevailing belief in our society that all and any kind of change in our social systems should be viewed as beneficial, and that no change means a static, dead system. This belief or myth needs to be examined, in relation to both positive and negative efficacious changes in systems and over a period of time. As students of change, we know that generally change produces some anxiety and fear. Change may have a positive effect upon a health system, or it may cause problems and never be particularly helpful to patients, health system, or staff. Generally, changes in a large health system are difficult to make and require persistence by group leaders and a willingness to take risks and face unknown consequences.

It is always interesting to note the ways in which systems resist or facilitate changes. For example, in one hospital, nursing-service administrators have traditionally employed only nurses who have been prepared from a particular school of nursing—"their favorite graduates." They are afraid to employ nurses from another school as it may change or "rock" the system too much and thus require the nursing administrators (supervisors and head nurses) to cope with different ideas and different nursing-care values.

How staff and patients and social system respond to changes should be observed and evaluated. Do staff "get up-tight" with any new changes? How do patients and their families react to changes in hospital visiting rules; nursing-care practices; new nurses in the system; different way of helping patients; etc.? The nurse should also be interested in knowing if the health system is generally rather a slow-change system, or if it is constantly adjusting to changes and has a capacity to respond rather rapidly to inside and outside changes. Societal forces play a definite role in changes in nursing practices, health-care systems, and health practitioners' values.

The nurse can promote and facilitate changes in health systems providing he is cognizant of questions such as the following: (1) What needs to be changed and why? (2) What have been my past behavioral tendencies about changes? (3) What are my strengths and capabilities to be an effective agent of change? (4) Which persons in the system should be involved to facilitate change? (5) What role will I play and what role will others play in the change? (6) What factors must we consider to evaluate if the change was effective over a short or long period of time? (7) How does one sustain the beneficial changes desired over a period of time? These questions and others are critical in planning for and implementing change. Being a change agent can be one of the most exciting and rewarding experiences for a nurse. It can challenge him to use his full professional skills, intellectual and creative abilities, and interpersonal skills, as well as all available resources in the community. The nurse can and should be a positive change agent to bring about better nursing care. Most of the time, he lives and works with change but is not always fully aware of the dynamics and consequences of his influence on changes in a system, a community, and our society. Beginning students have little chance or power to effect marked change, but can prepare for their eventual role by becoming astute observers of system changes and their behavioral consequences.

WHO IS OBSERVED AND EVALUATED BY THE NURSE

Throughout the discussion in this chapter, it is clear that the nurse observes and evaluates the following in relation to social system behavior and for plans of action: (1) the patient or client, (2) the nurse, (3) other staff members, e.g., psychologists, social workers, physicians, pharmacists, nonprofessional staff, and others, (4) the family, group, and community who affect the patient and health system.

Observation, study, and evaluation of any social and cultural system requires a *gestalt,* or a *holistic* view of all components of people interacting and living in the system. If the nurse has "tunnel," or limited-object, vision, it will be difficult to grasp the total picture of system behavior as outlined in this chapter. The nurse has to "put the pieces of the puzzle" together, or to synthesize what he has observed, studied, and evaluated. This requires systematic observations made over a period of time, concentrated thinking, and sometimes verifying findings with others knowledgeable about system behaviors.

As the nurse observes the patient, nurses, other staff members, and the family and community, he focuses upon the major components already identified in this chapter about cultural social system behavior. In addition, the nurse may wish to consider these questions: (1) Who seems powerful or powerless in the system? (2) Who is responsible to whom and for what areas of care or treatment? (3) Who makes decisions in the system, and how effective are these decisions? (4) How are problems solved in the system, and do patients participate in solutions to the problem? (5) Who helps evaluate the care of the patient? (6) What is the general affective, or emotional, climate of the system, e.g., helpful or less helpful, impersonal or personalized, kindly or hostile, competitive or noncompetitive, trustful or distrustful, autocratic or democratic, human-centered or task-centered, service-ori-ented or job-oriented? (7) What kind of group feelings, values, and patterns exist inside and outside the system? These questions and others may be used as valuable guides to observe and evaluate any social and cultural system. The data from these questions can provide rich sources of information to design, implement, and assess nursing-care practices.

SUMMARY

In this chapter, the author has defined and discussed the basic ideas related to cultural and social systems. The major components that the nurse needs to observe, study, and evaluate were identified and briefly discussed. Throughout the presentation, the nurse's role in system behavior and operations was discussed to help him understand the significant aspects of system behavior and of his own role as he functions in social and cultural systems. Understanding system behavior was discussed as one of the most essential areas of study for the nurse of tomorrow, as it is vital to giving effective, successful nursing care. The nurse when performing this role lives in a social and cultural system, makes decisions to maintain or change the system, and can achieve the highest kind of professional skill and insight about human behavior through system experiences. System behavior directly affects the patient-client, nurse, and all professionals living and working in it. It is, indeed, the significant factor in changing health-care practices and in maintaining effective health practices.

REFERENCES

King, Stanley H., The Hospital: An Analysis in Terms of Social Structure, in *Perceptions of Illness and Medical Practice,* Russell Sage Foundation, New York, 1962, pp. 307-348; 349-392.

Leininger, Madeleine M., Health Institutions as Cultural and Social Systems, in "Nursing and Anthropology: Two Worlds to Blend," John Wiley & Sons, Inc., New York, 1970, pp. 83-96, 145-165.

Taylor, Carol, "In Horizontal Orbit: Hospitals and the Cult of Efficiency," Holt, Rinehart and Winston, Inc., New York, 1970, pp. 1–18, 63–95.

ADDITIONAL READINGS[1]

Caudill, William, et al.: Social Structure and Interaction Process on a Psychiatric Ward, *American Journal of Orthopsychiatry,* **22**:314–334 (1952).

Leininger, Madeleine M.: The Significance of Cultural Concepts in Nursing, *Minnesota League for Nursing Bulletin,* **16**(3):3–12 (1968).

———: The Use of Cultural Concepts in Patient Care, *Minnesota League for Nursing Bulletin,* **16**(5):3–9 (1968).

———: Cultural Differences Among Staff Members and the Impact on Patient Care, *Minnesota League for Nursing Bulletin,* **16**(5):5–9 (1968).

———: "Using Cultural Styles in the Helping Process and in Relation to the Subculture of Nursing" *Psychiatric Nursing Bulletin* of the Illinois Psychiatric Institute, Chicago, Illinois, 1972.

Smith, Alfred G., "Communication and Culture: Readings in the Codes of Human Interaction," Holt, Rinehart and Winston, Inc., New York, 1966.

Wooden, Howard E.: The Hospital's Purpose Is the Patient, But . . ., *Modern Hospital,* **92**:90–96 (1959).

[1] Several cultural readings are included in Chapters 7 and 9.

The Process of Diagnosis and Intervention

Most people think of *diagnosis* as a term which applies only to a physician's determination of the nature of an illness. Its meaning is broader, however, and it can be used in any field in which systematic methods are used to determine the nature of something. Educators speak of diagnosing learning problems; mechanics diagnose the source of engine failure; and nurses have begun to speak of diagnosing patients' nursing problems (Chambers, 1962; Durand and Prince, 1966).

The purpose of this section is to provide a detailed framework for diagnosing the need for nursing care and for providing this care. The framework is based upon the method of identifying and solving problems which is common to all scientific disciplines—the "scientific method."

Nursing cannot claim to be a scientific profession unless its practitioners utilize a rational, systematic method in defining and providing services to its consumers, as well as in discovering new knowledge. Much nursing practice in the past has been based on intuition and pragmatic use of "whatever works." Criteria to determine what "works" have often been weak or lacking, and the lack of such criteria has hampered the development of a well-defined science of nursing.

For the practitioner to evaluate the benefits of his therapeutic program in a scientific manner, he must be able to utilize a system to define the need for the program, propose various solutions, choose and try a solution, and evaluate the results. Such a system is presented in these pages, with the emphasis on its use to define a patient's or client's problems which can be solved with nursing help.

The processes described in Part 2 are presented to provide the student with one system for using the scientific method in nursing care. Consistent use of such a systematic approach to analyzing and providing nursing care will ultimately free him from the need to think about each step as it is used, enabling him to perceive more subtle data and to think of more creative approaches.

The analysis and solution of problems take place within the context of a collaborative interpersonal relationship or transaction between the nurse and the patient-client. Without this personal transaction, the process of diagnosis and planning will be a most impersonal exercise and can result in little lasting help for the patient or client. The scientific method and its interpersonal aspects are artificially separated in these chapters in order to facilitate identification of the components of the process. In actual use, they are inseparable.

REFERENCES

Chambers, Wilda: Nursing Diagnosis, *American Journal of Nursing,* **62**:102-104 (1962).
Durand, Mary, and Rosemary Prince: Nursing Diagnosis: Process and Decision, *Nursing Forum,* **5**(4):50 ff. (1966).

Interpersonal Relationships in Nursing

Pamela Mitchell

The nurse-patient relationship is the essential process of involvement with another person. It is the core—the heart—of nursing which gives the process greater meaning to both nurse and patient.   JUDITH GOLDSBOROUGH   (1969)

The following chapters in Part 2 will present the mechanics and tools with which a nurse can help a patient-client. However, unless the *person* who is the nurse becomes involved with the *person* who is the patient-client, the nursing process described becomes merely a mechanical, intellectual exercise in collecting, sifting, and analyzing data. Too often, the humanistic notion of "person" gets lost in the scientific notion of "data," and students in the helping professions become detached "scientists," rather than the compassionate people they once meant to be.

Why does this change in attitude occur? Is it because the human aspects of practice are not

really important in helping people get better? Is it because involvement with the person in the patient's role is too uncomfortable or threatening for the professional? Or is it because students and practitioners do not know how to go about relating to their clients in a personal way? Most likely all these factors are involved when students in the health professions change from compassionate, idealistic people to uninvolved, "hardened" practitioners.

Aside from the purely humanistic reasons for being kind, there is growing evidence that the quality of interpersonal contacts has an influence on a person's becoming ill, coping with illness, and becoming well. What "significant others"—which would include health professionals—do and say (or do *not* do and say) affects a person's definition of and reaction to his health problem and thus, ultimately, its solution (Wooldridge et al., 1968). It seems, therefore, that it *is* important to establish a personal relationship with the people who are patient-clients. Despite this professional "norm," social scientists who have studied the process of becoming a doctor or nurse have documented that many of the students they studied became less "idealistic" and more detached from patients as they progressed toward graduation. Curricular emphasis is often more on the technical and less on the human aspects of illness. Students often see teachers, supervisors, and practitioners acting in an impersonal way with patients, find it emotionally difficult to become "involved" themselves with some patients, and thus tend to imitate the impersonal behavior they see around them.

The impersonal approaches which every student sees and the widespread lay assumption that involvement is hazardous might suggest that close interpersonal relationships with the patient-client are indeed to be avoided, if only for the mental health of the practitioner.

Certainly there *are* dangers to the self-esteem of the person who is the practitioner when he exposes himself to the person who is the patient-client. People who are ill or have continuing health problems often have many fears and anxieties to share. Seeing their suffering, hearing their fears, and being able to do nothing to dispel them can be a most disturbing experience, particularly for the novice in a health field who may never have been exposed to suffering, nakedness, or "crazy" behavior. Each of us must have some means of protecting himself when continually exposed to the miseries of others. If we do not, we become lost in these emotions and, indeed, cannot help others. Some persons simply leave the situation and change their career goals. Some avoid the emotions of others by developing an impersonal shell which generally prevents one from seeing, or prevents the patient-client from sharing, suffering. Others develop their own self-esteem and confidence to the point where they can share the emotions of the other person without becoming lost in the other person's emotional state. This is not to say that these people do not become uncomfortable or feel helpless in the face of the patient-client's difficulties, but they are able to work directly with their own reactions and then with the patient-client's reactions.

The purpose of this chapter is to help you, the person who is a practitioner, to analyze your relationships with the people who are your patient-clients, so that you may become involved enough to help them and yet maintain your own emotional integrity. We can state time and again the importance of interpersonal relationships in helping people cope with their health problems, but unless you have some means to protect your own identity in these relationships, you may either avoid close relationships or leave them altogether.

Some persons come to professional education with skill and security in dealing with people who have problems. More persons do not, and need help to develop these skills. Common sense is simply not enough to enable most beginning nurses to help a person deal with his reactions to illness while simultaneously dealing with his own reactions to that patient-client's situation. In order to become therapeutically involved (i.e., with the goal of helping), the nurse needs to learn about the nature of interpersonal relationships and the parts which both he and the patient-client play. He needs to learn to analyze his interactions and relationships in order to assess what happened, why it happened, and why it was helpful or not. In the same context, he needs to examine his own reactions to the contact: where he felt comfortable, where he felt uncomfortable, and, most important, where to turn for help when he does not know what to do next.

Most of this learning will not occur while reading this textbook. The only way to learn how to interact helpfully with patient-clients is to be with them under the supervision of a skilled person, analyze the experience, and try again. This chapter will present some concepts, some examples, and some ideas for you to use as you try to establish therapeutic relationships.

INTERPERSONAL RELATIONSHIPS

The terms *interaction* and *relationship* will be used frequently in this chapter. Therefore, it is important to define them.

Interaction

A social interaction is a situation in which two or more persons *act upon each other.* Verbally or nonverbally, they exchange behavior, so to speak. Each stimulates and responds to the behavior of the other. This stimulation and responsiveness are the *sine qua non* of interaction (English and English, 1958, p. 220). Small children may play side by side for many minutes but never interact, for they do not respond to each other's behavior. If one child takes the other's toy, however, a loud and active interaction will most likely occur!

Relationship

English and English define relation in terms of the *influence* objects have on one another. The relationship becomes somewhat of an entity, at least partly independent of the related objects (p. 454). Relationships are apt to extend over a longer period of time than interactions, and usually consist of many interactions. A single, prolonged interaction may become a relationship, however. The actors in a relationship evolve a series of emotional responses to each other (positive or negative), and will continue their actions in the light of these emotional sets.

To express what occurs simply, they become important to each other.

A *professional relationship* is one in which the professional purposely tries to help by using the special knowledge or skill which he possesses. Hofling, Leininger, and Gregg (1967) define the therapeutic nurse-patient relationship as "an interaction process between two persons in which the nurse offers a series of purposeful activities and practices that are useful to a particular patient." [1]

Interpersonal Relationship

The interactions and relationships between nurse and patient-client are interpersonal ones—occurring between people. Whether the persons involved have a single, one-minute interaction or an extended relationship, the behavior of each participant during this time has some meaning and importance to the other, even if it does not make sense to an observer. The meaning of a person's behavior may not be readily apparent—in fact, may not be known to the person himself.

However, the more that is known and understood about the motivations and needs which the behavior expresses, the more fully the problem will be recognized and met. The behavior of the nurse, as well as that of the patient-client, is motivated by these factors. The nurse must analyze his own and the patient-client's behavior in these interactions in order to understand what is happening. Some helps to analyzing one's own behavior are given in the following pages.

FACTORS IN OVERT BEHAVIOR

Behavior and the meaning attached to it are influenced by several factors. Past experiences in similar situations, the situation at hand, the physical and psychosocial needs are all determi-

[1] Charles Hofling, Madeleine Leininger, and Elizabeth Gregg, "Basic Psychiatric Concepts in Nursing," 2d ed., J. B. Lippincott Company, Philadelphia, 1967.

nants of a person's responses and behavior toward others. If the nurse does not realize that behavior in any interpersonal contact is affected by all these components, he may find his own or a patient-client's behavior inexplicable in terms of the situation. Thus, he may fail to analyze the interactions sufficiently to discover the real problem.

Past Experiences

The following examples illustrate the influence of past experience on behavior:

A hospitalized five-year-old shrieks with fear when a nurse brings his dinner tray to him. This seems a strange reaction to food. However, nurses have also brought "shots" on trays, and the child is probably associating the tray with being hurt. Hence, his unusual reaction to food is most likely based on a painful past experience with trays.

In another situation, a nurse may find that he avoids a certain patient without apparent reason. When he analyzes his behavior, he may realize that the patient reminds him of his grandmother, whose death he has not fully accepted.

Simply recognizing the past experiences which are affecting present relationships with patient-clients will not magically result in therapeutic interaction with them. However, recognition of these past experiences is the first step in dealing with the present situation. For example, rather than dismissing the child's reaction as "silly," the nurse can let him see what is on the food tray and stay with him until he has calmed down. Then he can plan some later doll play in order to help the child act out his fears and anger about the shots. The nurse in the second example can begin to examine his reactions to his grandmother's death and seek help, if need be, to resolve his feelings. This may not help him care for the present woman, but can help him be more effective in future similar situations.

Present Situation

The situation at hand will, of course, influence much of the overt behavior of nurse and patient-client. The stresses and emotions inherent in many health situations are often sufficient to explain behavior; e.g., joy at the birth of a healthy child, anxiety prior to major surgery, shock at hearing the diagnosis of cancer. Nevertheless, the responses of both patient and nurse to these common situations will be affected by their own needs and past experiences.

Needs

The third factor affecting behavior in interpersonal situations is the person's needs, both psychosocial and physiological. Psychosocial needs include the need for approval, self-esteem, safety, and personal growth. Physiologic needs include the need for food, shelter, oxygen. Part 3, Chapter 9, contains an expanded discussion of needs and their origins.

Needs are generally defined in terms of a lack; i.e., something which is missing and by its absence leads to tension in the organism. When the lack is supplied, tension abates.

Maslow (1962) feels that there are two types of needs: deficiency-motivated needs (described above) and growth-motivated needs. An example of the growth need would be the need of an artist to express himself through a painting, or the need of a person to achieve his highest potentials.

Maslow ranks needs in a hierarchy from basic physiologic to self-actualization (1954, pp. 80-106). According to his schema, higher needs do not fully emerge until lower ones are met. If the lower needs are not fully satisfied, higher ones will be only partially met. For example, the man who can barely feed his family will have little time or energy to meet his growth needs. In fact, he may not even be aware of these higher needs (see Fig. 4-1).

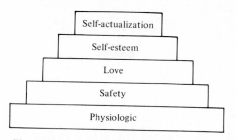 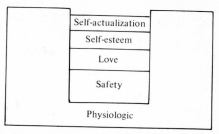

Figure 4-1 Hierarchy of needs. The more basic needs form a foundation upon which the fulfillment of higher needs rests. If basic needs are not fully met, the foundation for higher needs is not complete. Thus the higher needs may be submerged or engulfed by lower-level needs.

Most nurse-patient contacts in a hospital are initiated by physiologic needs of the patient, because most illness is defined in physiologic terms. However, the patient's behavior may reflect the assault of the institution on his self-esteem. In addition, he may covertly express fears for his safety (survival), engendered by his physiologic problems. His energies will necessarily be centered on meeting lower-level needs and stabilizing the foundation of his self-esteem. Hence, he may behave "unreasonably" in an attempt to stabilize his foundational needs. He may order personnel about, trying to bolster self-esteem; or he may make *no* demands, attempting to foster his safety by avoiding staff displeasure. These motivations may be completely outside his conscious awareness.

The nurse too has needs which will influence his relationships with patients and his ability to forget self in helping another. If the nurse's need for love and approval is great, he may be reluctant to set necessary limits for a manipulative patient. His need to "cure" people may prevent him from working effectively with people who do not get well. His need to be appreciated may prevent him from seeing the underlying needs of the "demanding" person. Again, these need motivations may be outside the nurse's awareness; e.g., he doesn't know *why* he cannot set limits, *why* he dislikes working on a rehabilitation unit.

TOOLS IN THE INTERPERSONAL RELATIONSHIP

There are some important tools and skills which the nurse must bring to a relationship between himself and a patient-client. These include his knowledge, his communication skills, his technical or mechanical skills, and himself.

Knowledge and Communication Skills

Knowledge includes his factual knowledge about health and illness, human behavior, and the patient-client's health problem and resulting therapy. Concepts related to these areas of knowledge are discussed elsewhere in this book and will not be repeated here. Communication skills are discussed in Part 2, Chapter 6, and Part 3, Chapter 9.

Technical Skills

People who are hospitalized for their health problem, or who require physical nursing care in their homes, expect their nurse to provide competent technical care (Fig. 4-2). The person who is physically ill or quite dependent often establishes his trust with the nurse on the basis of skillful physical care. Thus, a nurse who is working with patient-clients who require physical ministration must possess competent mechanical skills as well as verbal communication

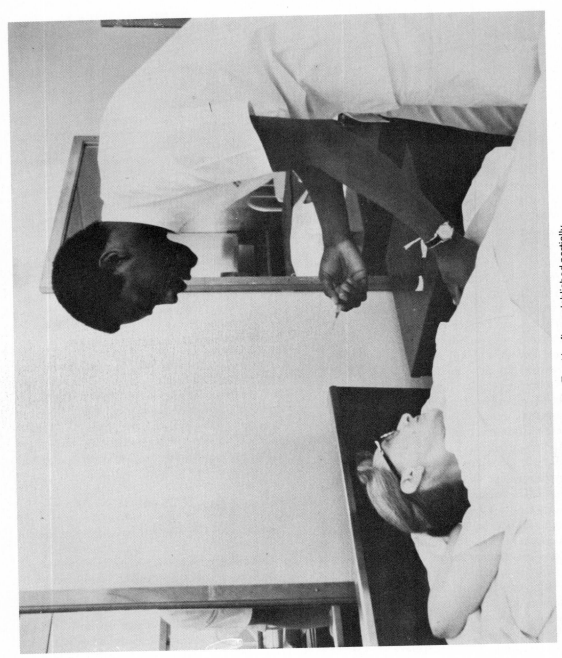

Figure 4-2 Technical skill as a tool in the relationship. Trust is often established partially upon the basis of skillful physical care. *(Photograph courtesy of University of Washington Medical Photography, Health Sciences Division.)*

skills. He is communicating nonverbally by means of these technical skills. Beginning practitioners require time to acquire these skills, and may reasonably wonder if they can establish trust when they are still "fumbling around." Most patient-clients do not expect the level of skillfulness from a beginner which they expect of a graduate practitioner. However, they do expect that a nurse will not attempt a procedure beyond his level of competence. If a nurse is having difficulty with a technical procedure and says, "I need to get some help with this; I'll be right back with someone more experienced," he is being honest and will probably not lose the patient-client's confidence. If, however, he persists in the procedure, becoming more anxious by the moment, the patient-client may empathize the anxiety and become distrustful of the nurse's judgment and ability. Children are often more open than adults in telling a nurse, "You're shaking," "You don't know how to do my bandage." Nurses, particularly beginners, may become flustered and defensive when confronted so frankly with the obvious. The best approach in this type of situation is to be just as honest as the child: "Yes, I'm nervous. I wonder if you have ever felt that way when you did a new thing."

Self

The most important tool the nurse brings to the relationship is *himself.* The phrase, "therapeutic use of self," has become a cliché in nursing. It simply means that the nurse helps the patient-client through the way that he is, rather than through the application of medications, treatments, or other external tools. It also implies that the nurse as a person is involved with the patient-client as a person, rather than relating to him as an object or thing.

If the nurse is to use his behavior in a deliberate way to help the patient-client, he needs to have thought about himself—who he is, who he would like to be, how he thinks others see him, what motivates his actions. These deliberations are summed up in the phrase, "insight into self"—literally, looking into oneself.

Everyone forms his self-concept through interactions with others. From these interactions a person gains some idea of how others see him. In addition, each person has his own ideas of what he is like; these ideas may or may not coincide with the opinions of others. One's own ideas and the opinions of others cannot be separated in the formation of the self-concept.

If a person has a positive self-concept and a feeling of worth, he is most likely to interact with others as he is, without attempting to influence their concept of him. He presents more of himself, as he sees himself, and less of his façade. However, if he has a negative self-concept or low self-esteem, he may present a façade to others, either trying to show them that he is better than *he* thinks he is or trying to convince them of his lack of worth (e.g., trying to make their concept conform to his). See Part 3, Chapter 9, for an expanded discussion of the formation of the self.

Both the patient and the nurse have their own personal self-concepts, based on social interactions with others. In addition, each has developed a self-concept related to his role as nurse or patient-client. We shall refer to this as the "professionalized self-concept." The nurse's educational and work experiences shape his professionalized self-concept. The patient-client's interactions with health-care personnel shape his professionalized concept of himself as a successful or unsuccessful patient.

The Personal Self-concept People are often not conscious of their self-concept. However, a person may be able to define his concept of self if he thinks about it. Sometimes a person's self-concept is such that he becomes anxious when thinking of it, and psychological defenses begin to operate to decrease that anxiety. A façade, or false presentation of self, is one kind of defense against the potential anxiety of thinking about one's low self-esteem. (See Part 3, Chapter 9, for discussion of the concept of anxiety.)

Because anxiety is such a vague feeling, a person cannot deal directly with it until he finds its source. He unconsciously takes measures which keep this unpleasant feeling within tolerable limits. These measures may stabilize relatively unhealthy or ineffective personality traits. The following example illustrates this.

Mr. J., a 40-year-old salesman, may unconsciously feel that he has little to offer anyone, but has put on a façade of self-reliance and bravado for so long that he sees himself this way. He has a coronary thrombosis and is hospitalized. He is suddenly in a position of forced dependency, with control exerted by others over his every action. His concept of self-reliance is greatly threatened, and he attempts, again unconsciously, to control the resultant anxiety by ordering personnel about, demanding immediate attention, and becoming generally obnoxious. The nursing staff, whose professionalized self-concepts are ones of helpers, find themselves rebuffed and chastised by Mr. J. Eventually, their frustration at being unable to do anything to please him turns to anger, and they avoid him whenever possible. The avoidance is a defense to protect themselves against further assaults on their self-concepts. Unfortunately, this behavior only reinforces Mr. J.'s original unconscious feeling of little worth, and he becomes even more demanding, as he tries to reestablish his concept of a self-reliant person who is in control.

In this example, both Mr. J. and the nurses responded to threats to their self-images with anxiety and with behavior which tried to reduce the anxiety. Since both reacted automatically, with no conscious recognition of the process or attempt to deal with the emotion directly, a cycle of mutual withdrawal occurred. Mr. J. would certainly profit from some insight into his behavior, in order to achieve a more positive self-concept, but not at this time of acute physiologic and psychologic stress. The aim at this point is to restore his equilibrium so that healing can occur.

An attempt to change Mr. J.'s self-concept now would only cause further disequilibrium. Therefore, it is incumbent upon the nurse to look at *his own* reactions, in order to stop the cycle of mutual withdrawal.

If the nurse in this situation is to help Mr. J., he needs to recognize his frustration because Mr. J. cannot be pleased. He must also recognize that this frustration occurred because his own professional and personal self-concepts were threatened. Further, he needs to realize that his subsequent anger is a defense against further anxiety. Anger is a concrete emotion with a specific object (Mr. J.); thus, it is more easily vented and objectified than anxiety. This nurse can apply his understanding of the self-concept and of anxiety to Mr. J.'s behavior in order to try to see how Mr. J. views the situation, what *his* feelings are. He can then try to bolster Mr. J.'s apparent need to have some control by letting him make decisions whenever possible.

The Professional Self-concept Closely related to the personal self is the professionalized self. Krikorian (1963) categorizes the nurse's professional self-concepts into three classes: the absolute authoritarian, the accepting authoritarian, and the supportive resource person. The absolute authoritarian approaches the patient (never client) with the attitude, "I know what you need, and I expect you to accept my help passively." The accepting authoritarian acknowledges that the patient has some ideas of his own but still sees himself as the sole judge of the patient's needs. He may encourage independent activity, but only when he (the nurse) deems it wise. The supportive resource person sees himself as a partner with a client, as they solve a problem together. He essentially helps the patient-client find his own solutions. This textbook is designed to help students gain a professionalized self-concept of the supportive resource person.

Even the newest student has some professionalized self-concept. This may have been derived from movies, television, books, or from actual experience in health-care settings. He needs to examine this concept to see if it is potentially helpful or harmful in the nurse-patient relationship. Frequently, beginning nurses see themselves as providing comfort to happy, grateful patients. When they are faced with the reality of miserable, complaining sick people, these nurses become frustrated—they find their professional self-image badly tarnished. At this point, one can either avoid much contact with patients who do not "appreciate" him, or he can look at his professional self-concept and try to change it. When a nurse can move from focusing on what response the patient gives to him, such as gratitude, to what he and the patient-client can do together, a truly helpful relationship has begun.

Patient-clients, too, develop a "professionalized" self-concept in their role. Professional and ancillary personnel covertly let them know what is expected of a "good" patient. The person who is pleasant to be with finds that personnel are warm with him; the one who makes many demands or is "grouchy" may find that his requests are filled but that there is an air of antagonism.

Patient-clients, particularly in institutions, rarely learn directly what the nursing personnel expect of them. This is unfortunate, for it leaves the patient in the position of having to guess what his role is, and usually of getting feedback only if his guess is wrong. Certain limits to the patient's role are imposed by an institution or by the nature of a nurse-patient relationship. It is only fair that the patient know these limits. This is not to say that the nurse tells the patient how to behave in order to be considered a "good" patient (usually a stereotype of a passive, noncomplaining person). It means that the nurse tells the patient in word or action how he can use the nurse's services and work with the nurse.

For example, the nurse may say, "I will be with you every Tuesday from nine to ten in the morning to . . . [talk about whatever you want; play with you; help you learn to dress yourself]." This orients the patient to the time limits of each contact (if there is such a time limit), the purpose of the contact, and their roles in it. Orienting the person to his role vis-à-vis the institution cannot be done in one sentence, but includes telling him of the time schedule, any limitations to his movement (e.g., if he can be out of bed, off the ward), how to call a nurse, the kinds of people who will be helping him.

The Nurse as a Model The example of Mr. J. showed how a nurse could use insight in dealing with a problem situation. The nurse need not wait for problems to arise, however, in order to use his understanding of himself and of human behavior. The more he understands and accepts himself and his feelings, the more effective he can be as a model of healthy interaction to his patient-clients. The person who accepts and knows himself is more open and honest in his relations with others. The nurse who is like this does not need to rely upon technique to help the patient-client articulate or act out his concerns. He is more able to establish a trusting relationship with the patient-client, for he does not "use" the patient to meet his own need to be needed.

How does a beginning nurse learn to look at himself? Hofling et al. gives some helpful guidelines:

1 Acquire as much knowledge as possible about human beings, human behavior, and human relations.

2 Observe carefully, and keep an open and questioning mind about one's own behavior and the behavior of others.

3 Try consciously and frankly to face one's own behavior, feelings, attitudes, and responses to various problems and situations.

4 Discuss and exchange observations and experiences with persons skilled in the field of human behavior and human relations.

5 Explore, test, and appraise one's understandings, insights, observations, and feelings in different situations.[2]

In a practical sense, this means that you think about your conversations and actions with patients, with instructors, with family, and with friends. Some interactions make you comfortable and pleased, some make you very uncomfortable. You need to analyze both kinds to help you find out why you felt as you did. Some pertinent questions are: What things make you feel good after being with patients or clients? What things make you feel bad? What things generally bother you; are these operating in experiences with patients? Can you identify the emotions that you felt in problematic or satisfying situations? Can you accept these feelings, whether they are positive or negative? Many nurses feel that they should not have negative feelings about patient-clients. However, being human, you *do* have these feelings. If you ignore or avoid them, they will influence the relationship outside your awareness. If you acknowledge and accept them, you can begin to find out where they come from and how you can use them to help the patient who evokes them.

You did not form your self-concept in isolation; neither can you look at yourself alone. Formal courses will aid in gathering knowledge of human behavior. However, a real look at your own behavior will require some assistance. Part of a student's clinical experience should be the discussion with a skilled person of the student's interactions with patient-clients. Faculties have different ways of offering these opportunities; but if you need them, seek them out *when* you need them. Informal talks with friends and family also form a large part of learning to know one's self.

Ujhely sums up the challenge of looking at your emotions:

With a great deal of support from others until one has gained sufficient inner security and skill, one can learn to welcome every occurrence of anxiety (instead of avoiding it as a threat) as a challenge to look at what is happening. . . .[3]

CHARACTERISTICS OF THE NURSE-PATIENT-CLIENT RELATIONSHIP

We now turn from a general discussion of the meaning of behavior and the role of self in relationships to some specific characteristics of relationships between people who are nurses and people who are patient-clients. The discussion is intended to present some concepts which may be applied to help move these relationships from impersonal ones between "nurse" and "patient" to personal ones between two persons.

Tasks in the Relationship

Because this relationship is a professional, as opposed to a social, one, there is work to be done. Each person in the relationship has some tasks which he must perform if the relationship is to be helpful. These tasks are outlined in Table 4-1. The nurse must establish trust with the patient-client and, therefore, must be trustworthy. This means that the nurse is not using the relationship to meet his own needs but honestly wants to help the patient-client with his problems. Second, the nurse must support the patient-client in his coping abilities and supplement him in areas of disability. In order to do this, the nurse must gather as much information as possible about the person's abilities and disabilities and his state of emotional and physical development.

Illness is a crisis, and crises bring a certain amount of psychological and physical regression or disorganization. Developmental conflicts not previously completely resolved may come forth

---

[2] Ibid., pp. 42–43.

[3] Gertrude Ujhely, "The Nurse and Her 'Problem' Patients," Springer Publishing Co., Inc., New York, 1963.

Table 4-1   Tasks of the Nurse and of the Patient-Client in a Therapeutic Relationship

Nurse	Patient-client
1 Establish trust	1 Develop trust and confidence in the helping person
2 Support abilities, supplement disabilities	2 Learn to identify and accept changes which health deviation has created
3 Foster a positive integration of crisis into life	3 Learn to make most of capabilities; value coping over adaptation
4 Function as a model of a healthy person, physically and emotionally	4 Maintain or learn effective ways to cope with crisis situations

once again (see the discussion of developmental tasks in Part 3, Chapter 9). Therefore, the third task of the nurse is to foster a positive integration of the crisis event into the person's life. This involves recognizing the degree of regression and helping the person resolve the conflicts characteristic of that stage of development. This is what Peplau means when she says that illness can be a learning experience in personal social growth (1952, p. 19).

Finally, the nurse needs to be or become a model of a healthy person, physically and emotionally. This means not that he must be a paragon of perfection, but that he must recognize his limitations and function effectively within those limitations. He tries to present himself, rather than his façade, to his patients.

The patient-client's tasks are complemental. In order to be helped, he must have trust and confidence in the helping person. He is in a state of relative crisis because of his deviation from health. Therefore, he must learn to adapt his life to changes created by his health deviation. This implies accepting the changes and making the most of his capabilities. In order to make the most of his capabilities, he needs to value or learn to value actively dealing with problems

(coping), rather than passively submitting to, or avoiding, difficulties (adaptation).

Finally, if the relationship is to have a lasting therapeutic value, he must maintain, or learn, effective ways to cope with future crisis situations.

Movement in the Relationship

There is a describable process or movement in the relationship between nurse and patient-client. Some authors describe this movement in terms of phases and the behavior characteristic of each phase. Our opinion is that this approach leads the beginning nurse to focus on identifying a phase, rather than looking at the movement or process which is occurring.

The following description of process in the therapeutic relationship is general. It leads from a superficial level to a personally involved level; no specific relationship will resemble it in all aspects. Some relationships will end at a superficial level, because the patient-client has received the help he wants, because he leaves, because the nurse leaves, or because one or both cannot progress to a more involved level. Others will become very close, person-to-person experiences.

An increasing amount of current nursing literature is devoted to the need for compassion and involvement of the self in the nurse-patient relationship. This emphasis is based on the premise that the self-aware, compassionate nurse is more sensitive to the patient's needs and is not expending most of his energy unconsciously meeting his own. Empirically, it appears that this type of nurse is more helpful to his patients, though this hypothesis has not been well substantiated by any published nursing research. Rogers (1961) and Jourard (1971) summarize research in the field of psychotherapy which suggests that the open, client-centered therapist is more successful with his clients than the impersonal, technique-centered person. Orlando's (1961) description of helpful nurse-patient interactions, and the studies supporting her work, support the view that a deliberative, validating approach to the patient is more effective than other approaches. However, there is no published work which demonstrates the personal attitudes which are necessary for the nurse to use this approach in the best way. On the basis of empirical evidence alone, we hypothesize that the patient will be most helped by a relationship at the involved, compassionate level. The nurse can be helpful at any point along the continuum, however, as long as he attempts to see how the patient views the situation and validates action with him. Figure 4-3 presents a model of movement in the relationships.

At the most superficial level, nurse and patient-client are strangers to each other; they perceive each other as their stereotyped roles and must begin to learn what they can expect of each other. They begin to gather information and clarify the need of the patient-client for help. The nurse begins to clarify his role with regard to the help he can offer and the services available.

As the relationship continues, nurse and patient further clarify roles and begin to respond to each other in terms of actual and symbolic roles, rather than stereotypes. The identity or person of the nurse and patient may begin to emerge, if allowed to do so. The nurse, as he gathers more information and acquires more understanding of the patient, begins to develop empathy toward him. The patient-client begins to trust the nurse, as he learns more about him and his attitudes. This time of beginning trust and empathy may also be marked by testing and conflict, particularly if either the nurse or the patient has had previous difficulties with close interpersonal involvement.

If the relationship proceeds to the level of involvement, empathy leads to compassion and testing yields to trust. Nurse and patient-client shed their roles and work together as themselves.

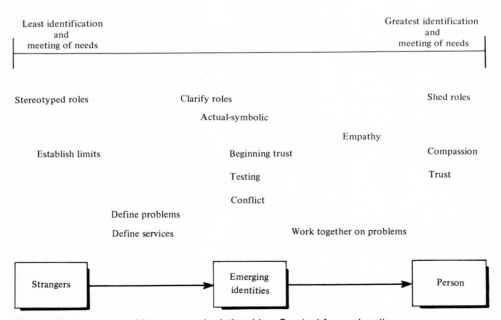

Figure 4-3 Movement of interpersonal relationships. See text for explanation.

Stereotyping Roles In their first contact, nurse and patient-client are strangers to each other and will interact in terms of their roles and what they perceive as the role of the other person. Both patient and nurse have certain ideas as to what behavior is acceptable in their own and the other's role; e.g., the "good" nurse, the "good" patient. Therefore, their early orientation to each other will tend to be an estimate of how well each fits the role the other ascribes to him. These responses to role are stereotyped responses and may halt the development of a therapeutic relationship unless nurse and patient move past them.

In the film, "Mrs. Reynolds Needs a Nurse,"[4] the head nurse's first encounter with Mrs. Reynolds occurs when the woman is brought to the unit, followed by a cart stacked with personal items. The ward is crowded; Mrs. Reynolds must be temporarily housed in the hall, and this "clutter" is the last straw as far as the head nurse is concerned. Her face mirrors her feeling that this woman may become a "problem."

The head nurse has responded to Mrs. Reynolds in terms of her concept of the good patient—one who does not add problems to an already difficult situation. In terms of the head nurse's stereotype, Mrs. Reynolds will not "need" so many personal things; she will not use them and they will be "in the way." Mrs. Reynolds as herself *does* need them, for they give her security in a frightening and unknown place.

Mr. Reynolds remains with his wife in the makeshift cubicle in the hall. A supervisor arrives to see how they are doing, and he complains bitterly about the lack of attention and concern over his wife's discomfort.

Mr. Reynolds is responding to the situation in terms of his stereotype of good nurses—ones

who show concern for his wife—and he has not perceived anyone who has done this. He does not care that the unit is running efficiently despite great odds, or that critically ill patients are being given excellent physical care (activities consistent with the head nurse's concept of her role). He knows only that he has found no one who fits his image of a good nurse.

Because nurse and patient-client can respond to each other only in terms of stereotyped roles until they get to know the individual in the role, one of the nurse's tasks is to establish his role with the patient. This may be done deliberatively, or it may be established covertly through the nurse's automatic activities. The head nurse covertly established her role as efficient manager with Mr. Reynolds by immediately telling him to take his wife's things home. She did not tell him her role in so many words, but Mr. Reynolds had a fair idea what to expect of her from that first encounter.

The approach to the assessment interview described in Part 2, Chapter 6, is an example of deliberative establishment of role. The nurse tells the patient that he will be asking some questions which will help him and the patient-client work together. This begins to establish a partnership role for the nurse, rather than an authoritarian one. A nurse in a pediatric unit may decide to try to discover a child's needs through play with him. Even if the nurse does not tell the child, "I'm your play nurse," the child will know that this is what to expect from this nurse. These are both examples of deliberative orientation to role, the first is verbal, the second nonverbal.

The patient-client is also establishing his role, both in his own terms and from the cues given him by the nursing personnel. The executive who brings briefcases to the hospital and asks for a private telephone is indicating that his concept of the patient role does not include relinquishment of his usual responsibilities. The need for nursing personnel deliberately to orient patient-

[4] Smith, Kline, and French.

clients to their role was discussed earlier in this chapter.

Sharing Information   A second activity during the early relationship is determining what the patient-client needs and the extent of his need for nursing help. A separate chapter is devoted to this process (Part 2, Chapter 6). During this process, the patient will become less a stranger to the nurse, as he shares some information about himself. The nurse's interactions and response during this time give the patient some idea of the person in the nurse's role. The nurse who feels he must hide all emotional response gives the patient no clues as to whether he can appreciate the patient's feelings. In addition, he gives no clues as to whether the patient can trust him for help.

Clarifying and Changing Roles   As nurse and patient-client begin to define problems and plan action, the nurse is clarifying his overt role. He is explicitly or implicitly defining the services which he can offer, as well as other services available.

The nurse's role may change throughout the relationship, in terms of both his approaches to the patient-client and the roles in which the patient places him. Ideally, both nurse and patient-client progress from dealing with each other in terms of roles and become people to each other. This does not always occur, however. The patient-client is often under a great deal of psychosocial and physiological stress because of his health problem. He may not be able to invest the energy necessary for a truly open, person-to-person relationship, or to reveal himself as he sees himself to the nurse. He will continue to cast the nurse in various roles which meet his needs, and try to remain hidden in the patient's role or behind the façade which he presents to the world.

Many times nurses are not able or willing to open themselves either, and remain hidden in

their roles. When this occurs, the relationship cannot exist at any but the most superficial level. The nurse (at least theoretically) is the healthier of the two participants and, thus, is the one who has the responsibility for progressing the relationship to a therapeutic one of open, person-to-person relationships. If the patient cannot open himself, the nurse can at least learn as much about him as possible and be a model of open communication.

There is potential for a great deal of conflict as roles are clarified. The patient-client may prefer to have a passive, dependent role, rather than a more active partnership which the nurse sees as advantageous. He may express this by refusing to do even the activities of which he is capable or by berating the nurse for being lazy. The nurse's task is to know the patient-client well enough to recognize stress-induced dependency needs and to allow him to be dependent until his coping abilities are back in order. Working as a partner with the patient does not mean that he is made to take sole responsibility for his decisions; it means that he has as much voice in what happens to him as he is able and willing to take.

Another potential area of conflict surrounds the roles themselves. The patient-client may perceive the nurse's role at two levels—actual and symbolic. The actual role is the one which the nurse tries to define to the patient: counselor, comforter, technical expert. The symbolic role is the one in which the nurse symbolizes some other important figure in the patient's experience. The patient tends to react to the nurse on the basis of his feelings toward that other person. Psychiatry calls this the transference phenomena.

The patient commonly casts the nurse in a mothering role. If his mother was authoritarian, he may look for this behavior in the nurse, either rebelling against the nurse or trying to elicit more structure and authority from him. Conversely, he may expect nurturing motherly behavior and remain passive in expectation of such behavior. Conflict occurs if the goals of the relationship require a different role for the nurse than the symbolic role given him by the patient.

The nurse may react to the patient-client on a symbolic level also. He may be similar to another patient-client or may be like a family member. If a nurse relates to all elderly men in terms of the "grandpa" role, he loses the opportunity to know this particular man. More important, he will not learn the individual cues needed to help this specific man.

Developing Trust A third area of potential conflict occurs as trust begins to develop. The patient-client who has had generally satisfactory interpersonal relationships will feel little need to test the nurse's trustworthiness. He will probably establish trust on the basis of the nurse's stereotyped role alone. This trust can, of course, be lost if the person in the role proves untrustworthy.

People who have had many unhappy interpersonal experiences are less able to take the risk of establishing a relationship unless they test the trustworthiness of the other person. A patient may repeatedly reject the nurse, testing whether the nurse really cares enough to return. He may continually test limits to see if the nurse thinks they are important enough to abide by.

Each person has his own criteria, often unconscious, as to who is to be trusted. The nurse may never know what these criteria are, and may find this testing emotionally and physically trying. A person who must test at length has probably had a number of assaults on his self-concept. He tests people as a means of protecting himself from the risk of further anxiety inherent in any close interpersonal relationship. Understanding this may help the nurse find the patience to establish trustworthiness with this person.

Developing Empathy and Compassion As nurse and patient begin to know each other better, their identities become more apparent to each other. They begin to see something of the person who is in the role. As this occurs, nurse and patient-client begin to develop *empathy* for each other's emotions and reactions.

There is no complete agreement in psychiatric literature about the definition of empathy. In general, it refers to one person's ability consciously to appreciate or understand the emotions of another.

In order to empathize, one must put himself emotionally in the place of the other and imagine what it must feel like to be in the other's shoes. Some authors view empathy as the ability to *experience* another's feeling, and relate it to compassion, or "feeling with" another (Hofling, 1967; Baumgartner, 1970). Travelbee (1966), however, differentiates empathy and sympathy (sympathy is similar to compassion, as used here). She feels that empathy connotes an intellectual comprehension of an emotional state, whereas sympathy goes further and is characterized by an emotional sharing of feeling and a desire to help (pp. 139–148). English and English support Travelbee's interpretation of the terms (1958, pp. 178, 540).

Regardless of whether one uses the term empathy, compassion, or sympathy, the important concept is that the nurse begins to appreciate what the patient *feels* in his experience and then moves into a real sharing of the emotional impact of the experience. The nurse becomes *involved* in the patient's experience, and both shed their roles. They then share an interpersonal rather than an inter-role relationship.

An important part of the nurse's compassion is the ability to share in the emotional experience without losing sight of his intent to help the patient-client cope with the experience. This is involvement in the professional sense: "to participate with the patient in the meaning and impact of his situation but to maintain a conscious recognition of one's part so as not to shift focus and begin to participate in the emotion itself" (Holsclaw, 1965).

The following incident shows how empathy and compassion helped a patient:

Mr. B.K. was hospitalized with pneumonia and had developed delirium tremens. He had been having hallucinations all day, shouting at the ceiling and warning away anyone who came near him. To protect him and others, he had been secured to his bed with a waist restraint. During the evening, he had to be moved to another room, and two nurses went to move his bed. "Get away, get away; save yourself, missy," he shouted. He became more and more agitated as the nurses wheeled his bed down the hall. He was shaking more violently than ever, and one nurse thought, "Why, he's frightened to death." She told the other nurse to stop; she put her arm around Mr. K. and began to talk to him in a quiet voice, soothing him as she would a frightened child. After a few minutes he quieted down and agreed to proceed to the new room. The nurse sat with him for awhile, telling him she would not let anyone harm him. He soon fell asleep.

The words the nurse used were not important. The important thing she did was to empathize his fear and actually participate with him in the experience by holding and staying with him until he was no longer afraid.

Instead of responding to the meaning of the fear, the nurse might have responded to the fear itself, perhaps becoming anxious that Mr. K. would not go to the new room or fearful that he would assault her. If this had been the case, her response would most likely have been some kind of withdrawal from the anxiety of the situation. She might have actually run away if her own fear had been great enough. More likely, she would have become authoritarian or punitive toward Mr. K. in an attempt to deal with her own anxiety. These defenses would not have helped either nurse or patient, for the source of the anxiety was the patient's impending panic.

Separating the two processes—sharing the meaning of the person's emotion and becoming enmeshed in the emotion itself—is difficult. It involves a continuing ability to look at and evaluate one's own behavior and emotions, preferably with the support and help of a skilled person. Nearly every nurse has had more than one experience in which he found himself caught up in the emotion, rather than in the meaning of it, and was of no help to the patient. These experiences may be useful to the nurse if he looks at what happened and why.

The patient-client empathizes also. He may overtly or covertly respond to the emotions of the nurse. If his response is overt—e.g., if he says, "You look angry, nurse; are you angry with me?"—they can discuss it, and the event will pass or perhaps strengthen their relationship as people. If, however, the patient-client senses the nurse's emotion, becomes uncomfortable, but does not deal directly with this discomfort, tension may result which covertly affects the relationship.

It is not the patient's responsibility to use his empathy to help the nurse with the nurse's problems, even though he may be quite aware of the nurse's anxiety, sadness, or whatever. The nurse, however, must realize that his own emotional state can be empathized by the patient-client. If he feels his emotional state may be harmful to the patient, he may need to make arrangements for someone else to see the patient-client this time, and withdraw to resolve his own problem. In most instances, he simply needs to be alert to any cues that the patient is empathizing the nurse's emotion and the patient's response to it. He can then discuss the situation directly (I'm rushing you this morning, aren't I? I'm afraid I'm a little tense about my exam today."), or withdraw until he has his feelings under control.

Terminating the Relationship   Many relationships will end before a person-to-person involvement has been reached. This may occur because the patient's need for help has been met, because patient or nurse physically leaves the health-care system, or because either one cannot develop a deeper relationship.

Either patient-client or nurse may initiate the termination. When the nurse terminates the relationship, he should prepare the patient-client for this whenever possible. Particularly when the relationship is at a person-to-person level, a sudden unannounced termination may leave both nurse and patient emotionally vulnerable, and may make it difficult for the patient to develop trust in further relationships.

If the nurse knows that there will be a time limit to the relationship, he should let the patient know this as early as possible. In addition, he ought to remind the patient-client of this time limit as the time for termination draws near. Nurses need to tell their patient-clients when they are going to have days off from work, or vacations. The relationship is not really terminated but is being interrupted. To an ill, dependent person, the sudden disappearance of "his" nurse may cause much distress.

RELATIONSHIPS WITH CHILDREN

The foregoing discussion of the nurse-patient relationship applies generally to relationships with children as well. However, there are some qualitative differences in children which are of significance in achieving helpful relationships with them.

First, children are going through periods of rapid growth and change. Their development is characterized by periods of crisis, disorganization, and reorganization (see Part 3, Chapter 9). A nurse dealing with children needs to know the characteristics of these periods in health and the effect of illness or other "accidental" crises upon normal developmental tasks. The nurse's task in the relationship is not only to help the child cope with the current health crisis but to support him in his developmental potential.

Certainly illness will lead to some regression in children, just as it does in adults. One of the nurse's tasks is to help parents and the child accept this regression as normal, and then help the child back to his developmental level when the crisis is past. For example, a nurse might provide bright objects overhead for the four-month-old to support his developing sensory exploration. A three-year-old may have regressed in toilet training during a temporary illness. A nurse can help his parents understand the commonality of this regression, and encourage them to avoid pushing the child until his illness has passed.

It is just as difficult for an active child to accept enforced dependency as it is for the executive or other independent adult. Once acute illness is past and the child feels relatively well, he may have great difficulty understanding why he must be inactive even though he feels fine. Children tend to view illness as a punishment for "bad" thoughts or deeds, and may see convalescent limits on activity as further punishment. Mastery and control of the environment are such an important part of child development that health workers and parents need to find as many activities as possible which the child can do for himself within the illness-imposed limits on activity and independence.

Growth and development take energy. Therefore if the nurse is to support the child's developmental potential during accidental crises, he must help the child conserve necessary energy. Since each interaction with a new adult uses emotional and physical energy, the staff are wise to limit the interactions which a child must have. In a busy hospital, even the minimum number of contacts for a child amounts to a great many: at least two nurses in each working shift, physician, and numerous persons in laboratories and other special areas. When a child is in acute crisis, every effort must be made to provide the security of a small number of adults in his world. Many hospitals allow the mother to stay and be the source of support.

A second difference is that the relationship is more often a multiple one among nurse, child, and parents (or parent substitute). The family's reactions are important in the care of adults as well, but the nurse can help an adult solely through the primary relationship with him. Because the important persons in a child's life are his parents, they must be a part of the nurse's relationship with the child. The relationship with family shapes a child's subsequent relationships with all others. Therefore, the nurse's role is to help the parents as they help their child. In an institution, the nurse may become a temporary or permanent parental substitute. In this situation, the nursing staff must provide the same consistency of approach as the parents would if the child were home. A child who is hospitalized is fearful and anxious, and will become even more so if there is no stability and constancy in his new environment. Again, a stable, limited number of personnel will help provide this security.

In situations such as pediatric offices, community health centers, and developmental clinics, the nurse may have the primary relationship with the parents rather than with the child. In such situations, the nurse's role is to educate and support the parents in fostering their relationship with their child.

A third differing characteristic of relationships with children is that their ability to understand and express ideas is not fully developed. Blake et al. (1970) list three determinants of the meaning which a child attaches to a situation: (1) the concepts which he has mastered, (2) his degree of understanding of cause and effect, and (3) his thinking processes. The preverbal child can express his feelings only through action (crying, running, hitting), and has only a rudimentary idea of cause and effect. The older child may know that it is the needle and syringe which cause the hurt, whereas a younger child may associate the hurt only with the *person* who does the hurting.

A child's emotional expression and control are related to his developing abilities to understand and express his feelings and thoughts. Consequently, children tend to be less controlled and more labile in their emotions than adults. They have not yet been socialized into the adult expectations of what is and is not appropriate emotional expression. The kind of feeling expressed and the control exerted vary with the child's age and language development; however, a number of generalizations about children's emotions may be made.

First, a child's emotions are intense and short-lived. One minute he may be crying bitterly and the next running happily off to play. Dramatic changes can often be caused by introducing an interesting new game or diversion.

Adults frequently attempt to hide their emotions; children usually express them freely, either verbally ("I love you," "I hate you") or nonverbally (crying, hitting, laughing). A very young child may not have the words for the strong emotions which he feels, and so he resorts to action. One of the tasks of parents is to help a child learn the verbal language of emotion—e.g., "happy," "sad," "angry."

Finally, each child has his own way of expressing his emotions and of responding to attempts to help him. Parents learn the patterns of their child through day-to-day contact. A nurse will need to learn from the parents and from observing the child. Play is an excellent tool in assessing both the emotional and cognitive development of a child. If a preschooler is given a set of dolls (dressed, for example, as a family or as hospital workers), he will assign roles to each doll and usually one to himself. He may scold the child just as he is scolded, or hit the baby just as he would like to hit the real baby. Often negative emotions are primary in such play, for such emotions are frequently suppressed in our society. The stories he makes up about the dolls may reveal much of his notion of cause and effect.

Play is also an effective way to help a child with problems occasioned by illness or hospitalization. Faulkner (1971) describes the use of a baseball game with an eleven-year-old boy who was withdrawn and communicated only by screaming and crying. The game provided some achievable goals, helped him express some of his feelings in words, and helped him form a relationship with the staff. Play is a child's work and his way of mastering the environment. Nurses can use it both diagnostically and therapeutically.

REFERENCES

Books

Baumgartner, Margaret, Empathy, in Carolyn E. Carlson (ed.), "Behavioral Concepts and Nursing Intervention," J. B. Lippincott Company, Philadelphia, 1970, pp. 29–38.

Blake, Florence, F. Howell Wright, and Eugenia H. Waechter, "Nursing Care of Children," 8th ed., J. B. Lippincott Company, Philadelphia, 1970.

English, Horace, and Ava Champney English, "A Comprehensive Dictionary of Psychological and Psychoanalytic Terms," Longmans, Green & Co., New York, 1958.

Hofling, Charles, Madeleine Leininger, and Elizabeth Gregg, "Basic Psychiatric Concepts in Nursing," 2d ed., J. B. Lippincott Company, Philadelphia, 1967.

Jourard, Sidney, "The Transparent Self," 2d ed., D. Van Nostrand Company, Princeton, N.J., 1971.

Maslow, Abraham, "Motivation and Personality," Harper & Row, Publishers, Incorporated, New York, 1954.

———, "Toward a Psychology of Being," D. Van Nostrand Company, Inc., Princeton, N.J., 1962.

Orlando, Ida, "The Dynamic Nurse-Patient Relationship," G. P. Putnam's Sons, New York, 1961.

Peplau, Hildegard, "Interpersonal Relations in Nursing," G. P. Putnam's Sons, New York, 1952.

Rogers, Carl, "On Becoming a Person," Houghton-Mifflin Company, Boston, 1961.

Thomas, Mary Durand, Trust in Nurse-Patient Relationships, in C. Carlson (ed.), "Behavioral Concepts and Nursing Intervention," J. B. Lippincott Company, Philadelphia, 1970, pp. 117–128.

Travelbee, Joyce, "Interpersonal Aspects of Nursing," F. A. Davis Company, Philadelphia, 1966.

Ujhely, Gertrude, "The Nurse and Her 'Problem' Patients," Springer Publishing Co., Inc., New York, 1963.

Wooldridge, Powhatan, James K. Skipper, Jr., and Robert C. Leonard, "Behavioral Science, Social Practice, and the Nursing Profession," The Press of Case Western Reserve University, Cleveland, 1968, p. 47.

Periodicals

Faulkner, Betty: From First Base to Home Plate, *American Journal of Nursing,* **71**:2331–2333 (1971).

Goldsborough, Judith: Involvement, *American Journal of Nursing,* **69**:66–68 (1969).

Holsclaw, Pamela A.: Nursing in High Emotional Risk Areas, *Nursing Forum,* **4**(4):36–45 (1965).

Krikorian, Diana: What Is a Nurse? a Patient? a Relationship? *Journal of Psychiatric Nursing,* **1**:452 (1963).

ADDITIONAL READINGS

Books

Dodson, Fitzhugh, "How to Parent," Signet Books, New American Library, New York, 1970 (paperback).

Francis, Gloria, and Barbara Munjas, "Promoting Psychological Comfort," Wm. C. Brown Company Publishers, Dubuque, Iowa, 1968.

Ilg, Frances, and Louise Ames, "Child Behavior," Harper & Row, Publishers, Incorporated, New York, 1955 (paperback, Perennial Library, 1966).

Ujhely, Gertrude, "Determinants of the Nurse-Patient Relationship," Springer Publishing Co., Inc., New York, 1968.

Wiedenbach, Ernestine, "Clinical Nursing, a Helping Art," Springer Publishing Co., Inc., New York, 1964.

Periodicals

Christman, Luther: Assisting the Patient to Learn the Patient Role, *Journal of Nursing Education,* **6**:17–21 (1967).

Erickson, Florence: Nursing Care Based on Nursing Assessment, in Betty Bergerson et al. (eds.), *Current Concepts in Clinical Nursing,* **2**:171–177 (1969). (Excellent summary of children's needs and methods of communication by age levels.)

Fagin, Claire: Therapeutic Intervention with Adolescents—The Nurse and the Adolescent, in Betty Bergerson et al. (eds.), *Current Concepts in Clinical Nursing,* **2**:116–125 (1969). (Good summary of normal adolescent behavior.)

Geach, Barbara: Gifts and Their Significance, *American Journal of Nursing,* **71**:266–270 (1971).

Goldsborough, Judith: On Becoming Nonjudgmental, *American Journal of Nursing,* **70**:2340–2343 (1970).

The Scientific Method in Nursing

Pamela Mitchell

DIAGNOSIS AND INTERVENTION AS A SCIENTIFIC ENDEAVOR

Definitions of *diagnosis* imply the scientific or analytic nature of the process. Nonmedical definitions are in terms of investigation, analysis, and conclusions regarding the nature of situations, problems, or phenomena ("Webster's New World Dictionary," 1970; "Webster's Seventh New Collegiate Dictionary," 1971).

Diagnosis is also defined in terms of critical investigation and the decisions resulting from that investigation. Therefore it seems logical to assume that diagnosis of nursing problems must be based upon a systematic method, and not be someone's guess or opinion about the matter. The *scientific method* is the name commonly given to the investigative approach used by

scientists. Classically, this method is a logical sequence of steps used in investigating phenomena (see Table 5-1). When he explores a general area which puzzles him, the scientist first surveys the available information to see what is known about the area. He uses this information and his "hunches," or empirical impressions, to define a specific problem or ask a specific question which he would like to study. He again surveys the literature or other sources, this time to see what research has been conducted about the problem, and to discover what theoretical framework exists which might be relevant to the problem. The theoretical background helps him predict what the outcomes of his testing "ought" to be, or to explain how a number of observations in the problem area relate to one another. All of the inquiry to this point has been an attempt to

Table 5-1 The Relationship of the Scientific Method to Nursing Diagnosis and Intervention

Scientific method	Nursing diagnosis and intervention
1 Recognize general problem area	1 Recognize general problem area (patient's need for help)

a Survey pertinent information (literature, observation)	**a** Survey pertinent information
	    (1) Assess patient-client status
	    (2) Review pertinent information

b Develop "hunches"	**b** Develop impressions
2 Define specific problem	2 Define problem requiring nursing help
3 Review related information (research already done, theoretical formulations)	3 Review related information (literature, theoretical knowledge, empirical observation)

4 Propose hypotheses	4 Propose hypotheses
	  a Goals and objectives
	  b Proposed actions

5 Test hypotheses
  a Establish base-line data
  b State criteria for acceptance or rejection
  c Collect data
	5 Implement intervention
	  a Establish base-line data
	  b State criteria for evaluating effectiveness
	  c Observe results

6 Analyze data—interpret results	6 Analyze results—interpret effects of intervention
7 Terminate or modify study	7 Terminate or modify intervention

gather sufficient preliminary data or information so that the scientist may propose reasonable hypotheses—possible answers to his questions which make sense in terms of his observations.

The next step is to test the hypotheses by trying them out, in a relatively controlled situation. This situation may vary from a rigidly controlled laboratory experiment to a constantly changing field, or natural setting. The testing of hypotheses usually constitutes an intervention or change in the situation being investigated. Therefore, the scientist must record some data about the base line, or preintervention state. He determines what he will accept as evidence that the intervention is successful, and then actually intervenes. The measurements and observations which he makes before and after intervention form the data used to test the validity of the hypotheses.

Once the scientist has analyzed or evaluated the data in terms of his preset criteria, he can interpret the results of his testing in light of the theoretical framework of the study. The framework may offer clues as to why the results did or did not support the hypothesis. He may end his research here, if he is satisfied with the answers he has, or if he has run out of time, patience, or money. Or he may modify the study on the basis of his results. He may try another approach if he could not verify his hypothesis, or he may move to another aspect of the problem which he is studying.

Because the foregoing series of steps lends itself as well to solving problems as to conducting experiments or describing phenomena, fields such as nursing which deal with practical problems often use an adaptation called the *problem-solving method.*

In the past nursing has been almost exclusively concerned with the application of scientific facts to practical problems of illness and health. Recently there has been increased involvement of nurses in research within their own field, and the scientific method is gaining increased use in clinical research as well as in patient-care problems. The average practitioner may never design a research study, but he will certainly need to evaluate the application of these studies to his practice. He therefore needs to be familiar with the method used. More basically, the same systematic evaluation of data, statement of problem, formulation and testing of hypotheses, and evaluation of results are the basis for his planning of nursing care.

Therefore, rather than speak of both problem solving and the scientific method, the term scientific method will be used here to mean the framework for both the clinical diagnosis of and research about nursing problems.

APPLYING THE SCIENTIFIC METHOD TO CLINICAL NURSING PRACTICE

The scientific method can and must be applied rigidly to research about nursing practice; it will be applied much more loosely to the actual practice of nursing. An example of research about practice is an attempt to prove that intervention *A* is more effective than intervention *B* in alleviating postoperative pain. In this case we must adhere carefully to the research method in order to be sure that it really *is* intervention *A*, not variables *XYZ*, which alleviated the pain.

When our primary goal is to alleviate a particular patient-client's pain, rather than study

Table 5-2   Use of the Scientific Method in a Clinical Problem

Method	Clinical problem
1 Define the general problem 　**a** Survey pertinent information	Acute pain (patient-client expresses need for help)
1 Assess patient-client status	In relation to pain: 　Subjective description: location, quality, duration, extent, precipitating factors 　Objective factors: appearance, autonomic response (pulse, perspiration, blood pressure)
2 Review related data	Nature of surgery, nature of expected pain, previous reactions to pain, other factors which might cause pain
b Develop impressions	Expected postoperative incisional pain—reaction in normal range
2 Define the specific problem	Postoperative pain, moderately severe
3 Review related information	Knowledge of pain source, means to alleviate, delegated medical therapy available, supportive nursing measures, expected efficacy of measures
4 Propose intervention 　**a** Define goals, objectives	Patient-client goals: relief and sleep Nurse goals: alleviation of pain, relaxation to allow sleep, support during experience
b Proposed action	Medication to decrease pain to tolerable level Back rub, position change to help relaxation
5 Implement intervention 　**a** Review base-line data	Patient-client tense, focused only on pain, "miserable"
b Establish criteria for effectiveness	Relaxation, sleep, subjective relief within 30 to 45 min
c Observe results	Patient-client sleeping in 20 min, relaxed appearance
6 Analyze results	This type of pain does not disappear spontaneously; thus assume sleep is result of relief. Do not know if medication or comfort measures most effective
7 Evaluate method	Use same approach when pain returns

methods of alleviation, we engage in practice. The practitioner may not be able to follow the scientific method to the letter. Table 5-2 shows how the nurse might use the scientific approach to provide a systematic framework in which to approach the problem of pain. There are, however, some important differences between the use of the scientific method in research and in clinical practice. The practitioner must be aware of the differences lest he think he is more "scientific" than he really is, or expect an exactness in the practice field which does not exist.

The example in Table 5-2 of an approach to a patient-client in acute pain implies one important difference between scientist and practitioner. This difference is time. The patient-client in acute pain cannot wait several hours or days while the nurse assembles all the theoretical information which he might want about the management of pain.

In many clinical situations, the practitioner must make speedy decisions, based upon whatever pertinent information he carries in his head or can obtain from others. Too many nurses, however, make all their decisions on the basis of their own store of knowledge, rather than using the other resources at their disposal.

The second difference between the use of the scientific method by scientists and its use by practitioners is the multiplicity of variables in the "real world" as opposed to the controlled research model. Even if the scientist is studying in a natural environment, he seeks to structure the situation so that "contaminating variables" are minimal. Contaminating variables are those over which he has no control but which may affect the outcome of the experiment. The practitioner, by contrast, has little control over variables other than his own interventions. Simply following the steps of the scientific method does not assure that unforeseen consequences will not enter the situation.

The nurse attempting to help a person who is in pain may know that certain measures help relieve pain in selected experimental conditions. However, he has no way of knowing if these measures will work equally well with this particular person, whose personality, reaction to pain, and type of pain may be quite different from those studied by the scientist. Benne, Chin, and Bennis (1969) point out the necessity of the practitioner to see "incomplete predictability" as a part of his work, rather than to become discouraged by his inability to be completely scientific.

The breadth of problems to be solved constitutes another problem for the practitioner when he attempts to use the scientific method. Application of the method to the research problem demands that the problem area be narrowed to a very small portion—the *one* question or problem to be studied. People who are ill rarely present only one problem for study or solution; rather their illness poses a multiplicity of problems, several of which may demand equal priority. Nevertheless, the diagnosis and management of their nursing problems must proceed by defining and planning for *each* problem. Several problems may relate to one another and cannot be treated in isolation, but the entire process can be followed for each of the definable problems. Lawrence Weed, in discussing an approach to medical problems, acknowledges this difficulty in relation to the physician confronted with the complexities of clinical care. He states, "The physician can act as a scientist, however, if he is able to organize the problems of each patient in a way that enables him to deal with them systematically."[1]

A final problem in utilizing the scientific method for nursing practice is the paucity of theoretical background in nursing per se. Nursing is an applied field, using concepts from the natural, physical, and behavioral sciences and concepts from medical practice to derive princi-

---

[1] Lawrence L. Weed, Medical Records That Guide and Teach, *New England Journal of Medicine*, **278**:593–595 (Mar. 14, 1968).

ples for action. Because we borrow concepts from so many fields, it is difficult for the student and the practitioner to know which are useful and which are not. And because these theories and concepts have been formulated in settings very different from nursing practice, they cannot be translated wholesale into a theoretical basis for nursing practice.

Essentially, the "borrowed" concepts point to *possible* relationships between observations made by the practitioner and by the scientist; they suggest hypotheses to be tested. The purpose of Part 3 of this book is to present some concepts which we believe are basic to the practice of nursing. These concepts are not intended to substitute for actual testing of interventions by the practitioner. In the last analysis, nurses, like all other practitioners, will use "whatever works." However, using the working tools within a scientific framework will help us pass on to others our useful approaches and to discard the outworn ones.

REFERENCES

Benne, Kenneth, Robert Chin, and Warren Bennis: Science and Practice, in W. Bennis et al. (eds.), "The Planning of Change," 2d ed., Holt, Rinehart and Winston, Inc., New York, 1969, pp. 113-123.

Selltiz, Claire, Marie Jahoda, Morton Deutsch, and Stuart Cook: "Research Methods in Social Relations," rev. ed., Holt, Rinehart and Winston, Inc., New York, 1966.

"Webster's New World Dictionary," 2d College Edition, World Publishing Company, New York, 1970.

"Webster's Seventh New Collegiate Dictionary," G. C. Merriam Company, Springfield, Ill., 1971.

Weed, Lawrence L.: Medical Records That Guide and Teach, *New England Journal of Medicine,* **278**:593-595 (Mar. 14, 1968).

The Process of Diagnosis

Pamela Mitchell

The process of diagnosis is a complex intellectual exercise involving collecting, sifting, and analyzing data; making decisions about the importance of data; relating data to standards and norms; and finally, making decisions about the client's need for nursing help. This chapter describes this process in some detail, dissecting it into component parts. As a result, the student may lose track of the whole in reading about its parts. Figure 6-1 summarizes the process as a pictorial model.

The patient-client and the nurse produce the raw data for analysis. The nurse seeks the data through the activities of interview, observation and examination, and consultation. Others in the nurse-patient environment (family, social and work groups, health professionals) may contribute to this raw information.

The raw data provide the "evidence" from which nurse and patient-client make their estimates of functional disability (areas of deviant function). They do this, together or independently, by analyzing the patient-client's status in terms of normative standards, i.e., what the "healthy" or "normal" person should be able to do. Nurse and patient-client compare the functional abilities with some norm; thus they are using comparative standards.

Comparative standards and perceptions of the nurse and of the patient are applied to these data to determine areas of deviance in functional ability. These standards, or norms, may vary depending upon the frame of reference of nurse and of patient.

The nurse compares standards to the data,

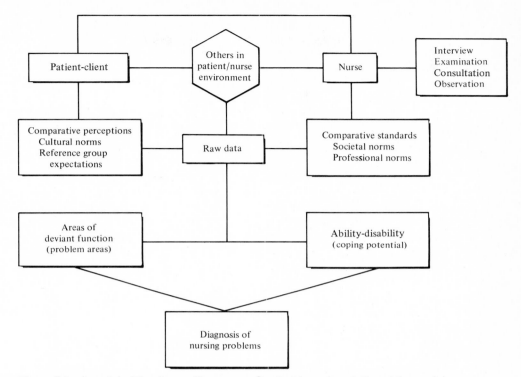

Figure 6-1 A model of the diagnostic process. See text for a description of the model.

comparing measurements of the patient-client's function and behavior with professionally and socially set limits or standards. The patient-client does not usually have the benefit of knowledge of health-care-system norms and tends to compare perceptions of his own function with his perception of the abilities of others, and with his reference group's expectations of "normal" function. A reference group is the group with which an individual identifies and whose values and norms he shares.

Finally, the nurse uses comparative standards to determine the patient-client's abilities and disabilities in potentially coping with daily life in each area of deviant function. Similarly, he analyzes the patient's perceptions of his own ability and disability to determine how well the person actually *is* coping with his life. This analysis of patient-client function in coping with deviance from health leads to the final step—the diagnosis of the nursing problem.

Nursing was operationally defined in Part 1 as a service to people whose deviation from health has impaired their ability to cope with the changes in daily living which result from that deviation. The general goals of nursing care are to prevent disability and to restore, maintain, or rehabilitate ability. Problems with which nursing is concerned, then, are a patient's or client's problems in coping with daily living which have occurred because of his deviation, or potential deviation, from health. Note that these are a *patient-client's* problems in his daily life, not the nurse's problems in dealing with him. For example, the classical "problem" patient is one who makes constant demands for seemingly trivial things. The problem is not that he is a "demanding" patient. The problem is whatever concerns, fears, or discomforts underlie his behavior and make him unable to cope with the situation in a more direct manner. In order to decide the exact nature of the problem, more information (data) must be gathered about the person and his health problem.

COLLECTING THE DATA— ASSESSMENT OF FUNCTION

Assessment in nursing diagnosis is done through a process of collecting data about the person's present and past health status. Nursing deals with the person's abilities to cope with daily living; therefore, the focus of this assessment is upon his abilities and disabilities in daily activity. These are his *functional abilities*—the ability or disability to operate in a normal manner. The nurse's and patient's definition of "normal" will depend upon his reference groups and may not coincide. Lack of congruence of these definitions will have to be taken into account when planning management of diagnosed problems.

In order to appreciate what changes in his coping abilities the person's present deviation from health has effected, the nurse needs to know something of his previous abilities and coping patterns as well as his current status. This information about the patient is referred to as a nursing history (Little and Carnevali, 1969; McPhetridge, 1968; Smith, 1968) or a nursing assessment (McCain, 1965). Because the term *history* denotes a recounting of past events more than present status, the term *assessment* will be used in this textbook. It connotes a critical appraisal of all factors, past, present, and future.

The term nursing assessment as used by R. Faye McCain refers to a systematic appraisal of the patient's status, "physiological, psychological and social behavior or functional abilities of a patient."[1] The collection of data includes information about usual habits and abilities prior to the health problem, as well as current functional abilities and disabilities.

The key point of collecting data from which to make a diagnosis is that it be done *systematically.* In the past, nurses have been taught to be good observers of the patient's behavior, and of signs and symptoms of disease. However, these observations have been implicitly or explicitly designed to be made while the nurse is engaged in care of the patient—"on the run," so to speak. This tends to result in incomplete, scattered data. In addition, it requires that the nurse assess the need for care while giving that care. This practice is no more consistent with nursing diagnosis than it would be for a mechanic to begin repair of an engine before deciding what is wrong with it.

In order for a nurse to assess a patient's status systematically, there must be an orderly means for collecting and evaluating information. The nurse must decide (1) from what areas of daily living information will be sought, (2) what methods of collecting information are most appropriate to this situation, (3) what priorities exist in collecting data and instituting therapy, and (4) what means will be used for organizing the data and analyzing the existing problems.

This chapter discusses a framework to help the beginning practitioner formulate a systematic process for diagnosis. The assessment outline given is a composite of several published in the literature which have been modified by the author's own clinical experience. The outline and the methods used to gather data are not inflexible patterns. Rather, they are intended to

---

[1] R. Faye McCain, Nursing by Assessment, Not Intuition, *American Journal of Nursing,* **65**:82–84 (1965).

guide the student in developing his own style of assessment by giving him a detailed example. Part 2, Chapter 7, gives an example of a completed assessment, diagnosis, and care plan.

Areas of Daily Living to Be Assessed

The outline in Table 6-1 includes all the areas of daily living with which nurses are concerned. It is applicable to people and groups with health problems in any setting—home, hospital, mental health center, industry, physician's office. The setting will tend to determine which areas as-sume primary importance, and will thus modify the amount and kind of data collected in each area. For example, the nurse working with a client in a community mental health center may focus more on his abilities in the psychosocial, mental-emotional, and possibly sensory-motor areas than on the condition of his skin (integument). However, the nurse who is working with a paralyzed person in a hospital will need to focus equally on abilities and disabilities in all 13 areas of daily living. No matter what the setting, the nurse must consider patient-client functioning in all the areas, lest important data be

Table 6-1   Data Which May Be Collected in Each Assessment Area*

I   Psychosocial.   This area deals with the person's roles in relationship to others about him—his family, work group, health professionals. If the nurse is attempting to diagnose the nursing problems of a group of persons, this area would include the social relationships within that group—patterns of leadership, methods of resolving conflict. However, beginning practice generally deals primarily with individuals, and the outline of data needed will focus only on that needed for an individual.

  A   General Social Status
    1   Ethnic background
    2   Occupation—status or position in that occupation
    3   Economic status
    4   Religious practices
      a   Religious affiliation
      b   Practices or beliefs which might affect reaction to health care (proscriptions against immunization or blood transfusion, dietary laws, beliefs about the cause of disease)
    5   Type of housing accommodation
    6   Contacts or previous referrals to social agencies
  B   Family or Peer Group Social Status
    1   Position in the family (father, mother, etc.)
    2   Others in family
    3   With whom the person lives; whom he considers close if he lives alone
    4   Marital status
    5   Role in family (e.g., source of support during crisis, "black sheep," etc.)
  C   Social Developmental Status
    1   Age
    2   Sex
    3   Marital status
    4   Degree of dependence and independence (prior to and during health deviation)
    5   Diversional and recreational interests
    6   Sexuality
      a   Reproductive data (number of pregnancies, live births, living children, age of menarche, contraceptive methods, menstrual pattern)
      b   Attitudes toward own sexuality
      c   Level of sexual development

* The outline is meant to serve as a guide to data collection, not as an exhaustive outline. The guide was developed from those published by R. Faye McCain and Associates (1965), L. Mae McPhetridge (1968), and Dorothy Smith (1968), and modified by this author's own clinical experience.

Table 6-1   Data Which May Be Collected in Each Assessment Area

II   Mental and Emotional Status.   These are considered as one category since one's intellectual growth bears on reactions to self and others, and vice versa. There is overlap between the psychosocial area and the mental-emotional area, but the student need not waste energy trying to fit a piece of data precisely into one category. The important thing is to note the information *somewhere*.

   A Mental Status

     1 Level of consciousness (response to verbal stimuli, response to noise and light, response to touch and painful stimuli, spontaneous activity)

     2 Orientation to time, place, and person

     3 Intellectual development relative to age

     4 Mental skills (level of education, ability to read and write, vocabulary, ability to comprehend and follow directions, attention span, memory span, ability to understand abstraction)

     5 Perception and understanding of health problem and goals of medical and nursing therapy

     6 Beliefs and attitudes about disease

     7 Previous experience with and reaction to illness and hospitalization

   B Emotional Status

     1 Affect (general mood and emotional response)

     2 Reactions to stressful situations (includes kinds of situations person considers stressful)

     3 Patterns of relating to others

     4 Special concerns or fears

     5 Concept of self—self-esteem (prior to and in relation to current health problem; body image)

     6 Substances taken to alter emotional response (includes prescribed medications—tranquilizers, sedatives, mood-elevating drugs; alcohol; mind-expanding drugs; amphetamines)

III   Environmental Status.   Factors in the patient-client's home, work, or institutional environment are assessed in several other areas. However, some factors, related to safety, control of infection, and environmental effects upon illness, need to be assessed in their own right.

   A Safety Factors

     1 Age

     2 State of mobility

     3 Arrangement of objects in physical environment; other potential safety hazards

     4 Sensory deficits

     5 Orientation-disorientation to environment

     6 Use of restraining devices—bed rails, restraints

     7 Use of prosthetic and other supportive devices—crutches, artificial limbs, mechanical lifting devices

   B Infection Control

     1 Presence of infectious disease or infected wounds in patient, family, or others in proximity

     2 Barriers to cross-infection (isolation techniques, hand-washing facilities, distance from infected persons or infectible persons)

     3 Patient and family understanding and beliefs about transfer of pathogens

     4 Equipment potentially harboring pathogens (isolettes, humidifiers, pulmonary therapy equipment)

   C Environmental Effects on Illness

     1 Patterns of activity, light, noise, color (varied, steady, excessive, absent)

     2 Arrangement of environment in relation to functional abilities or disabilities (Are pictures and reading material placed where bedfast person can see them? Are implements placed where handicapped person can reach them?)

IV   Sensory Status.**   This area refers to the state of the perceiving senses—vision, hearing, smell, taste, touch. Speech perception and formation are categorized here although they are dependent upon both sensory and motor function.

   A Visual Status

**Areas IV and V, which deal with sensory-motor status, evaluate the individual's ability to perceive the world about him, and to act on those perceptions. Functions in these areas are mediated by the central nervous system, and their status is one clue to the intactness of motor and sensory nerves and tracts. Deficits in one modality often correspond to deficits in the other. For example, the person who is hemiplegic (paralyzed on one side) often has decreased sensation to touch on the paralyzed side. For this reason, the two areas should be assessed in relation to each other, although a systematic evaluation is made of each.

      1 Visual acuity (ability to distinguish objects at a specified distance)
      2 Field of vision (lateral, horizontal, vertical)
      3 Known deficits (myopia, presbyopia, astigmatism, color blindness, blindness)
      4 Corrective or prosthetic devices (glasses, contact lenses, artificial eye)
      5 Unusual sensations (rainbows around lights, blind spots, flashing lights)
   B Auditory Status
      1 Ability to distinguish voice (distance, loudness)
      2 Known deficits (extent—i.e., one ear, both ears, complete, partial)
      3 Corrective devices
      4 Unusual sensations (ringing, buzzing, dizziness)
   C Olfactory Status
      1 Ability to discriminate odors
      2 Unusual sensations (lack of smell, heightened sensitivity to smell, smelling odors with no stimulus present)
   D Gustatory Status
      1 Ability to discriminate sweet, sour, salt, bitter
      2 Unusual sensations (lack of taste, aftertaste, substances taste alike)
   E Tactile Status
      1 Ability to discriminate sharp and dull, light and firm touch
      2 Ability to perceive heat, cold, and pain in proportion to stimulus
      3 Ability to differentiate common objects by touch (stereognosis)
      4 Intactness of body image
      5 Aberrant sensation (lack of pain, touch, heat, cold sensation; increased or decreased pain in proportion to stimulus; diffuse burning, pricking, or pain)
   F Speech Perception and Formation
      1 Intactness of speech organs (mouth, teeth, tongue, palate, larynx)
      2 Deficits in phonation (stammering, lisping, repetition, jargon, mutism, staccato speech)
      3 Ability to understand and initiate speech
   G Sensory Environment
      1 Intensity
      2 Pattern
      3 Variety
      4 Appropriateness to developmental level

V   Motor Status.** This area evaluates the ability of the person's nervous system to initiate action in response to stimuli perceived by the sensory organs. Much of the data centers around the state of the structural organs of movement—the muscles and the bones.
   A Medical Restrictions on Activity (physician's prescription for bed rest, bed rest with bathroom privileges, etc.)
   B Musculoskeletal Status
      1 General movement (coordination, ease, stability)
      2 Muscle strength, tone, and mass (all extremities, trunk and abdomen; symmetry; prior to and during health problem)
      3 Range of joint motion (all joints, active and passive motion)
      4 Posture
      5 Handedness
      6 Deformities (intactness of extremities, prosthetic devices)
      7 Abnormal innervation to muscles (paralysis, weakness)
   C Mobility
      1 Method of ambulation (unassisted, with supportive aids such as cane, crutch, wheelchair)
      2 Gait (mode of walking, coordination, stability)
      3 Endurance (amount of activity tolerated)

**Areas IV and V, which deal with sensory-motor status, evaluate the individual's ability to perceive the world about him, and to act on those perceptions. Functions in these areas are mediated by the central nervous system, and their status is one clue to the intactness of motor and sensory nerves and tracts. Deficits in one modality often correspond to deficits in the other. For example, the person who is hemiplegic (paralyzed on one side) often has decreased sensation to touch on the paralyzed side. For this reason, the two areas should be assessed in relation to each other, although a systematic evaluation is made of each.

Table 6-1   Data Which May Be Collected in Each Assessment Area

VI   Nutritional Status.   This area deals not only with obvious data about intake of foods, but also with attitudes toward eating and toward special diets.

   A Dietary Habits
     1 Usual eating habits (number and timing of meals, inclusion of "basic four" categories of food, preferred foods, excesses)
     2 Appetite
     3 Changes related to health problem (appetite changes, special diet prescribed by physician or by patient-client)
     4 Person responsible for preparing food at home
   B Adequacy of Diet
     1 Height, weight; gain-loss pattern
     2 General appearance (obese, normal, thin; appearance of skin, hair, nails)
   C Attitudes toward Eating
     1 Importance of food to feeling of well-being
     2 Religious dietary restrictions
     3 Symbolic meaning of food—reward, love, punishment
   D Factors in Food Ingestion
     1 State of teeth (dentulous, partially or completely edentulous; disease of teeth and gums; oral hygiene habits)
     2 State of mouth (intactness of mucous membranes; disorders of salivary glands; moistness; odor; presence of debris)
     3 State of consciousness
     4 Ability to swallow
     5 Gastrointestinal motility
   E Digestion
     1 Ease of digestion
     2 Nausea, vomiting, retching
     3 Eructation (belching)
     4 Medications affecting digestion and metabolism of foods
   F Non-oral Means of Feeding
     1 Parenteral fluids; hyperalimentation
     2 Nasogastric tube, gastrostomy

VII   Elimination Status.   This category includes elimination via the urinary and gastrointestinal tracts.

   A Normal Patterns (frequency, amount, color, consistency of stool)
   B Aids to Elimination Normally Used (beverages, laxatives, position)
   C Changes Due to Health Problem
     1 Character of urine (color, odor, specific gravity, unusual constituents)
     2 Character of stool (color, odor, consistency, presence of unusual constituents)
   D Method of Eliminating (toilet, commode, bedpan)
     1 Artificial orifices (ileal conduit—urine; colostomy, ileostomy—bowel)
     2 Method of care for excretions from artificial orifices
   E Special Problems
     1 Incontinence (urine, stool; ways of coping)
     2 Urinary retention
     3 Constipation
     4 Diarrhea

VIII   Fluid and Electrolyte Status.   Maintenance of a balance of body fluids and electrolytes is essential to homeostasis and to life. Although the physician has primary responsibility in restoring this balance, nurses' observations often provide key data for the medical management. In addition, the nurse may play an important role in helping to maintain this balance.

   A Normal Patterns of Fluid Intake and Output
     1 Ingestion of food and fluids (amounts in 24 hr, types preferred)
     2 Output (urine, stool, perspiration)

B Changes Due to Health Problem (increase or decrease in intake or output)

C Measurements

    1 Oral and parenteral intake (includes type of solid foods)

    2 Output (urine, liquid stool, number of formed stools, drainage from wounds, occasionally perspiration and respiratory loss)

D Indirect Data

    1 State of hydration, dehydration

      a Weight

      b Thirst

      c Skin turgor, dryness

      d Condition of mouth, mucous membranes (dry, moist, coated, presence of crusts)

      e Edema

    2 Venous state (distended, flattened, filling time)

    3 Level of consciousness

    4 Depression or elevation of fontanels in infants

    5 Neuromuscular flaccidity or irritability

    6 Laboratory values of electrolytes, pH

    7 Medical therapy (drugs, parenteral fluids, blood)

IX Circulatory Status. These observations give indirect data about the state of the heart and blood vessels.

A Pulse

    1 Rate

    2 Quality (thready, weak, bounding, strong)

    3 Rhythm (regular, irregular, paired beats)

    4 Apical-radial differences

    5 Response to activity, emotional stress

    6 Medications which alter heart rate or rhythm

B Blood Pressure

    1 Systolic, diastolic

    2 Lying and standing

    3 Discrepancies between arms

    4 Factors altering accuracy of reading (obesity, cuff size)

C General Appearance

    1 Color (skin, lips, nails)

    2 Evidence of volume depletion or edema

    3 Urine output, fluid intake

    4 Warmth and color of extremities

    5 Undue fatigue after exertion

    6 Pains in legs after walking

    7 Chest or epigastric pain, precipitating factors

D Special Observations. If the patient has acute cardiac disease and his condition is being specially monitored, the list may also include data from monitoring devices such as the character of the electrocardiogram, central venous pressure, arterial pressure.

X Respiratory Status. The state of the respiratory function may be assessed both directly and indirectly. The indirect measurements give some clues to the state of cellular respiration.

A Direct Measurements

    1 Patency of the airway

    2 Respirations

      a Rate, rhythm, depth, ease, use of accessory muscles

      b Factors altering character (position, emotion, cough, humidity, air pollution)

    3 Cough

      a Patterns (upon arising, continuous, random, after smoking)

      b Productive of sputum

      c Character of sputum (color, viscosity, odor, hemoptysis)

B Indirect Measurements

    1 Smoking history

Table 6-1 Data Which May Be Collected in Each Assessment Area

    2 Medications affecting respiratory rate, patency of bronchial tree
    3 Color (skin, lips, nails)
    4 Clubbing of nails
    5 Posture, skeletal defects such as kyphosis
    6 Level of consciousness (increase or decrease)
    7 Anxiety or apprehension (diffuse or specific regarding breathing)
    8 Laboratory values (Po_2, Pco_2; pH)
  C Supportive Devices
    1 Nebulizers, aerosols (patterns of use, effectiveness)
    2 Positive-pressure breathing
    3 Tracheostomy
    4 Assisted or controlled ventilation with respirator

XI Temperature Status
  A Subjective Feeling of Warmth and Cold
  B Usual Measures for Temperature Comfort
  C Body Temperature
    1 Oral
    2 Rectal
    3 Axillary
  D Perspiration
    1 Presence or absence
    2 Pattern (night, day, intermittent)
  E Environmental Temperature and Humidity
  F Methods of Altering Temperature
    1 Convection, conduction, radiation, evaporation
    2 Special equipment (hypo-hyperthermia blanket)

XII Integumentary Status. This area refers to the condition of the skin and underlying tissues, nails, and hair.
  A Skin Condition
    1 Color, turgor
    2 Intactness (presence of wounds, incisions, ulcers, pressure cores, diaper rash)
    3 Character of any lesions present (dry, draining, infected)
    4 Areas of ischemia
    5 Factors predisposing to skin breakdown (prolonged pressure, lack of position change, unprotected bony prominences, incontinence, age, hyperactivity, self-destructive tendencies)
  B Condition of Nails and Hair
  C Habits of Personal Hygiene
  D Odors and Excretions (oily, perspiration, abnormal)

XIII Comfort and Rest Status
  A Sleep
    1 Normal sleep pattern (number of hours, time, feeling of being rested)
    2 Alterations due to health problem
    3 Aids used for sleep (beverages, warm bath, medications)
  B Comfort
    1 Presence of pain or discomfort (location, duration, degree, extent, character, precipitating factors)
    2 Use of aids to relieve pain or discomfort (prior to and during current health problem)
    3 Changes in pain or discomfort with current health problem

overlooked because of focusing too much on the nurse's own area of specialization.

The kinds of information which may be collected are outlined in each assessment area. This outline may appear overwhelming to the beginner, who wonders when he will have time to care for the patient. However, not all these data must be collected for every patient, family, or group with whom the nurse comes in contact. The outline is presented simply to give an idea of the direction which assessment may take. It is the function of faculty and nurse specialists to help students and beginning practitioners know what specific information to gather for people with particular presenting health problems. Beginners will tend to focus on the broad aspects of data collection; they will add more details as they gain knowledge and experience.

Simply collecting data is not enough to make a systematic assessment. The data must be stated and recorded in specific terms. For example, the observation that a patient is "hard-of-hearing" tells us little about how this deficit affects the person. It is more helpful to know that the person "states he has 50 percent hearing loss in the right ear; can distinguish normal conversational tones when approached from the left side." It is most important to describe the patient-client's abilities and disabilities in enough detail so that anyone could have a clear picture of his health status.

Methods of Collecting Data

There are four major means of collecting the data needed for assessment of the patient's condition: *interview, examination and observation, consultation,* and *review of the literature.* The primary source of data is the patient or client himself. Secondary sources include persons within the client's life (family, friends, employers, teachers), other health professionals, the written records of the person's present or past health problems, and scientific knowledge about his general kind of health problem.

No one method or one source is sufficient to gather all the data needed. The nature of the situation and the time available for data collection will determine which methods and sources will receive priority. For example, the majority of information about a well infant will come from interviewing the mother of the child and from direct examination of the baby. In contrast, the fifty-year-old man with a chronic illness will probably relate his own history. His previous clinic and hospitalization records will also be an important source of data.

Time may be a factor in determining methods, as in an emergency situation. The nurse in the emergency room, confronted with a badly injured person, will have to make a very rapid assessment by examination and observation, supplemented with a brief interview of family members or witnesses to the accident. Perusal of medical records, consultation with other health workers, and extensive interviewing have to wait until the crisis is past.

THE INTERVIEW

The interview has been defined as a conversation with a purpose (Fenlason, 1962, p. 2). As such, it is one of the primary means of obtaining information about a person's usual habits, values, and norms regarding health, perceptions of illness and therapy, and perceptions of himself. If the patient's age and mental ability allow it, he is interviewed directly. The family or other knowledgeable persons may be interviewed to gain additional data. These persons may be the primary source of information for the child, the unconscious person, or the disoriented person.

Several aspects of interviewing are relevant to the assessment interview: (1) the purpose of the interview, (2) the roles of the interviewer and the interviewee, (3) the structure of the interview, and (4) the setting, or climate, in which the conversation takes place.

The Purpose of the Interview

The purposes of an interview may include (1) gathering information, (2) diagnosing problems, (3) teaching, (4) evaluating progress, (5) attempting to understand another's point of view, (6) counseling, (7) providing support, (8) providing therapy. The purpose of the assessment interview is *to gather information* (data) in order *to diagnose* nursing problems. Because people who are in need of health services generally do not separate their health data from their fears or concerns, the assessment interview may also have some elements of the supportive and therapeutic interview as well. It is important to remember, however, that the primary purpose at this point is data collection, not therapy. It is hardly sensible to begin providing therapy when the need has not yet been clearly defined.

For example, the patient may say that he is very much worried about who will care for his elderly mother while he is in the hospital. Simply to make note of this fact (gather information) and then pass on to other topics ignores the importance of this situation to the patient-client. Further, it may make him feel that the nurse does not realize his concern. The nurse might inquire further about his mother (the extent of her disabilities, what arrangements have been made or could be made with family or friends) and then tell the man that immediately after the interview the nurse will contact a social worker, who will help make arrangements for the patient's mother. In this way, the nurse has engaged in limited supportive therapy (recognition and acceptance of the patient's concern) while gaining further data as a basis for definitive action. It is most important to let the patient know when he can expect the help for which he has directly or indirectly asked.

The Roles of the Interviewer and Interviewee

Roles are patterns of behavior which people assume by virtue of being in certain situations—the role of student, of teacher, of patient, of nurse. They are also the responses and behavior which people assume by virtue of interaction with others in specified situations. Thus, the role of student is shaped not only by society's definition of student behavior but also by the interactions of student with teachers and peers.

The interview situation assigns certain roles to interviewer and interviewee. The extent to which they conform to these specified roles will depend upon their expectations of each other and the interaction they have during the interview. Although the roles discussed here are in relation to the assessment interview, they are essentially the same as those in therapeutic communication (see Part 3, Chapter 9).

The major roles of the interviewer are to clarify the purpose of the interview, to set the focus, to maintain the momentum, and to create an atmosphere in which the interviewee will feel free to talk. Bermosk and Mordan (1964) define

Table 6-2 Intentions of the Nurse Interviewer

1 To encourage the communication of ideas, feelings, and data from the patient in an effort to identify both his immediate and long-term health needs
2 To communicate to the patient the nurse's desire to understand the patient's ideas, feelings, and personal data so that, together, patient and nurse may come to a common identification of the patient's health needs
3 To identify and clarify the patient's health needs and to communicate the kinds of information (facts, knowledge, resource people, services, and facilities) which will enable the patient to formulate a solution for meeting the identified health needs
4 To direct the communication so as to allow the patient an opportunity to explore and discuss the information presented and to arrive at his own solution for meeting the identified health need

Reprinted by permission of The MacMillan Company from "Interviewing in Nursing," by Loretta Bermosk and Mary Jane Mordan. Copyright, The MacMillan Company, 1964, pp. 9-10.

four intentions of the nurse interviewer which fit within this role. These are presented in Table 6-2.

Clarifying the Purpose and Focus   No matter what the purpose of the interview, it is the obligation of the interviewer to clarify the purpose to the interviewee. The public image of the nurse does not generally include formal interviewing. Therefore, the nurse who simply begins the interview without explaining the purpose to the patient is not only being discourteous to him, but may also find him guarded in his responses as he does not know why the information is being sought. One approach is to tell the patient or other informant that you are going to ask him some questions about his normal habits and his health problem which will enable you and him to plan his nursing care (in a hospital), to help him stay healthy (in preventive situations), to make the return to work easier (in industry), or whatever is appropriate to the situation.

Maintaining Momentum   This approach helps the interviewee know what is expected of him, sets the focus of the interview, and lets him decide if your request for information is legitimate in his eyes. If he feels that the help you offer is worth the disclosure of personal information, the interview will proceed. Your next task is to keep the conversation moving. Some people tend to ramble or go off on tangents when discussing themselves or their health. The nurse's role is to help them organize their thinking. This can be done by tactfully directing the discussion back to the central purpose. Statements such as, "You hadn't finished telling me about . . . , could we go back to that?" are helpful here. Be alert, however, for important cues in the patient-client's "ramblings," and do not cut off all elaboration. For example, an elderly gentleman may make frequent tangential references to his sister. Asking the man to tell about her may lead him to

disclose that she died following an illness with symptoms similar to his. To have dismissed these references might have caused the nurse to miss his fears that his illness is terminal.

The line between redirecting tangential conversation and not cutting off important elaboration is difficult for beginning students to draw. Experience in gathering information and in interviewing in general will make the differentiation easier. Until that experience is gained, it is probably better to lean toward encouraging too much rather than too little elaboration.

The nurse's own comfort in interviewing, his reactions to the patient-client's ideas and expressions, and the nurse's own emotions are all factors in the degree to which he can keep the interview moving. The importance of self-knowledge in the nurse-patient relationship is amplified in Part 2, Chapter 4, and the student is advised to read that chapter before beginning to interview patients and clients.

Nurses who have had little experience in interviewing are often *not* comfortable in their new role. They feel they must "get lots of information" or "fill up the history sheet," primarily for the benefit of instructor or supervisor. They frequently feel that they are prying into the private life of the patient-client and wonder if the patient feels that way also.

There are many possible sources for this discomfort. The novice nurse is suddenly expected to discuss many subjects with a total stranger—subjects which his culture generally considers private and personal. It is therefore no surprise that he might feel uncomfortable.

Second, he often has no idea what to do with the information, once he has it. This is a common feeling of the inexperienced nurse; it tends to diminish as he gains more knowledge of nursing and medical care. It often helps to remember that the purpose in exploring all these areas of daily living is not simply to get lots of "answers" on paper, but to get as complete a picture as possible of your patient-client, how his health problem affects his life, and how you can help him. Another source of discomfort for the nurse is the patient-client's response to his situation. The person with a health problem may be miserable, angry, or unhappy—types of behavior which our predominantly Western culture encourages us to hide. Therefore, it may be hard for the patient-client to express these feelings, and hard for his nurse to be comfortable in allowing him to do so. It takes a lot of conscious effort to allow a person to express feelings or to behave in ways which our own upbringing has taught us to suppress. However, the purpose of the assessment interview is to see how the patient-client sees his situation *at this time,* whether or not we agree with his interpretation of it or his reaction to it. Therefore, the nurse needs to work at overcoming his own discomfort with tears, or with anger, or whatever behavior bothers him, in order to see the patient-client's view of the situation.

Opening Communication

Another role of the interviewer is to create an atmosphere favorable to the disclosure of information by the patient. He is being asked to tell a total stranger many things about his personal life. Therefore, this stranger (the nurse) must convey enough acceptance and trustworthiness that the patient will allow him to assume the role of confidant.

Establishing an Unhurried Atmosphere

Initially, the interviewer establishes an unhurried atmosphere (see Fig. 6-2). This is one reason why the assessment interview is not particularly satisfactory if conducted while carrying out nursing ministrations. Not only are the data apt to be incomplete, but the patient begins to feel that the nurse has many other things to do and must not be detained by "just talking." Because hospitals are busy places, nurses working in institutions need to plan time for interviewing, just as they plan time for giving medications.

Listening

Secondly, the interviewer must convey a willingness to listen to the patient-client. Listening is an active process and involves hearing, analyzing, and responding to the speaker's message. Nodding one's head, comments such as, "Go on," or "Tell me more about that," convey that one is listening. However, no number of verbal techniques will cover up the nonverbal cues that one is not really listening. The nurse needs to listen not only to the words (content) but also to the pitch, tone, harshness, or softness of the person's voice. All these factors may give clues to topics about which the person feels comfort or discomfort.

Use of Language

The language that the nurse uses will either help or hinder the communication between himself and the interviewee. The use of medical terminology may be confusing or intimidating to many lay persons. This is particularly true if the nurse uses it to bolster his own feelings of insecurity. A few minutes of talking to the patient-client will tell the nurse if the interviewee is speaking in simple, concrete terms or on an abstract, intellectual plane. The sensitive nurse will adjust his language accordingly, neither "talking down" to the less-educated person nor oversimplifying for the medically sophisticated one.

People of different cultural and socioeconomic levels use different terms for ordinary body function. Learning those common to the clientele which the nurse serves will help him communicate better with them. For example, many working-class people may greet the request to "void" with a blank look, whereas they would readily comply with a request to "pass your water." Similarly, one needs to learn the terms a child uses for bodily functions if one is to help him.

The assessment interview is one kind of starting point for the relationship in which nurse and patient-client seek to discover and to solve whatever problems of daily life the client's health

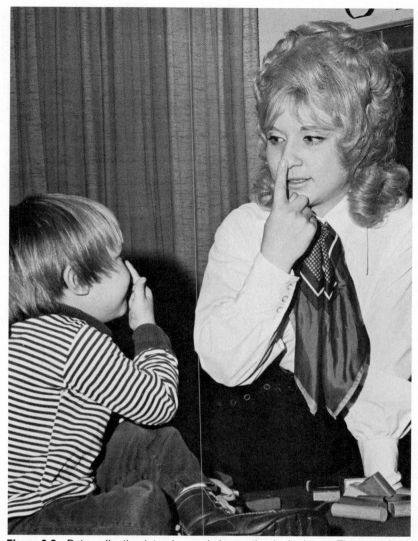

Figure 6-2 Data-collecting interview and observation in the home. The nurse is playing with the child both to set an accepting atmosphere and to observe the child's development. *(Photograph courtesy of University of Washington Medical Photography, Health Sciences Division.)*

problem has created. Rogers (1961) reviews a number of studies analyzing attitudes basic to a helpful or growth-producing relationship. Again and again, the desire to understand, sensitivity to the client's feelings, and concern without loss of one's own emotional integrity characterize attitudes of successful relationships.

Understanding, Acceptance, Compassion
Finally, the atmosphere created must be one of

understanding, acceptance, and compassion. The interviewer who simply records the patient's responses, or who sits impassively while the patient-client talks, gives no feedback to the interviewee. Communication is facilitated only when there is feedback to the speaker that his message is understood. If there is no feedback at all, the speaker may either cease to talk or may cast about for something, no matter how extreme, that will evoke some response from the other person. In either case, he is not able to give a clear picture of the situation as he sees it.

The nurse may indicate that he understands by nodding or by asking that the patient-client validate the understanding ("Am I correct that you mean . . .?"). If the nurse does not understand, he should quickly seek clarification ("I don't understand what you mean when you say. . . .").

Understanding implies not only understanding the content of the patient's conversation (what he says) but making an attempt to understand the emotions underlying it. Comments such as, "That must have been hard for you," "You must have been very frightened," convey this attempt to understand. A word of caution about telling a person, "I understand just how you feel"; unless you really do understand (i.e., have had the same experience and emotion), the patient-client will sense that this is a false attempt to reassure.

Acceptance means to accept the interviewee's perceptions, feelings, and statements as the way *he* views and reacts to the situation. It means to accept him as a person worthy of listening to, whether or not one accepts the appropriateness of his behavior or attitudes. It does not imply that one gives approval to the action or the behavior itself. For example, if a teen-age boy says, "I was so mad at my Ma that I slugged her in the belly," the nurse is not obligated to either condemn or praise the action of hitting the mother. The anger which preceded the action is what one accepts as the emotion that the boy felt

at the time. If a goal of therapy is to help him find a way of talking out his anger, subsequent therapeutic interviews (or conversations) will be used to help him find other means of venting his emotion.

Compassion is literally a "feeling with" another. It involves having enough security in one's own feelings to permit oneself to experience the meaning of an emotion to another.

Most people enter nursing because they have some notion of wanting to help others; this caring and concern for another form the basis of compassion. The terms *sympathy, empathy,* and *compassion* appear frequently in professional literature; all refer to the attitudes showing the patient-client that the nurse cares what happens to him. If the patient knows that the nurse is concerned and is willing to be open, he will be more apt to open his own feelings to view. Basic to compassion is an involvement with the person and his feelings, an appreciation of the meaning of the feelings to him. However, if the nurse is to help the patient-client, this appreciation will stop short of becoming enmeshed in the emotion itself. For example, if the emotion is anxiety, the compassionate nurse knows what it is to be anxious and cares that this is upsetting to the patient. If the nurse becomes anxious himself, however, he cannot help the patient to become less anxious.

The Role of the Interviewee The obvious role of the interviewee in a data-gathering interview is to supply the desired information—to describe his perceptions of his health problems and to tell of his approaches to them. However, several factors may modify the extent to which he accepts this role. His previous experience with interviews, what he perceives as the expectations of the interviewer, and his understanding of the purpose of the exchange will all affect how he fulfills the interviewee role.

If the patient-client has participated in a questionnaire interview, he may expect to answer only "Yes" or "No," or to pick one of several alternative responses. Thus he may feel it is not his place to elaborate on his feelings or to bring up topics not posed by the interviewer. His previous experience with nurses probably does not include an information-gathering interview, and he may need clarification of the use to which the information will be put in order to feel free to talk.

Just as the interviewer watches the interviewee for unspoken cues as to his reactions, the person being interviewed will try to pick up cues as to the expectations of the interviewer. For example, if the nurse invites elaboration with an open-ended question ("Tell me more about your family") and then proceeds to ask specific questions in this area ("How many children do you have?", "How old are they?"), the interviewee will quickly sense that the real expectation is that he answer only the specific questions asked, without elaboration. Thus, he will deal with the incongruence of stated purpose and expectations by responding to the actual expectations.

The Structure of the Interview

The structure of the interview will also influence the interviewee's perception of what is expected of him. There are two basic interview structures—the *directive* and the *nondirective* or *permissive.*

The directive interview is highly structured, with specific information sought and expected. It is frequently used in surveys, such as public opinion polls and research about the demography of disease. Respondents may be asked to give a yes-no response, to choose one of several responses, or to respond in their own words. In all cases, the direction of the interview is set by the interviewer. The questions above about the number and ages of children are examples of directive questions.

In contrast, the interviewee sets the focus of the nondirective interview, as developed by Carl Rogers (1942). The interviewer and interviewee may or may not agree upon the area of content. The interviewer's role is to clarify statements, to encourage elaboration, and to help the client come to his own solutions. The open-ended statement, "Tell me about your family," sets a general focus but is nondirective in the sense that the interviewee may determine what aspect of the family he wishes to discuss. This structure is particularly well suited to counseling and to therapy. It helps keep communication open because the interviewer does not proceed with preconceived notions of the client's concerns or problems. Nursing has taught the use of nondirective conversation, emphasizing its value in keeping communication open and in identifying covert (concealed or hidden) nursing problems (Matheney et al., 1964, p. 78).

A combination of these two interview types is most appropriate to the assessment interview. Although one desires a great deal of specific information in many of the assessment areas, a constant barrage of questions may put the patient-client on the defensive and lead him to believe that he must not elaborate beyond the specific information requested. Much of the data needed to make a nursing diagnosis refers to the person's perceptions of his health problem, his feelings about it, and the disruption that it has caused in his life. These cannot be discovered by questions which are answered with a "yes" or "no," nor can one get an accurate description of the person's perceptions unless he is allowed to describe them himself. Therefore, nondirective techniques are essential in the context of a relatively structured interview.

The structure derives from the need to gather data in 13 areas of daily living and serves to guide the discussion if the informant gets far afield. The nondirective aspect of the interview is the technique used to elicit information about feelings, perceptions, and relationships with others. Nondirective structure is also useful in discussing areas of physical function about which the informant is uncomfortable. In addition, some nondirective structure offers flexibility in the order of data gathering, and allows the patient-client some initiative in discussing what he sees as major concerns.

The Use of Technique   Throughout the interview, the interviewer uses certain techniques to keep the interview moving and to keep communication open. These techniques are simply ways of talking and responding which facilitate, rather than stifle, the openness of the interviewee. They are not ends in themselves, but rather are tools to further the purpose of the conversation. Sidney Jourard, a psychologist, feels that reliance on technique leads to stereotyping of responses to the patient, and to lack of openness in the therapist [interviewer] (Jourard, 1971). His concern is valid, but there is a place for deliberate use of certain ways of responding to the interviewee (technique), particularly for the inexperienced interviewer. Techniques give him tools to use while he is developing skills in facilitating communication. Some people use these techniques in their everyday conversation, having learned openness of communication in their families. However, a great many persons who come to professional education do not have these skills, and must learn them in order to help people more effectively.

Beginning interviewers are often uncomfortable when deliberately using an interviewing technique. They feel that they are being artificial and that they are "tricking" the respondent into revealing things about himself. It may help to overcome this feeling if you remember that no one can be forced to reveal himself—he will declare only as much as he feels comfortable revealing, no matter how much "technique" the interviewer employs. The genuine interest in helping and the openness of the interviewer himself are the most important tools in helping the patient-client talk about himself. The purposes of the techniques described here are to

prevent cutting off the respondent's conversation, and to help the respondent organize and clarify his thoughts. Only a few of the more common facilitating techniques will be described here. The student should consult the readings given at the end of this chapter for a more extensive discussion of interviewing techniques.

Techniques Facilitating Communication

1 Giving information. "I'm Miss Jones, and I will be your nurse while you are in the hospital. I'd like to ask you some questions about yourself and your health which will help me to plan your care while you are here. May I sit down?" This series of statements not only states the purpose of the interview but orients the respondent to his interviewer and begins to set an unhurried atmosphere (the nurse sitting down).

2 Using open-ended statements. These are questions which require more than a yes-no answer and invite elaboration. They allow the respondent to take the lead in the interview. Such statements or questions include: "Tell me about why you came to the hospital"; "Johnny is having a great deal of trouble in school, can you tell me about it?"; "How are things going with your baby?"

3 Expressing acceptance and understanding. Listening attentively, nodding, occasionally saying, "Uh-hum," "Yes," or "I follow what you're saying," suggest that the respondent is being understood.

4 Verbally recognizing feelings. This technique requires that the interviewer verbalize what he thinks the respondent may feel or may have felt in a particular situation. The respondent may or may not be consciously aware of the feeling, and use of this technique can help him put into words what has been bothering him. Some examples of this type of statement are: "Many people feel angry when no one listens to them; is that how you felt?"; "That must be very painful for you"; "It must be lonely to be without your children." It is essential to this technique to allow the patient-client to validate your assumptions about his feelings. Therefore, he must be allowed time to respond to your statement.

5 Consensual validating statements. After making an observation about the interviewee's mood, possible feelings, or appearance, one essentially asks, "Is this how it seems to you?" There need not be an actual statement of this question. The nurse could make one of the statements in example 4, above, and follow it with silence. This silence allows the respondent to validate the accuracy of the nurse's perception. If the patient-client does not respond, the nurse may ask, "Does your silence mean that you have a different feeling about this?" If the respondent has expressed an idea, rather than a feeling, the interviewer might say, "Is this what you mean by . . . ?" or, "Tell me if my understanding of what you say is correct."

6 Clarifying. Clarification is used when the interviewer does not understand what the respondent means; it provides immediate feedback if the speaker is not understood. Clarifying statements include: "I don't quite follow you," "Could you explain what you mean by . . . ?"

7 Exploring. Exploring is simply seeking more information. It is different from probing or prying in that the interviewer is not merely seeking to satisfy his curiosity. He has the purpose of completing the picture of the patient's health problem by adding information. If the respondent feels that exploring has become prying, he will show evidence of discomfort, become evasive, or simply cease talking altogether. If this occurs, the interviewer needs to discuss the halt in communication with the interviewee, and establish again the use to which the information will be put.

8 Making observations. This is simply stating aloud what the interviewer observes about the respondent. For example: "You look very uncomfortable when we discuss this"; "That seems to please you"; "I notice that you are restless." Allow a bit of time for the interviewee to respond to these observations and validate or refute them.

The choice of words may be important in stating observations about the client's emotional state. Words such as "angry," "anxious,"

"afraid," and "depressed" often carry negative connotations. The patient-client may therefore feel that he should deny anger, even though it is evident. He may introduce a less emotionally charged word, such as "annoyed," to describe his behavior. The nurse will do well to follow his lead. Alternately, the nurse may have to find a more neutral word if the patient flatly denies the validity of the observation and offers no other interpretation.

9 Reflecting. The mirroring back to the respondent of what he has just said is reflection. Its purpose is to keep the interviewee talking freely once he has begun. It provides feedback that he is being heard, yet does not introduce any extraneous or threatening material from the interviewer.

Patient: My mother's death was a tremendous blow to me.

Nurse: Your mother's death was quite a blow.

Patient: Yes, she . . . (proceeds to elaborate his relationship with his mother).

This technique, as any technique, may be overused until the respondent feels that he is being parodied. It is one which beginners find particularly artificial. However, it soon becomes a very natural part of conversation if used to help the respondent keep talking.

10 Silence. Silence is a nonverbal technique which can be effective in allowing the respondent time to collect his thoughts or to gain control of his emotions. Many persons are uncomfortable with silence, particularly if they are in the position of "helping" someone else, as the nurse is. It takes practice to become comfortable enough in interviewing to allow periods of silence to occur. Silence is not helpful if it is used by the interviewer when the interviewee is talking and asking for feedback.

Techniques Not Facilitating Communication There are a number of ways in which the interviewer can cut off patient-client responses and hamper the communication. These include such expressions as, "Everything will be all right," and "Don't you worry about that." Such statements constitute false reassurance. They minimize the patient-client's concerns, by implying that there *is* nothing to worry about or that he is foolish to be concerned. This statement cuts off any means for the patient-client to discuss his fears or concerns with the nurse, for the nurse has implied that they are not important. Other nonhelpful techniques or ways of response include persistent direct questioning, giving advice, and minimizing expressed feelings. All these techniques tend to prevent the patient-client from describing his position as *he* sees it.

Following is an actual conversation with a hospitalized woman. It illustrates several techniques and their effect in encouraging expression of an emotional reaction. The right-hand column identifies the technique. Cover it with your hand while you read the conversation, and see if you can identify the techniques used.

N.: I see the foot of your bed has come down. (It had been elevated to prevent further thrombi from forming in legs.)	Stating observation (Nurse aware that medical therapy precluded lowering foot.)
P.: Yeah, I put it down last night. I took off my elastic stockings, too. I'm gonna get M. B. to be my lawyer and sue those doctors at X Y Z hospital [said vehemently].	
N.: Oh? [matter-of-factly].	Encouraging patient to elaborate (Nurse felt defiance of medical therapy and threat to sue were part of some as yet unclear problem.)
P.: I never did trust Dr. X. The clots never came from my legs in the first place. They probably came from the needles when my veins were collapsed. He said he could prove it in court, too.	
N.: Who is "he"? The lawyer?	Clarifying vague pronoun
P.: No, it was Dr. L. I haven't called Mr. B. [the lawyer] yet.	
N.: Have you thought about suing long?	Exploring
P.: No, just since last night when Dr. L. told me I never had clots in my legs. I never did trust Dr. X. anyway. You know Dr. M. said I should have a heart catheterization, and I think they'd better do that 'cause if they don't and it comes out in court that I should've had it then *they*'ll get sued, too [rapidly and angrily].	
N.: You're pretty angry about this.	Verbally recognizing the patient's feeling
P.: I sure am! Maybe I won't actually sue when it comes down to it, but I sure am mad enough.	
N.: (Silence)	(Allowing time for further expression)
P.: I don't get mad often, but when I do I really blow!	

(Further discussion of her anger followed. The patient-client eventually stated that she felt better after "blowing my stack," and felt that she would not sue anyone. She also put on her elastic stockings, and allowed the nurse to elevate the foot of her bed.)

The Setting of the Interview

The last factor to consider in successful interviewing is the setting in which the conversation takes place. The physical setting may vary considerably, from clinic waiting room, to hospital bedside, to a home or factory. However, any of these settings may be favorable if the interviewer creates an unhurried atmosphere.

Privacy is an aspect of the interview setting. This is not always easy to achieve, particularly in an institution or an outpatient clinic. If a private area cannot be found, it is well to remember that some of the information given may be altered by lack of privacy. If possible, try to return at a more private time to discuss areas in which you suspect lack of privacy made the informant reluctant to talk freely.

A final aspect of the setting is the recording of information. Nurses vary in their comfort in taking notes while talking with a patient-client. Some feel it hampers the openness of the discussion, and prefer to record the data immediately after leaving the interviewee. If the information is not recorded immediately, however, much distortion and memory loss may occur.

Other interviewers, who find it impossible to remember all the facts and impressions, make notes as they talk. Interviews may also be tape-recorded. This is particularly helpful for beginners, who can use the recording to evaluate their interview technique. Most patient-clients readily accept an explanation for the note taking or tape recorder and are not bothered by them after a few minutes.

Terminating the Interview

The interview may be terminated by either the nurse or the patient-client. An assessment interview is usually terminated by the nurse when the information is complete. The nurse indicates that he has the information he needs and that he will return later to discuss with the patient-client the help he can offer. At other times, it may be obvious that the interviewee is becoming tired or resistant to further discussion. In such situations, the interviewer may voice this observation: "You look as though you're becoming tired. Would you rather that I come back when you are more rested?" On occasion, the patient-client may request that the nurse come back later, thus terminating the interview himself.

Evaluating Interviewing Skills

Interviewing is a skill which requires much practice. Not only is practice important, but so is an evaluation of the interviews one conducts. Beginners need to develop the habit of constantly evaluating the interviews they conduct, noting where communication is free and where it slows down, and trying to decide why. This evaluation involves observing the responses of both the patient and the nurse, and the feelings and reactions of both. Bermosk and Mordan have published an excellent guide to the evaluation of a nursing interview. It is reproduced in the appendix at the end of this chapter (Bermosk and Mordan, 1964).

EXAMINATION AND OBSERVATION

The second aspect of data collection is assessment by examination and observation. These activities are carried out concurrently with the assessment interview and are used to collect data which can be seen or objectively measured. History and subjective data (the person's perception and feelings) are obtained by interview.

Examination is used in the sense of inspecting or investigating; observation is used in the sense of noticing or perceiving. Thus, examination implies some activity on the part of the ex-

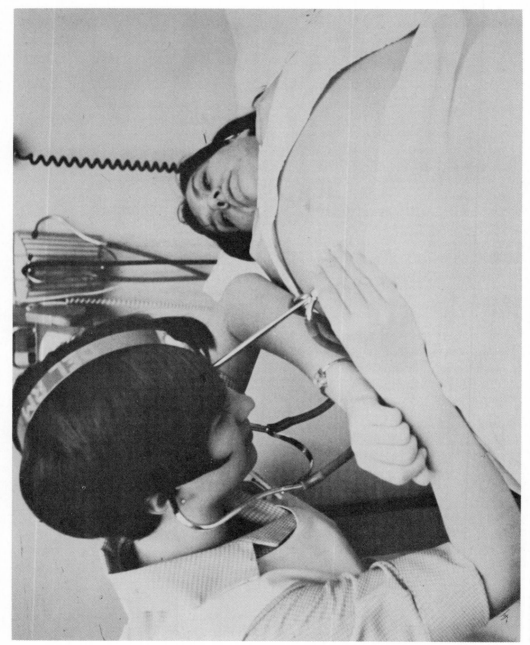

Figure 6-3 Examination as a means of collecting data. The nurse is listening to the fetal heartbeat to gather data about the effect of labor on the baby's circulation. Prior to this she has determined the baby's position in the uterus by palpating the woman's abdomen. *(Photograph courtesy of University of Washington Photography, Health Sciences Division.)*

aminer—testing hearing, taking a blood pressure, testing taste. An example is shown in Fig. 6-3. Observation is obviously a part of examination, and is also important in its own right. Examples of observation include noting the color of the skin, noting the character of respirations, and observing mannerisms suggestive of anxiety. The nurse in Fig. 6-2 is both observing and interviewing.

Much of the data in the areas of physiological functioning can be collected through examination and observation. It is important not to rely only on the patient-client's statement of function when that function can be objectively measured. For example, the patient may state, "I don't have any trouble with my walking," but the nurse should verify this by watching him walk. Most people have never considered whether they have full range of joint motion. Therefore, this is another area which the nurse should examine for himself.

In addition to data regarding physiological functioning, some data about emotional reaction can be obtained through observation. We all communicate nonverbally through our mannerisms and by the way we use our bodies. During the interview, the nurse should observe not only what the patient-client says but what he does as he says it. Perhaps he says, "I don't worry about this being cancer," but has smoked three cigarettes in half an hour, fidgets restlessly, and has repeatedly changed the subject when his current symptoms are referred to. All these observations point to anxiety or discomfort, perhaps because of a fear of cancer. Frowns, clenched fists, and rigid posture are some of the nonverbal kinds of behavior associated with anger or discomfort. Smiles, pats on the back, and a relaxed manner are associated with happiness or comfort. Nonverbal cues to psychological distress are discussed in more detail in Part 3, Chapter 9.

In general, nonverbal behavior is a more accurate clue to an adult's feelings than his words. Socialization has taught most of us to control our spoken feelings (except in the height of emotion); nonverbal control is not always so well developed. Therefore, as in the above example, when actions are not congruent with words, the nurse may want to explore the area of apparent discomfort further.

CONSULTATION

Once one has left the patient-client, data collection is not complete. Consultation of resources other than the patient-client constitutes the final aspect of data collection.

Health records are one source of additional data. They may be current or old hospital records, clinic or physician's office records, or records from community health or social agencies (public health department, welfare department, adoption agency). Among the data available from these records are laboratory data, results of physician's examination, patterns of hospitalization, previous levels of functioning, and ways in which problems were handled in the past.

Verbal consultation with other professional workers is also a source of information. These workers may include the patient's physician, chaplain, physical therapist, or workers in agencies where the person has previously sought help. These persons may be able to give perspective on how they see the patient-client's problems, how he has coped or is coping with them, and resources they have for helping him.

A final source of consultative information about the patient-client is made up of the people in his normal world—his family, friends, teachers, coworkers. They can give valuable perspective on the person's functioning in his everyday life.

REVIEW OF THE LITERATURE

Review of the literature is actually a form of consultation. It does not give further data about the individual patient but is necessary to expand the nurse's factual knowledge about the presenting health problem, related medical-care problems, nursing problems common to this group of people, and possible nursing intervention. The literature includes textbooks and periodicals in nursing, medicine, and the social and biological sciences.

Some of the review of the literature will serve to expand or refresh one's knowledge about a specific type of health problem or disease, its usual course, and treatment. For example, if a particular patient-client has diabetes mellitus, I might want to read in medical and nursing texts to see what is known about the disease, how physicians commonly treat it, what nursing problems are usually associated with it, and how they are managed. This will give me a better understanding of the usual medical therapy in this disorder and some ideas about potential nursing problems. I can then compare this information with what I know about Mrs. X. to see if she is indeed experiencing some of these common problems.

However, Mrs. X. is not a composite of all the people with diabetes and will therefore not "fit" the textbook picture. This initial review can serve only to give clues as to her possible disease-related problems. She herself will provide the clues as to whether these problems actually exist.

Another function of the literature review is to expand one's conceptual knowledge. Concept refers to a general idea based on related observations. For example, we speak of a "concept of immobility"; certain known changes in body function are commonly based on lack of ability to move around. We speak of the "concept of poverty"; certain ways of thinking and of acting relate more to low-income status than to ethnic or other common denominators.

Conceptual knowledge is an important part of professional nursing practice. It is not enough to know the facts about a disease or the nursing care directly related to the medical treatment of that disease. Nursing seeks to help the *person* who has the disease, a person whose reaction to the crisis rarely fits any textbook description of pathologic change.

We can return to Mrs. X., the woman with adult-onset diabetes, to illustrate this point. Suppose that Mrs. X. has a fourth-grade education, is the mother of six small children, has no husband to help her, and is very poor.

The facts say that she will need to follow a careful diet to control her diabetes. Failing that she may need to have oral or injectable drugs. These facts do not tell us anything about whether she will be able to adhere to the diet, whether she will be able to afford it, whether she will understand what to do, or whether she will even try to do it.

Therefore, we must try to find concepts which will give clues to the way in which we can help this woman adapt the health prescription to her own life. We can use the concepts of poverty, of motivation, and of learning to help diagnose her potential coping problems and to design a plan which has some possibility of success. Part 3 of this book is intended to introduce some of the concepts basic to nursing practice.

Setting the Priority and Order of Assessment

There is no set order to the assessment of a patient's status. It is best to take one's cues from the physical state of the person or from his opening responses. If he is in a life-threatening situation, the assessment must be limited to vital areas—airway, breathing, circulation. Further assessment is deferred until action has been taken to assure his physiologic stability. If he is in physical distress which is not life-threatening, such as pain or vomiting, the nature of that distress needs to be explored and the condition alleviated before further assessment is attempted. Similarly, if he is in acute emotional distress (anxiety bordering on panic, active hallucinations), action must be taken to relieve that distress before making a detailed assessment. In such situations, observation and consultation may precede the interview.

The majority of persons whom the nurse meets, however, will not be in these assessment categories. In these situations, let the patient's response guide the order of assessment. If the patient-client wants to discuss the hospital meals first, by all means let him.

Nurses working in specialized areas will probably give more weight and priority to those categories which are most pertinent to their area of specialization. For example, the nurse in the prenatal clinic will probably begin with reproductive data and collect more detailed information in that area than will the nurse seeing a geriatric client. No matter what the specialty area, however, the nurse should take note of patient-client functioning in each assessment category. Otherwise, he may find, for example, that the hostility of his psychiatric patient is aggravated by the ingrown toenail which no one knew about.

The Continuing Nature of Assessment and Diagnosis

The diagnostic process is one which is never completed as long as the nurse and patient-client are in contact with each other. When initial data collection is complete the nurse makes a diagnosis. These diagnoses are usually tentative, and many of them will require further assessment for confirmation. As long as the patient-client has his health problem, he will continue to define the situation for himself, adapt to it, and change in his functional abilities. Consequently, the nurse has to assess these changes and adapt the nursing diagnoses and interventions to them.

ANALYSIS OF THE DATA— INFERRING PROBLEMS

When the initial assessment is completed, it is time to evaluate the data, determining where the person's abilities and disabilities lie, and to decide which of these disabilities constitute problems for the patient-client.

Collaborating with the Patient-Client

At this point we must emphasize the *collaborative* nature of nursing care. Problems which concern nurses are the *patient-client's* problems in coping with daily life; therefore he should have some say in defining these problems. Far too often, this is not the case. Nurses decide what they think a person's needs are, what problems bother him, and how these problems should be solved. Anyone who has received advice for which he has not asked and which he does not want will appreciate how frustrating it is to have others anticipate his problems without checking their perceptions with him. Ida Orlando writes that unless the nurse validates the accuracy of his perceptions of needs with the patient-client, the nurse is engaging in automatic nontherapeutic activity (Orlando, 1961). Several studies have shown that nursing actions based on consultation with the patient at each step of the process (from diagnosis to evaluation) are more effective than actions based on assumption of what the person's wants and needs are (Dumas and Leonard, 1963; Meyers, 1964; Tryon and Leonard, 1964).

Why should this be so? Nurses have spent several years learning what patients' needs are and how to meet those needs. Is it not therefore more efficient to plan care for the patient, rather than consulting with him as a client? Not necessarily.

First we must accept the premise that professional nurses are helping people who have difficulty coping with some aspect of daily life. Therefore the nurse is either temporarily coping for the person (e.g., as when he feeds or bathes a helpless person) or helping the person change some aspect of his behavior so that he can cope himself. In either case the nurse is helping the patient-client to effect some *change* in his life.

Bennis, Benne, and Chin (1969) make a good

case for the collaborative relationship as an essential component of successful change. In both editions of their book of readings about planned change, they show how the most successful changes are brought about through collaborative relationships between change agent and client-system (single client or complex organization). Long-lasting change and growth do not occur unless the client has a real stake in the outcome, and thus actively participates. Change which is forced by coercion or passive submission is often short-lived.

These editors offer three reasons why the collaborative relationship is basic to change:

1 Working together is basic to a trusting relationship; without trust, the data which the client provides (or which the change agent perceives) may be distorted or invalid. If the data are not valid, the diagnosis may be inaccurate.

2 Change is difficult and risky, and people tend to resist it. Therefore, the trusting relationship offers the client an anchor and support as he takes these risks. Certainly in health crises, the risk which the patient-client perceives may involve life itself.

3 The collaborative relationship implies mutual influence. The client cannot establish a real stake in the change unless he feels that he has some influence in the means by which it is effected. Therefore, he must be able to influence the change agent, as well as be influenced by this same agent. In practical terms, this means that the nurse listens to the patient-client's ideas and perceptions and acts on them, in addition to performing services and offering suggestions.

Certainly there are situations in which the patient-client is unable to participate in the diagnosis of his needs. Such situations include acute, life-threatening situations, acute physical or emotional distress, unconsciousness, and prostrating illness. However, anyone who is willing and able to participate actively in the diagnosis and treatment of his nursing problems should be encouraged to do so by the nurse.

Initial involvement occurs when the patient-client is interviewed and examined and when he relates his perceptions of the difficulties which he is having. His participation ought not to end here, however. When the nurse has looked over the data and drawn some conclusions about the nursing problems, he may return to the patient-client and discuss his findings. When a period of time will elapse before the next contact (as in a home visit, clinic, counseling session), these impressions need to be discussed at the first contact.

One approach is to say something like: "I've looked over the information which you gave me about the difficulties that you've been having. You told me that ——— was bothering you, and it seems to me that ——— and ——— are other things we need to help you with while you are here. Does this seem right to you?" If the nurse will not see the person again for some time, the approach might be: "As we've talked, it seems to me that ——— and ——— are the main things we might work on together. What do you think about this?"

Notice that the word "problem" is not used in either example. Problem is an emotionally charged word which connotes negative judgment to many persons. It is best avoided until one knows what connotation it carries to the patient-client.

The extent to which each patient-client and his family can participate in defining their difficulties varies considerably. The discerning nurse will utilize much of his assessment data to determine the intellectual and emotional readiness of the patient-client to participate, and to determine how completely he may be willing to participate. Almost every patient-client can be involved in some aspect of planning his nursing care; it is up to the nurse to allow him to be.

It is not always easy to form a collaborative relationship. The more insecure and inexperienced the nurse, the more he may feel that he must be "in charge." Alternatively, he may abandon his position of expertise, leaving the patient-client to make all the suggestions, and to wonder why he came to this nurse in the first place. Carl Rogers (1961) feels that one's own growth and security determine how well he can help another to grow or change. He sees this as a challenge to develop one's own potential.

Applying Norms to the Data

The patient-client applies his own ideas about what is "normal" (his standards) to the raw data when he decides in what areas of living his problems exist, and when he defines what constitutes a disability in those areas. Because the patient-client's perceptions of and attitudes toward his problems affect his subsequent response to nursing help, the nurse must learn the patient-client's standards and take them into account in defining and solving his problems with him.

The nurse also applies comparative standards to the raw data in order to define problem areas (areas of deviation from health) and the functional abilities and disabilities of the patient-client. These standards with which the patient-client's function and behavior are compared are derived from norms determined by health professionals and from societal norms of health behavior.

Medical science has defined a certain range of weight as normal and desirable for a given height and bone structure. Middle- and upper-class society has accepted this norm for both its health and aesthetic values. Since most health professionals come from middle-class backgrounds, they are apt to apply both the professionally derived height-weight tables and their subcultural norms proscribing obesity in their analysis of data on their patient-client's height-weight ratio (i.e., decide if the person is underweight, normal, or obese).

Many professional norms are influenced directly by cultural and societal values. For example, acceptable middle-class behavior involves talking about one's anger rather than taking violent action. Similarly, one professional norm for emotional stability is the ability to verbalize anger rather than acting it out. There are, however, subcultures in our society where acting out anger (e.g., hitting the other fellow) is the norm.

The bulk of nursing education is devoted to teaching the professional norms which the nurse uses to determine the patient-client's areas of deviance. The nurse needs to be aware that cultural influences are operating in some of these norms. He needs to be equally cognizant of the operation of his own norms in defining the patient-client's problems. Otherwise, the nurse may find that he is trying to help the person with a problem that does not exist for that person.

The patient-client compares his perceptions of his situation with his perceptions of societal norms and expectations. His own reference group (those with whom he identifies) is most influential in shaping his concepts of illness and wellness. This group in turn derives its value from the culture or subculture to which it belongs. (See Part 1, Chapter 1, for further discussion of perceptions of health and illness, and Part 3, Chapter 9, for influence of culture on values.)

Client and nurse may or may not hold similar norms for health behavior. If they do, the diagnosis is more likely to be arrived at mutually, and cooperation of the patient-client and the nurse will characterize attempts to resolve the nursing problem. If the patient-client and the nurse apply different standards to the data, they are more apt to disagree about the nature or even existence of the nursing problems. Efforts by the nurse to help the patient-client in such a situation may be frustrated or may even fail. This is not to say that the nurse cannot diagnose or aid in the nursing problems of people with backgrounds different from his own. He must be cognizant, however, of the perceptual base of the patient-client if he wishes to offer this person help in terms which can be accepted and utilized. References regarding various cultural and subcultural groups are included in Part 2, Chapter 7; Part 3, Chapter 9; and as appropriate in other chapters in Part 3.

Organizing the Data

The first step in analyzing the data is to organize it into areas of deviance. Within these areas of deviance, or problem areas, abilities and disabilities must be identified, and gaps in the data noted. When these gaps have been reasonably filled, conclusions are drawn as to the nature of the nursing problems. These conclusions are the diagnoses or impressions.

Categorizing Problem Areas   Part of the process of diagnosis is the naming of the conclusions reached. However, there is no standard nomenclature for nursing diagnoses, as there is for medical diagnoses. Abdellah, Martin, Beland, and Matheney have proposed a system for classifying nursing problems which is helpful in naming general groups of problems. These broad groupings might be considered areas of deviant function. Many of the 21 problem areas defined by these nurses reflect the categories of assessment used in this textbook. The 21 problem areas, stated as objectives for the nurse, are:

1 To maintain good hygiene and physical comfort.

2 To promote optimal activity, exercise, rest and sleep.

3 To promote safety through prevention of accident, injury or other trauma and through the prevention of spread of infection.

4 To maintain good body mechanics and prevent and correct deformities.

5 To facilitate the maintenance of a supply of oxygen to all body cells.

6 To facilitate the maintenance of nutrition to all body cells.

7 To facilitate the maintenance of elimination.

8 To facilitate the maintenance of fluid and electrolyte balance.

9 To recognize the physiological responses of the body to disease conditions—pathological, physiological and compensatory.

10 To facilitate the maintenance of regulatory mechanisms and functions.

11 To facilitate the maintenance of sensory function.

12 To identify and accept positive and negative expressions, feelings and reactions.

13 To identify and accept the interrelatedness of emotions and organic illness.

14 To facilitate maintenance of effective verbal and nonverbal communication.

15 To promote the development of productive interpersonal relationships.

16 To facilitate progress toward achievement of personal spiritual goals.

17 To create and/or maintain a therapeutic environment.

18 To facilitate awareness of self as an individual with varying physical, emotional and developmental tasks.

19 To accept the optimum possible goals in light of limitations, physical and emotional.

20 To use community resources as an aid in resolving problems arising from illness.

21 To understand the role of social problems as influencing factors in the cause of disease.[2]

Although this classification is general and does not state specific nursing problems, it may be used to group data about deviant function before stating the specific problem. For example, the inability to swallow solids is a specific problem in the general area of maintaining nutrition to the cells.

Identifying Ability and Disability   The raw data may be inspected to note where the person's

[2] Reprinted by permission of The Macmillan Company from "Patient-centered Approaches to Nursing," by Faye Abdellah, Almeda Martin, Irene Beland, and Ruth Matheney. Copyright, The Macmillan Company, 1960.

abilities and disabilities lie. It is most helpful to analyze these areas under each group of deviant functions, using the assessment outline or Abdellah's nursing-problem groupings. What is classified as ability or disability is determined by applying the standards of "normal" function which are part of professional education. A note should be made if there is disparity between nurse and patient-client perceptions of ability-disability. Separation of the data into these two categories in each area of function is an aid to visualizing gaps in the data, and is most important in identifying coping abilities when planning help for the patient-client.

Identifying Gaps in the Data Gaps in the data need to be identified before defining specific nursing problems in order to avoid making diagnoses on assumptions rather than on actual data.

The first step in determining gaps in the data is to visualize or simply look at the data in order to find obvious omissions. The following data about comfort and rest illustrate this method.

precipitating events, and any methods that he has found to ease it. Since he has described the pain as constantly dull, it may have a bearing on his sleeping difficulties; thus, we need to know if he feels the pain is keeping him awake or wakens him.

More data are needed about the person's sleep, also. We need to know what he sees as contributing factors to his loss of sleep—pain, worry over diagnosis, environmental noise. Does he feel that the lessened amount of sleep is a problem? What does he do at home when he cannot sleep? How rested does he feel after the sleep he does get?

How do we know when more data are needed? How do we know that gaps exist in the data given in the example above? The assessment outline shown in Table 6-1 is one aid to identifying gaps. It provides ideas about needed data in areas of daily living which the patient-client has mentioned only briefly.

Another aid to identifying gaps is the review of the literature, which was discussed earlier in this chapter. Reading about the concept of pain

Assessment area	Problem category	Ability	Disability
Comfort and rest	Promote physical comfort		Rectal pain; constant, dull, occasionally sharp
	Promote sleep	Falls asleep easily Normal 8 hr sleep	Fitful sleep Sleeps only 4–5 hr now

In the example given above, we can see that the person has problems in getting adequate sleep and in maintaining physical comfort. A diagnosis of a nursing problem should be specific enough to give some clue to dealing with it. Therefore, it is clear that more data are needed about both the pain and the sleeping problem.

We know only that the person has rectal pain, varying from dull to sharp. Information is needed about the duration of the pain, any

and the concept of sleep gives clues as to information which we need to determine the nature of pain or sleep problems. Reviewing the literature also expands our knowledge of potential problems of the patient-client. We can then scan the data to see if these problems are or are not present, or if we need more data to determine whether they are present.

Although each person has his unique problems, certain constellations of nursing problems exist in a large number of persons within the category of a presenting health problem. For example, if we read about paraplegia, we learn that people who are paraplegic (paralyzed from the waist down) sometimes have severe muscle spasms of the legs. These spasms are frustrating and often painful. In addition, they increase the chance of developing contractures of the legs. The nurse can use this knowledge to observe for spasms or evidence of contractures during the assessment. If the written data make no reference to spasms, he can return to the patient-client in order to see if they are or are not present.

Similarly, people with head injuries may have specific changes in the level of consciousness, breathing difficulties, and deficits in motor abilities. The knowledge of these specific potential problems guides the nurse's observations during the assessment and while checking the data for gaps. The experienced nurse may have this knowledge at the time the assessment is made, and can fill in the gaps during interview and examination. The inexperienced nurse may begin to consider some potential problems only while he is reading about the presenting health problem in the literature. He would then have to fill in the gaps by further assessment.

Stating the Nursing Problems and Impressions

Tentative diagnoses or statements of impressions can be made even while gaps in the data exist. Each contact between the nurse and the patient-client will contribute more knowledge about him. One could never plan his care if this necessitated waiting until all the data were in. "Working diagnoses" are in order as soon as the initial data are collected. If large gaps exist in some areas, however, it is best to return immediately to the patient-client and fill in these gaps.

When working diagnoses are made, the terms *diagnosis* and *impression* tend to be used some-what interchangeably. An impression is a vague notion or feeling retained from the encounter, and connotes a tentative conclusion. The diagnosis is the definitive conclusion. Thus, an impression is less concrete or decisive than a diagnosis. In many cases there is not enough initial information to do more than state impressions, if one is to avoid unwarranted assumptions about the patient's condition. This is true in the following situation.

> Mr. L. is a 52-year-old man in a full body cast because of a nonhealing femoral fracture. He is myopic, and he responds to questions only if they are spoken loudly. He knows that he is "in a hospital," but not which one. He knows who he is, but does not know the month or year. He often confuses the nursing personnel with one another, or calls them "Maude" or "Milly."

Without more data, one can only state impressions about Mr. L.'s mental state, such as "confuses identity of personnel, not oriented to time." He cannot be labeled as "confused" or "disoriented" without more specific information collected over a period of time. Mr. L. may be showing signs of sensory deprivation (decreased sensory input from vision, hearing, touch), mental deterioration, organic brain disease, or the effects of certain medications. The medical and nursing approaches to each of these conditions will vary, and it is therefore important not to jump to conclusions as to the nature of his difficulty.

Diagnoses or statements of nursing problems may be considered conclusions made about one or more impressions of the patient-client. These diagnoses should be stated as specifically and concisely as possible in order to provide clues to dealing with the problem (Little and Carnevali, 1969, p. 60). In the preceding example, if enough data are gathered to support the hypothesis that Mr. L.'s disorientation is due to lack of sensory input, the diagnosis might be stated as, "Disorientation to time, place, and other persons secondary to sensory deprivation." A conclusion has been drawn as to the nature of his disorientation, and the diagnosis is specific enough about the extent of disorientation to guide efforts to reorient him.

Diagnosis is not simply a summary of all the abnormalities found during the assessment. Because it is a statement of conclusions about the areas in which the person needs *nursing* help, the nurse and patient-client must decide whether the noted deviations from the norms constitute nursing problems. Recall that a nursing problem is a patient-client's problem in *coping* with daily life secondary to his deviation or potential deviation from health. A person may have disability or illness and yet manage his daily life quite well. He therefore does not require nursing help. An example is the person with an amputated leg who has learned to use a prosthesis and who carries on all his usual activities. The fact of his amputation and prosthesis would be noted in a nursing assessment, but no diagnosis of difficulty is indicated because he manages his life in this area without help.

Because diagnosis is an ongoing process, the initial statement of problems will probably be a mixture of impressions and concise diagnoses. When only impressions or vaguely worded diagnoses are initially stated, these statements must be revised as more data become available. For example, it may appear obvious that a woman is "anxious," but the source of her anxiety is not readily apparent to the nurse during the first visit to the family. Therefore, the nurse can only state the impression of "anxiety; source undetermined." When the nurse has been able to identify the source of the anxiety, he can revise his original statement into a more definitive diagnosis: "anxiety about ability to measure up to her own standards as a mother."

REFERENCES

Books

Abdellah, Faye, Almeda Martin, Irene Beland, and Ruth Matheney, "Patient-centered Approaches to Nursing," The Macmillan Company, New York, 1960.

Bennis, Warren G., Kenneth Benne, and Robert Chin (eds.), "The Planning of Change," 2d ed., Holt, Rinehart and Winston, Inc., New York, 1969, pp. 147-153.

Bermosk, Loretta Sue, and Mary Jane Mordan, "Interviewing in Nursing," The Macmillan Company, New York, 1964.

Fenlason, Anne, "Essentials of Interviewing," rev. ed., Harper & Row, Publishers, Incorporated, New York, 1962.

Jourard, Sidney, "The Transparent Self," 2d ed., D. Van Nostrand Company, Inc., Princeton, N.J., 1971, p. 148.

Little, Delores, and Doris Carnevali, "Nursing Care Planning," J. B. Lippincott Company, Philadelphia, 1969.

Matheney, Ruth, Breda Nolan, Alice Ehrhart, Gerald Griffin, and Joanne Griffin, "Fundamentals of Patient-centered Care," 2d ed., The C. V. Mosby Company, St. Louis, 1971.

McCain, R. Faye, et al.: "Guide to the Systematic Assessment of the Functional Abilities of a Patient," The University of Michigan School of Nursing, 1965.

Orlando, Ida, "The Dynamic Nurse-Patient Relationship," G. P. Putnam's Sons, New York, 1961.

Rogers, Carl, The Characteristics of a Helping Relationship, in "On Becoming a Person," Houghton-Mifflin Company, Boston, 1961, pp. 39-58.

———, "Counseling and Psychotherapy," Houghton-Mifflin Company, Boston, 1942.

Periodicals

Dumas, R., and R. C. Leonard: The Effect of Nursing on the Incidence of Post-operative Vomiting, *Nursing Research,* **12**:12 ff (1963).

McCain, R. Faye: Nursing by Assessment, Not Intuition, *American Journal of Nursing,* **65**:82-84 (1965).

McPhetridge, L. Mae: Nursing History; One Means to Personalize Care, *American Journal of Nursing,* **68**:68–75 (1968).

Meyers, Mary: The Effect of Types of Communication on Patients' Reactions to Stress, *Nursing Research,* **13**:126 ff (1964).

Smith, Dorothy: A Clinical Nursing Tool, *American Journal of Nursing,* **68**:2384–2388 (1968).

Tryon, Phyllis, and R. C. Leonard: The Effect of the Patient's Participation on the Outcome of a Nursing Procedure, *Nursing Forum,* **3**(2):79–89 (1964).

ADDITIONAL READINGS

Bozian, Marguerite: Nursing Care of the Infant in the Community, *Nursing Clinics of North America,* **6**:93–101 (1971). (Examples of assessment of the newborn and family.)

Coles, Robert: A Fashionable Kind of Slander, *Atlantic Monthly,* **226**:53–55 (1970). (Demonstrates how political and social values can influence professional norms for behavior.)

Griffith, Elizabeth Welk: Nursing Process: A Patient with Respiratory Dysfunction, *Nursing Clinics of North America,* **6**:145–154 (1971). (Example of data collection and diagnosis.)

Hayes, Joyce Samhammer, and Kenneth H. Larsen, "Interacting with Patients," The Macmillan Company, New York, 1963.

Wilson, Lucille, Listening, in Carolyn E. Carlson, (coordinator), "Behavioral Concepts and Nursing Intervention," J. B. Lippincott Company, Philadelphia, 1970, pp. 153–170.

APPENDIX: Guide for Evaluation of the Interview[1]

I. PATTERN	PRINCIPLES	ACTION
1. Long-term goal	1. The climate the nurse creates within the patient-nurse interaction influences the substance of the interview.	1. Observing
2. Immediate goal	2. Professional attitudes of warmth, acceptance, objectivity, and compassion are essential for effective interviewing.	2. Listening
3. Plan of interview	3. Defined needs and goals, for the patient and for the nurse, determine the purpose of the interview.	3. Responses
4. Interview	4. The identification and clarification of conflicting thoughts and feelings of the patient and of the nurse lead toward a harmony of goals in the interview.	4. Verbal, nonverbal
5. Evaluation	5. Continuous and terminal evaluation of the interview are made in terms of behavior changes in the patient and the nurse related to defined needs and goals.	5. Interpretation of data
		6. Reporting and recording of data

[1] Reprinted with permission of The Macmillan Company, from Loretta Bermosk and Mary Jane Mordan, "Interviewing in Nursing," pp. 170–172. Copyright, The Macmillan Company, New York, 1964.

II. Brief description of patient—who, what, where, and when
Brief description of nurse—who, what, where, and when
Statement of long-term goal
Statement of immediate goal

[The following portion of the evaluation might involve substituting what you and the interviewee actually said and did, and your interpretations of this material based on the questions in the evaluation column. P.H.M.]

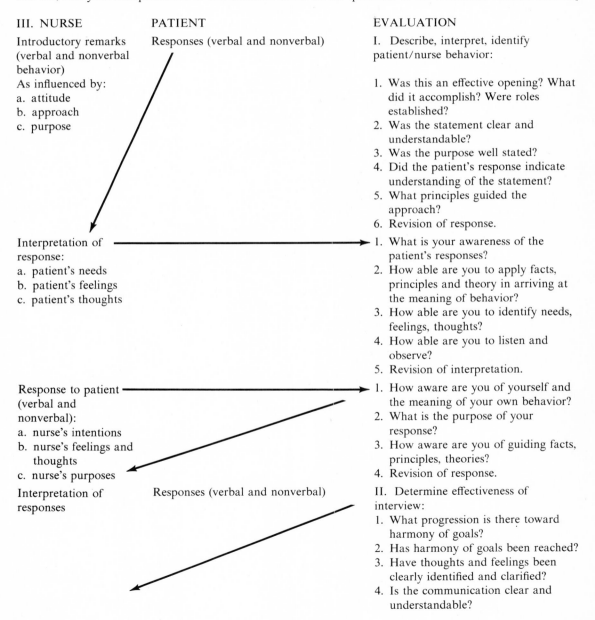

III. NURSE	PATIENT	EVALUATION
Introductory remarks (verbal and nonverbal behavior) As influenced by: a. attitude b. approach c. purpose	Responses (verbal and nonverbal)	I. Describe, interpret, identify patient/nurse behavior: 1. Was this an effective opening? What did it accomplish? Were roles established? 2. Was the statement clear and understandable? 3. Was the purpose well stated? 4. Did the patient's response indicate understanding of the statement? 5. What principles guided the approach? 6. Revision of response.
Interpretation of response: a. patient's needs b. patient's feelings c. patient's thoughts		1. What is your awareness of the patient's responses? 2. How able are you to apply facts, principles and theory in arriving at the meaning of behavior? 3. How able are you to identify needs, feelings, thoughts? 4. How able are you to listen and observe? 5. Revision of interpretation.
Response to patient (verbal and nonverbal): a. nurse's intentions b. nurse's feelings and thoughts c. nurse's purposes		1. How aware are you of yourself and the meaning of your own behavior? 2. What is the purpose of your response? 3. How aware are you of guiding facts, principles, theories? 4. Revision of response.
Interpretation of responses	Responses (verbal and nonverbal)	II. Determine effectiveness of interview: 1. What progression is there toward harmony of goals? 2. Has harmony of goals been reached? 3. Have thoughts and feelings been clearly identified and clarified? 4. Is the communication clear and understandable?

Response to patient at ————————————————————▶ III. Describe, identify results of
end of interview   interview:
                                                                   1. How was the interview terminated?
                                                                   2. Was the immediate goal
                                                                      accomplished?
                                                                   3. What are the ongoing plans?
                                                                   4. What patient learning occurred from
                                                                      the interview?
                                                                   5. What nurse learning occurred from
                                                                      the interview?
                                                                   6. What is the restatement of the
                                                                      immediate goal?
                                                                   7. Regarding the content and clarity of
                                                                      written and oral reports:
                                                                      Was continuity of care provided?
                                                                      Was confidentiality of content
                                                                      maintained?

Intervention: Planning Nursing Care

Pamela Mitchell

Nursing intervention consists of those activities which the nurse initiates to help the patient or client resolve his nursing problems. These activities may be performed by the nurse alone, by nursing personnel acting under the professional nurse's direction, or by patient and nurse (or nursing personnel) acting together. They may be performed in direct contact with the patient or carried out on his behalf elsewhere. Lastly, these activities may be initiated independently by the nurse or may be delegated to him by the physician's plan of care. Often, the activities are a combination of independent and delegated action.

In this context, examples of interventions include:

Bathing a man the first day after surgery	Performed by the nurse
Instructing the nurse's aide to give a man a glass of fluid every two hours	Performed by other nursing personnel
Helping a woman who is hemiplegic learn to dress herself	Performed by nurse and patient
Playing checkers with a teen-age boy	In direct contact with the patient
Contacting a volunteer group to provide visitors for a home-bound woman	On behalf of the patient
Relieving pain by helping a woman in traction to change position	Independent action
Relieving pain in a man by administering morphine	Delegated medical action

Nursing care is the sum of the interventions which are planned in the nursing problems of the patient or client. Planning implies that actions or interventions are designed to solve specific nursing problems defined, that they are performed to meet specific goals, and that their efficacy is evaluated.

The planning process is a continuation of the diagnostic process and follows the scientific method. The process consists of the following steps:

1 The nursing problems are defined.
2 Related information is reviewed.
3 Goals and objectives are defined.
4 Priorities of problem solution are determined.
5 Interventions are proposed for each problem.
6 Interventions are implemented and tested.
7 Results are evaluated.
8 The plan is modified.

The model in Fig. 7-1 summarizes the process of intervention in one problem.

DEFINING PROBLEMS

The final step of the diagnostic process, discussed in Chapter 6, was to state the nursing problems or impressions. Little and Carnevali point out that the more succinct and specific the problem statement is, the better one is able to devise specific action to meet the problem (Little and Carnevali, 1969, p. 60).

REVIEWING RELATED INFORMATION

When the scientist has defined the problem which he will investigate, he reviews the literature a second time (the first review was a part of data collection prior to defining the problem—see Part 2, Chapter 6). The purpose of this review is to determine what is known about this specific problem, to see how others have approached it,

and to determine from what theoretical or factual base he may form hypotheses. Because nursing intervention is also a testing of hypotheses, the nurse needs to review what is known about the specific nursing problem and review concepts and theories relevant to it in order to set achievable goals and propose workable interventions.

Nursing is considered an applied science, because it uses facts, concepts, and theories from basic sciences to formulate ways to accomplish its goals. The field of engineering is analogous—the engineer uses or applies concepts from the basic sciences of chemistry and physics in order to build a bridge. In the same way, the nurse derives principles for nursing action from sciences such as physiology, anthropology, and psychology. Some of the interventions so derived have been tested scientifically and found to be consistently useful. Many others have not been so tested and have been empirically accepted in nursing education and practice. Because each nurse should critically evaluate the interventions he uses and because such appraisal is necessary to formulate a true science of nursing practice, we will indicate whenever possible those nursing interventions of which the basic principles have been validated by scientific study.

The Relationship of Scientific Generalizations to Practice

When the nurse reviews information related to the patient-client's problem, he must go beyond what has been written about the problem. He must combine the generalized concepts and principles from the literature with his own experience in similar situations, with the observations he has made of other practitioners, and with his observations of his specific patient-client.

Most of the literature deals with generalizations. Statements such as, "One of the common manifestations of anxiety is a narrowing of perception," or "Most people with adult-onset

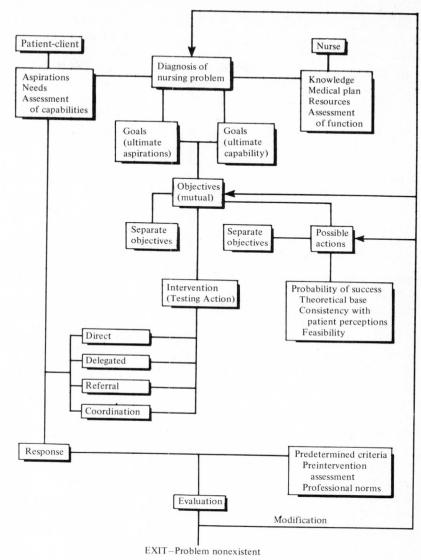

Figure 7-1 A model of the intervention process. See text for explanation.

diabetes respond to oral hypoglycemic agents," are generalizations. The individual patient-client may or may not fit the picture given in the generalization. Therefore, the literature serves to guide the practitioner to the *possible* relationship between his patient-client's problem and "the one in the book." It helps him generate hypotheses as to what help might be effective.

Weidenbach (1970) calls the potential interventions derived from the literature "nursing lore" and emphasizes that this knowledge must be pooled with "nursing wisdom"—the experiences of oneself and others in helping people. If the nurse is able to do this cognitively (i.e., by reasoning and thinking), as opposed to intuitively, he can build a rational framework for practice which will enable him to be consistently effective. In Weidenbach's words:

> Unless she can communicate the essential factors that caused her to obtain desired results with the particular patient, not only may she be unable to contribute to the improvement of another's practice [by transmitting the means of successful action], but there is no assurance that she will be able to have the same outstanding success the next time.[1]

Levels of Knowledge Used

How then can we use the scientific literature to build a rational framework for practice? First we must clarify the kinds of knowledge which we seek—facts, principles, concepts, and theories.

A *fact* is a thing which is accepted as true. For example, it is a fact that hydrostatic pressure in the capillary must be greater than that in the cell for nutrients to pass from the capillary to the cell.

A *principle* is a statement of relationship between facts. It also forms a basis for explanation of phenomena and enables one to predict outcomes. The principle that fluid flows from areas of higher pressure to areas of lesser pressure is the basis for the above fact about cellular nutrition, and allows prediction that changes in capillary-pressure relationships will affect cellular nutrition. The terms fact and principle are often used interchangeably; however, a principle implies relationships of facts to one another.

A *concept* is a label for a set of things that have something in common. Concepts enable one to classify such things as objects, behavior, and phenomena. The concept "pressure sore" relates observations about prolonged pressure, skin ulcers, and cellular nutrition to one idea which is

comprehensible to those who have the same knowledge of the observations, facts, and principles subsumed in the concept.

To conceptualize is to abstract common elements from many separate facts or events. It allows us to talk with others who also know these commonalities without having to describe the whole structure or range of events.

A *theory* is a systematic ordering of related concepts or principles. By means of a set of logically connected, confirmed or partially confirmed hypotheses, it explains the relationships among the concepts or principles. For example, the theory regarding the origin of pressure sores ("bedsores," or decubitus ulcers) relates the concept of cellular nutrition, principles of hydrostatic pressure, and observations of the effects of prolonged pressure on the skin and subcutaneous tissues. Experimental evidence substantiates that pressure on the surface of the body which is greater than capillary hydrostatic pressure prevents nutrients from reaching the cells underlying the area of pressure. If this pressure is prolonged beyond a critical point, cell death ensues. Death of many cells in the skin and subcutaneous tissues produces an ulcer or sore.

Among the sciences from which nursing borrows, the biological and medical have the greatest stock of well-founded facts, theories, and principles. These frequently relate to particular diseases and modes of therapy. For example, the principles for producing and maintaining sterile supplies were derived from microbiologic facts about the nature of pathogenic organisms.

Writers of most medical and nursing textbooks select certain facts and principles which relate to certain diseases or pathologic states, and which serve to guide intervention specific to those states. Professional journals generally report studies which attempt to substantiate or disprove the theoretical basis for management of specific diseases or patients' problems. Nursing journals often contain a mixture of textbook-like articles and reports of studies regarding practice.

---

[1] Ernestine Weidenbach, Nurses' Wisdom in Nursing Theory, *American Journal of Nursing,* **70**:1058 (1970).

There are no well-defined facts in the biological sciences for many of the problems with which patient-clients and nurses deal. These are the problems involving behavior, relationships with people, and adjustments to illness; we must turn to the behavioral sciences for concepts and theories relevant to them. The theoretical basis for principles from these fields is not so well proved as in the natural sciences; thus the practitioner will find fewer well-outlined approaches to practice from the behavioral sciences. He will often find it necessary to derive his own principles from the general concepts in these fields, and then test them with his patient-clients.

The Review of Information as a Guide to Planning

We can use scientific knowledge both before and after the fact, so to speak. It can be used to form goals and plans which "ought to work" in a specific problem, or to explain why some approach actually did work. Using knowledge to predict outcomes is preferable in the strictest scientific sense. However, as Samuel Butler put it; "Life is the art of drawing sufficient conclusions from insufficient evidence." There are many occasions in which the practitioner acts or must act without time for reflection. Whether his action worked or not, he needs to find out why. Therefore, he may review the literature or other information after the fact, and relate his experience to it.

Reflection after action is, at best, a trial-and-error method. At worst, it is subject to many distortions of data and reasoning as the nurse tries to find principles which "fit" the action. One of the objectives of professional education is to teach the learner a way of thinking, as well as to provide him with a stockpile of facts. It is hoped that he will learn to think before acting most of the time, and will build a conceptual and factual background sufficient to help him in those instances when there is little time for reflecting.

The process of building concepts is discussed in more detail in Part 3, Chapter 8.

Knowledge from the second review of the literature can be used in all the aspects of planning and evaluating intervention. It can be used to (1) explain the nature of the problem, (2) guide further data collection, (3) define realistic goals, (4) form a basis for successful intervention, and (5) define criteria for evaluation of the effect of intervention.

The following example will show how the concept of sensory restriction (see Part 3, Chapter 11) can be used to design a plan for nursing care. The remainder of this chapter describes in detail each step of the process.

Explaining the Nature of the Problem In Chapter 6, Part 2, we used an example of Mr. A. L., an elderly man in a body cast, who was myopic and hard of hearing. Mr. L. was confused, disoriented to place and time, and spent much time sleeping. We could only state impressions of confusion and disorientation, for we did not know why he behaved this way. If we apply the concept of sensory restriction to these impressions, we begin to make some sense of our observations.

His body cast decreases tactile and kinesthetic sensation; his myopia decreases visual sensation; and his hearing impairment alters auditory input. Confusion, disorientation, and decreased responsiveness to the environment are some of the types of behavior seen in hospitalized people in restricted sensory environment. Thus the concept of sensory restriction suggests some possible explanations for Mr. L.'s behavior.

We must emphasize the hypothetical nature of this "diagnosis," as we do not know if his confusion occurred only after the body cast was applied, or if it is a chronic feature of his behavior. Nevertheless, we can postulate sensory restriction as the basis of his problem and design a plan to both help him and substantiate our hypothesis.

Guiding Further Data Collection A second function of the conceptual framework is to guide further data collection. Once we have decided to look at Mr. L.'s behavior as a possible consequence of sensory restriction, we need to gather more data about the extent of his sensory deficits, the nature of his sensory environment, the timing of the onset of confusion in relation to sensory restrictions, and the character of his behavior in a normal environment. This will help us determine if sensory restriction is a tenable hypothesis.

Defining Realistic Goals Some studies of clinical sensory restriction suggest that enriching the sensory environment can clear up the behavioral abnormalities. On this basis, it seems reasonable to try to reorient Mr. L. to his environment.

Forming the Basis for Intervention If sensory restriction is the basis for Mr. L.'s confusion, then increasing the quantity and meaning of sensory input might help him. Actions which would accomplish this might include having him wear his glasses, helping him wear his hearing aid, increasing social contacts, increasing tactile contacts (back rubs, bathing). The evidence for this approach is scanty but sufficient to make it worth testing.

Defining Evaluative Criteria The concept of clinical sensory restriction suggests some criteria for substantiating the hypothesized diagnosis. These include association of behavioral abnormalities with the onset of sensory restriction, lack of organic or drug effects which might explain the behavior, and association of increased sensory input with clearing up of the behavior. The criterion for evaluating the actions designed to increase sensory input is simply whether or not the confusion and disorientation diminish or cease. For many clinical problems,

the literature provides specific criteria for evaluating the effect of intervention.

Selecting Concepts from the Literature At this point it is reasonable to ask how one selects a concept or theory to guide planning. If you have identified a specific problem of a patient (such as pressure sore, anxiety, dehydration), you can turn to textbooks and periodical indexes to find sources of information related to the problem area.

In the example of Mr. L., however, no specific problem had been identified. How did the nurse consider sensory restriction as a possible cause of his problem? Perhaps he had been reading about the concept as a course assignment, or as part of his general reading, and Mr. L.'s symptoms seemed similar to those in the readings. More likely, an instructor or graduate nurse suggested that the concept of sensory restriction would be worth pursuing. Wide reading and consultation with nurse experts will help the novice practitioner accumulate the ideas which will help him select appropriate concepts when he is faced with similar ill-defined impressions.

DEFINING GOALS AND OBJECTIVES

Once the problem has been stated as clearly as possible, nurse and patient-client must decide what is to be accomplished; goals and objectives must be defined. Goals are defined here as the ultimate result or behavior; objectives are the operational or working goals in day-to-day management of the nursing problem. Both nurse and patient-client have goals which they have set within their own perceptual framework. If nursing care is to be most effective, they must somehow bring these goals together in defining objectives.

The nurse sets his goals in terms of what he sees as the ultimate capability of the patient-client in the context of his problems of daily living. Essentially, he is estimating a prognosis of benefit from nursing care. To arrive at this prognosis, he applies to the diagnosed problems his knowledge of the usual course of the health problem, the medical plan of care, the resources of the patient and of the health-care system, and his assessment of the patient-client's current abilities. Patient-client resources include such things as his motivation, ability to participate actively in management of his problems, financial means, and living circumstances. Health-care-system resources may include the philosophy of care (collaborative or custodial), the availability of specialized therapists, and the kinds of mechanical equipment used.

The patient-client also has goals in terms of the ultimate results; however, these tend to be in terms of aspirations. He often does not have knowledge of the usual course of his health problem or of the resources available; indeed, this is one of the reasons why he seeks health care. His goals are formulated on the basis of his needs and aspirations for himself, and on his assessment of his capabilities. His perceptions of his capabilities may vary considerably from those of the nurse, particularly if the person's aspirations exceed or are less than these capabilities. It is important to know the patient's goals and the factors which lead to them. Only then can the nurse have some idea of the congruence of goals set by the nurse and those set by the patient and the potential acceptability of the nurse-defined objectives and actions to the patient-client.

Once goals are set, objectives are defined in order to meet them; the objectives become the operational guides in attempting to solve one or more nursing problems. Whenever possible, objectives should be mutually set by the nurse and patient-client. If they are not defined together, the objectives of nurse and patient-client may be in conflict, and little progress will be made (see Part 2, Chapter 6, regarding the collaborative nature of helping relationships). Mutual setting

of objectives may take many forms, depending upon the mental, emotional, and physical capabilities of the patient and/or his spokesman (e.g., family, parent, spouse). The nurse may discuss the goal and actively work on defining objectives with a motivated, capable person. In another situation, the nurse may need to define possible or desirable objectives and then ask the patient if they are agreeable to him. The patient-client may lack the energy, knowledge, or skill needed to help design specific objectives to meet his goals. In situations where enduring behavior changes are essential, the nurse may need to find ways to motivate the patient-client to *want* to collaborate.

It is possible that the nurse and patient have conflicting or differing goals and yet will be able to come to agreement about operational objectives. For example, Mrs. G., a 22-year-old mother, is paraplegic (paralyzed from the waist down). If the usual course of her type of paraplegia is complete and permanent loss of function, the nurse may feel a feasible long-term goal is for this woman to function independently from a wheelchair. The patient, however, may hope to walk again, regardless of what her doctors tell her. Thus, her goal is independent life as it was before. However, she can see that she is paralyzed now and would agree that being able to sit in a wheelchair, to dress herself, and to regain bowel and bladder control are intervening objectives. Eventually she will need to come to grips with permanent loss of function, and the nurse will probably define this as an objective separate from their mutually set ones.

Objectives may be long-term, intermediate, and short-term. The specific activities which fall into each of these categories are relative, depending upon what phase of the health problem the patient is in. Moving from bed to chair unaided might be a long-term goal for Mrs. G. while she is in an acute-care hospital immediately after the accident. The same activity might be a short-term goal in a rehabilitation hospital. The patient, too, may hold objectives which are separate from the mutually defined ones. If these are in conflict with the nurse's objectives, progress may be slow. If the nurse has not tried to define mutually acceptable objectives with the patient and the objectives of nurse and patient are in conflict, an impasse will result.

> A public health nurse visited Mrs. L., a 35-year-old woman with renal disease. Mrs. L.'s doctor had prescribed a 500-mg low-sodium diet in an effort to control her edema and sodium retention. However, Mrs. L. continued to have pitting edema in her legs and sacrum; and her weight fluctuated rapidly, suggesting fluid retention secondary to dietary indiscretion. The nurse defined the problem as "fluid retention secondary to excess sodium ingestion," set a goal of dietary understanding and "adherence to 500-mg sodium diet," and proceeded to teach Mrs. L. what she could and could not have on the diet. Despite Mrs. L.'s ability to outline a day's menu and to tell the nurse how she could prepare foods with spices to add flavor, she continued to have edema. Finally, Mrs. L. disclosed that she understood the diet but did not adhere to it and had no intention of doing so. She felt that it did not prevent her disease from worsening, and she planned to have some pleasure from life while she was still alive.

Clearly, Mrs. L.'s goal of a pleasurable existence (defined as having good food in this case) was in conflict with the nurse's goal and objective of dietary understanding and adherence. The nurse's failure to define objectives with the client led to a great deal of wasted time for them both.

There are situations in which the patient's or client's goals and objectives do not seem to be in his best interest, and the nurse feels he must knowingly set conflicting ones. An example would be the patient whose goal is to kill himself. The nurse's immediate objective is to prevent him from harm. The long-term goal is to help him find a life worth living. In a less dramatic situation, the nurse may have an objective to have all the children in a family immunized; the mother's goals for her family do not include this. The nurse may try to help the mother see her

need for adopting this value but cannot force her to do so.

SETTING PRIORITIES AMONG PROBLEMS

People who have deviations from health generally have a number of problems posed by that deviation, any or all of which may become nursing problems. There are many times in any nursing setting when the nurse cannot deal with all the nursing problems presented by the patient; therefore, some choices must be made. The determination of priorities of problems will foster wise choices.

Abraham Maslow's hierarchy of basic human needs is one aid to ordering priorities. He describes some needs as most basic, and says they must be met before higher-level needs become important to the person. He ranks the hierarchy in five levels of need—physiologic, safety, love and belonging, esteem, and self-actualization (or self-realization) (Maslow, 1954, pp. 80-106). Thus, when the patient's problems involve breathing, pain, eating, he will tend to devote his energies to solving these problems before being concerned with feeling wanted (love and belonging) or pursuing creative interests (self-actualization). These categories are not meant to be mutually exclusive. Anyone who has read romantic novels knows that the spurned lover's need for love subsumes all interest in eating and sleeping. In general, however, the hierarchy serves as a general guide to the ordering of priorities of problems.

Setting priorities not only aids in a logical approach to the multiplicity of each individual's problems, but enables the nurse to make decisions about the priorities of care among several patients or clients. For the nurse in a hospital, this may involve postponing teaching one patient about diabetic foot care (safety need), because another patient's acute respiratory insufficiency (physiologic need) requires almost constant attendance. The public health nurse may postpone a visit to one client whose major problem is insecurity with her new baby (self-esteem need), because another is having suicidal thoughts (safety) and needs to talk.

If the patient or client is at all responsive to his environment, he will have his own ideas as to the priority of his problems. Unless the nurse finds out what these priorities are and sets mutually acceptable priorities with him, they may be working at cross purposes.

PROPOSING INTERVENTION

Devising a Wide Range of Potential Solutions

The next step in planning nursing care is to propose a number of possible actions to solve a problem. The objectives serve as a guide to proposing actions. In the example of Mrs. G., who was paralyzed, an objective is to move from bed to chair unaided. Therefore, actions should be proposed that are within the range of this objective and do not extend to ways in which she might learn to cook from her wheelchair. At this point, one should be as inventive as possible and not be limited to one or two possible actions. This is a time to "brainstorm" a number of possible solutions. Some may be impractical or far-fetched, but do not exclude them from your thinking until you have assembled a whole range of possibilities. With a man who is hard-of-hearing, possible actions to improve communications with him might include shouting at him at all times, teaching him to read lips, using sign language, writing all communications, speaking in low-pitched tones, having only men care for him (low voices), turning up his hearing aid, getting new batteries for his hearing aid, speaking slowly while facing him so that he can try to read lips.

Selecting Actions to Test

From the range of possible actions, one or more will be selected for actual use. This selection, or decision making, involves an identifiable intellectual process. A probability of success is assigned to each potential action, on the basis of several criteria. These criteria are (1) the sound-ness of the factual and theoretical base, (2) compatibility of the action with the patient-client's perceptions, goals, and values, and (3) feasibility in the situation.

If numerical value were assigned to the probability of success of each proposed action, one could quantitate this decision-making process and propose action on the basis of a truly objective method. However, the state of nursing knowledge is not advanced to the point where we can say, for example, that shouting at the hard-of-hearing man has a probability value of 0.50 (effective in 50 of 100 similar situations), whereas speaking slowly while facing him has a value of 0.70. This inability to assign exact probability value is partly due to the number of variables in individual situations. In addition, nursing has not compiled sufficient research about the effects of given actions in given situations. Researchers are attempting, however, to quantitate the results of nursing actions in order to facilitate choosing interventions in a less empirical manner (Hanken, 1966; Finch, 1969).

Until nursing research is able to provide analytical models of the effects of specific actions, the practicing nurse has to rely on considerably cruder estimates of the probability of success of proposed actions. The student can use any method which suits him to assign estimates of success to the proposed actions. These methods might include assigning arbitrary numerical value, assigning pluses or minuses, or using terms such as "little chance," "some chance," "most chance." Many people automatically weigh alternatives "in the head," so to speak; others commit the process to paper. Whatever way it is done, this weighing of alternatives is a necessary step before testing one or more actions.

Soundness of Theoretical Base A successful intervention is usually based upon facts, concepts, or theories which suggest why it works. The fact that people with presbycusis (deafness associated with old age) hear low-pitched tones best suggests that the action of speaking in a deep voice will be more effective than shouting in a higher voice. Knowledge of the function of his hearing aid suggests that the actions related to improving amplification may also be effective. However, it is possible that increasing amplification may create distortion of the sound and thus nullify the effect of this action. Given these two opposite effects based on the known facts, the nurse must test the solution before accepting it as the best one.

Part 2 is based upon the collaborative or transactional concept of change. Much of the research supporting this conceptual model is from analysis of change in industry and of change brought about by counseling (Bennis et al., 1969; Rogers, 1961; Jourard, 1971). Orlando and others at Yale University have used this collaborative model specifically in nursing, finding that nursing intervention is most effective if the nurse's observations, conclusions, and proposed actions are validated with the patient. Orlando cites many observations which support this theory (Orlando, 1961), and subsequent research has tended to confirm her hypotheses (Dumas and Leonard, 1963; Tryon and Leonard, 1964; Moss and Meyer, 1966). This concept constitutes the theoretical framework for teaching that the plan which is made *with* the patient-client will be the most effective one.

Compatibility with the Patient-Client's Beliefs, Attitudes, and Perceptions Actions which have the greatest probability of success are those which consider the patient-client's perception of the situation and are compatible with the beliefs, values, and attitudes which have shaped those perceptions.

Beliefs are ideas or tenets which a person or cultural group accepts as true; values are one's standards or principles, and are grounded in one's beliefs. Attitudes are the feelings or emotional commitments one has toward an idea, belief, or value. Beliefs and values are cognitive (on the thinking level), although not necessarily rational. Attitudes are affective, on the feeling level. A person views his current situation and others in it (including health professionals) on the basis of his belief system, sets his goals in terms of his values, and reacts to attempts to introduce change in his behavior on the basis of his attitudes. The nurse's behavior and action which does not take these factors into account may result in overt rejection of proffered help or failure to produce any lasting help for the patient-client.

For example, nurses and others who have done health work with Mexican-American and other Spanish-speaking people have learned that profuse admiration of the babies can lead to rejection by the Mexican-American of the proffered health services. The belief system of these people supports the idea that praise of a baby, without touching it, will inflict the "evil eye" on the child (Leininger, 1967). Thus, failure to understand the beliefs of this culture can lead to rejection of the nurse and his help.

An example of the effect of patient-client attitudes on nursing intervention occurs in family-planning clinics. A nurse may help a woman select a contraceptive method which is understood and accepted by the client. However, the method may never be used if the woman's husband feels that the number of children he fathers is a sign of manliness, and induces his wife not to use the contraceptive.

How can health workers help people whose beliefs, values, and attitudes differ from his own, or are in conflict with the help he offers? First, he must learn what the patient-client's beliefs and attitudes are. Writings by anthropologists and social psychologists, people who study the belief systems, habits, and customs of cultural and social groups, can provide generalizations about the specific group from which the patient-client comes. Selected references are noted at the end of this chapter, in Part 1, Chapter 3, and in Part 3, Chapters 9 and 13. The patient-client will provide the important information by which the nurse can determine if the generalizations are true for the particular patient-client.

Once we have determined what the general and particular attitudes of the person are toward his problems, we can decide which of the proposed nursing interventions are apt to conflict with these ideas and feelings.

Beliefs, values, and attitudes tend to stabilize the individual and group position in life. They provide some things which are relatively unchanging in one's relationships to others and to the environment. If most citizens believe it is wrong to steal, they do not have to ponder over whether or not to pay for each item, or how to get items too expensive for them. In addition, the society does not have to expend great sums of money enforcing laws against stealing.

Any threat to change the system of beliefs or attitudes is usually resisted strongly by those who hold them. Similarly, action which is incongruent with one's beliefs and attitudes is often perceived as critical of or threatening to the system, and is also resisted. Therefore, nursing interventions which can be adapted to the belief and attitude system of the patient-client are less apt to be resisted than those which require change in attitudes, values, or beliefs.

An example is the way in which one group of public health nurses adapted their explanation of the need for hospitalization to the value system of a group of Mexican-Americans in the Southwest United States.

Many Spanish-Americans do not believe in the germ theory and the communicability of disease. Instead, they believe that illness is, among other things, *castigo,* or punishment for disobeying God. Consequently, traditional attempts in the control of tuberculosis by isolation of the ill and protection of contacts have not been particularly successful (Baca, 1969). Paynich reports a study in which attempts were made to have public health nurses alter their advice and teaching methods to conform to the common points between public health and Spanish-American belief systems. (See Part 1, Chapters 1 and 2, for further discussion of belief systems about health.) The investigators found

that a tuberculous patient was more likely to agree to hospitalization if he was told, "It would be best for you to be admitted to the hospital to get rid of your sickness," rather than, "You should get treated at the hospital so that you won't spread your sickness to others in the family and in the village" (Paynich, 1964). The first statement suggests the benefit to the person himself and is more aligned with his cultural belief that disease is a punishment to *him.* The second statement stresses the communicability of the disease, a concept which he does not hold.

Sometimes, however, we cannot help the patient-client without basic changes in his attitudes or those held by others in his environment. The husband who feels his wife's use of contraceptives destroys his virility is an example of a person in the patient-client's environment whose attitudes prevent effective nursing help. If his attitudes can be changed, his wife can be helped to avoid further pregnancies; if his attitude cannot be changed, the nurse cannot help his wife.

Attitude change is marked by some degree of strain, disequilibrium, or conflict. As long as attitudes perform their function of providing stability to a personal or group position vis-à-vis others, there is no incentive to change them. If, however, the actions of others important to the person suggest that he is "out of line," his stability is threatened. He may reject the implied or stated observations of the other, and thereby restore his equilibrium. Or he may begin to examine his attitude or belief and seek to restore equilibrium by changing the attitude.

The man in the previous example who prevented his wife from using a contraceptive reacted to the threat to his attitudes about manliness by rejecting his wife's attempt to change her ability to be impregnated. If the wife does nothing further, her husband's attitude toward contraception will not change. If she refuses to have further intercourse with him, he is faced with a new conflict. He will have to change his behavior and perhaps his attitudes if he is to continue to have sexual activity. Either he will have to seek new sexual partners (which may be contrary to his values) or accept his wife's use of contraceptives. The wife's tactics are definitely coercive, and will result in an attitude change only if the conflict so induced leads her husband to take a new look at information and feelings about contraception.

At this point, the nurse might be able to help effect an attitude change. Schein (1969) defines two processes of attitude change—cognitive redefinition of the situation through (1) identification, and (2) scanning. Once people have become motivated to change, they become open to new information. This information may come from one person or institution (identification) or from many sources (scanning). If the husband in the example knows the nurse who is helping his wife and respects this nurse's opinions, he might be ready to listen to the arguments for contraception which this professional has to offer. He may, however, reject the nurse as incompetent and feel that the nurse is responsible for his current predicament. On the other hand, he may be more alert and sensitive to information about contraception in the newspapers, on television, or in general conversation. Scanning these sources may lead to an attitude change.

The above example is one in which the nurse might have used the conflict which naturally occurred to effect change. He can also deliberately create conflict in order to motivate people or groups to change attitudes. This technique requires much skill and careful planning to avoid unexpected and potentially disastrous consequences. It is *not* recommended for novice practitioners.

Another way in which health professionals can help bring about attitude change is to *reduce* the conflict accompanying proposed change. This is effective when the person already has some desire to change but is in conflict with his own beliefs or attitudes or those of others important to him. Schein terms this approach the removal of barriers or the creation of psychological safety. To accomplish this, one might give moral support to the person as he faces the conflict, help him identify the source of the conflict, support him in enduring the anxiety, and help him see how the end result is worth the present discomfort (Schein, 1969, p. 101).

If the husband in the above example has some inclination to limit his family but fears ridicule from his peers, a health professional whom he respects might be able to help him face the potential conflict. He might be able to rationalize the use of contraception if he could tell his friends, for example, that the doctor has said it would be bad for his wife's health to have any more babies. Underwood (1971) describes role playing with the nurse as an effective way to help people whose backgrounds differ from that of the nurse. In these "practice sessions," the person can work out an approach in his own style before confronting the source of his conflict.

Feasibility The feasibility of the proposed solution is a third factor to consider. To illustrate, we return to the example of the man who is hard of hearing. If he has no ability to read lips, it would be very helpful for him to learn. However, most nurses working in a hospital would have neither the time nor the skill to help him do this. Moreover, if he is hospitalized with an acute illness, he would probably be discharged before he could learn to read lips. He may have some ability to read lips if the speaker faces him and speaks slowly. In this case, a feasible action is to have nursing personnel address him slowly while facing him.

The potential solution of having only men care for him is based on scientific fact, since men have lower voices than women, but is probably not feasible in many hospitals where most workers are women. Writing all messages to him is a solution which has merit, but it is time-consuming and may serve to isolate him more. It should be reserved until other solutions have been tried and evaluated.

Each potential solution should be weighed in terms of its probability of success. Some solutions will appear more promising than others and may be tried first. Others will be rapidly excluded as first choices but are there to try if the first approaches are not effective.

Selecting Criteria to Measure Effectiveness of the Action

Fundamental to the intervention chosen is some means to evaluate its effect in relieving the patient's problem. If the goal is that he be able to hear conversation directed to him, then we must find some way to measure or note whether he actually does hear us. His initial assessment should give some data to use as a base line for evaluation.

Before action was initiated, he wore a hearing aid and responded only to a very loud voice. His responses included: frequently asking the speaker to repeat, statements which did not fit the question or statements of the other person, misinterpretation of words, and not complying with spoken directions or requests. He was able to comply with written requests. These observations may be used to set criteria for evaluating the effect of intervention in his hearing problem. If he hears better, his responses to the speaker can be expected to become appropriate, to be in compliance with requests, and to occur with less frequent or no requests to the speaker to repeat.

Planning for Multiplicity of Nursing Problems

Initially, we defined the nursing-care plan as the sum of interventions designed to help the patient with his nursing problems. By implication, most patients or clients have more than one nursing problem, and more than one problem may demand attention at any one time. Each problem must be analyzed in its own right, but actions appropriate to one problem may also be effective in solving another. For example, getting the postoperative patient up to walk is an action which is effective in the problems of preventing hypostatic pneumonia. It also helps prevent peripheral venous thrombosis, muscular atrophy and contractures, and pressure sores, while pro-

moting the movement of gas and flatus. This action may cause incisional pain, however, and the plan will have to include other actions to deal with that problem.

IMPLEMENTING INTERVENTION— TESTING APPROACHES

At this stage, the nurse actually tries the proposed solution to the problem. The necessity to evaluate the results of the intervention dictates that the action taken be considered in two parts—what is *done* and what is *observed* about the patient-client response.

Nursing intervention may take many forms, depending upon the problem, the role of the particular nurse, and the needs of the patient. The professional nurse diagnoses the nursing problems, proposes possible solutions, and evaluates the results of the actions taken. This nurse may or may not actually carry out the proposed intervention. There are several means by which the professional nurse may choose to implement the plan of care. He may act directly with the patient or client, delegate care to and supervise the work of other nursing personnel, refer the patient to other professionals for specialized services, or coordinate the efforts of several health workers in helping the patient.

Direct Service to the Patient or Client

The nurse often chooses to give direct service, whether the intervention is in the realm of physical ministration, counseling, teaching, or assisting with the medical plan of care. There are many situations in which the professional nurse is the only member of the nursing team with the technical or communication skills to implement the plan of care for a particular patient. In other situations, the nurse may wish to use direct care of the hospitalized patient to establish a firmer rapport with him, corroborating the patient-client's concept of the nurse as a "doer," in order to move to a concept of the nurse as one who helps him find his own solutions to his problems.

Intervention through Other Nursing Personnel

When the professional nurse is responsible for service to a number of patients or clients, he often must utilize other nursing personnel to implement the nursing actions which he has proposed. In this case, it is essential that the proposed actions take written form as *nursing directives* or *nursing orders*. Many agencies and institutions use terms such as "nursing approach" or "nursing action" synonymously with nursing directive or order. However, Little and Carnevali point out that the term "nursing order was selected to . . . convey responsibility, a specified behavior and content area and . . . a greater urgency about implementation than other terms currently in use."[2]

When intervention is implemented by several nursing personnel, it is essential that each person understand exactly what is to be done, how it is to be done, when it should be done, and what results must be noted. A simple example is seen in a problem of fluid intake.

Problem: Inadequate fluid intake due to inability to feed self

Objective (immediate):
  3,000 cc free fluid every 24 hr
  1,500 cc—day shift
  1,300 cc—evening shift
    200 cc—night shift

Nursing Directives:
  1 Use bent glass straws as patient likes them best.
  2 Elevate head of bed 60°—patient chokes if too flat.
  3 Feed patient; offer 200-300 cc fluid between meals; likes 7-Up, orange juice, ice water, ice cream.
  4 Observe: total intake and output each shift; state of hydration—skin, hair, eyes.

Vague directives such as "tender loving care" have no place in nursing orders. The nurse must specify exactly *how* one is to provide loving care. If the goal is to let the anxious patient know that

someone is readily available to him, then specify, "At least every hour, ask patient if there is anything he needs." If you are trying to show the patient that he is important as a person, specify, "Discuss hobbies and interests while giving other care—likes skiing, sports car racing, model cars."

Referral to Other Professionals

Referral to other professionals is action taken on behalf of the patient or client. There are many problems a person may have which are outside the scope of nursing practice, yet which adversely affect a person's coping with his daily life. The woman who needs teaching about special therapeutic diet may be referred to a dietitian; the man whose marital problems divert his ability to cope with his recovery from an automobile accident could be referred to a social worker or psychologist who specializes in marital counseling; the family whose child seems to be mentally retarded could be referred to a diagnostic center. The nurse needs to continue contact with the professional to whom his patient-client was referred in order to coordinate his plan of nursing care with their efforts at dealing with the referred problem.

Coordination of Activities

Coordination of nursing actions with the activities of other professionals involved with the patient-client is the last major type of intervention. The nurse and other professionals may or may not be working as a formal health team. If they are, the team goal will have been set with the patient or client, and the nursing objectives are a part of this overall goal. If the other professionals' activities are not directly health-related or if these professionals are not associated with the nursing institution or agency, it is up to the nurse to determine whether his goals and those of the others are compatible. If they are not, he needs to work with these other workers to form compatible goals and modes of treatment. Ultimately, it is the patient-client who

[2] From Delores Little and Doris Carnevali, "Nursing Care Planning," J. B. Lippincott Company, Philadelphia, 1969, p. 174.

suffers if several professionals working in his behalf are not working together.

EVALUATING THE INTERVENTIONS AND THE PLAN

Criteria for evaluating effectiveness need to be specific and measurable, either qualitatively or quantitatively. This is relatively easy if one is interested in determining the amount of fluid drunk in eight hours, the number of hours slept, or the quality of the pulse. It is not so simple, however, when trying to determine whether pain has been lessened or relieved, or whether anxiety has decreased. In essence, such questions require the quantitation of a subjective experience, a task which is never easy.

Probably the best way to go about measuring subjective responses is to recall the observations which led to the diagnosis of the problem, i.e., the patient's behavior which led you to believe that he was in pain or was anxious. Once these behaviors have been documented, one may observe whether or not they have disappeared or lessened in frequency.

For example, the person with abdominal pain may have some of the following signs and may exhibit some of the following behavior:

Elevated pulse
Rapid respiration
Excessive perspiration
Lies in bed with knees drawn up
States he is in severe pain
Focuses only on pain
Grimaces
"Guards," or maintains rigid posture of
　abdomen and trunk
Is irritable
Moans

Criteria to measure effectiveness of nursing action to relieve the pain would consist of statement of relief, relaxation, decreased pulse and respiration, cessation of perspiration, increased interest in surroundings, absence of guarding.

The foregoing is an example of an acute nursing problem in which observations of effectiveness of the action can be made in a short time. Many of the persons whom the nurse serves have more chronic or long-term problems, and evidence of change in their behavior is not immediately apparent. It is even more important in these situations to have good criteria for measuring the effect of nursing intervention.

A school nurse visited the G. family in relation to George, their 7-year-old son who required special schooling. One of the problems which the nurse and Mrs. G. identified was Mrs. G.'s inability to express negative feelings directly to the person with whom she was in conflict. She frequently told the nurse of her disagreement with the approach of George's teacher, but had never discussed this with the teacher. Further, Mrs. G. felt this was the pattern of her relationships with most people, and she wanted to change. This change in behavior became Mrs. G.'s goal. The objective set by Mrs. G. and the nurse was for Mrs. G. to tell the teacher directly when she did not agree with the things the teacher asked her to do with George. Each time Mrs. G. told the nurse of her frustration with the teacher's advice, the nurse planned to ask if Mrs. G. had discussed this with the teacher. In addition, she would help her "role-play" her approach to the teacher.

The nurse visited the family every month and planned to note whether or not Mrs. G. had actually discussed her disagreements with the teacher. As a second criterion measure, she planned to talk with the teacher and determine how effectively Mrs. G. had communicated her disagreement.

For the next three months, Mrs. G. continued to complain about the teacher's approach, but each time she said she hadn't discussed this with the teacher. Each time she and the nurse tried role-playing a hypothetical discussion with the teacher. When the nurse visited the fourth month, Mrs. G. greeted her, saying, "I actually did it!" She had talked with the teacher and was pleased that they had come to a compatible approach to George. She also discovered that she had misinterpreted the teacher's intent. A subsequent visit by the nurse with the teacher corroborated Mrs. G.'s perception of the conference. The teacher commented that she had known something was bothering Mrs. G. and was glad it was now out in the open.

In the example given, the nurse evaluated her plan on the basis of two observations: Mrs. G.'s behavior and the teacher's perception of Mrs. G.'s action. In this case, she felt the plan had worked.

MODIFYING THE PLAN

Had the plan for Mrs. G. not been successful, the nurse would have had to think back to her initial proposals for action and try another approach. If she had not originally used role playing, she might have tried that next, reasoning that Mrs. G. might want to talk to the teacher but might not know how.

Even though the plan was successful in accomplishing the immediate goal, it will still need to be modified, for the teacher is only one of the many people with whom Mrs. G. finds it hard to disagree. She and the nurse need to modify the plan to help her find ways to express negative feelings and thoughts to others. Thus, they have accomplished one short-term objective and are modifying the plan to reach longer-term goals.

A plan for nursing action may require modification whether or not it accomplishes the initial objective. Modification is indicated when (1) more data are available which better define or change the problem; (2) new problems appear or old ones are solved; (3) one or more of the short-term objectives are met, indicating the need to move on to long-term objectives and the goal; (4) the initially proposed action is not successful; (5) the patient or the nurse modifies goals, setting them higher or lower; or (6) new resources become available, or former ones are no longer available.

RECORDING THE PROBLEMS AND PLAN FOR INTERVENTION

Sometimes a nurse may have one brief contact with a patient or client, and the process of assessment, diagnosis, action, and evaluation is accomplished in his head. In most instances, however, there will be more than one contact with the patient, necessitating a written record of the diagnostic and therapeutic process. When only one nurse serves the client, he needs the record to refresh his memory with each contact. When many health workers, such as nurses, physicians, physical therapists, serve him, a written record is essential for communication between them and within each health discipline.

The following discussion of health records is confined to the *problem-oriented* record, as defined and popularized by Lawrence Weed (1968, 1969). This type of record is organized around the patient or client's health problems, as seen by him and by the professionals helping him. Traditional records are source-oriented, i.e., the data are recorded and categorized according to their source. The physicians' notes are in one place, the laboratory data in another, the nurses' observations and the graph of vital signs are in still other portions of the chart. Thus, if the physician or nurse wishes to see what progress is being made in a patient's problem of edema, he must look in four or more different places in the record to obtain the data needed to evaluate changes. In the problem-oriented record, all this information would be identified in one place, categorized by the problem of edema. Because the focus of each health discipline is somewhat different even in the same patient's problem, a problem-oriented record immediately provides a comprehensive picture from several viewpoints of the client's response to therapy and of his ability to cope with the problem. In a source-oriented record, such perspective is often lost or overlooked.

Use of the problem-oriented record promises to help coordinate efforts of several professionals for any one client. It is by far the most logical recording tool for the approach to nursing care described in this book.

Many agencies throughout the country are adopting Weed's approach, modified to suit their own needs. In some areas, the problems identified by nurses and the observations they make in relation to patients' problems are part of a general progress record used by all health workers. In others, each discipline may keep separate problem and progress notes. Because nursing and medical focuses in health problems overlap so frequently, the integrated record is preferable to coordinate care of the patient-client. Examples of both integrated and separate records are shown in Figs. 7-3 and 7-4.

Characteristics of the Problem-oriented Record

The specific mechanics of recording in such a record varies among and even within agencies using it, and are best learned in each agency. Consequently the following discussion is of general characteristics of the problem-oriented approach.

Basically, the record consists of the data base, the problem list, the initial plan, the progress notes, and the final summary. The *data base* is comprised of the objective and subjective data gathered by interview, examination, observation, and diagnostic tests. In the true problem-oriented record, members of any health discipline contribute to the data base. In source-oriented records in which some professionals use a problem approach, the data base will be scattered among sources—e.g., physician's history and physical examination, nursing history and assessment, social worker's history, laboratory and x-ray data.

The *problem list* is formulated either by the health team or by individual professionals after the data base is analyzed (see Part 2, Chapter 6, regarding analysis of data). Thereafter, all plans, further data, and notes regarding progress are organized around the defined problems or potential problems. When problems are resolved, they are not removed from the list, but the date of resolution is noted. New problems are added to the list at any time. Thus the problem list is, in Weed's words, a "dynamic table of contents" (1968). Important potential problems may be added to the list in order that ongoing observation is planned. Yarnall and Libke (1972) propose listing only major problems, and identifying problems secondary to these in the progress notes.

Initial plans are recorded in relation to identified problems and potential problems. Revisions of plans are incorporated into the progress notes. In institutions medical and nursing plans must often be implemented by and communicated to large numbers of personnel. It is often not possible for each worker to refer to the record for details of daily care; therefore a bound card file (Kardex) is frequently used to provide easy access to the information. An example is shown in Fig. 7-2.

Problem	Directives	Date	Observe for
L hemiparesis (pot. disuse)	Position in normal alignment	2/2	Hips, shoulders 90° to spine
	Passive ROM TID	2/2	Base line: full ROM all limbs; note any ↓ or pain
	Resistive, isometric exercises R side, trunk, abdomen (schedule at bedside)	2/8	P.T. will assess
Pot. pressure sores	Turn L side 1 hr; R side 2–3 hr	2/2	Redness, absence of blanching on bony prominences
	Teach to turn self (turn him if 3 hr any position)	2/4	Q2H, note position
Incontinence	Note time of voiding; offer urinal Q2H	2/2	Record bedside flow sheet; record continence

Medications	Treatments—scheduled care	Problem list	
		Date	Problem
	2/2/72 Passive ROM TID	2/2/72	1. RMCA–CVA
	2/2 Turn 1 hr L; 2–3 hr R		(a) L hemiparesis
	2/2 Elastic stockings		(b) Recent memory loss
	2/2 Offer urinal Q2H		(c) Expressive aphasia
	2/8 Resistive exercise		(d) Bladder incontinence
		2/4	(e) Depression

Name	Physician	Diagnosis	Hosp. Number	Room
Doe, Harold	J. Smith	RMCA–CVA	1–002–72	662–4

Figure 7-2 Example of Kardex form. Forms vary among institutions but are generally folded, with space for identifying data, medications and other treatments, and problems and approaches. In this example, the problem list from the health record is incorporated, and the directives are a combination of nursing and medical orders regarding the problems.

Information is transcribed from the record and usually consists of identifying data, medical directives (orders for medication and treatment), and nursing directives. Use of a Kardex does not substitute for writing care plans in the record, however, for Kardex plans are rarely permanent documents.

Progress records are of two types: narrative notes and flow sheets. Figures 7-3, 7-4, and 7-5 show examples of forms used for each.

The narrative note is a written description of data (both objective and subjective), impressions, plans, actions, and results about each identified problem. The frequency with which these notes are written depends upon the stability of the problem and the relevancy of observations which any worker has made. Frequency varies from once a week to several times a day. In the past, nurses in hospitals have felt that they must make some notation in the nurses' notes several times a day, regardless of whether the patient's status has changed. These repetitious, meaningless observations ("good day," "without complaint") have no place in progress notes.

There are times when frequent observations of patient or client status must be made, for example, when status is changing rapidly, when observing for potential problems, or when teaching

a new skill. In such situations, the flow sheet is a logical recording device. The observations to be made are listed on the vertical coordinate of the flow sheet and the frequency of observation or learning session on the horizontal coordinate. A summary of change, stability, or progress as analyzed from the flow sheet is then written periodically in the narrative notes. Flow sheets, too, may be of two types: the bedside sheet for recording frequent data, and the long-term flow sheet.

Bedside graphs are currently used everywhere to record fluctuating data such as vital signs, neurologic status, and laboratory data. However, long-term flow sheets are used less frequently by nurses to record data about potential problems or teaching plans. Use of flow sheets for such data could help reduce the repetition and unrelated data characteristic of present-day progress records.

The last portion of the record is the *final summary,* written when the patient or client leaves the health-care system. Such a summary includes the status of each problem identified (e.g., resolved, still active, still potential), summary of effective or ineffective intervention of all disciplines, and recommendations for further help. In the source-oriented record, the physi-

Subjective and objective data, assessment & plan	Orders	Time/init.

Problem: Right middle cerebral artery thrombosis #1
Date/Time: 2/2/72   10 A.M.

Source: pt's. wife; pt. seems confused as to place & time.

During past *6 months,* periodic "dizzy spells," did not persist, not associated with any specific activity. *Last night,* went to bed c/o "headache"; woke about *6 A.M.* wet with urine, "talking nonsense," and unable to move L arm; L leg moved only side to side (15° on physical exam).

See physical exam and neuro exam on physical form.

Impression: L hemiparesis secondary to R middle cerebral artery thrombosis.

Related problems:

(a) Memory loss for recent events

(b) Expressive aphasia

(c) Bladder incontinence

Plan: Bed rest until condition stabilizes; neuro VS. Refer for P.T., speech therapy when stable.

_____ MD

1. Bed rest c̄ footboard.   10a   MD
2. Passive ROM TID.   MD
3. Neuro VS Q2H til stable.

#1, c; Bladder incontinence
2/2/72;   12 P.M.

Was incontinent at onset of CVA, according to wife, and upon admission.

Incontinent of urine again at 12 P.M.; was banging on siderails and pointing to wet sheet; seemed upset; kept repeating, "I need, I need"; could not name urinal; nodded when I asked if he needed to pass water.

Impression: Incontinence due to inability to make his needs known.

Plan: Make urinal available frequently.

_____ RN

1. Note time of voiding.
2. Offer urinal Q2H, oftener if needed.   12p   RN

2/5/72   10 A.M.; #1—L Hemiparesis

Arm: Still does not move spontaneously or on command; able to put through full passive ROM, no edema.

Leg: Improved, able to move side to side 30°; can lift heel about ½ in. off bed, no edema, some tightening of hip extension.

Impression: Improvement in leg, slight loss of full ROM L hip.

Plan: Consult with Dr. _____ and P.T. re more vigorous exercises.

_____ RN

Doe, Harold
1-002-72
662-4

NURSES' AND PHYSICIANS'
**PROBLEM-ORIENTED
PROGRESS NOTES & ORDERS**

Figure 7-3 Example of an integrated progress note. Both physician's and nurse's observations are on one record. A nursing assessment (see example in Fig. 7-4) and medical history and physical examination would be included in the data base elsewhere in the record. A computerized data base would provide most of the data needed by either nurse or physician. (*Forms courtesy of Stephen Yarnall, M.D., and Medical Computer Services Association.*)

Nurses' Record

Date	Time	
2/2/72	11 A.M.	Data: 52-yr-old man admitted via ambulance; awoke this A.M. "talking funny," wet with urine, and unable to move L side. Physician's diagnosis: CVA-R middle cerebral artery thrombosis. See nursing assessment form re current functional status. Problems: 1. L hemiparesis secondary RMCA-CVA (a) Memory loss for recent events (b) Expressive aphasia (cannot name objects, uses jargon) (c) Potential: edema L side, muscle atrophy 2nd bed rest, venous stasis, ↓ sensory input, pressure sores, difficulty coping with dependence. Plan: 1. Frequent neuro check until stable as per physician's plan. 2. Position in normal alignment, frequent position change to prevent disuse phenomena, pressure sores. 3. Institute passive ROM when physician feels is safe. 4. Gather more data when stabilizes as to extent of memory loss and expressive aphasia. 5. Support wife in coping with husband's disability. _____ RN
	12 P.M.	Problem #1 (d)—bladder incontinence Data: Was incontinent at onset CVA (according to wife) and on adm. Presently lying in wet bed, banging on siderails, and pointing to wet sheet; repeated "I need, I need." Could not name urinal; nodded when I asked if he needed to pass water. Impression: Incontinence due to inability to make need to void known. Plan: Note frequency of voiding; offer urinal Q2H or oftener as indicated. _____ RN

Doe, Harold
1-002-72
662-4

Figure 7-4 Example of separate problem-oriented progress notes. Both the nurses' record and the nursing assessment are in a separate portion of the health record.

Nursing Assessment

Area	2/2/72 Data
Psychosocial	Informant: wife 52-yr.-old house painter; lives with 45-yr.-old wife; 2 married daughters live out of state. Has never been ill before, according to wife; she defines illness as "not being able to get about." Wife asked repeatedly (in front of Mr. D.), "Will he be a cripple?"
Mental/Emotional	Subjective: Wife says he has always coped c̄ problems by himself, never asks for help; says he is "stubborn"; 8th grade education; wife states, "He's good with his hands; he's not so good with words." Objective: alert, oriented to person—thinks today is "January"; knows he is not at home, but cannot name where he is; recognizes wife. Follows single action command (move your R hand). Cannot assess his perception of situation fully as he is having much difficulty expressing himself; cannot name objects, using jargon ("is-a-is-a-flup").

Neuro/Sensory/Motor	Subjective: States "Can't move" and points to L arm.
	Objective: L arm flaccid, no spontaneous movement, no response to touch or pinprick.
	Some spontaneous movement L leg (foot 15° side to side), no response to touch or pinprick.
	Moves foot slightly in response to command; does not raise it off bed.
	Attempts to turn himself but cannot.
	No visual field defects noted.
	Pupils =, reactive to light and accommodation (PERLA).
	Headache prior to onset, none now.
	Speech: cannot name simple objects; able to say "I want," "I am," but cannot finish sentence. Yes and no answers appropriate, but cannot elaborate.
	L facial droop; slurring of speech.
Circulatory	BP 150/70/68 on adm., 140/70/70 1 hr later; pulse stable 88. No edema L arm or leg.
Respiratory	R = 16; spontaneous; takes deep breaths on command, no abnormal chest sounds; oral moist "blowing" sounds when mouth breathing.
Temperature	99°F rectally
Nutrition/Fluid	170#, normal fat distribution; prefers Italian-American food.
	Able to swallow $\bar{o}$ choking; saliva and food collect in L side of mouth.
	Normally drinks fluid only with meals, plus one P.M. beer.
	Could not reach bedside fluids without help.
Skin/Integument	No areas of redness or breakdown.
	Prefers to lie on back; may be problem to position on sides.
	Strong odor of urine.
Elimination:	No hx of problem with either bladder or bowels.
	Incontinent of urine at onset of CVA.
	Normally has BM daily, in A.M.
	No patent medicines taken to aid bowel movements.
Comfort/Sleep	Subjective (per wife): Normally sleeps 7 hr (11^P–6^a).
	No aids used for sleep.
	Sleeps on stomach.
	Rarely takes medications for discomfort; occasional aspirin.
	Feels medication "is for sissies."
	Impressions: Independent man (wife's perceptions) who may have difficulty coping with enforced dependency of partial paralysis. Appears to understand others, but marked difficulty expressing self.
	Problems:
	1. L Hemiparesis.
	(a) Memory loss for recent events.
	(b) Expressive aphasia.
	(c) Potential disuse phenomena—edema, muscle atrophy, venous stasis, ↓ sensory input, pressure sores.
	(d) Potential difficulty coping with dependence.
	(e) Potential rejection by wife.

Doe, Harold
1-002-72
662-4

Nursing Assessment Form

Date		2/2/72	2/3/72	2/4/72	2/5/72	2/6/72	2/7/72	2/8/72
Vital Signs	Weight	170	170	169.5	169	168.5	169	168.5
	Syst/Diast.	150/70 to 140/70	140/80/80	152/78/70	150/70/68	140/68/68	148/74/72	140/70/70
	Pulse Rate	120–88	90–100	80–90	82–84	80–84	78–82	82
	Resp.	22–28	18–24	16–24	16–18	16–24	16–18	16–20
	Temp.	99 R	98.8 R	98.4	98	98.6	98.4	98.2
L hemiparesis		Adm. Phys. (see Exam.)	Unchanged	Unchanged	Arm unchanged leg improved	Unchanged	Unchanged	Arm improved leg improved
ROM		See adm.	Full	Full	L hip ↓	Same as 2/5	Full	Neck ↓ Other full
Muscle atrophy		0̄	X	X	X	X	X	0̄
Edema		0̄	0̄	0̄	0̄	L arm	Same	↓ in L arm
Pressure sores		0̄	0̄	0̄	0̄	Redness L hip	0̄	0̄
Bladder incontinence		All day	Cont. X 2	0̄	0̄	0̄	Incont. X 1	0̄
Bowel movements		0̄	i (incont.)	i	i	i	i	0̄
Self-turning (turn = by staff self = by self)		X	X	Demonstrated turn X 4 self — 0	Turn X 4 Self X 2	Turn X 1 Self X 4	Self	Self
Fluid intake		700 cc	1,000 cc	1,500 cc	2,000 cc	1,800 cc	2,000 cc	2,200 cc

Doe, Harold 1–002–72 662–4	NURSES' AND PHYSICIANS' **PROBLEM-ORIENTED FLOW SHEET**

Figure 7-5 Flow sheet. Flow sheets are used to record observations about long-term or rapidly changing problems. In the above example, potential problems are noted in terms of criteria defined by the physician or nurse. The Kardex in Fig. 7-2 shows some criteria for potential problems. Whenever change is noted, a descriptive note is written in the narrative progress record. For example, see the note written on Feb. 5, 1972 in Fig. 7-3 about changes in ROM (range of motion of joints) and L hemiparesis. Teaching plans can be incorporated into flow sheets, as shown in the observations about self-turning. More frequent observations can be noted on bedside flow sheets for such data as vital signs, fluid intake, and neurological status. Daily summaries can be added to the flow sheet above. (Forms courtesy of Stephen Yarnall and Medical Computer Services Association.)

cian most commonly writes a discharge summary. Summaries by other professionals may or may not be found.

ADVANTAGES OF THE PROBLEM-ORIENTED APPROACH

There are a number of advantages to the "Weed method."

1 The patient-client and his problems become the focus of health care; the method of recording data requires that one approaches the client in terms of health problems, rather than in terms of disease, procedures, or specific professional orientation.

2 The approach provides a system for logically organizing data so that all professionals reading the account can see what is happening in resolution of any problem. The data are clustered logically, and conclusions as to the nature of problems are supported by data. Evaluation of efficacy of care is easier if data are well organized. The systematic nature of this approach makes it easily codified for computer storage and retrieval. This type of storage, in turn, makes the data more accessible for statistical studies, research about the effects of health care, and permanent communication among health workers.

3 Problem orientation provides a common language among health disciplines and may help bridge the gap between nursing and medical approaches to the patient-client.

4 Last, this type of recording should help improve communication within nursing. Nurses too frequently record an apparently random hodgepodge of data which is primarily related to medical procedures. Conclusions are left totally to the reader. At one time nurses were taught that objectivity demanded that they draw no written conclusions. That time is past, and nurses must commit themselves to their conclusions, on the basis of available data. The problem-oriented record offers a logical way to organize the data and to support one's conclusions.

REFERENCES

Books

Bennis, Warren G., Kenneth Benne, and Robert Chin (eds.), "The Planning of Change," 2d ed., Holt, Rinehart and Winston, Inc., New York, 1969.

Jourard, Sidney, "The Transparent Self," 2d ed., D. Van Nostrand Company, Princeton, N.J., 1971.

Little, Delores, and Doris Carnevali, "Nursing Care Planning," J. B. Lippincott Company, Philadelphia, 1969.

Maslow, A. H., "Motivation and Personality," Harper & Row, Publishers, Incorporated, New York, 1954.

Orlando, Ida, "The Dynamic Nurse-Patient Relationship," G. P. Putnam's Sons, New York, 1961.

Rogers, Carl, "On Becoming a Person," Houghton-Mifflin Company, Boston, 1961.

Schein, Edgar H., The Mechanisms of Change, in Warren G. Bennis et al. (eds.), "The Planning of Change," 2d ed., Holt, Rinehart and Winston, Inc., New York, 1969.

Weed, Lawrence L., "Medical Records: Medical Education and Patient Care," The Press of Case Western Reserve University, Cleveland, 1969.

Yarnall, Stephen, and Albert Libke, "A Problem-oriented System for Patient Care and Medical Records," University of Washington School of Medicine Syllabus, 3d ed., Seattle, 1972. (To be published in book form by Medical Computer Services Association.)

Periodicals

Baca, Josephine: Some Health Beliefs of the Spanish-speaking, *American Journal of Nursing*, **69**:2173–2176 (1969).

Dumas, R., and R. C. Leonard: The Effect of Nursing on the Incidence of Post-operative Vomiting, *Nursing Research*, **12**:12ff. (1963).

Finch, Joyce: Systems Analysis: A Logical Approach to Professional Nursing Care, *Nursing Forum*, **8**(2):176–190 (1969).

Hanken, Albert F.: Pain and Systems Analysis, *Nursing Research*, **15**:139–143 (1966).

Leininger, Madeleine: The Culture Concept and Its Relevance to Nursing, *Journal of Nursing Education*, **6**:27–37 (1967).

McKay, Rose: Theories, Models and Systems for Nursing, *Nursing Research*, **18**:393–399 (1964).

Moss, Fay T., and Burton Meyer: Effects of Nursing Intervention upon Pain Relief in Patients, *Nursing Research*, **15**:303–306 (1966).

Olson, Edith: The Hazards of Immobility, *American Journal of Nursing*, **67**:780–796 (1967).

Paynich, Mary L.: Cultural Barriers to Nurse Communication, *American Journal of Nursing*, **64**:87–90 (1964).

Tryon, Phyllis, and R. C. Leonard: The Effect of the Patient's Participation on the Outcome of a Nursing Procedure, *Nursing Forum*, **3**(2):79–89 (1964).

Underwood, Patricia: Communication through Role Playing, *American Journal of Nursing*, **71**:1184–1186 (1971).

Walker, Virginia, D. A. McReynolds, and E. Patrick: A Care Plan for Ailing Nurses' Notes, *American Journal of Nursing*, **65**:74 (1965).

Weed, Lawrence: Medical Records That Guide and Teach, *New England Journal of Medicine*, **278**:593–600 (Mar. 14, 1968).

Weidenbach, Ernestine: Nurses' Wisdom in Nursing Theory, *American Journal of Nursing*, **70**:1057–1062 (1970).

ADDITIONAL READINGS

Health Records

Bloom, Judy T., et al.: Problem-oriented Charting, *American Journal of Nursing*, **71**:2144–2148 (1971).

Recording the Home Visit, *Nursing Outlook,* **15**:38–40 (1967).

Rosenberg, Marvin, Bernard C. Glueck, Jr., Charles F. Stoebel, Marvin Reznikoff, and R. Peter Ericson: Comparison of Automated Nursing Notes as Recorded by Psychiatrists and Nursing Service Personnel, *Nursing Research,* **18**:350ff. (1964).

Walker, Virginia, and Eugene Selmanoff: A Study of the Nature and Use of Nurse's Notes, *Nursing Research,* **13**:113–121 (1964).

Culture and Social Group

Agee, James, and Walker Evans, "Let Us Now Praise Famous Men," Houghton-Mifflin Company, Boston, 1939; Ballantine Books, Inc., New York, 1966. (The author's impression of the life of tenant farmers, written while he lived among them.)

Cleaver, Eldridge, "Soul on Ice," McGraw-Hill Book Company, New York, 1963.

Cohen, Yehudi (ed.), "Man in Adaptation: The Cultural Present," Aldine Publishing Company, Chicago, 1968.

Coles, Robert, "Children of Crisis: A Study of Courage and Fear," Atlantic Monthly Press, Little, Brown and Company, Boston, 1967. (Effects of integration on black, low-income children.)

———, "Migrants, Sharecroppers, Mountaineers: Volume II of Children of Crisis," Atlantic Monthly Press, Little, Brown and Company, Boston, 1971.

———, "The South Goes North: Volume III of Children of Crisis," Atlantic Monthly Press, Little, Brown and Company, Boston, 1971.

——— and Jon Erickson, "Middle Americans: Proud and Uncertain," Atlantic Monthly Press, Little, Brown and Company, Boston, 1971.

Glazer, Nathan, and Daniel P. Moynihan, "Beyond the Melting Pot: The Negroes, Puerto Ricans, Jews, Italians, and Irish of New York City," M.I.T. Press, Cambridge, 1963.

Gordon, Milton, "Assimilation in American Life," Oxford University Press, New York, 1969. (Oriental Americans.)

Irelan, Lola M. (ed.), "Low-income Life Styles," U.S. Department of Health, Education and Welfare, Welfare Administration Publication, 1968.

Leininger, Madeleine, "Nursing and Anthropology: Two Worlds to Blend," John Wiley & Sons, Inc., New York, 1970.

Lewis, Oscar, "Five Families: Mexican Case Studies in the Culture of Poverty," Basic Books, Inc., New York, 1959. (Introduction of the concept of a cultural pattern to being poor.)

———, "La Vida: A Puerto Rican Family in the Culture of Poverty; San Juan and New York," Vintage Books, Random House, Inc., New York, 1966.

McCabe, Garcia S.: Cultural Influence on Patient Behavior, *American Journal of Nursing,* **60**:1101–1104 (1960).

McGregor, Frances C.: Uncooperative Patients: Some Cultural Interpretations, *American Journal of Nursing,* **67**:88–91 (1967).

Mead, Margaret: Understanding Cultural Patterns, *Nursing Outlook,* **4**:260–262 (1956).

Paul, Benjamin (ed.), "Health, Culture and Community: Case Studies of Public Reactions to Health Programs," Russell Sage Foundation, New York, 1955.

Reissman, Frank, "The Culturally Deprived Child," Harper & Row, Publishers, Incorporated, New York, 1962.

Steiner, Stan, "The New Indians," Harper & Row, Publishers, Incorporated, New York, 1968.

Storlie, Frances, "Nursing and Social Conscience," Appleton-Century-Crofts, New York, 1970.

Wright, D., "They Harvest Despair," Beacon Press, Boston, 1965. (Observations of East Coast migrant workers made while the author lived with them.)

Part Three

Concepts Basic to Nursing Practice

Part 2 of this book describes the *process* by which nurses and clients work together to determine what help is needed, how that help will be provided, and, later, whether the help has met the need. However, without basic knowledge (content), the nurse's ability to diagnose need and to provide and evaluate help would be limited indeed.

The remainder of this book, Part 3, is devoted to just such knowledge. It is presented in terms of concepts which encompass maintenance of functional ability, prevention of disability, and provision of sustenance and comfort in the face of health problems.

These selected concepts are organized in relation to the data-gathering outline presented in Part 2. Pertinent data are outlined at the beginning of each chapter in order to help the student to interpret and use information which he collects. When appropriate, problem areas common within the concept and nursing interventions that should be considered are identified at the end of each chapter.

Conceptualizing, a Nursing Skill

Doris Carnevali

The knowledge that a nurse uses in a nursing situation is at least as important as the action taken. Without knowledge, the welter of cues in the environment may make no sense, or may be misinterpreted, while the actions become those of a programmed robot. The validity and reliability of the concepts that a nurse applies are the essence of her professional competence.

However, the information explosion of our times makes it difficult to have readily available the ideas that should influence observations and decisions. Thus, the ability to organize knowledge as it is stored so that it becomes quickly retrievable is an increasingly important thinking skill.

CONCEPTS AS AN INFORMATION RETRIEVAL SYSTEM

Conceptualization is an information storage and retrieval system. It is like a filing system within one's head where the words form the label on the pull tab for a whole file of related ideas and experiences, as shown in Fig. 8-1. The entire file can be pulled out when some unit of input signals the need for this package of ideas. This is

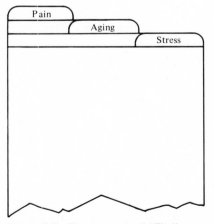

Figure 8-1 The conceptual "file."

much more efficient than having to search for facts and ideas as single units of information.

AWARENESS AND CONCEPTUALIZING

Through experience and exposure to ideas, one can develop the ability to form concepts without real awareness of the process. For example, most people in developed countries have a concept of telephone that enables them to identify the instrument regardless of variations in color, location, or shape; to understand its use; and to behave appropriately in using it to make or to receive calls. The concept of telephone may never have been formally taught, yet it is learned and used.

The nurse, however, is expected to develop purposefully those conceptual packages that will be needed in nursing situations. They will become the basis for:

1 The interpretation of the dynamics of a given situation
2 The direction of additional data gathering
3 The prediction of possible or probable outcomes
4 The taking of effective action
5 The setting of criteria for evaluating responses

Concepts are woven through every aspect of nursing behavior.

CONCEPTUALIZING AS A PERSONAL ACTIVITY

Developing conceptual packages is a very individualized activity, one that each person must do for himself. Some of the ideas may come from other persons, but the form in which they are organized and stored, the words that are used, the content stored in each package, and the plan for using the concept can be chosen only by the person himself.

It follows, then, that when different persons develop the same concept, their concepts will have commonalities but also will have unique features. Thus one may never take for granted that one person's concept is a replica of another's, even though the persons may have read the same books, attended the same lectures, or had some of the same experiences. Nor can one assume that one's own concepts will be unchanging over periods of time. Concepts tend to be responsive to new experiences and input of knowledge; they are dynamic, growing, and evolving.

Let us look at the way in which a single concept, *heart,* might be used. A child may think of heart as a red paper shape associated with Valentine's Day. For a bridge devotee, it may be one of the four suits of cards. A coach urges the team, "Get out there and put your heart into it," meaning, "make a personal investment." A business man says, "Let's get to the heart of the matter," when he wishes to deal with the essence or core of a situation. Physiologically, an adult with a normally functioning heart tends to take the concept of heart as a cardiac pump for granted—it is an unimportant concept as long as the pump is competent. But for the person with a damaged heart, the concept has changed to include predictable or unpredictable pain and other disturbing symptoms, uncertainty, and even a threat to life. Heart could also be a nursing concept developed by an advanced clinical practitioner in a coronary-care unit. This would be a highly developed concept incorporating both knowledge and experience. It would include many subconcepts such as coronary anatomy, physiology, and pathophysiology—ischemia, edema, arrhythmia—and their effect on the patient's ability to cope with living. This nurse would respond in terms of her concept when she made discriminating judgments about almost indiscernible changes in the patient or his electrocardiographic tracing, knowing when to take action and what action to take—quickly!

The patient and his family are part of the concept, as are medical and nursing therapy. The coronary-care nurse's concept of heart is both broad and deep. *Your* current concept of heart may incorporate portions of each of those described. It will undoubtedly move toward more depth in the clinical area within the next few years.

All these concepts of heart had something in common, yet much that was different, because of experience, knowledge, and orientation. Each person would communicate and respond to "heart" on the basis of his own concept. As a nurse, one needs to be aware of his own concept, yet be prepared for differences from the concepts of others.

BUILDING A CONCEPTUAL PACKAGE

The development of a conceptual package initially involves four major steps:

1 Determining the identifying properties
2 Organizing the ideas within the concept
3 Testing the concept in situations for usefulness
4 Developing responses related to the concept

Before one can purposefully develop a conceptual package, there must be an awareness that a variety of objects, phenomena, or ideas have something in common. Chairs, for instance, come in many shapes, sizes, and colors, yet have enough attributes in common so that one becomes aware that a common concept is applicable to all of them. Until one begins to create a concept of chair and to describe the common properties and discriminating features in actual words, "chair" means very little.

Description of Identifying Properties

Once the awareness of commonality or pattern emerges, the next step is to state specifically the common attributes or patterns that enable one to identify variations in stimuli (events, phenom-

ena, ideas) that fall within the concept, at the same time discriminating from those which do not.

This process may be as concrete and simple as specifying the four equal sides and 90° angles that are necessary to categorize a shape as square. Such a description of properties of the concept of square would enable any viewer to identify a square shape regardless of size, substance, or location. And it certainly would enable him to discriminate between squares and other geometric shapes, such as triangles, circles, and even rectangles or parallelograms, where the approximation is close. To be sure, not all concepts are so concrete or so explicit.

In nursing, the practitioner will be concerned with physiologic concepts such as fluid balance, shock, sexuality, and functional concepts such as immobility, sensory deprivation and overload, anxiety, and many others that are discussed in this section. Eventually, discrimination will be needed between such closely related concepts as acceptance and tolerance, sickness and disability, health and illness, just as it could be necessary to discriminate between square and rectangle.

Whether a concept is concrete or abstract, decidedly distinct from others or tending to overlap, the goal in beginning to define a concept is to state as precisely as possible the attributes that characterize stimuli to be recognized as falling within the concept. This description includes:

1 The characteristic commonalities of attributes (all spiders have eight legs)
2 The range or variability that still falls within the conceptual package (e.g., the age range of children that still falls within the concept "infant")
3 Characteristics which do not influence inclusion or exclusion from a concept (e.g., color, size, material, and location neither exclude a piece of furniture from the concept "chair" nor indicate its inclusion)

For some examples of criteria which nurses have set up for identifying and organizing data within nursing situations, see Witt's description of the characteristics of anxiety or of displacement, in Part 3, Chapter 9. Other books in which concepts are similarly developed include *Developing Behavioral Concepts in Nursing* (Zderad and Belcher, 1968), *Behavioral Concepts and Nursing Intervention* (Carlson, 1970), or *Advanced Concepts in Clinical Nursing* (Kintzel, 1971).

Look up the concept of anxiety. See if you can identify the attributes that would enable you to categorize responses in yourself or others within this concept. Does it put them into perspective? Try to develop some identifying criteria for a concept of your own choosing. (It is best to begin with a fairly concrete, simple concept, since this type of thinking is difficult at best.)

Organizing Ideas within a Concept

The second step in developing a usable conceptual package is to organize the ideas and subconcepts that fall within the package. This may be done in several ways. Engel used a sequential pattern in describing the stages of grief and mourning in which the loss of a valued love object is followed first by shock and disbelief, then by the development of awareness of the loss, and finally by restitution (Engel, 1962). Another way of classifying and grouping ideas within a concept was used by Carnevali and Brueckner in their development of the concept of immobilization. They grouped ideas and data according to areas and causes of immobilization, extent, duration and direction of change, side effects, and the degree of volition involved in the immobility (Carnevali and Brueckner, 1970).

This organization of ideas within a concept helps the user to make more discriminating observations and responses. For example:

A nurse came to care for a patient-client and noticed wet, wheezy-sounding respirations, and cough, new symptoms in this patient. Because this patient had cardiac pump problems, the nurse immediately considered the concept of edema, specifically pulmonary edema (see Part 3, Chapter 15), as possibly explaining the dynamics of the new symptoms. She set about to see if additional data would fit with this concept. The record showed more fluid intake than recorded output—but someone might have forgotten to chart some of the output. As she removed a supportive binder from the patient's trunk she noticed that there were deep ridges in rather doughy-feeling tissue on his back and abdomen. These signs reinforced the validity of edema as an explanatory concept. She examined the skin on his legs; it was taut and shiny. When she pressed her fingers into the tissue the imprint remained, additional verification of her original conceptual explanation of the situation. Her concept of "edema" enabled her to take two symptoms plus knowledge of the physiology of heart failure, pull a concept from her file, and use it to make additional systematic observations quickly as a basis for valid diagnosis and appropriate action.

Testing the Concept

The third step in concept development is that of testing the concept empirically (i.e., in "real-life" situations). It is all well and good to dream up a concept, but its practical value must be tested. Here the conceptualizer tries to apply the concept he has built in a variety of possible situations with the goal of testing whether he can:

1 Recognize and classify stimuli within the situation by using his identifying criteria
2 Exclude stimuli that do not fall within the concept
3 Explain the dynamics of the situation by using the organization he has developed within the concept
4 Accurately predict outcomes or responses within a situation based on the concept

The following situation is a real one for many students. It offers a potentially personal experience in which a concept may be tested.

It is early afternoon. Tomorrow you face an examination, one that carries real weight in your chosen career goals. You settle down with your books and notes to prepare for it. You begin to read and review, but your mind will not "stay put" . . . you get up . . . wander over and turn on the radio . . . hit the books again . . . get up and go to the kitchen for some food . . . come back, try again . . . put it down . . . phone a friend—the line is busy . . . you feel increasingly uneasy . . . the deadline is approaching . . . you make a trip to the bathroom . . . now maybe you can concentrate . . . unable to focus . . . cannot remember . . . shift position . . . try another chair . . . get up and walk about . . . say the words. . . .

In a sense you are *immobilized*—you are certainly not moving toward your goal of becoming adequately prepared for the test. Still, the concept of immobilization does not explain the dynamics of your situation very well. Try the concept of *anxiety*. The data: decreased intellectual function is associated with moderate-to-severe levels of anxiety; the restlessness and uneasiness also fit as signs of a state of anxiety. The test is a genuine threat to your continued status as a student in your chosen field and therefore fits with the attribute of threat to self that is the genesis of the concept of anxiety. Therefore you could feel secure in testing the concept further by determining whether the stated dynamics within the conceptualization explains the situation and offers potential outcomes and problem-solving options.

The concept of anxiety incorporates the idea that when a threat to self is perceived, the resultant sensation is one of discomfort ranging from mild uneasiness to absolute panic. In order to dispel these disagreeable sensations, relief-seeking behavior is undertaken. This may or may not result in removal of the threat and subsequent relief. If the threat is one of not meeting expectations (those of oneself or others), the options may take one of two avenues: (1) modify the goals to more achievable ones; (2) evolve more successful techniques that will permit achievement of present goals. Since mild anxiety is a helpful influence in learning, the goal in the present test situation is not to remove anxiety

entirely but to bring it down to a productive level—to make it work for you, not against you.

Now how could you operationalize these options to the situation that faces you on this afternoon before the examination? In lowering or modifying the goals, several options may be possible. You may have wanted to get an A on the exam; could you settle for a B or even less? Are there any other options for succeeding in the course such as outside work, papers? Should you extend the time within which you accomplish the set goal by withdrawing from the present course and taking it again in order to assure that you have adequate knowledge and skills? The second avenue of approach is to strive with more effectiveness to meet the goal. Could you find someone else who is less anxious with whom you could study, so that you will have an outside focusing force? Can you set up a time schedule and allocate smaller sections of what is to be reviewed so that the task is less global, more defined and manageable?

It would seem that a conceptualization of anxiety could be an effective means of explaining and dealing with the pretest situation described. Try to think of other situations, involving other threats to self, in which the concept would also be useful. Imagine the situation rather specifically, and again apply the concept. Through this vicarious experiencing, through reading, as well as in real life, concept effectiveness can be tested.

Developing Responses Related to the Concept

The final step in initial concept development is that of considering responses that are logically related to the concept. These responses tend to fall into two categories—verbal responses and behavioral ones.

The *verbal* response is that of applying the concept label to presenting stimuli, even though the few units of information represent only a piece of the whole situation. Seeing a patient in a cast and in traction, as illustrated in Part 3, Chapter 11, one may respond verbally with "immobilization," or "potential sensory reduction." On learning that a person is torn between two unacceptable alternatives, such as mutilating surgery or fatal cancer, one might also respond verbally with "immobilization." The nurse in the earlier paragraph responded to the wet-wheezing breathing and cough in her patient by diagnosing the condition as edema. Since in labeling, the response is to a few stimuli, the concept selected influences the direction of additional observation and interpretation. It follows, then, that the selecting of a concept that validly applies to the situation is very important.

The *behavioral* response is that of action. One often responds to "chair" by sitting on the piece of furniture, to "book" by opening it, turning the pages, and looking at the contents. In nursing most concepts are more complex, and so are the actions. In Chapter 18, for instance, you will read about the concepts of pressure and ischemia (lack of blood supply to tissues). You could respond in terms of these concepts when you see a patient who tends to lie in one position for several hours at a time. Perhaps he cannot move himself, or it hurts to turn. Noticing these cues becomes a signal to use the *pressure-ischemia* concept as a basis for moving the patient and examining the tissues at points of pressure for any of the cardinal signs of poor blood supply. Beyond this you might decide on other responses, such as setting up a turning schedule, teaching the patient, and continuing observation of pressure points. As Doby suggests in his chapter "Science and Concepts," one of the functions of concepts is to provide a tool that gives direction to activity (Doby, 1954, p. 25).

STAGES IN DEVELOPING SKILLS OF CONCEPTUALIZING

Becoming a skilled conceptualizer is a long-term project but one that can bring a continuing sense of achievement. In the beginning, one is hampered by the small number of personally developed "working concepts." You may notice, as you proceed through this section of the book, that upon reading about the concept of anxiety, you will apply that concept to many situations. Later the concept of immobilization may suddenly become preferable. This is a stage of your development, one that was experienced by all of us.

As you develop a larger store of working conceptual packages, you will find yourself quickly testing first one and then another, seeking the one with the best "fit." Even as you are working in a situation, when one concept becomes less productive as a source of direction in thinking and action, you will find yourself seeking more effective ones. This is the continuing dual challenge—developing a store of increasingly precise, well-organized concepts, and developing finesse in applying them.

REFERENCES

Carlson, Carolyn, "Behavioral Concepts and Nursing Intervention," J. B. Lippincott Company, Philadelphia, 1970.

Carnevali, Doris, and Susan Brueckner: Immobilization, Reassessment of a Concept, *American Journal of Nursing,* **70**:1502–1507 (1970).

Doby, John, "An Introduction to Social Research," The Stackpole Company, Harrisburg, Pa., 1954.

Engel, G. L., "Psychological Development in Health and Disease," W. B. Saunders Company, Philadelphia, 1962.

Kintzel, Kay Corman (ed.), "Advanced Concepts in Clinical Nursing," J. B. Lippincott Company, Philadelphia, 1971.

Reif, Kerry: "A Heart Makes You Live," *American Journal of Nursing,* **72**:1085 (1972).

Zderad, Loretta, and Helen Belcher, "Developing Behavioral Concepts in Nursing," Southern Regional Education Board, Atlanta, 1968.

Psychosocial and Mental-Emotional Status

Rosemary Witt and Pamela Mitchell

Data about a person's psychosocial situation and mental-emotional status are rather neatly separated in the assessment tool shown in Part 2, Chapter 6. The concepts related to these areas of function cannot be so nicely separated, however. Nor can the nurse readily segment the categories of information when he attempts to use them with any particular patient-client's problems. For example, Rosemary Witt presents the concept of anxiety in Section A of this chapter. Anxiety is a state of feeling (emotional) which is similar in most people. However, many of the situations which cause anxious feelings are peculiar to each person. A person's family, cultural, and social experiences (psychosocial area) largely determine which particular situations provoke anxiety in him. Consequently, to help a person who appears to be anxious, a nurse must be able to combine understanding of the feelings accompanying anxiety, the kinds of general social and environmental situations which may provoke anxiety, and the sociocultural factors which determine anxiety-provoking situations for a particular person.

The concepts presented in this chapter are only a few of the many relevant to a person's social, emotional, and intellectual function. The authors selected these concepts because we feel that they are common to the kinds of problems which beginning practitioners and their patient-clients face, and are basic to achieving a collaborative nurse-client relationship.

Much of the data collected in assessment of psychosocial/mental-emotional functioning is rather private. Beginning nurses often feel uncomfortable in discussing these "personal" areas

139

with patients or clients. When you have finished this chapter, we hope that you will see the importance of these data and will know how to use them, either to prevent problems for some patients and clients or to understand and work with the "problem behavior" of others.

Data to Be Assessed

General social status	Psychological status
Ethnic background	Placement in hierarchy of basic need fulfillment
Occupation	Development level achieved
Economic status	Level of anxiety
Religious practices	Defense mechanisms utilized
Type of housing accommodation	Mental-emotional status
Contacts or previous referrals to social agencies	Level of consciousness or awareness of self
Family or peer-group status	Orientation to time, place, and person
Position in family	Intellectual development relative to age
Others in family	Mental skills
With whom the person lives	Perception and understanding of health problem—
Marital status	goals of therapy
Role in family	Beliefs and attitudes toward health and illness
Social developmental status	Previous experiences and reactions to illness or
Age	hospitalization
Sex	Use of drugs to alter emotional or intellectual
Marital status	behavior
Degree of dependence and independence	
Sexuality	

Section A: Psychosocial Status[1]

Nursing is a service to people. To provide this service effectively, the nurse must have knowledge of the components which together make up the whole man. These components may be studied in varying degrees of specificity or generality. Usually the components are divided into two broad groupings: the *soma* and the *psyche*. The soma includes the physical or biological elements; knowledge of it is drawn from the natural sciences. The psyche is comprised of the psychological, social, and cultural elements which influence man. Knowledge of the latter is drawn from the social sciences, including psychology, sociology, and anthropology. Readings may be found which describe the various levels at which man functions within this broad classification. As

illustration, the student may read about man as an emotional being, a rational being, a social being, or a spiritual being. But while reading about these specific aspects one must not forget that man is more than a sum of all these parts. Also not to be forgotten is the idea that activity or change at any one of these levels will call for some sort of change or adjustment in other levels.

For clarity in presentation, however, the major focus of this section will be on the psychosocial elements. Attention will be given to factors which provide partial explanations as to why man, or the patient-client in particular, behaves as he does. The partial explanations will be achieved by looking at behavior learned in the process of growth and development; behavior suggested to the person by the family and cul-

[1] This section was written by Rosemary Witt.

tural group in which he is reared; and behavior frequently evoked by discomfort or anxiety. If the student gains knowledge related to these factors, he will then begin to see how they combine to give each person a unique way of responding to, or behaving in, various life situations.

The definitions given to the term *behavior* are many and varied. Wiedenbach has defined it as the individual's response, both verbal and nonverbal, to a stimulus (Wiedenbach, 1964). The response is based on the way the person is thinking or feeling. However, as nurses we are unable to observe what another person is thinking or feeling. What can be observed, by the use of all the senses, are cues which allow an inference to be made about the way the person is thinking or feeling. Inferences are the meanings attached to the cues observed, after comparing these observed cues to the knowledge gained in studying the various behavioral and biological sciences. For this reason it is of great importance that nurses cultivate keen observational powers.

IMPORTANCE OF PSYCHOSOCIAL ELEMENTS

As stated previously, the human organism functions as a total unit. Its physiological functioning is affected by its psychosocial functioning and vice versa. The clearest example of this unity is the physiological response to anxiety. When a person is anxious about a situation, such as marital difficulties, his body responds with what is known as the "fight-flight reaction." His body does not differentiate between a threat in the psychosocial field and one in the physiological area; it responds the same way in each situation. The details of this response will be discussed later in this chapter. In reverse, the person who is experiencing some physiological disturbance, such as impaired hearing, will be required to make adjustments in the psychosocial field. He may spend less time with other people, or he may not perceive accurately what has been said, thus causing misunderstandings in his interpersonal relationships. Some theorists suggest that many of the disease entities experienced by people have their roots in the psychological field of the person. Examples frequently listed are peptic ulcer, ulcerative colitis, asthma, and rheumatoid arthritis.

Psychosocial elements also play an important role in determining what a person defines as illness, when and if he should seek help or treatment, and, once help is sought, how much information he will share concerning his symptoms. Psychosocial elements will also influence how well he will cooperate with the suggested treatments, such as taking medications.

Knowledge of the psychosocial elements of behavior is also important because when a person becomes defined as a patient-client, he will continue to experience the same problems and concerns experienced prior to his illness. For example, if the patient-client is a small child he will probably continue or increase his attempts toward both physical and psychological growth and development. If he is in the stage of developing autonomy, he will probably display behavior which is self-asserting. This may be considered problematic by the nurse, unless he understands the reasons for, and importance of, continuing this behavior. If the patient-client is an adult, he may be involved in behavior which attempts to gratify his basic need for self-esteem. He may perceive his illness as a threat to this goal, and may therefore ignore or deny the treatments which interfere with meeting this need. The concerns of the person may be accentuated because of the individual's lessened ability to participate completely owing to his illness. Other areas of concern which may be accentuated include an increase in financial burdens related to the illness, and separation from the persons who provide him with love and a sense of belonging.

Many other factors could be enumerated, but the above examples were pointed out to emphasize the importance to the nurse of developing skills and attitudes which will help the patient-client to meet his continuing psychosocial needs. This is an area of care in which each nurse can make a significant contribution toward improving the patient-client's welfare; it is the area which recipients of health care most frequently claim is neglected. Because the nurse spends a great deal of time observing and interacting with patient-clients, it is his responsibility to recognize cues that indicate when psychosocial needs are not being met; to collect data which will help him to make inferences concerning which particular needs require gratification; and to provide interventions which allow the patient-client an opportunity to meet his needs.

BASIC OR MOTIVATING NEEDS

One of the motivating factors in a person's behavior is his attempt to fulfill his basic needs. Need is defined as a requirement of a person, which if supplied, relieves or diminishes his immediate distress or improves his immediate sense of adequacy and well-being (Orlando, 1961). Maslow compiled a list of needs which he considered basic to human growth and development. They include physiological drives and needs for safety, love, esteem, and self-actualization. They are usually emergent in that order (Maslow, 1943).

Physiological Drives

The physiological drives include the need for oxygen, food and fluids, elimination, rest and activity, shelter, and sex. This grouping of needs is also referred to as "survival needs," because they are vital for continuing physical existence. An exception to this statement is the need for sexual activity; as important as it is to people, it is not absolutely necessary for individual survival. The physiological needs are the most prepotent of all, and unless they are fulfilled, the person will be unable to move to the next higher level of motivation. However, when these needs are met, the person is motivated to move onward. Thus Maslow suggested that these human needs arrange themselves in a hierarchy of dominance; as one need is satisfied and thus becomes less dominant, another need becomes strong and demands satisfaction. This is a slow, gradual process. The person may never completely satisfy each of the needs, but will satisfy each to such an extent that he can move to the next level in the need hierarchy. As the person moves upward in this hierarchy he is also meeting growth and development needs.

The remaining needs that Maslow identified include those that are learned or acquired. This grouping of needs is sometimes referred to as "secondary motives" or "social motives" (Brennecke and Amick, 1971). The designation of secondary does not in any way suggest that they are less important than the primary, or physiological, needs. They are called secondary because they are not directly related to physiological drives. Probably in our society, where basic survival needs are easily fulfilled, the secondary needs are the main motivators of our behavior.

Brennecke and Amick (1971) have related the needs identified by Maslow to the chronological growth and development pattern of people. This relationship may make it more easy for the student to comprehend the motivating factors in Maslow's hierarchy of needs. For example, in infancy our primary job is to survive. The infant needs other things, too, but the major emphasis will be on meeting the physiological needs.

Safety Needs   When the person reaches childhood he has some confidence that his physiological needs will be gratified. At this time his emergent need is for security and safety. Safety means the need to experience the absence of threat or danger. The threat or danger may be perceived in either the internal or external environment. The child with this emergent need wants to explore his environment, to find out what is safe or unsafe. At this time, he will also be told by the significant others who are responsible for his care and protection, what he can or cannot do. By these two methods, he will develop patterns of thoughts and actions which will lead to a sense of safety. In working with an adult who has never had this need completely fulfilled, we may find that much of his behavior is motivated by attempts to establish a feeling of safety. This motivation is probably on an unconscious level, meaning that it is not at a level of awareness which the person can verbalize. In fact, most of the needs which motivate people are on an unconscious level. Even those persons who have had this need met to a great extent in childhood still seek safety, as indicated in the preference for the familiar and known, rather than the unfamiliar and unknown. Other indications of security needs are desires to maintain a savings account, to have insurance of varying kinds, and to have a job which has some permanence. These needs may become most prepotent in times of emergencies such as war, social disorganization, and illness. Thus some of a patient-client's behavior may be motivated by attempts to feel safe in an environment which is probably unknown and is no doubt perceived as threatening. In addition to this, an internal threat is related to not knowing what will actually be the outcome of an illness.

Love Needs When the physiological and safety needs are fairly well satisfied, the needs for love, affection, and belonging emerge. As Brennecke and Amick suggest, the person begins to seek out, discover, and test his relationships with others. The child wants to know the quality of his belonging and the depth of the affection of his significant others (Brennecke and Amick, 1971). In growth and development, emergence of affection needs also coincides with the time a child is experiencing interaction with his peer group and later the development of the chum

relationship. When this need is prepotent in either the developing child or in the adult, he actually feels the absence of the love of his family and friends, and the security he experiences by being a member of a social group. He also misses the opportunity to give love to those persons as well as receive it. One can easily see how this need may become dominant to the patient-client who is separated from the significant others in his life. This need also points out why so much stress is given to the development of the nurse-patient relationship.

Esteem Needs Once the individual has satisfied himself that he is able to love and be loved, he begins to be strongly impelled to discover who or what this loved and loving person actually is. The individual attempts to discover his self; to see how strong he is, how adequate he is, how independent he is, and what he can achieve (Brennecke and Amick, 1971). He evaluates himself as to his accomplishments, and is also evaluated by others. When the evaluation is based on realistic factors and accomplishments, the individual feels self-confident, worthy, and capable, and is also accorded praise, recognition, and status by others. If the esteem needs are not met, the person may feel inferior, weak, or helpless. Consider the blow that may occur to the patient-client when he finds out that activities such as a job, or athletic pursuits, which have led to esteem in the past, must be curtailed because of an illness. The nurse may witness behavior which is an attempt to gain esteem in other areas of life. Perhaps the patient-client will attempt to direct his own treatment or give advice to other patients as to how they should behave. He may attempt to increase his self-esteem by being more knowledgeable than the nurse about certain medical practices or procedures.

Self-actualization Needs Self-actualization is the desire for self-fulfillment, to make actual all the potential elements and facets of selfhood.

Types of behavior which will fulfill this need are diverse and unique to each person. It may be self-actualizing to be the best possible nurse, or wife, or husband. It may be self-actualizing to write books, or paint pictures, or compose music. It may be self-actualizing to appreciate the uniqueness of one's self and of other human beings, and to strive toward making more rich the life of one's associates. Unfortunately, most of us are too busy meeting our security needs, or love needs, or esteem needs to achieve our full self-actualizing potential. Maslow suggests that only about 1 percent of the population are really self-actualizing people.

Maslow adds two more needs to his list of basic needs: the need to know and the need to understand. He suggests that these needs are always present along with the others, and allow us to meet the others more efficiently. Brennecke and Amick suggest that these cognitive needs are more fully developed after an individual has achieved his potential, or become self-actualized. Jourard has added other needs to Maslow's list: the need for health, both physical and mental, the need for freedom, challenge, cognitive clarity, and varied experience. Jourard indicates that each person ranks needs in order of importance to himself, but that all are essential to human life (Jourard, 1963). He agrees with Maslow that to understand another person's behavior or motivation, it is important to know what basic need is most urgent at a given time.

SOCIOCULTURAL INFLUENCES ON BEHAVIOR

The sociocultural environment in which a person is reared has a potent influence on him; it provides a type of blueprint which regulates many aspects of his behavior. Through continued association with family members, kinship groups, friends, neighbors, and work associates, each person learns what should or should not be valued; which actions and kinds of behavior are considered normal, healthy, or permissible in any given situation; and which actions or kinds of behavior are considered abnormal, unhealthy, or unacceptable. Learning not only takes place through verbalization by members of the sociocultural groups, but also is transmitted through observation of, and participation with, the various individuals in these groupings. The blueprints, or rules and regulations, that are handed down might be thought of as sociocultural prescriptions, since they guide the individual. These sociocultural prescriptions have two functions: (1) they provide assurance of the maintenance of the environmental equilibrium, and (2) they provide for fulfillment of the needs of the individual. Variations in these prescriptions may be introduced by the person's place of residence, socioeconomic status, or level of education (Beland, 1970). The student is encouraged to read Part 1, Chapter 1, for a discussion of the effect of sociocultural influences on a person's perceptions of health and illness.

It is important for the nurse to be aware of the varying sociocultural prescriptions, so that he may understand the patient-client's behavior in context. The nurse may cause the patient-client anxiety if he expects behavior for which the patient-client has previously been admonished. Also, he may not be able to help the patient-client unless he can offer help which is acceptable within the client's social and cultural values. The nurse, too, is a product of various sociocultural factors, and may be indoctrinated with different values and standards than those of the patient. When the nurse is then introduced to behavior that he has classified as wrong, unhealthy, or deviant, he may also experience anxiety. It is helpful to recognize differences as just that; the fact that the behavior of another person is different does not make him unacceptable, inferior, or wrong.

Sociocultural factors and their related values which are generally thought to be significant and which would affect the behavioral responses of both the patient-client and the nurse have been identified by many authors. The following discussion is based on the values identified by Beland (1970) and Leininger (1970). Any attempt to detail the characteristics of each social and cultural group from which our clients come would be superficial. Therefore, the student is referred to the references at the end of this chapter and to Part 2, Chapter 7, for further readings in this area.

Value Placed on Life

Glaser and Strauss state that in the American culture "life is preferable to whatever may follow it." [2] This brief statement seems to summarize the beliefs and attitudes of most Americans. Evidence of this idea is apparent in the many efforts to prolong the length of life, sometimes without consideration of the fullness or richness of the life that has been prolonged. Technology has developed many ways of prolonging life, the prime example being the ability to replace diseased organs with more healthy transplanted organs or mechanical devices. Centers have also been developed where the deceased can "be quickly deep-frozen and placed in a special building of low temperature, awaiting the day when science and technology have advanced enough to defrost them, to return to life and back to society" (Kubler-Ross). [3]

In a society where life is so highly valued, it is not surprising that death is a frightening event and that attempts are made to avoid and ignore this reality. Attempts to avoid it are demonstrated by the facts that until recently death was not publicly discussed, and that when discussions did center on death, the participants usually exhibited signs of discomfort. It is no wonder that both the patient who is dying and the

nurse who is providing care find this normal life event overwhelming. Further discomfort is generated because death is an unknown; none of us has a chance to ready himself for something that is unknown.

Even with these factors in mind, we must recognize it as a reality that people do die and that nurses are given responsibility for providing care for the dying person. As beginning nursing students, you may not be providing care for persons when their death is imminent, but you will be caring for patient-clients who may be anticipating their death in the near future. The process of dying progresses through many stages, beginning with the first detection of symptoms by the patient to the terminal stage (Schoenberg, 1970). During this period the patient may experience times of well-being and times of acute distress.

The person who faces death, faces many problems and reactions. The reactions of the dying person have been studied extensively by Kubler-Ross. On the basis of interviews with 200 dying patients, Ross has proposed that the dying person goes through five stages in the process of accepting death. The five stages she conceptualized are (1) denial and isolation, (2) anger, (3) bargaining, (4) depression, and (5) acceptance. The student is urged to read her book, *On Death and Dying*, to gain knowledge of individual reactions within each of these stages, plus suggested interventions. Ross stresses the importance of allowing the patient to move through these stages at his own pace, and the helpfulness of listening at each stage (Kubler-Ross, 1969).

Students frequently raise the question about the advisability of telling the patient with a terminal illness the truth about his disease. No easy answer is available. Much has been written concerning both the positive and negative values in advising the patient of his approaching death. Kubler-Ross suggests that all patients *know* that they are dying, and also know *when* they are dying. Schoenberg believes that when the patient

[2] Barney G. Glaser and Anselm Strauss, "Awareness of Dying," Aldine Publishing Company, Chicago, 1965, p. 3.

[3] Reprinted by permission of The Macmillan Company from "On Death and Dying," by Elisabeth Kubler-Ross, copyright The Macmillan Company, New York, 1969.

is told the truth about his illness he is given an opportunity to settle financial affairs, resolve religious problems, express feelings to family members, and resolve differences with friends, and is also given a feeling of control because his knowledge allows him to make decisions and help make future plans for his family (Schoenberg, 1970). Other authors caution against this practice since the truth may precipitate a reaction of depression, emotional disorganization, and withdrawal from reality.

If it is decided to tell the patient that he is dying, this is usually done by the attending physician or the patient's family. Imparting this knowledge to the patient is not an all-or-nothing process but is a gradual one based on the patient's readiness to deal with this fact. When the patient is told, Kubler-Ross stresses the importance of emphasizing the aspects of the situation which can be controlled—especially pain. It is also important to allow for some hope—such as the fact that the condition was diagnosed early, or that new medications and techniques are being discovered each day, or that one really never knows definitely when death will occur. These explanations must be valid, not given as false reassurance. It is also important to convey to the patient that he will not be deserted. Many people have written about the loneliness associated with dying (Kubler-Ross, 1969).

Most patients seem to fear the process of dying more than death itself. The process of dying connotes decompensation, lingering debilitation, loneliness, emotional abandonment and isolation from relatives and friends, and the ultimate loss of control over one's own life (Robinson, 1968). It is in this process that nurses can be of greatest help. Since man throughout his life has needed people, there is no reason why he should not need someone more at this time of stress (Francis and Munjas, 1968). Because of our cultural attitude toward death, the nurse may find it difficult to share in another person's dying.

The difficulty is also complicated because in the education involved in becoming a nurse, one is taught to do everything possible to save human life. When a patient is close to death, the nurse may have a feeling of helplessness, and perhaps guilt that he has not done everything possible. The nurse, deprived of the usual gratifications of success, may also feel anger because the patient has not responded to his efforts. Frequently these feelings of helplessness, guilt, or anger may prompt the nurse to withdraw, either emotionally or physically, from the patient at the time when he needs him most—at the time when the patient fears abandonment. The sharing of the dying process may also be difficult for the nurse because it forces him to face the fact of his own eventual death. If the nurse has worked with the patient for any length of time, he will also be forced to deal with a personal and social loss. This loss is made more difficult if the death is unexpected, or if the person is young, perhaps a child or someone near the age of the nurse.

To anticipate and overcome some of these difficulties, each nurse must come to grips with his own thoughts and feelings concerning death and dying. This can be accomplished through discussions with classmates, instructors, families, and friends, and through pertinent reading. Once these feelings and attitudes are brought into conscious awareness, they may be modified, changed, or reaffirmed.

Current literature offers suggestions for care of the dying patient that may be helpful when planning intervention. Quint suggests that it is helpful for the nurse to switch from a recovery focus to a comfort focus; comfort must be of both a physical and a psychological nature (Quint, 1967). Physical care may be looked upon as challenging and active; such an attitude helps to overcome the feelings of helplessness experienced by both the patient and the nurse. The patient and the nurse together can decide how to handle such problems as pain, sleep, food, and rest. Robinson has set forth guidelines in providing psychological comfort:

1 Be available and humane. Make time to spend with this patient. His opportunity for friendship and reciprocal communication is limited.

2 Allow the patient to set the pace. If the patient utilizes denial, do not try to break down this defense. Should an actual choice be necessary, the patient's defensive operation must be supported. If the patient wishes to discuss his death, he should not be cajoled into changing the subject. This may comfort the listener, but it does not change the character of the patient's preoccupation.

3 Focus on the present. The future does not exist for the dying patient. Help him to cram all that is possible into today.

4 Keep communications open. When either patient or nurse feels that expression is no longer feasible, then the opportunity for supportive nursing care is lost. Within the confines of the attending physician's orders, every effort must be made to keep the channels of communication open.[4]

The people who love a person who is dying also need help in coping with feelings about the impending death, and in grieving after the death. Most of us expect that a family will grieve after their loved one's death, yet we forget that mourning occurs during the dying process as well. The stages which Kubler-Ross describes in conjunction with dying are similar to those involved in grieving. Part of dying involves mourning for the loss of oneself.

Engel (1964) describes the process of grieving in several stages. First is a period of disbelief, which parallels Kubler-Ross's stage of denial and isolation. Developing awareness, the second stage, may occur minutes to hours after the death. During the dying process, anger and bargaining represent a time of developing awareness. After death, crying, anger, or repression of crying may occur and should be accepted. The work of mourning comes in the third stage, that of restitution. Engel notes that the formal funeral practices of a culture help ease this recognition of the finality of death, and provide others to support the mourners. The major work occurs during the process of resolving the loss, or coming to grips with it. This resolution may take a year or more and is probably exacerbated each time a holiday or other period of seasonal memories occurs.

Initially, the mourner is preoccupied, as was the dying person, with himself and his loss. Gradually he begins to move out of himself and to regain interest in the world about him. At some point he probably idealizes the lost one and represses any negative feelings about him. In normal grief work this idealization is gradually replaced with a more realistic memory of both the desired and undesired attributes of the lost person. At this point grief work is considered successfully completed. This normal process may be arrested or altered at any point, and a pathological grieving may result.

The nurse and other professionals who are caring for a dying person must often deal with the grief work of the person's family as well as with that of the dying one himself. When a person dies, his family remains and may need considerable help. Engel suggests that news of the death be given to the family as a group so that they will have each other's support. Further he emphasizes the importance of allowing emotional expression as the impact of the news hits the family, and of providing a private place for them to express their grief.

Nurses may encounter people in the later stages of mourning either in the community or in health-care agencies if these persons have become patients themselves. In order to help such people, the nurse must first recognize that grief is present. People may grieve not only when they lose another person, but also when they have lost a body part, mobility, or anything which they hold central to their conception of themselves (Engel, 1964).

[4] Lisa Robinson, "Psychological Aspects of the Care of Hospitalized Patients," F. A. Davis Company, Philadelphia, 1967.

Once the nurse has recognized that a person is mourning, he can provide opportunities for the person to talk about his grief, to acknowledge it, and to work through the acceptance of the loss. The nurse must be patient, for such work may take much time. It is hard for people of our culture to talk about grief or loss, and many grieving persons will "cover up" unless they know that the nurse is really willing to listen.

Value Placed on Individual Achievement

In the American culture we have always given recognition and praise to the person who has achieved success, and even more recognition if he has achieved this success independently. These two factors can have great significance for the person who becomes ill. If success has been achieved, he may feel that his previous accomplishments will be threatened; or if the person is young, he may feel that his illness will limit his chance for future success.

Since we also place great importance on independence in our culture, it is frequently hard for the patient to accept the enforced dependency that often accompanies the sick role. As nurses we may understand the therapeutic benefits derived from accepting this dependent role, and may wonder why the patient fights it. However, to many patients acceptance of dependency also signifies loss of control. He is no longer able to make the common decisions of daily living, such as when and where to eat, and with whom and how long he will talk.

Nurses are not immune to the influence of this value related to individual success. Many nurses express a preference toward working with patients who are acutely ill and who will get well and go home. It is as though individual success can be measured only by the fact that the patient is discharged. Sometimes it is hard to have feelings of achievement related to helping the person understand one small part of his problem, making the person more comfortable, or helping the patient die a dignified death. Individual success is sometimes measured by the nurse according to how many activities he has accomplished during the day. Nurses frequently state with pride that they have given seven complete baths between 8 A.M. and noon. It seems to be hard for some persons to measure success in terms of planning or directing the care of a patient.

Values Placed on Time

In the American culture there may be various orientations concerning time, but the general tendency is to consider the future of great importance. With this orientation it is easy to understand why many patient-clients will be concerned about the long-range effects of illness or of various treatments. A patient may be hesitant, for instance, to take a narcotic for the immediate relief of pain, because he may be afraid of addiction in the future. Or a patient may not consent to a surgical procedure which is considered lifesaving because of the future disfiguring effect. For example, the chance of metastasis (spread) of cancer may be decreased if a breast is removed, but the patient may refuse because she feels the surgery would have devastating effects on her future.

In general, Americans who are future-oriented are desirous of early diagnosis and treatment so that they can look forward to a healthy future. Many persons feel they should have a yearly health examination. Middle- and upper-middle-class Americans also spend a great deal of money preparing for the future; they enroll in retirement plans and buy health and life insurance. Contributions are liberal to volunteer organizations such as the American Heart Association or American Cancer Society in the hope that our futures may be free of these diseases.

In contrast, low-income Americans as a group do not share this orientation toward the future and to what professionals consider preventive health care. A feeling of powerlessness, meaninglessness, and isolation characterizes the viewpoint of the poor. Attitudes of fatalism, resignation to the vicissitudes of life, and orientation to the present are a consequence of these perceptions (Irelan and Besner, 1968). Related to health, these attitudes are expressed by statements such as, "Nothin' you can do 'bout gettin' sick."

Disease, disability, and isolation from the health-care system are greater in this group than in the population as a whole. Yet even when free health care is easily accessible, persons of low income often do not avail themselves of care unless they are severely ill. Failure to keep appointments for regular health care is more common among this group than among upper-working- and middle-class people (Irelan and Besner, 1968). Many observers have interpreted this lack of use of health facilities and preventive care as evidence that low-income persons do not value health so much as do middle-income persons and health professionals.

Brinton (1972) suggests that the lower-income mother's definition of health is a greater factor in her behavior than are the values she professes to place on health. Brinton measured the priorities which community health nurses and low-income mothers placed on health, and the importance which they assigned to such behavior as getting immunizations, following physician's advice, and taking a child to the physician when the child is ill.

The nurses, when tested separately, predicted that the mothers would place low priority on health and would rank many kinds of health behavior as of low importance. This was not borne out by the mothers' rankings, however. The values regarding health and health behavior were quite similar in the two groups; only the nurses' perceptions of the mothers' values differed. The nurses probably responded in terms of the prevalent stereotype of the low-income person as devaluing health, and on the basis of their

knowledge that a large percentage of such mothers do not keep appointments for their children's care.

Many of the women in the study considered health as the absence of incapacitating illness; thus their definition of health differed from that of the health workers.

Another characteristic belief about time that permeates the middle-class American culture is the view that time itself has value. The lives of many persons tend to be dominated by a clock. Certain persons sometimes find it difficult to relax because they feel they are wasting time. This belief influences both the patient-client and the nurse. Patients may focus on the punctuality of medications, treatments, doctors' or nurses' rounds, or serving of meals. If the nurse is prompt, she is considered to be both efficient and caring. Also related to this factor is the importance that nurses give to getting activities done on time. Even though there may be several good reasons why some patients may not require a bath in the morning, many nurses seem to cling to the idea that this is the proper time for all baths to be given. Some nurses are also afraid that they will be accused of wasting their time if they talk with patients at times other than when providing some physical treatment.

It is important to the nurse to recognize the significance of these time values to many of his patients. Even more important, he must recognize his own values and behavior regarding time, preparing for the future, and preventive health care. Most nurses and physicians come from backgrounds in which the above-described middle-class attitudes and types of behavior are dominant. Some or many of their patients and clients are from groups which may hold health, achievement, and security as important, but do not behave in the same way about achieving goals related to these values. These differences may be associated with differing definitions as to what constitutes health, security, or "making it," or with a feeling of helplessness in realizing goals. Nurses who do not recognize these differences may find themselves critical of and unable to understand a client's lack of interest in keeping appointments, being on time, or seeking regular health care.

Value Placed on Cleanliness

Probably in no other culture is such stress placed on the importance of cleanliness. We seem to believe that cleanliness is truly next to godliness. Nurses may be even more convinced of the truth of this tenet than other people because of our knowledge of the germ theory. But this belief is also shared by many persons who become patients. It becomes important to both the nurse and the patient-client that the patient receive a daily bath. In some instances, e.g., in caring for an older patient, this may not be therapeutic, since a bath each day may further dry out the skin. However, if a bath is not given, the patient-client and the nurse may both experience discomfort. The patient may have been conditioned by his upbringing and also by advertisement to believe that he will be offensive if he is not bathed each day. The nurse may feel that he is not providing good nursing care if the bath is missed. Related to these feelings is our need to maintain a neat appearance. Patients will spend a great deal of time applying makeup or combing their hair, and their condition is often judged by others to be improving when they engage in such activities.

The value of cleanliness is also associated with the cultural beliefs concerning the eliminative processes. People have been so indoctrinated with the importance of washing their hands after going to the bathroom that they may experience discomfort if unable to carry out this task. Nurses may sometimes forget the importance of this attitude, and fail to offer material which allows for cleanliness after the patient uses the bedpan, thus causing the patient to experience unnecessary discomfort.

Americans usually place more emphasis on modesty than those in some other cultures. The patient-client may experience embarrassment at the shortness of his gown, or if the nurse must remain in the room when he is using the bedpan. Almost all patients have feelings of discomfort associated with intrusive procedures, such as enemas or pelvic examinations. The nurse must be aware of these feelings and always strive to provide as much privacy as possible.

Value Placed on Religious Beliefs

Almost everyone has some form of belief system which guides many of his life decisions, and to which he turns in times of distress. Often this belief system is based on the teaching of some formalized religious group, such as Judaism, Catholicism, or Protestantism. The beliefs that a person adopts from his association with any one of these groups will be motivating factors in his actions or behavior.

A person's religious beliefs frequently help him give meaning to his suffering and illness; they also may be helpful in his acceptance of future incapacities or death. At other times, however, an illness may be interpreted as God's punishment, and this feeling increases the patient's discomfort.

Within some religious doctrines, specific practices or beliefs may influence the patient-client's care. For example, a Jehovah's Witness is by doctrine not permitted to accept a blood transfusion. A member of the Church of Christ, Scientist, is taught to believe in spiritual healing, and thus will experience guilt or hesitancy in seeking the aid of a physician. Restrictions may be placed on the eating of certain foods, such as pork and shellfish for a person practicing Judaism. A member of the Church of the Latter-day Saints will not drink coffee or tea. The degree of importance given to rites varies according to personal beliefs. For instance, for a Roman Catholic and for some Protestants it is important to be baptized before death; however, this belief is not a part of the Jewish faith (Du Gas, 1972).

It is important for a beginning nursing student to become acquainted with the various belief systems and to be sensitive to the patient-client's individual wishes. The patient, himself, is frequently the most reliable source of information in planning what modifications may be required to provide acceptable nursing care. It is also helpful to consult the clergy to gain knowledge of these various beliefs as they relate to providing nursing care.

Other Influencing Sociocultural Variables

Throughout this book emphasis has been placed on how the patient-client, and the nurse, are influenced by many other sociocultural variables. The student is referred to Part 1, Chapter 1, to review how sociocultural influences help the patient-client to determine when he is ill, to identify his responsibilities when he is sick, and to know the expectations of others when he accepts the sick role. The section in this chapter on the family identifies ways in which patterns of family organization influence the patient-client's behavior. Another variable of great importance is the method of communication that is predominant in a culture or social class. For example, middle- and upper-middle-class communication tends to be primarily verbal and more abstract than blue-collar and lower-class communication. Moles (1968) describes the language of the lower working class as simple, with short sentences and without shades of meaning. Abstraction and intellectualism are not a part of the everyday business of surviving. Consequently, persons from low-income groups may tune out the nurse who uses "fancy words."

The student should also be aware that in various cultures, there are differences in the importance placed on verbal and nonverbal behavior. For example, people of Latin descent are likely to use much more nonverbal behavior than people of Anglo descent. The nurse must also become aware of his own use of nonverbal and verbal communication and attempt to see how it influences the behavior of the patient-client.

THE FAMILY

As stated previously, it is within the family setting that the sociocultural prescriptions are transmitted to the individual. It is also within the family setting that each person is introduced into the social roles, which are patterns of expected behavior. Some of these roles he will be expected to perform immediately; others will be expectations for the future. Thus it is necessary for the nurse to have some knowledge of the patient-client's family before he can begin to understand the patient-client's behavior.

The family has been conceptualized and studied in several different ways: (1) as a group of individual members, with emphasis placed on the individual rather than the group; (2) from the viewpoint of the interpersonal relations between various family members, e.g., husband and wife, or parent and child; (3) as a group, or system, with emphasis on the interaction and reaction patterns of each family-group member on all other family-group members; and (4) as a group interacting with the external environment, with attention given to how individual members within the family, and the family as a whole, meet the expectations of society. Although research is continuing in each of these conceptual frameworks, no one theory has been established to show the definite relationship of each level to the other levels of conceptualization (Meissner, 1964). It is, however, agreed that each area is important, and that each will influence the reactions of a person who experiences illness.

Each family unit has its own unique characteristics, but some similarities of functions are found universally in family units. These universal functions include the socialization of the children, the satisfaction of sexual needs, and the psychological, biological, and material maintenance of each family member (Engel, 1962). There will be variations in the ways that these functions are carried out by each family. Variations will be introduced by the location of the family. For example, there are differences in urban and rural family life in America. The urban family tends to live in a separate residence away from members of the extended family; in rural America, the nuclear family residence may include members of the extended family or they may live in close proximity. In that respect, it might be anticipated that if illness were to strike in a rural family, they would have more resources available than an urban family.

Another factor which may introduce variations in family function is the social status of the family. The roles held by individual family members tend to be influenced by the socioeconomic level of the family. For example, in studies of American class structure, it is suggested that division of labor is much more specialized in the lower-class family than in the middle-class family. Child rearing is more apt to be shared by parents in a middle-class family, whereas it is more often solely the mother's responsibility in the lower-class one (Bloom 1965; Besner, 1968). One may speculate that when there is illness, it might be more difficult to fill the role of the absent or ill member in a unit with highly specialized divisions of labor than in a family structure where more sharing of labor occurs.

The number in the family and the developmental level of each family member will also cause variations in the family functions. If the mother in a family becomes ill, for example, it makes considerable difference whether she has several small children for whom she is responsible or whether her two children have reached adulthood. If there is a teen-aged daughter in the home to care for the smaller siblings, the mother may feel much less stress than if the oldest child is an eight-year-old boy. Variation in family

functioning would also be introduced if one member of the family was absent, e.g., if the father had died, or was away a great deal on the job, or if the parents had become divorced. Each of these absences would have different effects on the family, but any one of them would call for a realignment of roles within the family. Additional people residing in the family would also affect its functioning. For example, if a grandparent was staying with the family, a different style of living might need to be mediated.

Illness within the Family

When an individual family member experiences a disease, every other member of the family experiences ramifications of this illness. This is because the family system functions as a whole, and when part of that system changes, it requires that every other part in the system make simultaneous modifications to continue functioning. For example, if Mr. King becomes ill and is hospitalized, the family source of income may be jeopardized. In order to overcome this problem, Mrs. King may begin work to meet the ongoing needs of the family. Because Mrs. King is out of the house during the day, she may ask her elderly mother in to take care of the small children. The grandmother's method of discipline may be quite different from Mrs. King's, so that stress is caused among family members. Not only does Mrs. King have to assume the role of breadwinner, she must also continue with her previous roles of providing harmony and stability in the family. Since Mr. King is cut off from his family, from whom he receives a great deal of emotional support and a sense of belonging, he may make more demands on his wife because of an intensification of these needs. Mr. King may also be experiencing anxiety on account of his illness, and wondering if he can return to his previous job. Through this example, it is apparent that illness will affect the intrapsychic functioning of family members, as well as the interpersonal relationships between various members of the family. The different role requirements of family members will also affect the internal dynamics of each member and the family's relationship with the external environment. Previously it was Mr. King's job which had established the status of the family within the community.

In the foregoing example, the assumption of a new role by Mrs. King might be characterized as an additional burden which she will probably gladly relinquish when Mr. King is again ready to assume his role in the family. However, in some instances the modification of roles within the family may be perceived as a gain for a person. If this is true, the person may not be willing to relinquish his newly acquired role, and conflict may result in the family. For example, perhaps Mrs. King finds that she enjoys going out and meeting people on her job, more than she enjoys staying home. She may not be willing to resume her previous role in the home.

Bloom also suggested that the person occupying the sick role may be reluctant to give it up (Bloom, 1965). Sickness may bring relief to a mother who has many heavy responsibilities; or the passive, dependent role of illness may provide a father with relief from the strain that his occupation causes him. Children are sometimes hesitant to give up the sick role because it is seen as escape from the more exacting obligations of behaving as a grown-up. And finally, an elderly man who has previously felt alone and uncared for may wish to continue in the sick role to go on receiving the attention of his family or the hospital staff.

The family's reaction to illness will also be dependent upon the prognosis of the disease. Reactions will differ according to whether the prognosis is nonserious and known or serious and uncertain (Gordon, 1966).

Earlier in history, the family home was the place of care for the ill person; as society has progressed, the care of the ill has become centered in the hospital. This has been attributed to the great advances in technology; the hospital could provide the most modern equipment required for care. Today, attention is again being focused on the value to an ill person of remaining in his home. Regardless of where the actual treatment is carried out, it is imperative that there be understanding and cooperation between the health-care givers and family members. This cooperation and understanding affect not only the care of the acutely ill person but also the rehabilitative and preventive aspects of health care. To gain such cooperation, the nurse must have knowledge concerning the family and its dynamics.

DEVELOPMENTAL LEVELS

As a human being progresses through life, certain cognitive, psychological, and motor developmental tasks must be completed. These tasks are similar in the development of all people; but each individual masters the task in his own way, depending on his genetic inheritance and his environment. The behavioral patterns expressed by an adult are partially a reflection of how well he has completed the various developmental tasks. These tasks usually occur in a similar pattern and within a specific age range; however, the chronological age of an individual cannot be equated with his developmental age. The task accomplished in each stage of development is never completed permanently but must be reinforced or reaffirmed throughout the person's life. As with the basic needs of man, as defined by Maslow, each stage in development must be partially completed before the next is attempted. When stages are left before partial completion, the person is handicapped in his adjustment to the environment and his relationship with other people. If the person has deficiency in several areas, his behavior may be labeled as mental illness.

It is important for the nurse to be knowledgeable about the stages of growth and development. Although very little attention is given in the following discussion to physical growth, it is of great importance, and the student should acquaint himself with this process.[5] It is important to be knowledgeable because it is the responsibility of the nurse, and of other health professionals, to support normal mastery and development. The nurse should be able to help people, e.g., parents, to acquire and utilize knowledge of situations which promote or discourage normal development. This knowledge should extend to situations which occur in both health and illness.

Eric Erikson has described eight stages of development through which man passes from birth to death; these stages will be utilized as the basis for the following discussion (Erikson, 1955).[6] Erikson proposes that with each stage of development, the person experiences a central task or crisis which must be resolved before there can be continued healthy growth. A crisis period is marked by a physical, psychological, or social change, in which the individual experiences disturbances in thoughts or feelings. These disturbances occur because the individual's previous life experiences do not suggest an immediate resolution to the emerging problem. New kinds of behavior must be learned. A crisis may be of two types: developmental or situational. A developmental crisis is considered normal since all people experience such crises in the process of growing up. Examples of a developmental crisis are weaning or toilet training. A situational crisis is precipitated by a stressful external event such as the death of a loved one or being fired from a job.

[5] See M. S. Smart and R. C. Smart, "Children: Development and Relationships," The Macmillan Company, New York, 1967; this is a helpful reference for both physical and emotional development.

[6] This is a very brief discussion of the highlights of Erikson's theory. Each student is encouraged to do further reading to expand and enhance his knowledge of this and other developmental theories. Material that appears in quotation marks in this discussion is quoted directly, by permission of Dr. Erikson, from "Growth and Crisis of the 'Healthy Personality,'" pp. 185-225, in *Personality in Nature, Society and Culture*, edited by C. Kluckhohn, H. A. Murray, and D. M. Scheider, Alfred A. Knopf, Inc., New York, 1955.

Infancy

This period of life starts with birth and continues until the emergence of the capacity for communication through speech, usually around one and one-half years of age. The central task specific to this age range is the development of *trust* rather than *mistrust*. Erikson defines trust as "what is commonly implied in reasonable trustfulness as far as others are concerned and a simple trustworthiness as far as oneself is concerned." This basic trust is regarded as the "cornerstone of a healthy personality," and is the result of the infant's learning to count on others to gratify his needs and satisfy his wishes. Some of the needs which require fulfillment at this time are for nourishment, warmth, and stimulation. The infant at first is a relatively passive recipient in his need gratification. Later as he gains more control over his motor activities, he becomes more active in this process. For example, he learns to "grasp" objects and reach out with his arms. However, the infant is still dependent on his provider, usually the mother. If for some reason the mother is unable to satisfy the infant's needs or unable to demonstrate love, the infant may develop an attitude of mistrust. At the time of weaning, the infant experiences some "sense of basic loss," and recognizes his separateness from his mother. An impression which may follow is that of having been deprived or abandoned and such an impression may leave a residue of basic mistrust. Each person must maintain a ratio of trust and mistrust in his life. As an adult, each time we enter a situation we need to differentiate how much we can trust and how much we must distrust; in this way we can anticipate when discomfort or danger may be present. When a patient-client enters the hospital, he is confronted with a new situation and new people. He does not automatically trust everyone; he looks for behavior which suggests that a particular person merits his trust. When trust has developed, the individual will be willing to share his thoughts, feelings, and experiences; he will be confident and comfortable in asking for help or accepting help when it is offered. If the ratio of mistrust is high, the patient-client may be guarded in what he shares with you or other members of the staff.

Childhood

This period of life begins with the emergence of speech and ends with a beginning need for association with compeers, i.e., when the child begins to form relationships with people of his own level who share his attitudes toward authority, activities, and the like. The age range for this developmental stage is usually considered to be one and one-half years to six years of age, and Erikson defines three central tasks during this period. The first task is acquiring a *sense of autonomy,* rather than a sense of *shame and doubt.* During this phase the child learns to accept interferences with his wishes. This learning is achieved because the person providing care begins to place more demands on the child. For instance, since the child has increased his muscular maturation, he is expected to gain control of his anal and urethal sphincter muscles. He also experiences some control over the powerful adults in his environment. He can experiment with the social modalities of "holding on" or "letting go," and thus begins the continuing struggle for autonomy. The response to this stage must be one of mutual regulation; parental or outer control must not be too demanding or too rigid. Ideally, the child develops a sense of self-control without experiencing loss of self-esteem. With experiences of a loss of self-control and parental overcontrol, the child may develop a lasting sense of doubt or shame. The patient-client who has successfully completed this stage of development exhibits behavior which shows confidence in his own decisions, and he feels comfortable when questioning the decisions of others. If this stage has been problematic, the adult may hesitate to state his opinions or may insist that others make his decisions (Simmons, 1969).

The next crisis which must be faced occurs around the age of four and five, and is that of *initiative* versus *guilt.* Erikson states that the child is now convinced that he is a person but must find out what kind of person he is going to be. The role model that he uses is that of his parents, who present a combination of images. Parents may appear beautiful and powerful, but also dangerous. During this stage, the child is getting around with ease and also has a vocabulary which allows him to ask many questions. With these new activities he can investigate what the world is really like. Also when faced with communication or situations which he cannot fully understand, he has an active imagination which fills in the details. These imaginings, or fantasies, may prove to be frightening. The child perceives himself as being "big" and "almost as good as Father and Mother." The consequences which result are related to what Freud has called the Oedipus complex. The child attempts to compete with the parent of the same sex in several spheres; because of his smallness and lack of maturation he is unable to better his opponents in reality, but he may do so in fantasy. If the message conveyed to a child at this time is that someday he will be equal to his mother or father, or perhaps better, he will feel comfortable in continuing to initiate activities, engage in energetic wishes, and seek the pleasure of conquest. However, the fantasies may lead to a sense of guilt. Guilt is a feeling that one has committed a crime, or crimes, and deeds which may have harmed others. This feeling can lead the child to the conclusion that he is basically bad. This is the time when the child's conscience is developing; and as the result of this development, he may feel the need to stifle initiative. If he perceives his actions as bad, he is afraid to act for fear that he will be found out. Adults who have successfully completed this stage are characterized by originality, creativity, and a free sense of enterprise. If this stage of development is unsatisfactory, the individual may indulge in self-restriction. If he does originate activity, he may be very upset and feel embarrassment if it does not work out as planned.

The last developmental stage of childhood, sometimes called the juvenile era, is that of *industry* versus *inferiority*. The beginning of this period coincides with the time a child enters school, and experiences a need for compeers; it ends with puberty. The age range is usually from six to about nine or eleven. The child has developed the initiative to try things and now wants to be shown how to accomplish things by himself and with others. Many of the demonstrations of how to master various tasks are accomplished in the formal educational institutions in the form of instruction, but a great deal of learning also occurs in his experiences with persons in his social environment. The child's environment now has been expanded from the members of the family, to include the teachers and children in school. His relationships outside of school time are mostly with people who are his own age and usually of the same sex.

If in the family, the school, and his relationships with other children, he is provided recognition for his task accomplishments, he will develop a sense of industry. He will feel that he is able to make things and make them well, and he will derive pleasure from work completion. Since much of the work is accomplished with age equals, he also is learning a sense of competition, compromise, cooperation, and collaboration, as well as when to rely on these various skills.

If recognition is withheld, the child may develop a sense of inadequacy. This sense of inadequacy may be prompted because the previous steps of development have not been completed or because his significant adults, especially teachers and parents, are not attuned to the importance of recognizing the accomplishment of the child. The recognition may be withheld in the home if the child is from a subculture which does not value industry. Industry and achievement are values which are promoted by the middle-class, but they may not be so important

to the person from a lower socioeconomic background; thus, the child may experience conflicting reinforcement. He may be reinforced or praised for accomplishments at school but not at home. If the home environment is a stronger force, the child will probably take on the value system in operation there, such as need for immediate gratification and lack of sustained effort. If a sense of inadequacy develops, the child may decide that what he does, the task he completes, is not any good and will probably not be of value in the future; or he may not develop the ability to stay with a task until it is completed.

Adolescence

This stage of development is often an uncomfortable time for the person experiencing it as well as for the others in his environment. The task to be accomplished during this time has been labeled by Erikson as *identity* versus *self-diffusion*. It is difficult to place an age range on this period, but it usually begins with the first evidence of puberty (nine to twelve years of age) and ends with completion of the physiological changes related to puberty (twelve to fourteen years of age).

Adolescence is an uncomfortable time because the person begins to define exactly who he is and what roles he will play in the future. This process of definition is complicated by the physiological revolution going on within; the person begins experiencing new drives, thoughts, and feelings.

He may be uncomfortable with some of the thoughts which cross his mind, especially those related to his sexual awakening. He may be concerned even though the thoughts which he has are within the range of normalcy. He may be uncertain as to the accepted way to meet his sexual needs, and will probably be receiving conflicting information from his peers and his parents. The person also becomes more aware of the sociocultural prescriptions which regulate what is considered masculine or feminine behavior, and may experience conflict in accepting the proper role which is implied. Further complications occur because a great many alternative social roles now become available. The adolescent must try to align his previous childhood goals with his biological drives, and to evaluate his potential in relation to the opportunities which are now available. During this process, he may return to some of the previous developmental tasks and seek reaffirmation or make changes. For example, he may wonder if he really is trustworthy and may redefine which other persons he considers worthy of his trust. Hopefully, at the end of this period the adolescent will have developed a sense of self, with the conviction that he is taking effective steps toward a rewarding future and that he is developing a defined personality within the reality of the environment as he understands it.

When an individual does not come to grips with the question of who he is, he suffers from what Erikson describes as self-diffusion. This person may overidentify with other individuals or groups, attempting to take on their values, ideals, and sometimes even their appearance. Frequently the overidentification is with other adolescents and may have either negative or positive results, depending on the composition of the group. A positive factor which may result from this identification is the separation from his parents which encourages steps toward independence. The adolescent will begin thinking of himself in an adult-to-adult relationship with his parents, rather than in a continuing parent-to-child relationship.

Adulthood

Erikson has defined three psychological crises that occur in adulthood. The first is that of *intimacy* versus *isolation.* In some developmental schemes this crisis is considered to occur in late adolescence. This period of living begins with the completion of the physiological changes occurring in puberty and ends with the establishment of a desirable situation of intimacy. The age range varies with each person but is generally considered to occur from fourteen to twenty-one years of age.

Once the person has achieved a sense of identity, he then can devote more energy to developing interpersonal intimacy. Because he has experienced puberty, his interest has probably switched to an interest in the opposite sex. The intimacy that is established, however, is more than sexual intimacy, although this is an important factor. Intimacy may be expressed in friendship, devoid of sexual experiences; there is a need for closeness and sharing. Erikson defines this as a "fusion with the essence of other people."[7] When true intimacy is established, the individual is able to fuse his own identity with another without fear that he will lose something of himself. In reaching this stage the person engages in endless hours of exchanging ideas and views. Everything of importance gets discussed—including how one feels, and how others are perceived; plans, wishes, and expectations are shared. By the end of this period the individual may have decided whom he would like to marry. If both individuals have found their self-identity and are comfortable in an intimate relationship, the possibility of success is better than if the young person has married hoping that his identity will be defined by the other person.

When a youth does not accomplish this interpersonal comfort with others, he will suffer from a sense of isolation. The isolation may be a physical type, in which he avoids other people, or, even more prevalent, a psychological alienation. This individual may make repeated attempts to develop friendships and find suitable love objects, but is usually met with failure. The

[7] Eric H. Erikson, Growth and Crises of the "Healthy Personality," in C. Kluckhohn, H. A. Murray, and D. M. Scheider (eds.), "Personality in Nature, Society and Culture," Alfred A. Knopf, Inc., New York, 1955.

interpersonal relationships which he does engage in are usually highly stereotyped and formalized, in the sense that they lack warmth, spontaneity, and any real exchange of fellowship.

The second developmental crisis in adulthood is that of acquiring a sense of *generativity* versus *self-absorption.* This period of living begins when one is comfortable in interpersonal intimacy with another person and probably ends with the changes prompted by the physiological climacterium, or menopause, and the related psychological adjustments. When the person has established mutuality with a loved partner of the opposite sex, he may develop an interest "in establishing and guiding the next generation." If he is married, this is usually the time when children are born to the union. For unmarried persons, and for some married ones, generativity may also mean the creation and leaving of ideas, products, or works of art which will influence the future generations. Before the person desires to leave something to the future generation, he must see worth in society, in his community in general, and in himself in particular. If he does not see worth in any of these things, he may be pervaded with a "sense of interpersonal impoverishment and stagnation." This is the crisis of self-absorption. This person may estrange himself from his community and from truly knowing himself. He may indulge himself as if he were his one and only child, and engage in behavior which provides for a pseudointimacy with others. He shows very little concern for others or for future generations.

The last developmental crisis which a person faces is that of *integrity* versus *despair.* This period of life generally begins with the physiological and psychological climacterium. A few of the changes which may be occurring include change in physical capacity, retirement, having the children leave home, and having to accept care from others, such as children. These events prompt the person to engage in a life review, in which he reflects on what he has accomplished in his life and on what is yet to be accomplished. The individual achieves a sense of integrity when he can accept the responsibility for his own life and his life style, and be pleased with what he has accomplished. If during this life review, the individual is not accepting of his own life's cycle, he may wish he had his life to live over again, or wish that it could have been different. This individual may experience a sense of despair. Despair may be expressed in a disgust and displeasure with people or institutions, but it usually reflects the person's disgust with himself.

STRESS AND ANXIETY

Each person behaves in such a way as to meet his conscious and unconscious needs and to maintain a feeling of well-being in each situation in which he participates. These objectives are not always realized. Throughout each day, circumstances occur which may block fulfillment of needs or which might momentarily interrupt this feeling of well-being. When this occurs, the person is undergoing stress, and he experiences the feeling of anxiety.

What is perceived as threatening varies with each person and is dependent on several factors. Related factors include a need which is not being gratified, the person's perceptual equipment, his earlier conditioning influences, his sociocultural background, and the current situation in which he finds himself. Analysis of the current situation would include the physical environment, plus the psychological and physiological equilibrium, or balance, achieved by the person. An event that may seem trivial to one person may be very distressing to another. The meaning of an event to a person determines what his reaction will be; therefore, one cannot predict the degree of individual stress inherent in any given situation.

Definition and Causes of Anxiety

Anxiety is a subjectively experienced emotion which is characterized by feelings of vague, unexplained discomfort and apprehension. It is differentiated from the similar response of fear by the fact that the stimulus is not related to a specific object (Peplau, 1963). For example, the patient may experience fear when he sees a syringe and needle and is told the injection is for him. The same person might experience anxiety when going to the doctor's office, but be unable to state the reason for this feeling. Anxiety is an energy and as such cannot be directly observed. The energy is translated into observable behavior. These behavioral cues may be utilized by the nurse to infer the presence of anxiety.

As stated previously, the stimulus which causes the anxiety response is highly personalized. However, two generalized types of threats have been identified: (1) threats to biological integrity, and (2) threats to self-esteem (Engel, 1962).

Threats to biological integrity include actual or impending interference with the necessary satisfaction of basic needs, such as the needs for food, drink, sexual expression, and maintenance of bodily function. A patient-client who is experiencing pain or is contemplating surgery is having his biological integrity threatened. The use of medications may also be considered a threat to some people, since drugs alter the function of the body in some way. Threats to the self-system occur when events precipitate the anticipated or actual loss of something that the individual holds essential to his existence or to his personality (Engel, 1962). Examples of these types of threat which might occur are loss of health, status, prestige, independence, or satisfying relationships with other persons or groups. Examples of situations which might be perceived as threatening and which occur in respect to illness and hospitalization are many and varied. Each reader can probably describe many more than those covered in the following paragraphs.

Patient-clients frequently experience a loss of identity when admitted to a hospital. They are assigned to a specific room and bed number, and may be referred to as "the man in 216B." Since a diagnostic label is also given, they may become known as "the colostomy in 216B." Further feelings of loss of personal identity occur as the result of shedding of street clothes and being dressed in bedroom clothes.

Patient-clients are frequently forced to become dependent recipients of care, rather than partners in their care. Staff frequently make and enforce decisions related to what and when the patient-client will eat; what type of bath he will take; where and when he will sleep (in a room by himself or with another person); and when and with whom he will be allowed to interact. This loss of control related to decisions affecting oneself may be anxiety-provoking.

If a person has never been admitted to a hospital before, he will probably experience anxiety for he will be unfamiliar with the hospital bureaucracy and will not know what to expect or what is expected of him. Procedures and routines which are very familiar to the staff will be new to him. The anxiety level will be affected by the mental image held concerning the hospital. The patient-client may view the hospital as a place where suffering is concentrated, where bodies are mutilated, or where people are taken to die; or his view may be of a more positive nature which includes the relief of pain and cure for those who are desperately ill. Probably persons who are very ill will hold less fearful views of the hospital than those who are not so ill. Anxiety is also prompted because when hospitalized, the patient-client is separated from families and friends who provide support and comfort. He is usually not allowed to see his young children. Instead, he experiences lack of individualized attention and may feel psychologically deserted. Although many interactions occur during the day, most of them occur with strangers and lack meaning to the patient. Being away from his home also decreases familiarity with the physical environment and decreases the availability of recreational or diversional activities.

The patient-client also does not know what the outcome of the disease process will be; he experiences anxiety related to the many unknown factors. Will he be able to continue his present job? What will be the expense incurred during the illness? Will his relationship with family members be affected?

Levels of Anxiety

Four levels, or degrees, of anxiety have been conceptualized by Peplau. They form a continuum ranging from mild anxiety to panic (Peplau, 1963).

Mild Anxiety When a person is experiencing mild anxiety he is alerted and becomes more consciously aware of stimuli in his environment. He may see objects not previously noticed, or hear sound previously undetected. The understanding of a situation may become more complete, as he may grasp details which had previously eluded him. In general, his perceptive abilities are increased, as is his learning ability. The person can utilize his cognitive abilities and engage in problem-solving activities by intensifying purposeful behavior and focusing his attention. He may experience a feeling of restlessness.

Moderate Anxiety As the anxiety level of a person increases, his perceptual field decreases. He tends to concentrate on some specific part of a situation, but it is still possible to direct his attention toward other aspects of a situation or environment. The person may experience some of the physiological responses of increased anxiety, such as muscle tension, perspiration, "butterflies" in his stomach, or headache. Learning ability will be lessened, but with intervention of another person he can still engage in the problem-solving process and thus decrease the anxiety to the first level, where learning ability is increased.

Severe Anxiety In severe anxiety, the person's perceptual abilities continue to decrease. Attention may be focused only on specific details within any given situation, or on many scattered details in the environment. The person is unable to connect these details into a unified whole but instead reacts to each one separately. He will experience increased physical and emotional discomfort. Physiologically, he may experience such sensations as headache, nausea, trembling, and dizziness. Emotionally, he may feel dread, awe, or horror. When the person experiences such discomfort, he may be unable to rely on cognitive processes to relieve these feelings but instead will engage in automatic relief behavior to decrease his anxiety level. Examples of this automatic relief behavior will be discussed later, but the three main patterns identified include those of fight, flight, and somatization. The beginning nursing student may be helpful to the patient-client if he provides channels to decrease the anxiety level. This may be done by assisting the patient to find activities which burn up the excess energy associated with increased anxiety. A few examples of activities include allowing the person to talk with you, providing a simple task which he could complete, accepting the person when he is crying, and, if his condition warrants it, walking with him.

Panic When a person experiences panic, the perceptual ability is further reduced and may become distorted. The person may be able to perceive only one detail of a situation, and he may distort the meaning of this detail. He may give more importance to this detail than he would in a less anxious state. Many times the person is unable to communicate verbally what he is experiencing, and his nonverbal behavior may appear bizarre and incomprehensible to an observer. The automatic relief kinds of behavior mentioned in the last paragraph may appear in exaggerated forms. He may look as if he is "frozen to the spot," or he may engage in random, nonproductive movements and verbalizations. The person experiencing panic cannot be expected to engage in learning activities which would lessen his anxiety, but he needs immediate help in becoming more comfortable. The nurse can provide help to the patient-client by remaining with him during this terrifying experience. When remaining with him, attempt to do nothing which might further increase his anxiety, but remind him quietly that you are with him, and give him short directive statements to help him feel that at least you are in control of the situation. You might say such things as, "I'm here," "Sit down," "Talk to me." As a beginning student, you might increase your own comfort by seeking the assistance of a more experienced person.

Mechanisms Utilized to Relieve Anxiety

A person experiencing the unpleasant feeling of anxiety will make attempts to seek relief. The attempts may be on a conscious or unconscious level and may involve both psychological and physiological processes. Each person develops his own unique response pattern to anxiety, depending on what activities have been successful or unsuccessful in his past experiences, and on the present situation in which he finds himself. As previously noted, the relief behavior will also be related to the level of anxiety.

Some of the psychological processes utilized by a person to reduce anxiety are called "defense mechanisms" or "mental mechanisms." These mechanisms are employed by everyone in the course of daily life and are required to make living less stressful. The mechanisms are considered pathological when a person always resorts to them to decrease his anxiety, never attempting to use his anxiety in the process of learning, or when reality is denied. The use of a defense mechanism may be on an unconscious or conscious level of awareness and is rarely seen in a pure form; two or more mechanisms are seen together. Some authors refer to conscious efforts as "coping mechanisms." Some of the more

commonly identified mental mechanisms are defined below. These particular mechanisms were selected because of their visibility in everyday life. This listing should not be considered complete. The student is encouraged to delve more deeply into reference books to complete his knowledge of such mechanisms. The definitions have been adopted from those given in *A Psychiatric Glossary*, published by the American Psychiatric Association.

Denial This mechanism operates unconsciously and is utilized to avoid or reduce anxiety by disavowing thoughts, feelings, wishes, needs, or external reality factors which would be intolerable if perceived on a conscious level. For example, a person who has been hospitalized for a myocardial infarction may deny the reality of his disability and not make any adjustments in his patterns of daily living. Or a person who does not know how to cope with feelings of sexual excitement may deny that he has such feelings.

Displacement Displacement occurs when an emotion is transferred or displaced from its original object to a more acceptable substitute. The emotion may be any one of the human feelings, such as fear, anger, grief, joy, or love. The secondary object may be either animate or inanimate. For example, as a student you may become angry with your instructor when he appears to be criticizing your work, but being fearful of your future relationship with him, you check your feelings of anger. You then discover, later in the day, that you are expressing uncalled-for anger toward a friend.

Projection When something which is emotionally unacceptable to the self is unconsciously rejected and attributed to others, the process is known as projection. The something that is unacceptable may be feelings, ideas, or behavioral characteristics.

The others who may be the recipients of these projected elements may be individuals or groups of individuals. For example, a person who had engaged in sexual fantasies about another person might report to his associates that that person had made some very suggestive remarks to him.

Rationalization   This defense mechanism also operates unconsciously; it is utilized by a person when he attempts to justify or make tolerable feelings, behavior, and other motives which otherwise would be intolerable on a conscious level. The person verbally justifies his behavior in terms which will find approval by others. Some of the actual basis for the behavior may go unheeded or at least not be stated. For example, if a person has a specific task to complete but has failed to do so, he may give various socially approved reasons for this failure, such as that he is "not feeling well" or that company dropped in unexpectedly.

Regression   Regression is the return to previously learned more infantile methods of adjustment and reaction. Regression occurs unconsciously and may be observed in a variety of situations. It takes place when a person sleeps and when he engages in activities labeled as play. Some degree of regression is almost always seen when a person becomes ill. For example, a very self-sufficient man who is suffering from cold symptoms may allow himself to be cared for as he was when a little boy. Regression is also observable when a new baby is brought home from the hospital and an older sibling who has been toilet-trained begins having accidents.

Repression   The mechanism of repression operates automatically and involuntarily. It is by repression that a person keeps unacceptable ideas, desires, or impulses out of consciousness. Conflicts are buried in the unconscious so that they are not dealt with on a cognitive level. However, since the conflict is not resolved, it frequently seeks expression and modifies behavior. The ability to utilize this mechanism occurs

very early in life and is the principal defense in early years. It is sometimes considered the primary defense mechanism and frequently is used in combination with, or prior to, other mechanisms. An example of this mechanism is the repression by a child of hostility he feels toward a parent. If he allowed himself to become consciously aware of this hostility, he would not know how to deal with it, or with the reactions it might prompt from others.

Suppression   Suppression differs from repression in that it is on a voluntary, conscious basis and the material concealed is easily recalled. Material which may be suppressed includes unacceptable impulses, thoughts, feelings, or acts. For example, if when studying for an exam, a student finds his thoughts drifting away from the assigned material to the argument he had with his father earlier in the day, he may consciously decide that it is more important to consider the test now and put out of his mind, or not attend to, the intruding thoughts.

Sublimation   By the process of sublimation, consciously unacceptable instinctual drives are diverted into socially sanctioned outlets. Instinctual drives such as strong sexual urges or aggression are released in avenues which have social approval, e.g., sports, creative writing, and vocational choice. Sublimation is usually considered the most normal and healthy defense.

Adaptive Behavioral Patterns

If the use of the defense mechanism is successful, the person will experience a sense of well-being and his anxiety will be negated or at least lessened. If the defense mechanisms are not effective in restoring the person's psychological equilibrium, further attempts will be made. These attempts may include continued use of the same defense mechanism, use of a different mechanism, or use of several mechanisms in a combined or exaggerated form. It must be stressed here that this process is on an unconscious, automatic level. The person does not consciously think, "My use of rationalization was ineffectual, I will now try denial and projection." The behavior which results from increased defenses may be classified into three main adaptive patterns: (1) the person may attempt to overcome the source of anxiety, i.e., "to fight" off the stressor; (2) he may attempt to flee from the source of anxiety, i.e., to use flight behavior; (3) he may convert the vague symptoms experienced as anxiety into various physical complaints. By internalizing the anxiety he becomes no longer aware of the uncomfortable feeling but may now experience a headache, pain in his extremities, or stomach upset. The adaptive pattern that he utilizes will be related to his self-concept and to which adaptive patterns have been most successful in the past in satisfying his needs or reducing his anxiety. Behavior characterized by fight or flight patterns will be briefly discussed. The student is referred to Part 3, Chapter 19, for examples of how stress and anxiety are converted into the physical symptom of pain.

Fight Behavior   Fight behavior is characterized by a general alertness and vigilance, and includes actions which allow the individual to feel he has control. By his behavior he attempts to gain power over the situation or person(s) that he perceives as threatening. The perceived threat may be either to his biological integrity or to his self-concept.

Anger is the emotion felt by the person who is transforming the energy associated with anxiety into fight behavior. The behavior which accompanies this emotion may be observable in either an overt or covert form. Flynn describes the characteristics of anger as complex and as having a chameleon-like existence. She suggests that the nature, coloring, and form of anger may be disguised, distorted, or displaced (Flynn, 1969). From this statement, it is possible to infer that

many observable types of patient-client behavior are motivated by a feeling of anger.

The expression of anger in our society has been repressed in the past. Many individuals have been taught at an early age that it is "not nice" to express anger directly. Because of these early warnings, the expression of anger toward the situation or person causing the anxiety may be redirected toward other objects. The objects that receive the expression of our anger have been identified by Peplau as (1) direct—the person or situation causing the discomfort, (2) an object resembling the original object—e.g., a person who looks or acts very much like the person causing discomfort, (3) an object with little or no resemblance to the offending agent— an inanimate thing, a table, a chair, the food served, or, (4) the self (Peplau, 1952).

The expression of anger may be overt, and the bodily activity may include biting, tearing, crushing, breaking, squeezing, hurting (Engel, 1962). In most adults, however, the overt expression of anger is seen in yelling, glaring, and increased muscle tension. The thoughts of the person are concerned with driving away or destroying the external object which is causing discomfort. The person may also express covert anger in sarcastic or ironical remarks, excessive kindness and politeness when the situation calls for anger, and an indifferent or "I-don't-care" attitude (Richter, 1958).

When anger is expressed, the person may feel that he has gained power over the object causing his distress, either by destroying it or by driving it away. When this occurs, relief is felt. If the person still perceives the situation as threatening, he will not feel relief and may have to engage in similar behavior to attempt to relieve the remaining anxiety (Baker, 1966).

The following case history may make this concept of anger more clear:

Mrs. Hadley, a 57-year-old woman, was admitted to the surgical unit with the tentative diagnosis of carcinoma of the lower part of the intestine. Although the physician had noted on her chart that she was aware of her diagnosis, and the possible surgical intervention had been discussed with her, Mrs. Hadley continued to refer to her condition as "the normal dysfunction of the bowel as one grows older." Her conversations were sprinkled with comments about her many club activities and how she enjoyed sports. She frequently mentioned that she had "a darn good figure for a grandmother," and that she could put many younger women to shame if she entered a beauty contest. When attempts were made to discuss the approaching surgery, she would quickly dismiss the subject. It was noted by the nurses that Mrs. Hadley displayed some signs of anxiety, such as rapid speech and trembling. She requested that her husband remain with her most of the time, and when it was impossible for him to be there, she was observed to be talking on the phone to friends, usually making plans for the next major social event.

Surgery was performed, and Mrs. Hadley returned to the unit after having a colostomy. In the days immediately following the surgery, the colostomy was not to be irrigated. When care was being given to Mrs. Hadley, she refused to look at the incisional site. The nurses noted that Mrs. Hadley's behavior had changed; she complained to the nurses that her physician did not care about her, and insinuated that the nurses took care of her only because it was their job. Mrs. Hadley also talked frequently about the fact that her daughter, who lived in a distant city, had not come to be with her during surgery.

On the day that the first colostomy irrigation was to be performed, Mrs. Hadley appeared to be very much upset. She refused her medications and did not talk to the nurse assisting her with her bath. During her bath time, she frequently asked the nurse to leave the room as she had to make a personal phone call which could not be postponed. She told the nurse that if the hospital schedule had been better arranged, she would have already received her morning care and would not have to excuse the nurse. At the time the irrigation was scheduled, Mrs. Hadley had asked her husband to come and bring in the insurance forms. When her husband arrived, Mrs. Hadley insisted that the colostomy irrigation could not be performed until the insurance forms had been properly completed. When the nurse entered with the equipment, Mrs. Hadley verbally attacked her concerning the invasion of privacy, shouting, "You nurses have to know everything about patients, can't you even allow my husband and me to discuss money matters alone?"

When intervening in this situation, it is important for the nurse to recognize the steps leading up to the final angry outburst. By the use of denial, Mrs. Hadley had not allowed herself to deal with the anxiety prompted by a threat to both her biological integrity and her self-concept. In her past experiences, she had apparently handled anxiety by becoming involved in many detailed and controlling activities, such as club work; or had reduced anxiety by burning the excess energy in sports activities. Since the second option did not appear to be open to her following surgery, she attempted to increase her control over the situation. When the nurse approached Mrs. Hadley with the equipment to be used in the colostomy irrigation, she could see that she had been unable to gain control over her source of anxiety and that she must face the situation that she had attempted to avoid. Her anxiety was further increased and transferred into overt anger in an attempt to drive the nurse away. She was still unable to deal with the real cause of her anger, but displaced it to what she considered a more socially acceptable reason for anger.

It is unfortunate that someone had not recognized and dealt with Mrs. Hadley's increasing anxiety before this incident occurred. At this time, Mrs. Hadley would be described in stage three of the anxiety-level continuum (severe anxiety). Thus, intervention would be based on lessening of her anxiety to a lower level so that she could gain some understanding of her actions. To lessen the patient-client's anxiety, the nurse might engage in a number of activities. He might reflect the patient's feelings and state,

"Mrs. Hadley, you look pretty upset." By expressing her anger directly to the nurse, she would be dissipating some of the excessive anxiety. When the anxiety had been reduced, it would be helpful to include Mrs. Hadley in future planning. Together, the nurse and Mrs. Hadley could determine a schedule of activities; the interest displayed by the nurse would also encourage Mrs. Hadley to express her fears and reactions to the surgical procedure, gradually to learn the importance of the irrigation, and to discuss alternative life-style patterns.

It must be stressed that it is the nurse's responsibility, not the patient's, to modify his behavior to meet the needs of the patient as demonstrated by the patient.

Flight Behavior Flight behavior is a pattern in which the person attempts to flee or retreat from the threatening situation. The flight might be actual, such as leaving the situation, but more likely it is symbolic, a type of psychological withdrawal. The person who withdraws psychologically demonstrates little interest in interacting with his environment and appears to be guarding what internal resources he perceives as remaining.

As with fight behavior, the actual observable behavior which might be motivated by an attempt to withdraw from a threatening situation may appear in many and varied forms. Affects, or emotions, usually associated with flight behavior include *helplessness* and *hopelessness* (Engel, 1962). The person may utilize regressive behavior, he may appear overdependent upon others, or he may be described as being depressed. In each case, it is as if the individual has given up his attempt to overcome the threatening situation and will allow whatever is about to happen to occur. He may or may not have hope that others in his environment can provide relief. If he still holds on to this hope, he is described as feeling helpless; if the hope has been given up, he is described as feeling hopeless.

When a patient-client is utilizing a flight reaction from an anxiety-producing situation, the behavior may be overt and easily recognized. He may look sad and dejected, engage in very little motor activity, talk very little or not at all. He may complain of disrupted sleep patterns—either that he is unable to sleep at night or that he sleeps all the time. He may also complain of anorexia and constipation. On the other hand, the patient-client may make attempts to cover up his feelings of helplessness; he may put on a façade of gaiety, of independence, or he may not show any change in his affect but complain of many physical symptoms or increased pain. These types of behavior may covertly show his inner feelings. The behavior pattern that the patient uses will again be determined by his past experiences and by the way in which he perceives his current situation.

If the threat is very powerful, the person may flee from the situation to such an extreme that he loses contact with reality. However, since this book is designed for the beginning nurse practitioner, no discussion concerning psychotic behavior is offered. The student is referred to the resources available to him in this area.

As an example of a patient-client who utilized flight behavior from an anxiety-producing situation, Mr. Hunt is presented.

Mr. Hunt, a 33-year-old man who worked as a house roofer, was involved in a motorcycle accident. In the accident, his right arm was severed from his body. With the loss of his right arm he had undergone both a threat to his body integrity and also a blow to his self-concept, as he felt he could not possibly continue his previous work as a roofer. In the beginning of his hospitalization, his recovery was described as uneventful by the staff; all his injuries appeared to be healing well. The staff did note, however, that he talked infrequently about how the loss of his arm would affect his future life. When this subject was mentioned, he would turn away from the nurses and begin crying. Although he had full use of his left arm, he would not attempt to bathe or feed himself. When encouraged to be up and around, he would confine himself to his room and never venture out in the hallway. He requested that he have no visitors except his parents. His parents reported to the nurse that they were very much concerned about Mr. Hunt as he talked about his "whole life being ruined" since he had lost his arm. When they mentioned the use of an artificial limb, he appeared not to hear them or ignored their comments, saying that his life might as well be over.

When observing Mr. Hunt, the nurse could note many of the signs described as belonging to flight behavior. He was dependent on the nurses to feed and bathe him; he was showing regression in that he chose only to seek comfort from his parents; depression appeared to be the basis for his crying and his reduced motor activity. In assessing his anxiety level, the nurse might note that his perceptions and attention appeared to be limited to the loss of his arm and that he was unable to focus on the possibility of an artificial limb. Mr. Hunt's emotional tone seemed to be one of hopelessness.

In planning care for Mr. Hunt, the nurse must first determine if intervention is required or if this is the normal grieving period to be expected after a loss. If it is decided that intervention is required, the nurse would then initiate activity which would allow Mr. Hunt to experience less anxiety. For example, the nurse might go into Mr. Hunt's room and tell him that she had a few minutes to talk about whatever he would like to discuss. The nurse should be aware of cues indicating that Mr. Hunt is ready to discuss his recent loss. He may not talk at all, or he may choose to talk about something else. The nurse should remember that Mr. Hunt has chosen to flee from the anxiety-producing situation and so may find it difficult to discuss. If the nurse continues to make short visits demonstrating patience and persistence, Mr. Hunt may develop enough trust in the nurse to begin to discuss his loss. As the loss is discussed and Mr. Hunt's anxiety is lessened through verbalization, he will become ready to begin looking at various alter-

natives available to him. The nurse should be well informed on rehabilitation resources, so that the alternatives will appear more positive than his previous withdrawal. During this intervention period, it would also be helpful for the nurses to accept Mr. Hunt's dependency needs at first, and then, as he gains more hope, to help him move toward more independent functioning.

DIAGNOSING PROBLEMS REFLECTED IN BEHAVIOR

In the previous section of this chapter consideration was given to two categories of nursing problems which are diagnosed by observing the patient-client's behavior. Suggestions were offered as to how the stress or anxiety level of the individual client might be minimized. However, the nurse's responsibility includes more than minimizing the anxiety; he must also help the patient-client to define the cause of the stress and to decide on action which will prevent or deal with it. This latter action cannot occur until the anxiety level of the patient has been reduced to either the mild or the moderate level, at which increased perception and learning are possible.

The steps utilized in this diagnosis of the nursing problem in the psychosocial and mental-emotional areas are the same as in other areas. The nurse must remember that seemingly clean-cut behavioral responses may result from multiple, complex causes. The diagram in Fig. 9-1 shows how the nurse collects data, diagnoses an actual or potential problem, and plans nursing intervention. The remainder of this chapter is an explanation in narrative form of the same process.

When the nurse has formulated a tentative diagnosis based on observations of the patient's behavior, he should explore his perceptions with the patient-client. He may relate what he has observed and the verbal and nonverbal messages he has received from the patient. In this way, the nurse can determine if the patient is in distress

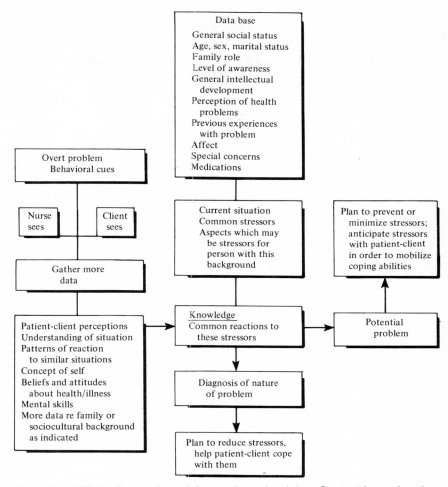

Figure 9-1 Utilizing the psychosocial/mental-emotional data. See text for explanation.

and if he perceives a need for help in relieving the distress.

When the patient-client confirms that he is experiencing distress, the nurse must help him explore the nature of this distress. He does this by asking questions or making statements which will allow the patient-client to provide descriptive data important to both the patient and the nurse in understanding the situation. Here are some examples of such questions and/or statements: "When did your wife visit last?" "Who is taking care of your children while you are ill?" "What exactly did the Doctor tell you?" or "I notice you are crying, tell me about how you are feeling." The nurse attempts to increase the patient's awareness of the factors related to his distressful situation. During this exploration, the patient-client may become aware of new or unrecalled elements in the situation, or may perceive the elements in a different way in light of the material discussed. The nurse may also be able to correct misinformation or provide new information to the patient.

When as many details as possible have been collected in relation to the specific situation, the nurse helps the patient choose an appropriate course of action. Included in this process is an evaluation of what the patient has done in the past when faced with a similar situation, and what alternatives are now available to either the patient or the nurse. Alternatives may include meeting a need in a different fashion than previously, restructuring the goal or choosing a substitute goal, or changing environmental factors that are interfering with the meeting of the need or goal.

When an alternative plan of action has been devised, it should be implemented by the appropriate person. This may be the patient himself, a relative or friend, or the nurse. The effectiveness of the action must then be validated by the patient. Validation may occur during the action or after the action is completed.

If the action has been successful, an account of the action and its outcome must be communicated to others significant to the patient. Such communication includes informing the staff verbally, as well as nonverbally by use of the nursing-care plan on the Kardex. These actions are never static but always constitute an ongoing, changing process.

Similarly, the nurse or the client may define potential problems. The current situation, in the light of the client's background and a knowledge of common human reactions to the same kinds of stress, may indicate potential difficulties in coping. Again, the nurse explores these observations with the client and they plan together to minimize the stresses or mobilize his coping abilities.

Section B: Mental-Emotional Status[8]

Two of the concepts selected for this chapter relate primarily to the mental and emotional function of the patient-client. These are the concepts of level of consciousness or responsiveness, and the concept of learning. The physical functioning of a person's brain is a prime factor in his state of consciousness. In addition, the social and emotional climate in which a person has been raised and functions also affects his awareness of his environment, how he responds to that environment, what he learns about it, how he uses what he learns, and how he responds to changes around him. His age is also a factor in his responsiveness and his learning, and in the expectations others have of him; we expect different kinds of response from children than from adults.

LEVEL OF CONSCIOUSNESS

Assessing level of consciousness is an important aspect in the care of many patients. The level of

[8] This section was written by Pamela Mitchell.

consciousness is the first item on the data list for mental function, and it is one piece of data needed to assess functional status in several other categories. Consequently, evaluation of this one function is extremely important in estimating the person's current physical and emotional state, any deterioration or improvement in status, and his ability to participate in the solution of his health problems.

Definition

Consciousness is a state of awareness of perceptual and physical stimuli—in short, of oneself and one's environment. The level of awareness ranges from simple perceptual discrimination to complex intellectual functioning and sensitivity to highly subtle sensory cues. Alterations in consciousness range from the purely subjective (e.g., changes in consciousness of self) to objective loss of consciousness (e.g., coma). Clinically, the term *level of consciousness* usually refers to objective assessment of the patient-client's awareness of and responsiveness to his environment (Adams, 1970). Alterations in awareness of self or of physical parts of oneself may be included in a description of level of consciousness if the person is able to describe such changes. These subjective components are not essential to the assessment of consciousness in the commonly defined medical sense. However, assessment of the client's state of awareness of self is important in many health problems. To avoid confusion in terminology, *awareness of self* will be used to refer to the subjective components of consciousness, *level of consciousness* to the objective aspects.

Causes of Alterations in Consciousness

A number of situations may precipitate alterations in the level of consciousness and in awareness of self. The most common physiological causes are (1) direct injury to the brain or its blood supply, and (2) metabolic dysfunction originating elsewhere in the body which subsequently interferes with brain-cell function. Brain cells are particularly sensitive to lack of oxygen and glucose; therefore any condition which results in hypoxia or hypoglycemia (decreased cellular oxygen or decreased glucose in the blood) can affect consciousness. Acid-base imbalance, vitamin deficiency, or disturbance of water balance can also affect brain-cell function and, thereby, level of consciousness. A number of drugs alter brain function temporarily or permanently and thus alter consciousness of self or the environment. Narcotics, barbiturates, alcohol, and hallucinogenic drugs are examples of these drugs.

Physical disorders involving loss of a part of the body, or of perception of a part (e.g., paralysis in which sensation is lost), may cause alteration in awareness of self. Absent, decreased, or disordered sensory stimulation may cause marked alteration in one's sense of self and perception of the environment. See Part 3, Chapter 11, for a more detailed discussion of this phenomenon.

A number of emotional reactions or states may also affect one's awareness of self or of the environment. The effect of anxiety on perception is an example of one such state. These effects are described in Section A of this chapter. Schizophrenia is an example of a psychiatric disorder in which alteration of self-perception and awareness often occurs.

Assessment of Level of Consciousness and Awareness of Self

Any statement regarding a patient-client's level of consciousness and awareness of self is an impression or conclusion based on subjective and objective data from the patient-client himself. There are at present no precise tools for measuring consciousness; consequently, estimation of a person's state of consciousness is just that—an estimate. It is therefore essential that the observer include his data with his impressions in order that other observers may verify or reject the conclusions on the same data base. Classifications or statements such as "alert," "comatose," "stuporous," "disordered body image," have no place in clinical assessment of level of consciousness or awareness of self. Such terms are not precisely defined; the meanings depend upon which observer or author uses them. Rather, one should state: "alert: oriented to person, place, and time; responds appropriately to questions"; "unresponsive to verbal stimuli or loud noise; draws away from painful stimuli; no response to touch" (see Gardner, 1968, for further examples).

Level of Consciousness If consciousness is awareness of self and environment, a person will respond in terms of the stimuli he receives from his internal and external environments. Alterations in his responses may then be inferred as alterations in his consciousness or perceptions. Assessment of the level of consciousness in terms of responsiveness to stimuli, plus measurements of motor status, of reflex status (pupillar, corneal, and plantar), and of autonomic activity (pulse, blood pressure, and respiration), can provide a great deal of information regarding the person's response to disorders affecting his brain, to the seriousness of his disorder, and to the degree to which the nurse will have to cope for him. The degree to which the nurse will have to cope or protect depends upon how fully the patient is able to respond appropriately to his environment.

Response may be considered in two categories: (1) level of sensory-motor response, and (2) level of intellectual or cognitive response. These categories must be evaluated as a base line in any individual patient-client, and then reevaluated against that base line when there are any apparent alterations in the level of consciousness. If the normal state is unknown for any patient, his presenting state is described and changes are compared with that.

Questions regarding sensory-motor responsiveness include:

1 How does he react to sound? To loud, soft, or sudden sounds?

2 How does he respond to bright light?

3 How does he respond to shaking, light touch, painful stimuli (pinching of the Achilles tendon, painful aspects of treatment, such as injections)?

4 Are responses appropriate, e.g., does he withdraw promptly or attempt to fight unpleasant stimuli, or are his movements random and without observable purpose?

5 Does restlessness or increased motor activity seem to correlate with internal sensation such as full bladder or need to defecate?

Evaluation of cognitive response may be based on answers to the following questions:

1 How does the patient respond to the observer's presence—verbally, nonverbally, not at all?

2 How easily aroused is he?

3 Does he remain aroused?

4 How does he respond to the observer's speech—verbally, intelligibly, in monosyllables? Does he have a motor response only?

5 Is his response appropriate to the content of the observer's speech?

6 Does he maintain attention to the observer? How much is he distracted by environmental stimulation?

7 Can he follow a simple command, e.g., "Hold up your hand"?

8 Can he follow more complex commands, e.g., "Pick up the glass; give it to me"?

9 Does he know where he is, who he is, the general time (day, month, year)?

10 Can he remember recent events? Past events?

More detailed assessment of the person's ability to interpret and to understand abstract ideas can be made by discussing with him the meaning of pictures or articles in a newspaper.

A great many of the above questions can be answered by apparently casual conversation with the patient or by noting his response to initial contacts with the nurse. If the level of consciousness is subject to rapid change or is rapidly changing (e.g., in a person with a head injury), systematic testing must be done frequently. Inexperienced nurses often think that they and the patient will feel foolish with this frequent testing. Indeed, the patient may well complain that he is tired and wishes to be left alone. However, when small changes in level of consciousness may indicate potentially fatal but reversible changes in the patient's condition, such frequent evaluation is fully justified and necessary.

Awareness of Self   Awareness of self is purely subjective. Some evaluation can be made from objective data, by observing whether the patient-client acts as if he is aware of all his body parts, or acts as if an amputated part is still present. People with hemiplegia (paralysis of one side of the body) resulting from certain kinds of stroke sometimes act as if the paralyzed side does not exist; indeed they often refer to it as someone else's arm or leg. Such people may also be unaware of one-half of any object placed before them; they do not eat food from half their food tray or stop reading midway across a page. Nurses and others working with such persons need first to recognize the existence of such a phenomenon in order to help the person compensate for his altered awareness of self. Specific details regarding help for such people are given in the references in the footnote below.[9]

The patient-client's way of referring to himself or of describing himself may give clues to his self-awareness. Such statements as, "I feel detached from my body"; "I feel as if I were floating"; "Someone gets in my mind and tells me what to do," suggest an altered sense of self. Children who are still developing a clear sense of self often refer to themselves in the third person. For example, "Robbie eats now." Adults who consistently refer to themselves in the third person may have an abnormal conception of self.

Nursing Responsibilities Responsibilities of the nurse to a person with an altered state of consciousness include assisting the physician to detect and reverse pathological states affecting consciousness, protecting the person whose response to the environment might result in physical harm, providing emotional support to the person whose altered perceptions are frightening or disturbing to him, and performing any activities of daily living (such as feeding, bathing) which the person's altered consciousness prevents him from doing himself.

LEARNING

The concept of learning is fundamental to the nursing process. Learning involves change and growth, and the basic goal of nursing is to help

people change and grow as they learn to cope with their health problems. People who have problems with their health and daily function often must make many changes in their ways of coping with life, in their attitudes toward health and illness, in their relationships with others. Whether or not they make these changes successfully, they are learning. If the client is to cope successfully with these changes in his life, he and the professionals who seek to help him must decide what new knowledge, skill, and values he will learn, how he can best learn them, and, later, whether his learning has achieved the goals set. The health workers who help the client with this learning may be considered teachers. However, as Carl Rogers (1969) points out, once we label a person "teacher," the focus shifts from what the learner is learning to what the teacher is teaching, with the implicit assumption that what is told or shown is that which is learned.

In Part 2, Chapters 6 and 7, we emphasized the importance of collaboration with the client in any plans which involve change in his life. People do not readily change just because someone, no matter how authoritative, tells them they must. They change when they see the need for the change, and when they are committed to and directly involved in planning the change. The same is true for learning. Learning is most meaningful and most lasting when it is actively sought by the learner and has relevance for him (Rogers, 1969). If we accept this approach to learning, the focus then shifts to what the *learner* is doing, and the "teacher" becomes one who facilitates learning. In the same way, when a nurse is helping a client to learn, all the nurse's contacts ultimately affect the outcome. If the client sees the nurse as an informed, caring person, he will be more willing to risk making major changes in his life, with that nurse's help. Conversely, if the nurse has seemed aloof and not understanding of the client's efforts to deal with his problems, he may not use the resources which the nurse could offer.

Most broadly, all nursing care is part of the

---

[9] R. Pigott and F. Brickett, Visual Neglect, *American Journal of Nursing,* **66**:101 (1966).

M. Ullman, Disorders of Body Image after Stroke, *American Journal of Nursing,* **64**:89 (1964).

client's process of learning. The plans which he and the nurse make to help him deal with his health problems are part of the learning and change he must accomplish. Therefore, if a nurse can plan care *with* the patient, he can facilitate learning. However, the nurse can be a more able facilitator if he has some knowledge of resources available to the client who has specific learning needs. The client's needs may range from advice as to where he may obtain free immunizations for his children, to better ways of solving his emotional problems, to management of hemodialysis (artificial kidney) at home. Beginning students are most apt to be involved with specific learning needs of individual clients or of small family groups. Nurses also help larger groups of learners, such as those in prenatal classes, school children in health classes, or nurses' aides in training. Resources and methods of working with larger groups of learners will not be discussed in this section. Redman (1972) and Rogers (1969) are good references for students who wish to study more at this point about group learning. These same references are also highly recommended for more depth in working with individual learners. Redman presents detailed and specific examples of each step of the learning process, as well as many good suggestions about resources for the learner. Rogers deals with a philosophy of learning; he speaks of having trust that the learner will learn what he needs if he is given the freedom and support to do so. He operates from the premise that learning is exciting and that people will learn if not stifled by too much teaching. In contrast, much of modern education (and, parenthetically, teaching of patients) is encumbered by the assumption that the student will not learn unless forced to. If the nurse's efforts to "teach" patients are characterized by telling the person what he needs to know, having him parrot back this information, and telling the other members of the team what to teach the patient, perhaps the patient as student will not want to learn, or will forget as soon as

the "exam" is over (i.e., when he goes home). Since most nurses have spent many years in school, have "learned" many facts, and have been told what they need to know, they in turn expect to teach patient-clients in the same way. Teaching approached in this manner is apt to be resisted and to fail, as are plans for any aspect of nursing care which are not made with the patient-client. If you have not recently read Part 2, Chapters 6 and 7, about the importance of planning care *with* the patient-client, it might help you to do so at this point.

Examples of Specific Learning Situations

As stated before, any change which the client must make is a potential learning situation. An obvious example is the person who must learn to manage a colostomy. A colostomy is an opening of the colon onto the abdominal wall, in a person who, for any of many reasons, must have the feces diverted from the rectum. Living comfortably with a colostomy requires regular evacuation of feces, usually by means of daily irrigations through the opening. However, learning to do this requires more than simply being shown how to irrigate the colostomy or even practicing the irrigation. A person who has recently had the colostomy performed also has to deal with his feelings about seeing a portion of his intestine on his abdomen, about handling his own feces, about being different, and about his sexual partner's potential revulsion. Often the colostomy is performed because the lower part of the intestine was removed on account of cancer. A person in this situation also has to deal with his fears of dying as well as his feelings about physical mutilation. Obviously, learning is not simply a matter of having information or of seeing a technique performed. If the emotional overtones surrounding the new skill or information are too great, learning will probably be incomplete at best. The person who is repelled by the whole idea of the colostomy may not even try to irrigate it himself. Therefore, the nurse who is trying to help him learn needs to be sensitive to his feelings, aware of his receptivity or resistance, and willing to try to find out where the difficulties lie. Recall Mrs. Hadley's complete resistance to colostomy care in Section A of this chapter.

Because learning should be actively done by the learner, the nurse must plan with him. In the example given, one might simply wait until the person shows some interest in the procedure of irrigation. He might say, "I wonder how I will manage that at home," or "Will a nurse come every day to do this for me?" The client and the nurse can then begin to talk about his perceptions of what is involved, how he thinks he can manage, what he needs to learn or change. Sometimes, the time factor makes it impossible to wait for the client to initiate the subject, e.g., he is to be discharged from the hospital shortly and has not even mentioned the subject. Here, the nurse might pose the problem: "I wonder if you've thought about how you will irrigate your colostomy at home," or, in Mrs. Hadley's case, "It's often hard to look at your incision, isn't it?" When learning is surrounded by a great deal of emotion, as in the example of Mrs. Hadley, it is extremely important that the person who is helping the learner be empathetic and understanding of the conflicts in the learner. Rogers states that any learning which involves basic changes in perception of self is threatening and apt to be resisted. However, reducing other external threats helps the learner to face the threatening task (1969, pp. 157–166). Thus if the nurse pushes the client, insisting that he *must* learn this skill, he only increases the external threats; conversely, empathetic support of the person will help him face what must be done.

In this context, consider your own reactions to many of the tasks which you have had to learn in becoming a nurse. You may have had to bathe adults, clean up their feces and urine, see people naked—all things which most young people in our society have rarely been exposed to, certainly not in public places. In addition to this, you may be expected to "act professionally," not showing your reactions to all this overtly. If you have had the opportunity to discuss your feelings with peers or your faculty, you may have found this helped you to become comfortable more rapidly. If not, you may still find these most uncomfortable experiences. Remember your feelings when you first entered clinical nursing the next time you help a client to learn something involving an emotionally charged area.

Planning for Learning

Planning for learning involves essentially the same steps as planning for dealing with one's health problem (Part 2, Chapter 7): (1) determine the learning needs (including potential learning strengths and barriers); (2) define objectives or goals; (3) select possible resources or activities; (4) choose resources; and (5) evaluate progress. Typically, this planning is done by the teacher for the student; it is hoped that after you have read this book and that of Rogers, you will do it *with* your clients.

In order to plan most effectively with his client, the nurse needs to know what resources are available for learning and which resources are apt to fit the learner best. For example, games, puppets, dolls, and activities which provide plenty of action are well suited for the preschool child; books which the child must read are obviously inappropriate, but so are stories, records, or television programs which present ideas in abstract form. In the same way, it is inappropriate to direct the adult who seldom reads to printed material dealing with his need, unless he indicates that he wants to find more in books or pamphlets.

Determining Need The client may come to the nurse or other health worker with his need specifically defined: "I want to know how to dress myself now that my arm is paralyzed." In other cases, the nurse may see a potential learning need which the client is either unaware of or has not chosen to discuss. In such cases, it is appropriate to pose the problem and see if the client sees that need also. Such an example was given earlier with the person who had a colostomy. If the nurse sees a need which the client does not, the nurse could still plan to "teach" the client but ought not be surprised if the client does not learn.

Defining Objectives   Once the need has been identified, client and nurse may proceed to decide just what the client wants to learn. Here the nurse often functions as a knowledgeable resource. If the client needs to learn how to give himself an insulin injection, or how to cook for his family while he is on a 200-mg sodium diet, he may have no notion of what specific tasks are involved. The nurse may suggest some goals, and the client may want to add to or revise them after he has begun learning. This is similar to experiences you may have had with a college course about a subject totally new to you. You did not know what you wanted to know, but once you started to explore the reading list, you found that you had many specific ideas.

If several health workers or nursing personnel may be involved in helping the client learn, the objectives and the rest of the plan should be in written form, in whatever format is pertinent to the agency. A written plan may be helpful, also, when only one nurse and client work together, for it will serve to help the client see if he is accomplishing his goals.

Objectives should be fairly specific, in order that the learner can see if he is making any progress. For example, if he states that his goal is "to learn everything there is to know about diabetes," he will never know if he has succeeded. If, however, he breaks this goal down into small subobjectives, such as "to name the food groups in the diabetic exchange diet," "to plan a day's meals using the exchanges correctly," he can measure his progress better. He

can still pursue his goal to know everything, but may also find successes along the way.

Selecting Resources   Traditionally, this step is called selecting teaching methods; however, since we are focusing on learning, rather than on teaching, we will focus on the resources to facilitate learning. Here again, the nurse is the informed resource and can use his assessment of the client's level of intellectual attainment, age, and interest to suggest some resources for learning. If the client wants and is ready to learn how to give himself an insulin injection, the nurse can show him, watch him do it, and provide feedback as to how he is doing. Certain principles of asepsis need to be followed if the patient is to prevent infection or complications. Therefore the nurse needs to help him incorporate this information into his learning of the motor skill. If the client wants to know more about a certain subject—diabetes, chronic respiratory disease, child care—the nurse may suggest specific books, films, persons, or community classes. Here again, the person's learning skills (reading ability, level of education, ability to understand abstractions, medical sophistication) are all important factors in choosing the resources to recommend. Many materials written for patients about various health problems were intended for people with at least a high school education; the majority of the persons given these materials have had considerably less education than this and do not understand many of the words used (Mohammed, 1964; Redman, 1972; Howell and Loeb, 1969). You might be surprised at the level of difficulty of the written materials used at the agency where you are currently practicing. Redman's textbook has excellent information on a variety of learning resources available to nurses and their clients.

Evaluating Progress   Traditionally, the teacher evaluates the progress of the student—through a paper-and-pencil test, through practical examinations in motor skills, or through oral examinations designed to test "understanding."

However, if the learner and his helper set the goals together, then perhaps they should set criteria to evaluate the progress together as well. If motor skills are involved, the nurse may help the client (for the client often cannot see himself) to see if he is contaminating sterile parts, or if he is using equipment efficiently. In turn, he is best able to evaluate his comfort with the skill, his confidence in doing it alone, how he will adapt it to his home life. When the "teacher" is the sole evaluator, or the prime one, the student often feels hesitant to admit that he is unsure or does not know, for he will get a "bad mark." If he is learning in an atmosphere where he is the primary evaluator, he may feel more free to ask for help.

This discussion of learning is not comprehensive and does not offer detail about learning resources or "methods of teaching." It is meant to offer an approach to helping patients meet their learning needs. Specific resources and theories about learning as they apply to health problems are well presented in the references. If you, the learner, feel you want to learn more about this aspect, I hope these resources will be of help to you.

REFERENCES

Books
Psychosocial Status

American Psychiatric Association, "A Psychiatric Glossary," 3d ed., American Psychiatric Publications Office, Washington, 1969.

Beland, Irene L., "Clinical Nursing: Pathophysiological and Psychosocial Approaches," 2d ed., The Macmillan Company, New York, 1970, pp. 208-216, 736-746.

Bloom, Samuel W., "The Doctor and His Patient," The Free Press, New York, 1965, pp. 119-141.

Brennecke, John H., and Robert G. Amick, "Significance: The Struggle We Share," Glencoe Press, Beverly Hills, Calif., 1971, pp. 52-58.

Du Gas, Beverly W., "Kozier-Du Gas' Introduction to Patient Care: A Comprehensive Approach to Nursing," 2d ed., W. B. Saunders Company, Philadelphia, 1972.

Engel, George, "Psychological Development in Health and Disease," W. B. Saunders Company, Philadelphia, 1962.

Erikson, Eric H., Growth and Crises of the "Healthy Personality," in C. Kluckhohn, H. A. Murray, and D. M. Scheider (eds.), "Personality in Nature, Society and Culture," Alfred A. Knopf, Inc., New York, 1955.

Francis, Gloria M., and Barbara Munjas, "Promoting Psychological Comfort," Wm. C. Brown Company Publishers, Dubuque, Iowa, 1968.

Glaser, Barney G., and Anselm Strauss, "Awareness of Dying," Aldine Publishing Company, Chicago, 1965, p. 3.

Gordon, Gerald, "Role Theory and Illness," College and University Press Services, Inc., New Haven, Conn., 1966, pp. 35-47.

Jourard, Sidney, "Personality Adjustment," 2d ed., The Macmillan Company, New York, 1963.

Kubler-Ross, Elisabeth, "On Death and Dying," The Macmillan Company, New York, 1969.

Leininger, Madeleine M., "Nursing and Anthropology: Two Worlds to Blend," John Wiley & Sons, Inc., New York, 1970, pp. 45-61.

Nordmark, Madelyn T., and Anne W. Rohweder, "Scientific Foundations of Nursing," 2d ed., J. B. Lippincott Company, Philadelphia, 1967, pp. 323-329.

Orlando, Ida J., "The Dynamic Nurse-Patient Relationship," G. P. Putnam's Sons, New York, 1961.

Peplau, Hildegard E., "Interpersonal Relations in Nursing," G. P. Putnam's Sons, New York, 1952.

———: A Working Definition of Anxiety, in Shirley F. Burd and Margaret A. Marshall, (eds.), "Some Clinical Approaches to Psychiatric Nursing," The Macmillan Company, New York, 1963, pp. 323-327.

Robinson, Lisa, "Psychological Aspects of the Care of Hospitalized Patients," F. A. Davis Company, Philadelphia, 1968, pp. 53-61.

Schoenberg, Bernard: Management of the Dying Patient, in Bernard Schoenberg et al., "Loss and Grief: Psychological Management in Medical Practice," Columbia University Press, New York, 1970, pp. 238-261.

Simmons, Janet, A., "The Nurse-Patient Relationship in Psychiatric Nursing," W. B. Saunders Company, Philadelphia, 1969, pp. 123-126.

Wiedenbach, Ernestine, "Clinical Nursing, A Helping Art," Springer Publishing Co., Inc., New York, 1964.

Mental-Emotional Status

Adams, R. D., in M. Wintrobe et al. (eds.), "Harrison's Principles of Medicine," McGraw-Hill Book Company, New York, 1970.

Redman, Barbara, "The Process of Patient Teaching in Nursing," 2d ed., The C. V. Mosby Company, St. Louis, 1972.

Rogers, Carl, "Freedom to Learn," Charles E. Merrill Books, Inc., Columbus, Ohio, 1969.

Periodicals
Psychosocial Status

Baker, Joan, and Nada Estes: Anger in Group Therapy, *Journal of Psychiatric Nursing,* **4**:50-63 (1966).

Besner, Arthur: Economic Deprivation and Family Patterns, in I. Irelan (ed.), "Low-income Life Styles," U.S. Department of Health, Education and Welfare, Welfare Administration Publication 14, 1968.

Brinton, Diana: Value Differences between Nurses and Low-income Families, *Nursing Research,* **21**: 46-52 (1972).

Engel, George: Grief and Grieving, *American Journal of Nursing,* **64**:93-98 (1964).

Flynn, Gertrude E.: Hostility in a Mad, Mad World, *Perspectives in Psychiatric Care,* **4**:153-158 (1969).

Irelan, Irene, and Arthur Besner: Low-income Outlook on Life, in I. Irelan (ed.), "Low-income Life Styles," U.S. Department of Health, Education, and Welfare, Welfare Administration Publication 14, 1968.

Lindemann, Erich: Symptomatology and Management of Acute Grief, *American Journal of Psychiatry,* **101**:141 (1944).

Maslow, Abraham: A Theory of Human Motivation, *Psychological Review,* **50**:370-396 (1943).

Meissner, W. W.: Thinking about the Family—Psychiatric Aspects, *Family Process,* **1**:1-40 (1964).

Moles, Oliver: Educational Training in Low-income Families, in I. Irelan (ed.), "Low-income Life Styles," U.S. Department of Health, Education, and Welfare, Welfare Administration Publication 14, 1968.

Quint, Jeanne C.: The Dying Patient: A Difficult Nursing Problem, *The Nursing Clinics of North America,* **2**:763-773 (1967).

Richter, Dorothea: Anger: A Clinical Problem, *Nursing World,* **132**:22-24 (1958).

Mental-Emotional Status

Aiken, L. M.: Patient Problems Are Problems in Learning, *American Journal of Nursing,* **70**:1916 (1970).

Gardner, M. Arlene: Responsiveness as a Measure of Consciousness, *American Journal of Nursing,* **68**:1034 (1968).

Howell, S., and M. Loeb: Nutrition and Aging: A Monograph for Practitioners, *The Gerontologist,* **9**(3):99, Part 3 (Autumn, 1969).

Mohammed, M.: Patients' Understanding of Written Health Information, *Nursing Research,* **13**:100-108 (1964).

Samora, J., L. Saunders, and R. F. Larson: Medical Vocabulary Knowledge among Hospital Patients, *Journal of Health and Human Behavior,* **2**:83-92 (1961).

ADDITIONAL READINGS

Books

Finney, J. C., (ed.), "Culture Change, Mental Health, and Poverty," University of Kentucky Press, Lexington, 1969.

Jourard, Sidney, "The Transparent Self," 2d ed., D. Van Nostrand Company, Inc., Princeton, N.J., 1971.

Kluckhorn, Florence, "Variations in Value Orientation," Row, Peterson, & Company, Evanston, Ill., 1961.

Skipper, James K., and Robert C. Leonard, "Social Interaction and Patient Care," J. B. Lippincott Company, Philadelphia, 1965.

Ujhely, Gertrude, "The Nurse and Her Problem Patients," Springer Publishing Co., Inc., New York, 1963.

Periodicals

Levine, Myra E.: The Intransigent Patient, *American Journal of Nursing,* **70**:2106-2111 (1970).

Schoen, Eugenia A.: Clinical Problem; The Demanding, Complaining Patient, *The Nursing Clinics of North America,* **4**:715-724 (1967).

Thomas, Mary D.: Anger in Nurse-Patient Interactions, *The Nursing Clinics of North America,* **4**:737-745 (1967).

Environmental Status

Barbara Innes

In today's world the public is very much aware of the environment and its effect on the health and comfort of human beings and animals alike. Environmentalists warn of the detrimental effects of air and water pollution; indiscriminate use of pesticides; and overcrowding of people, cars, and buildings with resultant lack of adequate housing, food supplies, recreational facilities, and privacy. Many persons, including legislators, health workers, urban planners, and private citizens, are working diligently to curb the ever-growing problems and reverse the unde-

Data to Be Assessed

Safety hazards
  Existing
  Potential
Comfort of environment
Convenience of environment
  For patient-client
  For family and visitors
  For health-team personnel
Medical orders for isolation
Causative organisms
Appropriate isolation techniques being used
Cleaning methods being used

Patient-client's and family's understanding of isolation
    procedure
Need for restraining devices
  Placement
  Tightness of application
  Skin condition underneath
  Bony prominences padded
  Key to lock available
Sensory stimuli being received
  Amount
  Variation
  Intensity

sirable trends. Progress is extremely slow because the known solutions often require large investments of time and money and, possibly most important, change in customs. People need to change long-established behavior patterns, such as their use of throw-away conveniences and of items that look nice regardless of their pollution index.

Nurses have a role to play in the environmental area—a role of which they are becoming more aware and in which they are increasingly taking part. They are filling positions on planning committees for health facilities; advising government agencies and private concerns about consequences of their projects on the health status of those involved; and assessing the health status and needs of certain groups of people (such as the aged, Indians, alcoholics) and reporting to the proper resources. Finally, nurses help educate people about existing and potential environmental hazards and about the essential behavior necessary to eliminate these dangers. All of this is part of a professional nurse's responsibility in providing and maintaining a healthful environment for his patient-client, using the broadest definition of the term "environment." The focus of this chapter, however, is environment in a somewhat limited sense—the patient-client's immediate environment.[1]

The nurse has an important role in regard to the immediate environment surrounding his patient-client. Nurses work in a wide variety of settings with persons who are at all levels along the health-illness continuum. These settings range from informal daily contacts in the community and the home to ambulatory clinics, hospitals, or other institutional facilities. The nurse's responsibility to each person differs according to that person's physical and mental capabilities. For example, a two-year-old child, who has very little ability to recognize a hazardous situation, needs more direct supervision than

a forty-year-old business executive. A newly blinded person requires almost constant assistance when he moves around his environment, while a person who has been blind for 10 years may need only a good initial orientation to his surroundings to avoid safety hazards. The setting also influences the degree to which the nurse needs to help the patient-client maintain his safety. As he is removed farther and farther from his normal environment, he may need more assistance. In his own home a person is familiar with his environment and the potential safety hazards in it. However, when that person leaves his home to enter a hospital, he may no longer be aware of where hazards are located or even of what constitutes a potential hazard in the new setting.

The nurse's capability to control the environment also changes in each situation. Whereas he may have great influence in room design and furniture selection in the building or remodeling of a hospital, the nurse may have very limited ability to effect a desired change in the home setting. For instance, the family of Mr. J., who is bedridden with terminal cancer, would like to continue caring for him in the home. After assessing Mr. J.'s condition and his environmental situation, the community health nurse decides it would be better for the family if the bed could be elevated to a more convenient height. Therefore he recommends the rental of a high-low hospital bed. However, because of their financial status and because Mr. J. has expressed a great desire to "be in his own bed," the family rejects the suggestion. In such instances, creativity on the part of the nurse can often provide an acceptable substitute. In this situation, the nurse arranges for the placement of notched wooden blocks under the legs of the bed to elevate it and also suggests using a padded box to help Mr. J. attain a comfortable sitting position.

In this chapter we will focus on three concepts regarding the immediate environment: safety, infection control, and environmental effects upon illness.

---

[1] See Jamann (1971) for a wider view of nursing and the environment.

SAFETY FACTORS

The broad use of the term "safety" includes both physical and psychological factors; however, this section will be primarily concerned with physical components. Certainly a person feels much more secure psychologically if he is confident that there is minimal danger in his physical environment.

Safety is of utmost importance to everyone. Accidents rank as the fourth cause of death among all age groups (*Vital Statistics of the United States,* 1969) and the first cause for children over the age of one year (Illingworth, 1968). Because of lack of reporting, the figures for nonfatal accidents are incomplete but are known to be high and thus a major health problem in the United States. Maintaining safety becomes even more critical when working with people who are ill or anxious and cannot exercise their usual control over their environment. Loss of strength, decreased sensory input, and disability often occur during illness. These changes may require modification of one's usual activity patterns, and adaptation to unfamiliar surroundings. In addition, the anxiety which accompanies many illnesses narrows the patient-client's perceptions and may thus cause him to react inappropriately to environmental cues.

Constant surveillance and alertness to potential hazards are important in maintaining environmental safety. The nurse must learn to look automatically at the environment in terms of safety factors. By concentrating his assessment in the following areas, he will better be able to predict and prevent situations with a high accident-causing potential.

Age

Each age level has its own particular safety problems which are related to the developmental skills and interests specific to that group. When the nurse knows the age-related ability of his patient-client, he can be more cognizant of specific potential dangers. However, it must also be emphasized that the age number itself has no magic qualities, since people mature at varying rates of speed.

Developmental changes are particularly rapid in the infant and preschool child. At birth, the baby lacks the ability for much physical movement or coordination and so is essentially not dangerous to himself. His safety hazards arise strictly from his external environment. Examples of such hazards include being dropped or held without proper support of his head, being poked with a safety pin, or being burned in his bath water. Because of his immature immunologic reactions, he is more susceptible to some infections. By the age of four months, he poses more hazard to himself since he is able to put things purposefully in his mouth, such as an open safety pin or a small button left within his reach.

Children develop physical capabilities and certain mental skills before they recognize a strong cause-and-effect relationship. Since personal investigation is their main mode of learning, they become potentially dangerous to themselves. They engage in such activities as touching hot items; playing with matches; sticking bobby pins into electrical outlets; consuming insecticides, cleaning fluids, and medicines; climbing to reach things in high cupboards; playing with knives and guns; chasing a ball into the street—the list is endless.

At the other end of the growth and development continuum, specific safety hazards are linked with loss of capabilities formerly possessed. For instance, because of decreased muscle strength and reflex speed, the elderly person is often unable to recover his balance when he starts to fall, an ability he had when he was younger. Other factors adding to the high susceptibility to falls among the aged are impaired sight and hearing and the inability to move rapidly (Peszczynski, 1965). Both factors make it difficult for the person to avoid dangerous situations such as collisions with other people, wheelchairs, or furniture. Therefore, important points in assessing the environment of the elderly include the amount of clutter, stability of rugs, placement of furniture, presence of stairs or other hazards, and the amount of lighting.

State of Mobility

The wider the range of a person's field of mobility, the more safety hazards are likely to be present. For instance, when a patient-client is confined to bed, the furniture arrangement in the rest of the room or an open door to the stairway does not directly affect his safety. (The extended environment will affect the nurse and other health-team members as well as the family and visitors who will be moving around.) As this patient-client starts to get up and increases his mobility, the area which will affect his safety expands. Examples of important safety devices include bed in the low height position, slippers with good soles, wheelchair in good repair, hot steam humidifier protected from a child's exploration, handrails installed in the bathroom, and proper night lighting.

In assessing the influence of mobility on the safety potential, the nurse would take note of any medical restrictions as well as the present condition of his patient-client. Such situations as use of a cast, decreased range of joint motion, weakness, or paralysis present their own specific problems and necessitate preventive measures by the nurse. Such preventive measures are presented in Part 3, Chapter 12.

The developmental level of the person also influences his mobility. Somewhat paralleling the expanded range of mobility of the convalescing patient-client is that of the infant as he grows and matures. At first he is essentially unable to move himself; then he gains the ability to turn over, crawl, pull himself up on things, walk, etc., each step increasing his access to safety hazards. The nurse may help mothers anticipate the increasing mobility of their infants and toddlers. He can also recommend measures to "child-proof" the home before accidents occur. Suggestions might include installing gates at the top and bottom of stairs, locking up medicines and cleaning articles, placing laundry detergent out of reach, and putting plastic covers over unused electrical outlets.

Persons whose mobility range has suddenly been restricted also need help in anticipating safety hazards. These people often are not fully aware of their new capabilities and may attempt to do things for themselves such as leaning out of their wheelchairs to pick up something from the floor.

Therefore, in predicting potential hazards, the nurse looks at the extent of his patient-client's field of mobility and his abilities or disabilities of movement within that field.

Arrangement of Furniture; Other Potential Hazards

The significance of the arrangement of furniture and other items in the environment has already been mentioned with regard to age and state of mobility, and it will again be mentioned in relation to sensory and orientation assessment. The great importance of this factor cannot be overstated.

Probably the most common hazard is clutter. Many falls are caused by litter on the floor, wet spots on linoleum floors, equipment crowded around the bed, chair legs sticking out, and short stools which are not easily seen when a person is walking. Excessive furniture and equipment are especially dangerous in hospital hallways, where weakened persons often use the walls for stabilization and where persons are just learning to manipulate mobility aids such as wheelchairs, crutches, and walkers.

The furniture itself can be a deterrent to accidents. Hospital furniture is designed to give maximum safety: beds can be lowered to a height which minimizes the potential of falls; chairs are made so that a person can get into and out of them as easily as possible; bedside stands are easily movable. This kind of equipment may not be found in the home, but acceptable substitutions can be made. It is up to the nurse to see that this equipment is in good condition and is used correctly. Proper arrangement of the furniture may also prevent accidents. One of the most important considerations is that wherever the patient-client is, he must have within easy reach a call bell or some other means of summoning help and that this equipment must be functioning properly. Placement of the overbed table or bedside stand so that the patient-client can comfortably reach the items on it may prevent falls. When getting the patient-client into a chair, obstructions in his path must be removed.

The nurse must also be aware of other hazards in the environment. Doors should not open out into hallways. Electrical cords should be placed out of the traffic pathway or, if this is not possible, they should be anchored securely so as not to cause falls. Cords should also be inspected for breaks and frays. When electrical beds and electronic monitoring equipment are being used, it is essential that all plugs and outlets be adequately grounded. Fatalities because of improper use of such equipment have been recorded (Hochberg, 1971). Nurses who have any questions about the adequacy of wall sockets and grounding should seek help from the institution's engineering department. Suggestions for further reading are given at the end of this chapter.

Sensory Deficits

Everyone depends on his sensory nervous system to apprise him of potential hazards; if any of this sensory perception is lost or impaired, the person loses part of his warning system. He then becomes more dependent on others to help him avoid dangerous situations, at least until he has learned to compensate for the impairment. A nurse working with these people must be aware of those safety hazards that increase in impor-

tance because of the person's particular sensory deficit. Hot packs must be applied with extra caution to a person with reduced sensitivity to heat or pain. Blind persons are particularly susceptible to the hazards of a changed environment; such a person must be carefully oriented to the position of furniture and equipment in his immediate surroundings, and then must be carefully informed of any changes that are made. Clutter must be avoided, and doors to stairways must be either closed securely or easily identified. Persons with hearing deficits may not be able to hear spoken warnings so that their attention must be reached through the visual or tactile senses; they may not hear carts or people coming toward them from behind or around the corner.

When the nurse finds that his patient-client has a sensory deficit, he must then assess the extent of the impairment and any compensatory mechanisms the person has developed.

Orientation-Disorientation

Orientation refers to a person's recognition of and familiarity with his surroundings, and his ability to adjust to changes in his environment. A disoriented person may not know where he is, the time or the day, or even his name, and is often described as being confused. Disorientation may be transitory, as when a person is first admitted to his hospital room or when children or the elderly awaken at night in a strange place. However, it is sometimes prolonged. Many factors connected with illness may increase the incidence and intensity of disorientation. Such factors include medications, high fevers, strange surroundings, loss of sleep, high levels of stress, brain damage, toxic substances, and marked alterations in sensory input.

In order to prevent accidents to the confused person, the nurse must assess the degree of disorientation, the times of its occurrence, and the incidents preceding the onset. Many of the problems can be avoided by completely orienting the patient-client to his surroundings on admission, i.e., showing him where to find things and how they work. Side rails and proper night lighting are used to prevent accidents during nocturnal wakefulness. Depending on the degree of confusion, it may be safer to keep toxic substances out of the person's reach, to securely anchor any tubes attached to the person, and to keep personal items well within reach. Recent memory may be impaired in disoriented persons, and explanations must often be repeated periodically.

Restraining Devices

Restraining devices are an important method of providing a safe environment for clients. They help keep the person from falling or climbing out of bed or a chair; prevent him from pulling at tubes, dressings, and monitor attachments; and hinder his attempts to scratch. One of the first assessments to be made about these devices concerns their necessity. The key factor is judicious use. When some type of restraint is needed to provide safety for the person, its utilization is imperative; however, too often restraints are applied merely so that the person will not have to be observed so frequently. Assessment of the patient-client's behavior, mobility, and state of orientation will help the nurse make an appropriate judgment.

Once the decision has been made to use some kind of restraining device, the proper type must be selected. The ideal choice would be one that applies the necessary degree of control without restricting the person's mobility too much. Side rails are the most common method used. Although these rails may prevent the person from falling out of bed, they often serve just as a reminder, since a person can rather easily crawl out around them. Side rails should be used when the bed is in high position or when the patient-client is confused, restless, or sedated. Many

hospitals have a policy requiring night use of side rails with persons age sixty-five and over. In general, side rails can be used freely and should be raised whenever the nurse has any suspicion that the patient-client may need the extra protection.

Many types of restraint are available. For instance, a folded bed sheet placed around the waist and back of a chair can help a person to stay in the chair. A more sophisticated type of waist restraint is a canvas belt with metal locks at the waist adjustment site and at the places where it is attached around the bed frame or chair. Limb restraints may be gauze or cotton strips around the wrist or ankle, with a clove hitch used and with the ends tied to a stable object. Cloth and leather cuffs, often with a lining of synthetic lamb's wool, are available.

The nurse's responsibility for safety continues after application of the restraint. He must be certain that the device remains properly placed and is functioning as desired. No restraining apparatus is perfect, and persons have been known to slip out of seemingly impossible situations. The nurse must also assess for constriction and skin irritation underneath the device. Involved bony prominences need to be well padded. If locked belts are to be used, it is imperative that the key be quickly available to personnel. Explanations to both the patient-client and his family will help them cooperate more fully with the method of protection.

Use of Prosthetic and Other Supportive Devices

As mentioned before, a patient-client using any ambulatory device (crutches, canes, walkers, or artificial limbs) is liable to particular kinds of accidents. Falls are again the paramount hazard. All equipment must be working properly and must be correctly fitted to the person. Crutches and canes should have jumbo-sized rubber tips. Wet spots on the floor and loose rugs are particularly dangerous, as are chair and table legs which stick out. Again, clutter is an acute problem.

Many hospitals and convalescent-care centers have mechanical lifting devices which are run by a hydraulic lift system and which can be employed to transport persons to and from bed, chair, bathtub, and toilet and to pick up fallen persons from the floor. If the person has to be lifted, the utilization of this apparatus reduces the use of poor body mechanics by both the nurse and the patient-client.

As may be surmised from the above discussion, falls and mechanical injury are the chief hazards in the patient-client's environment, with thermal injury in the form of burns also being very significant. The nurse must be continually evaluating the environment with an eye to potential accident-causing factors. Some conditions are dangerous to everyone. In addition, the preceding categories include hazards specific to certain clients or groups of clients. In general, it is much better to prevent an accident than to repair the results of one.

INFECTION CONTROL

There are microorganisms all around us. Most of them are harmless, and some are actually beneficial, such as those in the intestinal tract which aid in the fermentation and digestion of food. However, some of these organisms, called *pathogens,* are capable of causing disease in man.

Even though a person is invaded by a pathogen, whether or not he develops clinical illness is contingent upon several factors. Depending on his physical condition, his normal body defenses will be able to fight off a certain number of microorganisms. However, if the number of invaders is too great for the body to handle easily, the result is infection. The defense system, or body resistance, is influenced by factors such as age, state of nutrition, certain medications, presence or absence of concurrent disease, and

stress. The more of these that appear on the deficit side of the assessment for a particular person, the lower is that person's resistance to microbial invasion. One important means of boosting the body's ability to fight specific organisms is passive immunization against them; successful preventive agents are well known against poliomyelitis, rubella, mumps, tetanus, and diphtheria, among others.

Everyone normally has a certain number of pathogens living on his skin and in his nasopharynx and other orifices; yet he continues to live in a healthy state. However, if these organisms find their way in sufficient quantities into a part of the body usually free of them, infection is likely to occur. For instance, if a person who ordinarily has staphylococcal organisms in his nasopharynx breathes into a fresh surgical wound on his abdomen, a wound infection may result. Bacteria carried into the wound from the surrounding skin surfaces may have the same effect.

The concept of infection control is relatively recent when looked at in a historical perspective. *The Cry and the Covenant* (Thompson, 1949) tells of the almost futile struggles of Semmelweis (1818–1865) to persuade the medical profession that their practice of not washing their hands between examinations of cadavers and deliveries of pregnant women seemed to be the main cause of frequently fatal infections in these persons. Work of such people as Pasteur, who disproved the theory of spontaneous generation, and Lister, who claimed that wound infections were caused by microorganisms, helped bring our knowledge of microbiology and epidemiology to its present-day state.

Until the discovery of antibiotics, there was no effective treatment of most infectious diseases. Only by quarantine and other techniques designed to hinder physical transmission of organisms was there any hope of preventing spread of infectious disease. The antibiotics introduced in the 1940s were "miracle drugs" which could combat pneumonia and other infections dreaded at the time. Originally these drugs were used rather indiscriminately. At the same time, practitioners began to relax their control techniques, since, after all, medications easily took care of any ensuing infection. One of the main results of these practices has been the development of strains of pathogens that are themselves resistant to existing antibiotics. Now the pendulum is swinging strongly toward using antibiotics only as necessary and again employing meticulous infection-control procedures.

It has been documented that *nosocomial,* or hospital-acquired, infections have become a major health problem. A nosocomial infection is defined as one which was neither clinically present nor latent in a person prior to his admission to a hospital. Common sites for these infections include the skin, wounds, urinary tract, and respiratory tract. In the recent past the *Staphylococcus aureus* was most frequently found as the causative organism, but now gram-negative organisms, particularly the *Pseudomonas* strains, are rising in frequency. In 1967 there were 30 million hospital admissions, and it was estimated that at least 3 percent of these persons developed nosocomial infections (there were persons who probably developed infections following discharge from the hospital, and they were not included in this total). The fact that these infections affected approximately one million persons demonstrates the importance of infection control (Himmelsbach, 1970).

Consequently, an important responsibility of the nurse is to protect his patient-client against excessive microbial invasion. As suggested by the preceding discussion, this risk is greatest in hospitals and other institutional care centers where not only are persons housed in close proximity to one another, but where the persons so housed have markedly lowered resistance. As an added risk, hospitalized persons often undergo procedures which open usually sterile areas of the body to microbial invasion. Examples of these procedures are surgery, catheterization, and venipuncture.

Infection Chain

As has been discussed, the mere presence of a pathogenic organism does not assure that an infection will occur; several other factors are necessary. Figure 10-1 depicts these essential elements as a chain, all links of which must be present and intact.

1 Infectious agent. Pathogenic organisms must be present in sufficient numbers and virulence.
2 Reservoir. This refers to the place where growth and reproduction of the pathogens can take place. Reservoirs may include a person either about to develop the clinical symptoms, such as a child coming down with the chickenpox, or one who already has the disease. A reservoir may also be a person, known as a *carrier,* who has no clinical signs of the disease entity even though he harbors the organism; Typhoid Mary is a well-known example.
3 Portal of exit. This is the means by which the organism leaves the reservoir. Common exits from the human being are the gastrointestinal and respiratory tracts.

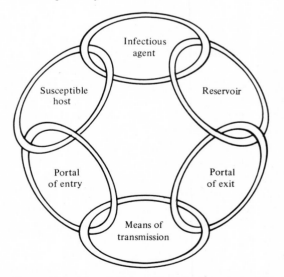

Figure 10-1 The six links of the infection chain. *[From V. W. Greene, Microbial Contamination: Control in Hospitals, Hospitals, 43:78ff. (1969). By permission of the author.]*

4 Means of transmission. The organism must have some way of traveling between the exit and entry sites. The methods may be direct contact with the infected part or its discharges, particularly exhaled droplets, or indirect methods such as contact with any object to which the organisms may cling, e.g., air, water, sewage, food, flies, and mosquitoes.

5 Portal of entry. There must be a means by which the organism gains entry into the new host. These portals often correspond to the portal of exit from the reservoir. Common entry routes include the respiratory and urinary tracts, mouth, and breaks in the skin.

6 Susceptible host. The susceptibility versus resistance of the host has been discussed. Everyone is a potential host—patient-client, family, visitors, and health personnel alike (Greene, October, 1969).

Controlling Spread of Infection

Control of the spread of infection is an objective hard to attain. Unlike other hazards in the environment, such as electrical cords and chair legs, microorganisms cannot be seen. Therefore, the problem of microbial invasion cannot be readily perceived unless it causes some visible response (e.g., purulent drainage). Integrity and steadfast awareness are key factors in the performance of nurses, as of others. Lister said, "You must be able to see with your mental eye the septic ferments as distinctly as we see flys, etc., with the corporeal eye." And this is a knack developed by practice.

Asepsis denotes being free from pathogens and is divided into two categories. *Medical asepsis* refers to procedures carried out to decrease the number of pathogens and to prevent the transfer of potential pathogens from one person to another. The object involved may still have nonpathogenic organisms on it, but it is considered that the patient-client can safely handle these. These practices are used for "clean" procedures, including many activities of daily living, and those procedures dealing with parts of the body not normally sterile. Examples of such procedures include bathing, administering oral medications, giving enemas. *Surgical asepsis* refers to those procedures designed to make an area or the objects within that area free of *all* microorganisms, not just pathogens. Such practices are employed in surgical suites and delivery rooms and during such procedures as catheterizations and venipunctures. These are called *sterile* procedures.

Techniques used to achieve asepsis constitute one means of controlling the spread of infection. In order to effect this prevention, the chain of infection must be broken, and the optimum place for breaking it is at its weakest link. To do this, the nurse must know the epidemiological picture of the disease process, e.g., symptoms, mode of transmission, incubation period, period of communicability, and susceptibility and resistance of the patient. In addition, he must also have knowledge of certain characteristics of the organism itself: (1) ability of the organism to survive outside the host—how long and under what conditions, and (2) how the organism can be destroyed. An excellent source book for such information is *The Control of Communicable Disease in Man* (Benenson, 1970). When he is aware of these factors, the nurse can begin to devise a system of barriers. A *barrier* is defined as anything which breaks contact with the organism or destroys it. The ideal barrier is not always feasible; when this situation exists, the "next best" method must be sought.

The nurse is only one of many health-team workers responsible for the control of infection. Others having a role include the physician, epidemiologist, laboratory worker, housekeeper, auxiliary worker, and the family. However, because of his knowledge and close contact with the patient-client and his family, the nurse is often the first to recognize an infectious process and to initiate the necessary procedures. For instance, a community health nurse visits a child with a sore throat, swollen glands, and a fever, and realizes the possibility of a beta-hemolytic streptococcal infection ("strep throat"). He has the family contact their physician, takes a throat culture, and delivers it to the laboratory. He instructs the child to cover his mouth when he coughs or sneezes and tells the family what precautions should be taken. Later he checks on the results of the culture. If it confirms the diagnosis, he follows up to make sure that the child and the rest of the family are adhering to the regimen of prophylactic antibiotics prescribed by the physician. He may also counsel the family about the time when the child can return to school without infecting classmates.

Many health-care facilities have an infection-control committee and an infection-control officer or epidemiologist. In a growing number of agencies, this epidemiologist is a nurse. The functions of these people vary from institution to institution but usually include such activities as setting infection-control policies, reviewing infection reports, tracking the origin of infection outbreaks, predicting and preventing potential sources of infection, and generally attempting to reduce the number of nosocomial infections within the institution. The epidemiologist works closely with the staff as a consultant.

In the hospital, the nurse is often the coordinator of measures recommended by the physician and the infection-control committee to set up barriers against the spread of infection. Some of the barriers in a system, such as adequate ventilation or the proper cleaning of special equipment, may be beyond the control of a beginning nurse. However, there are many barriers which he will be using frequently and for which he will be personally responsible from the earliest days of his practice. One of these is hand washing.

Hand Washing Hand washing is considered the most important barrier to infection. Two types of bacteria are found on the hands. *Resident* bacteria make up the rather stable flora present—stable in both type and number of bacteria. These kinds of organisms are deeply embedded, and it is essentially impossible to wash them off the skin. *Transient* bacteria are, as

their name implies, relatively transitory and usually are picked up in whatever task the person is presently engaged. These organisms are easily washed away, although if they are allowed to remain for a prolonged period, they may tend to become resident.

The three main components of an effective hand-washing technique are (1) running water, usually tap water; (2) soap, which reduces the surface tension of water and emulsifies the oils on the skin; and (3) friction. Friction is probably the most important, because it is this element that mechanically removes debris and organisms. There is no optimum washing time, since factors such as the presence or absence of rings and the degree of contamination will influence the amount of time needed. The major requirement is that the nurse establish a personal habit pattern so that he will be sure to wash completely every area every time. Since the skin is the body's first line of defense, a person's hand-washing technique should not be such that it causes excessive drying and cracking of the skin, thereby opening it to bacterial entry. Some precautions include using tepid rather than hot water, thus preserving more of the protective skin oils, and frequent use of hand lotion to replace the oils.

The frequency of hand washing depends on the situation in which the nurse is working. If hand washing is the best method of controlling cross-infection, it should be employed between physical contact with patient-clients and prior to handling stock supplies, such as the linen on the main cart. The nurse should immediately remove transient bacteria that he may have picked up during dressing changes or after handling soiled tissues. At the same time, he also needs to use good judgment, because hand washing done too frequently may unnecessarily break down the skin.

Isolation Technique *Isolation* is a procedure in which mechanical barriers are established to confine pathogens within a given area or prevent their entry into the area. Although the names assigned to different types of isolation techniques vary with the particular institution, the procedures employed are similar.

Contagious or *containment* isolation (Fig. 10-2) is designed to protect others from the patient-client. There are several gradations of restriction. *Strict* safeguards involve use of mask and protective garb by the nurse whenever he is in the patient's room. These protective measures are taken when dealing with conditions spread by droplets and of severe and moderately severe transmissibility and virulence, such as diphtheria, staphylococcal pneumonia, and acute bacterial meningitis (until antibiotic therapy has decreased the communicability). *Dressing,* or *hand and linen precautions* require special garb only when directly handling lesions which can be covered with a dressing and which then cause little or no environmental contamination. *Stool, needle, and urine precautions* involve special han-

dling of these items and are utilized against those organisms transmitted primarily through these exit and entry points, such as salmonella and viruses causing hepatitis.

Reverse, or *protective* isolation (Fig. 10-3) is intended to protect the patient-client from his environment. It is employed when the person's resistance to infection has been reduced by bone marrow failure because of radiation, leukemia, and anticancer medications; skin loss from extensive burns; or immunosuppressive drugs used after transplants. Under certain circumstances it may be necessary to combine the two major types of isolation.

The concept of isolation has always had its controversial aspects, especially in terms of specific techniques. Researchers and clinicians are looking at the set of restrictions in terms of its ritualistic features versus its scientific basis. Recently some major changes have been made in the procedure of active pulmonary tuberculosis

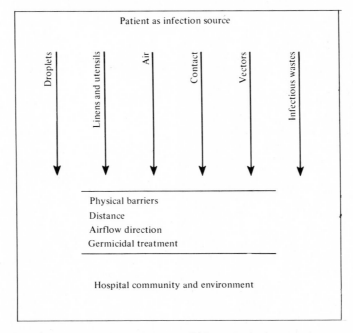

Figure 10-2 Contagious, or containment, isolation. *[From V. W. Greene, Microbial Contamination: Role of Nursing Services, Hospitals, 43:71ff. (1969). By permission of the author.]*

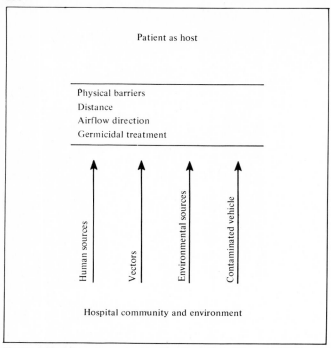

Figure 10-3 Reverse, or protective, isolation. *[From V. W. Greene, Microbial Contamination: Role of Nursing Services,* Hospitals, **43**:71ff. (1969). By permission of the author.]

isolation. Previously the nursing personnel wore gowns and masks (and sometimes caps) whenever working with the patient-client. This was based on the assumption that the tubercle bacillus would be carried via clothing and other objects. We now realize that although the bacillus can indeed survive on floors and clothes, it does not infect unless it is *inhaled.* Consequently, the patient-client now wears the mask if intimate face-to-face contact is necessary. Since the hardy bacillus can be carried via the ventilating system, more attention is being paid to this aspect of control (Weg, 1971).

When selecting the appropriate barrier techniques to be used, two questions need to be asked: "Who is being isolated from what?" and "How far do the restrictions have to go?" The answer to these queries will guide wise and practical choices. As discussed before, the decision about the use of these barriers needs to be a team one, and the nurse plays a major role. For instance, it is often on his suggestion that a potentially infectious patient-client is isolated to prevent spread of the organism to others in the environment. The nurse may also be the major adviser in the home situation, as in the case of the child with the streptococcal throat infection. Again, *The Control of Communicable Disease in Man* is an excellent source book for advisers.

The setting in which isolation procedures will be arranged varies from the home to a room on a general hospital ward to an elaborately designed room specific to that purpose. At home, restrictions will usually consist of any combination of hand washing; taking special care with dishes, tissues, and dressings; and restricting intimate contact with other family members (which is often difficult when there are small children). The essential requirements of a converted room on a general unit are that it be private and have running water; private toilet facilities are preferable. When no private rooms are available, persons infected with the same organism are often isolated in multiple-bed rooms. Staff use separate protective garb and supplies for each patient. Although necessity often dictates this arrangement, the risks of cross-contamination appear to be high. Isolation in multiple-bed rooms has not been adequately studied.

Each health-care facility has a well-defined procedure written out as to the specific techniques used within the isolation program. These techniques usually include the definition of clean and dirty areas; the kind of protective clothing to be worn and how to don and remove it; how to adapt certain nursing activities, such as taking vital signs, serving food and medications, and transportation of the patient-client; methods for *concurrent*, or day-to-day cleaning, and *terminal* disinfection after the patient-client is discharged; methods for collecting specimens; and visitor control. The nurse should always analyze these policies in terms of their scientific basis. Overelaborate techniques may be worse than none at all, since personnel may take short cuts. Such procedures should be the minimum necessary to ensure adequate barriers.

In addition to mastering these parts of the regimen, the nurse must also develop excellent work-organization habits. This will help him avoid being caught inside the isolation room without equipment he needs, resulting in unnecessary trips in and out of the room. Frequent movement in and out increases the risk of contamination and the necessity for hand washing.

Cleaning Methods These techniques are designed to remove pathogens from an object or area and are devised according to the characteristics of the known or suspected organisms present. The effectiveness of various methods of disinfection and sterilization depends on (1) concentration of the chemical or intensity of the physical agent used; (2) time allowed for the process; (3) nature of the material being treated, e.g., the presence of organic material, such as blood, on the object interferes with the process;

an enamel basin is easier to clean than a piece of rubber tubing; (4) the type of organisms to be destroyed, with spores being the most resistant; and (5) the number of microorganisms present.

Disinfection methods kill pathogenic organisms except spores; *sterilization* procedures destroy *all* microorganisms. Methods are of varying complexity and include use of soap and water, dry and wet heat, chemical solutions, steam under pressure, and gas sterilization. The latter is used on items such as plastic or rubber material or motors which cannot tolerate the heat of the regular autoclave. Packages which have been sterilized often have some kind of indicator showing that they have been through the sterilization process; the indicator may be masking tape which develops stripes, color patches which change color, or inserts placed inside the package. It is the nurse's responsibility to check these devices and to make sure that the wrapper around the package has not been punctured or damaged in any way.

The introduction of disposable items into health-care facilities has undoubtedly reduced the incidence of cross-infection. Because an item is used once or for one person only and then discarded, cleaning is not an issue. However, the accumulation of tremendous amounts of plastic waste is producing a different environmental problem.

Other Barriers The list of conceivable barriers could go on almost endlessly. Some examples of commonly utilized methods include increasing space between persons, closing doors or curtains, using soap, turning faucets off with a dry paper towel, muffling a sneeze with a tissue, and using a dishwasher.

In addition to assessing the need for and devising the appropriate barrier system for his patient-client and himself, the nurse must learn what the patient-client and his family know about the existence and transfer of pathogenic organisms. This needs to be done early so that the patient-client may be included in the planning of any restrictions deemed necessary. Not only does this enable him to take part in drawing up his own plan of care, but proper explanation will allow him and his family to cooperate better with the procedure. The importance of including both the patient-client and his family must be emphasized, since the patient-client will be depending on those family members for support.

It will be helpful to know what the family understands about organisms and how they cause infections, their knowledge about the infection chain, and their understanding of the purpose of the restrictions being placed on the patient-client and his family alike. Many times health workers falsely assume that their client's knowledge base in this area is the same as theirs. However, a whole realm of misconceptions is revealed when the client is asked how much he knows about the subject. It is also helpful to know what this infection means to the person—financial cost, loss of job time, expected prognosis, etc.

Using this assessment data, the nurse may begin his program of patient-client and family teaching. Careful and continuing explanations are necessary. The person with an infectious disease often feels that he is "dirty" and undesirable; therefore, enhancement of his self-esteem and demonstrated acceptance by others will help his psychological equilibrium.

Besides maintaining his own proficiency in the techniques discussed here, the nurse has the responsibility to see that others also follow proper procedure. Whenever he sees any break in technique, he must remind the involved person, whether doctor, nurse, laboratory technician, or visitor, of the degree of isolation regimen required.

Equipment Potentially Harboring Pathogens

Any equipment used in hospitals, if not cleaned properly between application to various patient-clients, is a potential source of cross-contamina-tion. However, some equipment is potentially more dangerous than others, mainly because it contains an environment conducive to microbial growth; warmth, darkness, moisture, and nutrients. Much research has been done to document the hazard of urinary tract catheters. Partial solutions to this problem include strict attention to sterile technique, and the use of sterile, closed drainage systems (Sanford, 1963; Santora, 1966).

It has been only rather recently that stress has been placed on the equipment used for inhalation therapy and the administration of anesthesia. Cultures of tubing leading from the patient-client to the machine produced colonies of gram-negative bacteria (Knight, 1967). Not only is this a potential source of cross-infection between persons, but it is also a hazard to the individual person himself, since a few bacteria left in the tubing after an intermittent positive-pressure breathing treatment may proliferate in the interim between treatments and be inhaled with the next treatment. If this process continues, the point will be reached when the number of organisms will overwhelm the person's defense system and will cause infection.

Isolettes in the nursery are also an excellent growth medium, as is intravenous equipment. The problem of hospital instrumentation infections will continue to grow as long as technology continues to provide new treatment modes; nurses must keep aware of the potential for infection so that intervention can occur.

Although nurses frequently recognize potential sources of contamination in equipment, they are rarely involved in the published research which documents such hazards. Nurses, as the handlers of much of this equipment and as the primary protectors of the hospitalized patient-client, must work more closely with epidemiologists to confirm their hunches. Such study does not require large-scale research. Recently, two nurses decided to follow up their hunch that bacterial contamination of urine occurred with the reuse of plastic catheter plugs. These plugs are commercially made to protect the ends of disconnected urinary catheters and drainage tubes from bacterial contamination. However, reuse of these plugs, which are not stored under sterile conditions, potentiates introduction of bacteria into the catheter and thus into the urine itself. These nurses cultured both the urine and the catheter plug of each of 20 patient-clients and found bacterial growth in both cultures for 80 percent of the patient-clients. Since organisms found on the plug were different from those in the urine, they concluded that the plugs were contaminated from outside the patient-client and that these bacteria represent a potential source of further urinary tract infection (Birum and Zimmerman, 1971).

ENVIRONMENTAL EFFECTS ON ILLNESS

The effect of our environment upon us is paramount. Research has shown that stimulation from the environment is essential for normal growth and development, and that patterns of sensory stimuli in infancy are closely linked with later functioning ability of that sensory modality (Waechter, 1969). We will all admit that elements such as the weather affect the way we feel. Environmental factors, such as color and noise, can also enhance or hinder the progress of a person's physical condition (Bartholet, 1968; Snook, 1964).

Although the areas of sensory deprivation and overload will be discussed in more depth in Part 3, Chapter 11, it is impossible not to include some aspects of them in our discussion of the environmental status. *Sensory* deprivation or overload is related to the amount or intensity of stimulation of the sensory organs; *perceptual* alteration deals with the patterning or meaningfulness of that stimulation. Deprivation in either of these areas may cause similar effects: confusion, hallucinations, difficulty in paying attention, impaired thought processes, and intense desire for stimulation, among other things.

The kinds of sensory stimuli this discussion is concerned with are the areas of the environment: light, noise, color, and patterns of activity, both of the person himself and of those around him. Disturbances which may occur are steady versus varied stimulation and excessive versus absent stimuli.

During health, most of us vary our sensory stimuli through our routine daily activities. Our systems require this variation, and we are able to meet this need. Illness alters this capability for diversification. Usually in the home situation, this means a reduction of stimuli, which may be advantageous for a time since the body is coping with the stress of illness. However, after an individualized length of time, the patient-client becomes restless, and the person caring for him must create ways to keep him occupied. These methods usually concern sensory stimulation, e.g., reliance on television, radio, toys, talking. These are all natural things to do.

Sensory and perceptual deprivation may progress to isolation, perhaps because of the restrictions of infection control. The dying person and the older person who is put in a private room because he is too noisy may also be isolated and avoided by the staff. Deprivation may occur in a person with a hearing loss, and most definitely occurs in the eye-patched patient-client. When caring for a person in isolation, the nurse must be particularly aware of what kind of stimulation he is receiving. Social stimulation is most certainly reduced because it is a chore to get ready to enter the person's room. However, this social interaction is extremely important for the isolated person, since his own self-concept depends on the reactions of others to him. Lack of contact with the staff is often interpreted by the patient-client as avoidance and rejection of him as an unacceptable person. Therefore, the nurse needs to plan for extra visits into the room just for the purpose of talking or other recreational activity.

The kind of stimulation must be varied in all senses: modality, pattern, and intensity. Otherwise the receiving sense organ becomes desensitized to the stimulation and may or may not seek a change.

The opposite of deprivation, or sensory overload, is also a frequent occurrence, especially in the hospital setting. Many studies have been done about the detrimental effects of the intensive-care unit with its constant light level, continuous noise, and activity. These conditions may also occur on the general ward. Most persons are more sensitive to excesses when they are ill and become very irritable and often unable to cooperate with the plan of care. This occurs because their body is already under the stress of illness or injury and does not have the energy to cope with added stimuli. The most common offenders are noise and patterns of activity. Because of hospital routines and prescribed medical and nursing regimens, patient-clients often do not have enough time to rest and recover the ability to absorb more stimuli.

There seems to be no easy answer to this problem, since no one can describe the happy medium. The nurse must carefully assess the condition of his patient-client and the effect the environment is having on him, and then make the proper adjustments.

The arrangement of the environment in relation to the person's functioning abilities and disabilities is also of vital importance. It will influence the amount of muscle activity he engages in and the joint range of motion he experiences. Many people need a period of dependence during their illness. However, as they convalesce, most people feel better when they can do as much for themselves as possible. This can be assured by arranging the environment so that the patient-client can help himself. Several suggestions made during the discussion of safety factors would also apply to this purpose, such as placing reading material and the television controls within easy reach and making sure the path is clear so that the person can get himself to the bathroom with his crutches.

Summary of Common Problems, with Approaches

Problem	Approach
Accidents	Eliminate existing and potential hazards.
Detrimental effects of restraints	Apply restraint properly, pad bony prominences, remove devices periodically to provide skin care.
Proper isolation procedure	Explain to patient-client and family, use proper technique and supervise technique of others, use good work organization, plan visits for socialization.
Sensory deprivation and overload	Vary stimuli, adjust stimuli as necessary, provide social interaction.
Patient-client independence	Arrange environment so that the patient-client can do things for himself.

REFERENCES

Bartholet, Mary: Effects of Color on the Dynamics of Patient Care, *Nursing Outlook,* **16**:51-53 (October, 1968).

Benenson, Abrams (ed.), "The Control of Communicable Disease in Man," 11th ed., American Public Health Association, New York, 1970.

Birum, Linda H., and Donna Zimmerman: Catheter Plugs as a Source of Infection, *American Journal of Nursing,* **71**:2150-2152 (1971).

Greene, V. W.: Microbial Contamination: Control in Hospitals, *Hospitals,* **43**:78+ (Oct. 16, 1969).

———: Microbial Contamination: Role of Nursing Services, *Hospitals,* **43**:71+ (Nov. 16, 1969).

Himmelsbach, Clifton: Nosocomial Infections, *Hospitals,* **44**:84+ (Feb. 16, 1970).

Hochberg, Howard: Effects of Electrical Current on Heart Rhythm, *American Journal of Nursing,* **71**:1390-1394 (1971).

Illingworth, Ronald, "The Normal Child," Little, Brown and Company, Boston, 1968.

Knight, Vernon: Instruments and Infection, *Hospital Practice,* **2**:82-95 (September, 1967).

Peszczynski, Mieczyslaw: Why Old People Fall, *American Journal of Nursing,* **65**:86-88 (1965).

Sanford, Jay: Hospital Acquired Urinary Tract Infections, *Proceedings of National Conference on Institutionally Acquired Infections* (1963).

Santora, Dolores: Preventing Hospital-acquired Urinary Infection, *American Journal of Nursing,* **66**:790-794 (1966).

Snook, Irving: Noise That Annoys, *Nursing Outlook,* **12**:33-35 (July, 1964).

Thompson, Morton, "The Cry and the Covenant," Doubleday & Company, Inc., Garden City, N.Y., 1949.

"Vital Statistics of the United States," Department of Health, Education and Welfare, 1969.

Waechter, Eugenia: Recent Research in Child Development,·*Nursing Forum,* **8**(4):374-391 (1969).

Weg, John: Tuberculosis and the Generation Gap, *American Journal of Nursing,* **71**:495-500 (1971).

ADDITIONAL READINGS

Amburgey, Pauline: Environmental Aids for the Aged Patient, *American Journal of Nursing,* **66**: 2017-2018 (1966).

Aranow, S., et al.: Ventricular Fibrillation Associated with an Electrically Operated Bed, *New England Journal of Medicine,* **281**:31-32 (July 3, 1969).

Bullough, Bonnie:·Where Should Isolation Stop? *American Journal of Nursing,* **62**:86-89 (1962).

Dyer, E., and D. E. Peterson: Safe Care of IPPB Machines, *American Journal of Nursing,* **71**:2163-2166 (1971).

Edmondson, Elmer B., et al.: Nebulization Equipment, *American Journal of Diseases in Children,* **111**:357-360 (1966).

Fierer, J., et al.: *Pseudomonas aeruginosa* Epidemic Traced to·Delivery-room Resuscitation, *New England Journal of Medicine,* **276**:991-996 (May 4, 1971).

How the Septicemia Trail Led to the I.V. Bottle Caps, *Hospital Practice,* **6**:35-45 and 151-154 (August, 1971).

"Infection Control in Hospitals," rev. ed., American Hospital Association, Chicago, 1970.

Jamann, Joann: Health Is a Function of Ecology, *American Journal of Nursing,* **71**:970-973 (1971).

Mertz, J. J., et al.: A Hospital Outbreak of Klebsiella Pneumonia from Inhalation Therapy with Contaminated Aerosol Solutions, *American Review of Respiratory Diseases,* **95**:454-460 (1967).

Roueche, Berton, "Eleven Blue Men and Other Narratives of Medical Detection," Little, Brown and Company, Boston, 1947.

Streeter, Shirley, et al.: Hospital Infections—A Necessary Risk? *American Journal of Nursing,* **67**:526-533 (1967).

Williams, R. Fraser: Clinical Infection 2: Environmental Factors, *Nursing Times,* **63**:1617-1619 (1967).

Sensory Status

Pamela Mitchell

Data to Be Assessed

Visual status
  Acuity
  Field of vision
  Known deficits
  Corrective devices
  Unusual sensations
Auditory status
  Ability to distinguish voices
  Known deficits
  Corrective devices
  Unusual sensations
Olfactory status
  Ability to discriminate odors
  Unusual sensations
Gustatory status
  Ability to discriminate sweet, sour, salt, bitter
  Unusual sensations

Tactile status
  Ability to discriminate sharp, dull, light, firm touch
  Ability to perceive heat and cold, pain
  Stereognosis
  Intactness of body image
  Aberrant sensation
Speech formation and perception
  Intactness of speech organs
  Deficits in phonation
  Ability to understand and initiate speech
Sensory environment
  Intensity
  Pattern
  Variety
  Appropriateness to level of development

SENSATION

Sensation governs our ability to perceive, define, and react to ourselves and our world. Consequently, deviation from normal sensory status has some of the most extensive consequences of any health deviation.

We first learn about the environment and begin to define ourselves as separate beings through our sensations. A newborn baby has no perception of himself as separate from his environment. Gradually, through his sense of touch, and later through vision and hearing, he begins to perceive the quality of the world. He turns toward noises, he follows light, he reaches for objects. His internal sensations play a part in defining self as separate from others. He is hungry (a visceral sensation) but not immediately fed, and eventually begins to realize that the food comes from "out there." He sees his hands and feet but does not recognize them as part of himself. Eventually he appreciates the sensations involved in moving his hands where he wants them to go (kinesthetic sensation).

Children use their senses to discriminate and generalize what they know about the world. They use sight, smell, and touch to discriminate "apple" from other somewhat round, red objects they see. They begin to sort out certain sounds and to imitate these sounds. From these efforts come language.

To be meaningful, sensations must be interpreted as well as perceived. The interpretation of sensations is the basis for response to the environment. Early response is primarily reflex. For example, the infant responds to hunger by moving his mouth toward any object which touches it (rooting). If something is put into his mouth, he sucks, regardless of whether he is hungry. Both these actions are reflex responses to sensation. Rooting is a response to visceral sensation, sucking to tactile sensation.

Later, our senses provide the cues for learned behavior. For example, we have learned to stop when we see a red traffic light. We also learn to respond to certain cues or partial information, rather than to the whole welter of sensory stimuli constantly about us. Carrying on a conversation in a noisy room is an example of such selective response.

People who suddenly lose sensory input from a major source cannot utilize these usual means to perceive and respond to environmental cues. For example, the newly blinded person may perceive all auditory stimuli as being of equal intensity. He can, however, learn to listen for cues. If he is trying to cross a busy street unaided, he can no longer see the traffic light, but he can learn to listen to the traffic patterns in order to know when cars are moving or stopped. He can learn to listen to the flow of pedestrian conversation in order to tell in which direction people are moving. And he can use his sense of touch (being jostled) to tell when the crowd begins to move across the street.

This example gives a brief idea of some of the kinds of changes which must take place in the perception and interpretation of stimuli when a deviation occurs in a person's sensory status. Because sensation is so basic to our perception and response to the environment, even minor alterations may make important changes in a person's life and his ability to carry on daily living.

CHANGES IN SENSORY STATUS

Sensory status is the person's situation in respect to all sensory modalities (specific sensory entities). It includes the functioning of the various sense organs and receptors, the normality or abnormality of perception of sensory stimuli, and the quality of the sensory-perceptual environment.

A wide variety of local or systemic diseases or structural defects can change sensory status. For example, disease or structural defect in the optic nerve can lead to varying states of decreased vision or blindness. A stroke (cerebrovascular accident) can destroy portions of central nerve pathways necessary for touch and proprioception. The person so afflicted "loses track" of where his arm or leg is, unless he is looking at it. Sometimes he cannot tell the shape of an object by simply feeling it, or he may stumble when changing from a grassy surface to the sidewalk because he cannot feel the difference in texture.

Categorizing and defining these specific consequences of changed sensory status are beyond the scope of this textbook, and are more appropriate to specialized medical and nursing books. Instead we will focus on the concept of sensory restriction and overload. This concept is broadly applicable to any patient-client who has a deficit or abnormality in sensory status.

The nurse's purpose in assessing sensory status differs from that of the physician. When a person has a health problem related to sensory function, the physician makes a detailed assessment of sensory organs, nerve pathways, and the person's interpretation of input in order to determine the cause of the sensory deficit. This cause may be in the sensory organ, the nerve pathway, or the brain itself.

The nurse may collect some of the same kinds of data, but he uses these data to determine the extent to which the abnormality affects the person's daily living. The cause of the deficit will certainly be of importance in determining whether the nurse and patient-client will focus on adaptation to the deficit (if it is temporary) or integration of it (if it is permanent), and how much it will affect growth and development. However, discovering the cause is not the primary purpose of the nursing assessment.

Data about the sensory environment form an important part of the sensory assessment. They are important in determining actions needed to support sensory development in infants and children, and in preventing or remedying effects of sensory restriction and overload in both children and adults.

One must assess not only the current sensory environment (kind, quality, quantity of stimuli) but also its quality in relation to the person's *usual* environment. Restriction and overload are relative terms: what constitutes a restricted or overloaded environment depends in part upon the usual amount and pattern of stimuli.

In some situations, much of the data regarding sensory status may be available in the physician's notes. However, the nurse still needs to determine, through observation and interview, the effects of sensory status upon the person's daily life.

SENSORY MODALITIES

There are a number of ways of classifying sensation, based upon the source of stimuli, the kind of sensory receptor, or the sense organ itself. None of these classifications is entirely satisfactory to encompass all the variants of sensation. For the purposes of this chapter, we will classify sensation on the basis of the origin of the stimulus—internal or external (see Table 11-1). This is an extremely broad and simplified grouping. However, since this chapter is concerned with broad problems of sensory restriction and overload, a detailed listing of sensory categories is not relevant.

Adequate stimuli (those sufficient to generate electrical potential in the specific sensory receptor) are external to the person for the classic senses of sight, hearing, taste, smell, and touch. Stimuli arise internally for the visceral and kinesthetic sensations. Visceral sensations are those arising from the hollow organs; kinesthetic sensations are those arising from muscles. These sensations allow us to tell where parts of the body are in relation to one another.

This broad classification of internal and external stimulation does not apply strictly even to these seemingly clear-cut sensory modalities. Astronauts report "seeing" flashes of light in the absence of any known external source. These

Table 11-1   Classification of the Major Sensory Modalities

Source of adequate stimulus	Modality*	Receptor	Sense organ
External	Visual		Eye
	Auditory	Exteroceptor	Ear
	Olfactory		Nose
	Tactile		Skin
	Gustatory (internal and external)	Enteroceptor	Tongue (taste bud)
Internal	Kinesthetic	Proprioceptor	Muscle
	Visceral	Interoceptor	Hollow organs (includes blood vessels)

* The visual, auditory, olfactory, tactile, gustatory, and kinesthetic modalities are most commonly involved in problems of sensory restriction or overload. The visceral modality is primarily involved in homeostatic regulatory mechanisms and the sensation of pain.

flashes may be caused by cosmic rays striking the retina and internally stimulating visual sensation. Disorders of the auditory nerve can stimulate "sound" when there is no external stimulus. Similarly, odors can arise from internal pressure on the olfactory nerve. However, in most instances, classifying stimuli by point of origin will be adequate for the purposes of this chapter.

The idea that sensation is stimulated both internally and externally is important, because stimuli from both sources contribute to the sensory information which is ultimately interpreted by the brain. An increase or decrease in stimuli from either the internal or external environment, therefore, only partially changes the total sensory input to the brain. The significance of this fact will be considered in discussing the implications of research in sensory restriction.

THE PERCEPTION OF SENSATION

This review of the transmission and perception of sensory stimuli is not intended to be a comprehensive treatment of this complex subject. It is intended to provide a synopsis of some of the current theories which attempt to explain the phenomenon of sensory deprivation. Several of the references at the end of the chapter provide more detail about these theories.

The process of sensory perception is initiated by an adequate stimulus which is generated either internally or externally. Adequate stimuli are generally quite specific for the sensory receptor—e.g., we do not "see" a noise or "hear" a light. The specific sensory receptor synapses with a nerve (peripheral, autonomic, or cranial) and transmits the sensory input (the electrical potential generated by the stimulus) to the brain. The nerve may directly synapse with areas of the brain, or it may synapse with sensory nerve tracts within the spinal cord. The spinothalamic tract is the principal such sensory nerve tract.

The exact mechanism by which the brain "processes" and thereby interprets sensory input is not known. There is evidence that the thalamus, hypothalamus, and reticular activating system (RAS) all play roles in assembling and integrating incoming and outgoing data. The input is relayed to the cortex, where it is interpreted, and conscious awareness of sensation occurs. Firing of neurons within the cortex itself can activate the reticular system and influence or alter the perception of external stimuli. This system of feedback circuits is complex and not well understood.

Lindsley hypothesizes that the reticular activating system is the major mediator of sensory input, serving as "a kind of barometer for both input and output level . . . regulating or adjusting input-output levels."[1] Sensory input is routed through the reticular activating system from the classical sensory tracts and from the hypothalamus. Although areas of the RAS respond selectively to input in specific sensory modalities, it appears that incoming stimuli and cortically generated impulses tend to act interchangeably as well in stimulating the RAS. Stimulation of the RAS creates an aroused state in the organism. Conversely, a decrease in stimulation leads to drowsiness and sleep. Arousal seems to be a necessary prerequisite to selective perception or response to cues (Schultz, 1965, pp. 15–19). For example, sensory stimulation in infant animals or human beings causes an aroused or alert state. However, the infant does not appear to discriminate among stimuli, but responds as if all environmental input is of equal intensity. As the nervous system matures, arousal of the RAS seems to facilitate the discrimination of a selective response to cues (Riesen, 1961; Schultz, p. 26). These cues are partial information from which the organism makes inferences about the nature of the environment.

The information which enables us to interpret or perceive the meaning of sensory stimuli is "stored" in the cortex. Arousal via the RAS appears to be an important factor in our ability to select and correlate this information. The physiologic and psychologic details of this process of perception and information processing are not at all well understood. Most theorists will agree that we somehow transform raw stimuli to rather complex understanding and inferences. They will also agree that sensory restriction, distortion, and overload somehow disorder this processing. They disagree as to the way in which this disordering takes place, and in the metaphors by which they attempt to describe the process.

[1] Donald Lindsley, Common Factors in Sensory Deprivation, Sensory Distortion and Sensory Overload, in P. Solomon et al. (eds.), "Sensory Deprivation," Harvard University Press, Cambridge, Mass., 1961, p. 177.

Sensoristasis

The abnormal behavior seen in developing and mature people and animals who have had sensory stimuli restricted has suggested to many behavioral scientists that there is a need or drive for sensory stimulation. Schultz calls this *sensoristasis,* relating it to Cannon's homeostasis, or dynamic physiologic equilibrium (1939). According to Schultz's hypothesis, an organism requires a level of stimulation, within a range, to function optimally. If sensory stimulation falls below that level, the organism seeks alternative stimuli, and becomes sensitized to stimuli as it seeks to restore equilibrium. Sensory stimuli greater than the optimal range would then lead to attempts to decrease input.

A decrease in optimal sensory level appears to affect the development of normal perception and response in the growing organism. For example, children and young animals reared in extremely restricted environments demonstrate abnormal social and perceptual behavior when placed in a "normal" situation. Despite subsequent normal environments, they often do not completely overcome these early deficits (Beach and Jaynes, 1954; Goldfarb, 1955; Sackett, 1970). This abnormal or slowed development may occur because the RAS has not been sufficiently aroused to facilitate normal cortical sensory development.

The mature organism seems to require a sensoristatic environment to maintain perceptual and responsive function. The adult subjects in experimental sensory deprivation often require one or more days to regain some preexperimental thinking and perceptual levels.

The concept of a need for sensory stimulation is not new, but research into the effects of sensory restriction and overload is not yet well enough developed to quantify the sensory input necessary for sensoristasis. Experiments with human beings show a wide variation in individual ability to tolerate and adapt to sensory restriction. Research conducted has not been designed to determine the limits of normal sensory stimulation. Therefore, the concept of sensoristasis is much less precise than the physiological concept of homeostasis. Despite its imprecision, the concept of sensoristasis has relevance to the consideration of the effects of sensory restriction and overload.

SENSORY-PERCEPTUAL RESTRICTION AND OVERLOAD

The concept of sensory restriction and overload is based upon research begun in the early 1950s. This research into the effects of reduced sensory input began in Canada, prompted by the "brainwashing" reported in Chinese and Russian prisons. Confessions and political conversions seemed to be accomplished rather rapidly by manipulating the sensory environment. Consequently, the governments of Canada, and later the United States, sponsored experimental work to determine what happens to human behavior under conditions of sensory deprivation. Long after the furor over brainwashing subsided, investigators continue to explore the effects of the sensory-perceptual environment on behavior, perception, and thinking.

Terms Used

A number of terms are used in describing the experimental conditions used in research in sensory deprivation. The term *sensory deprivation* is commonly used to refer to diminution in amount and pattern of sensory stimuli. More strictly, there are differences in experimental conditions involving sensory deprivation (or restriction), perceptual deprivation, perceptual monotony, and social isolation.

Sensory deprivation or *restriction* is usually defined as the reduction of all sensory stimuli to a minimum. There is no way to deprive an organism absolutely of sensory stimuli, as many stimuli are generated from within the organism. There is also an unavoidable low level of stimu-

lation due to experimental equipment. Thus, this condition is more properly termed sensory restriction. The terms are used interchangeably in the experimental literature.

Classical experimental conditions of sensory deprivation or restriction include absence of light and sound (via soundproofed room, or goggles and earphones blocking sound and light) and padded limb mitts to decrease tactile stimuli. Obviously, there is still some tactile stimulation from other areas of the body, as well as visceral and kinesthetic sensation.

Perceptual deprivation or *restriction* refers to the absence or decrease in *meaningful patterning* of sensory stimuli. Perceptual deprivation is produced experimentally by muffling the tactile sense with padded mitts and shoes, providing a constant and unchanging low noise level, and providing dim, unchanging light. Translucent masks and halved Ping-Pong balls over both eyes are two of the methods used to create an unchanging visual field.

Perceptual monotony occurs when the sensory stimuli have a normal pattern but are without variety. Staying in a windowless room for several hours would produce perceptual monotony.

Social isolation is a form of perceptual monotony. An unchanging environment and the absence of other people (or animals) creates the social lack of variety. Social isolation may occur in a group setting as well, provided there is no variety in social contact. Most of the information about the effects of social isolation is anecdotal, from recollections of prisoners and shipwrecked sailors. There have been a few experimental and field studies of isolated groups; most of these are military studies related to effects of submarine or Antarctic group isolation.

Studies in animals demonstrate the important effects of social isolation on the developing animal. Various animals reared in seclusion demonstrate asocial and abnormal social behavior when placed with other animals. If the early deprivation has been long enough, the animals never are able completely to learn normal social behavior (Beach and Jaynes, 1954; Sackett, 1970).

In this chapter, the term *sensory-perceptual restriction* applies to nonexperimental situations in which the normal amount, variety, and pattern of sensory input are diminished. *Sensory-perceptual overload* will refer to a marked increase in amount or intensity of stimuli to the point at which normal discrimination of pattern is lost. As pointed out before, the range of "normal" pattern of sensory input is not clearly defined. Thus, restriction or overload may be fairly marked before it is detectable in nonexperimental conditions.

Effects of Sensory and Perceptual Restriction

One cannot succinctly summarize the behavioral effects of experimental sensory-perceptual deprivation. Experimental conditions, tests and measurements used, and individual reactions are so varied as to preclude a concise listing of effects. The length of experiments varies from a few hours to as long as two weeks. Severity of the condition varies from simply lying on a bed in a room to being totally immersed in water with an air mask. Results are usually reported in terms of those who finished the experiments; yet the effects on those who could not tolerate the conditions and quit are of great interest in relation to conditions of clinical sensory-perceptual restriction.

Despite the wide variety of response and experimental procedure, there are some consistent responses to sensory-perceptual deprivation. Very little research has been conducted into the effects of sensory overload in human beings. However, researchers postulate that the effects may be similar to those of sensory-perceptual deprivation, because of similar disorganizing effects on the RAS regulator mechanism for sensory input (Lindsley, 1961).

Japanese investigators recently attempted to compare the effects of sensory overload and sensory deprivation. They postulated that sensory overload (experimentally produced by increased intensity of sound and light) would be more disorganizing to thought processes than sensory deprivation. The objective measurements did not support this hypothesis; however, the subjects of the overload experiments found the situation more uncomfortable and reacted with more anxiety, aggression, and sadness than did the deprived subjects (Studies in Sensory Overload, 1970).

Objective Effects In experimental situations, people whose sensory, perceptual, and/or social environment is markedly restricted have shown decreased ability to perform a variety of objective cognitive (thinking) and motor tests. These tests include mathematical problem solving, abstract reasoning, recall, eye-hand coordination, and general motor coordination. Deficits in perceptual abilities include decreased ability to reproduce a figure (see the example in Fig. 11-1), inability to reverse reversible figures, and changes in color perception. Other consistent effects are a decrease in physical activity and a change in the electroencephalogram that is characteristic of decreased alertness. These electroencephalogram changes become more pronounced as the duration of sensory-perceptual restriction increases.

The impairment of performance seems related to the duration of the experiment, the nature of the deprivation (primarily sensory or perceptual), and the kind of tasks performed. In general, longer deprivation leads to a larger number of impairments. The extent of impairment does not seem to increase after a certain amount of time, adaptation occurring in about twenty-four hours. Perceptual deprivation and immobility (kinesthetic deprivation) produce greater cognitive deficits than sensory deprivation alone. Subjects are better able to perform highly structured tasks, such as memorizing a list of words, than moderately structured or unstructured tasks. A

Presented figure   Perceived figure

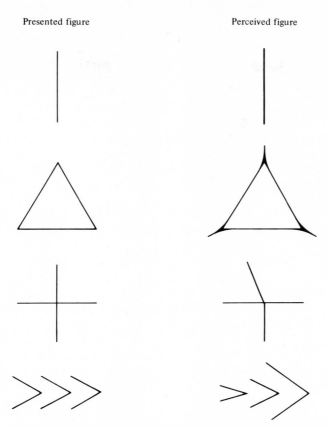

Figure 11-1 Figures used in a perception test with examples of perceptual distortion. *(From P. Solomon et al., "Sensory Deprivation," Harvard University Press, Cambridge, Mass., 1961. By permission of the publisher.)*

moderately structured task might be to make up a story about a specific picture; an unstructured task would be to make up a story about anything.

Subjective Effects People in the experiments consistently report difficulty in thinking and concentrating, but these subjective changes are not easily verified by objective tests. Because the subjective experience is extremely important in a patient-client's reaction to clinical sensory-perceptual restriction, we will discuss the common subjective reactions in some detail.

The commonly reported subjective reactions include difficulty in thinking and concentrating, drifting thoughts, daydreaming, disorientation to time, anxiety and apprehension, strange illusions about one's body (a floating feeling of parts or all of the body), restlessness, claustrophobia, somatic discomforts (backache, headache), feelings of persecution, hallucinations, and auditory and visual images. Specific reactions vary considerably with persons. Some find their fantasies and daydreaming rather pleasant; others become so much disturbed as to leave the experiment. Goldberger and Holt (1961) hypothesize that the decrease in environmental pattern and stimulation interferes with normal contact with reality and allows the release of "primary-process" thought—the kind of unreal or instinctual thinking which is usually experienced only in dreams or psychotic states. According to their hypothesis, people who are mature, with a strong ego, are better able to handle this primary-process thought and, therefore, adapt successfully to isolation and sensory-deprivation situations. Those who are threatened by these thoughts tend to become more severely anxious, find the experiment very unpleasant, or even quit.

Hallucinations or Visual Images   The occurrence of visual and auditory hallucinations (imagined events or objects) and illusions (distortions of the real environment) is a dramatic and much-publicized phenomenon of the sensory-perceptual deprivation experiments. Similar phenomena have been reported by truck drivers and jet aviators, both of whom are exposed to monotonous, perceptually restricted environments (Heron, 1957; Bennett, 1961).

These reported sensations range from flashes of light to complex scenes, such as squirrels marching across a landscape. Some experimental subjects experienced only visual or only auditory sensations; others saw images complete with sound. In some instances, the subjects felt the hallucination or illusion to be quite real; in others, they were aware that what they saw and heard "wasn't really there." The occurrence of visual and auditory sensation varies with the experimental condition, method of reporting (whether during or after the experiment), and the expectational "set" given the subject (e.g., whether he is told or knows to expect something unusual to occur). However, these phenomena do occur in some people in nearly all the experiments. There is no consistent correlation of any particular personality characteristics, levels of anxiety, intelligence, or amount of physical activity during the experiment with the occurrence of imagery. The phenomena occur in both sen-

sory and perceptual deprivation and in some experiments in social isolation. There seems to be a greater incidence in the first hours of experiments, with the number of experiences diminishing in frequency over time (Schultz, 1965; Zuckerman, 1969).

Individual Tolerance for Sensory-Perceptual Deprivation   A number of investigators have attempted to predict, on the basis of paper-and-pencil personality tests or psychoanalytic tools, the factors which contribute to individual tolerance to experimental conditions of sensory-perceptual deprivation. The findings are inconsistent at best, but tend to confirm what a sensitive observer of people's habits might predict; namely, that the person who becomes bored easily, wants a great deal of excitement, is impulsive, and needs to manipulate others endures a perceptually deprived environment poorly or not at all (Meyers, 1969). Conversely, the person who does not depend on the environment for intellectual or emotional satisfaction, who finds some pleasure in fantasy or imagery, can tolerate or even enjoy such conditions (Goldberger and Holt, 1961; Lilly, 1956). The many biographical accounts of solitary confinement in prisons or solitary sea voyages suggest that the people who survived were those who had inner intellectual and emotional resources for structuring their isolated environments.

CLINICAL PROBLEMS OF SENSORY-PERCEPTUAL RESTRICTION AND OVERLOAD

It is tempting to apply the findings of sensory-deprivation research wholesale to the clinical situation—to explain many behavioral oddities on the basis of sensory-perceptual restriction, or to expect anyone in a monotonous institutional environment to develop the same cognitive and behavioral impairments reported in the research literature. The experimental and clinical situations are not that comparable, however. Most sensory-deprivation experiments are conducted on young male volunteers, either college students or military personnel. Unlike the ill or clinically confined person, these experimental subjects were free to leave the experiment at any time, and they often knew its duration. The kinds of sensory deprivation employed, the psychological set of the subject, and the definitions of normal and abnormal behavior are considerably more defined in the laboratory than in the usual institutional environment. Finally, the clinical situations which we will consider include a variety of sensory, perceptual, and disease factors which are not constant; whereas the variables in the experimental situations are manipulated at the discretion of the investigators.

However, if we bear in mind the limitations of direct application of research findings to the "real world," the concept of sensory-perceptual restriction can be useful in examining the potential effects of many health problems on a person's sensory status.

Many clinical situations contain some of the elements of sensory-perceptual restriction or overload. The hallucinations of some people with bulbar poliomyelitis who were in tank respirators ("iron lung") prompted early clinical comparisons to sensory-deprivation research (Leiderman, 1958). Because of Leiderman's observations, tank respirators were used as the restrictive condition in a number of sensory-deprivation experiments (Solomon, 1961).

A person immobilized in a body cast or traction is somewhat comparable to those in the group whom Zubek and Wilgosh (1963) immobilized in a box. These young men had a normally patterned but obviously restricted perceptual environment. Nonetheless, they had the same perceptual and motor impairments found in previous sensory-perceptual deprivation studies. This led the investigators to hypothesize that immobilization, or kinesthetic deprivation, accounts for many of the perceptual and motor abnormalities.

The person who is acutely ill is usually anxious and afraid, and these emotions in themselves lead to narrowed perception. He may have decreased awareness because of drugs which have been prescribed by the physician or which he takes habitually. If sensory-perceptual restriction or overload is added to this state, it is reasonable to predict that he may exhibit many of the perceptual distortions, problem-solving difficulties, anxieties, or even hallucinatory behavior reported in experimental sensory and perceptual restriction. If this is the case, raising or lowering the level of sensory stimulation or providing meaningful pattern to the sensory input should decrease these symptoms in time.

The case presentations of "clinical sensory deprivation" tend to support these hypotheses. There are a few reports of people in restricted sensory-perceptual environments whose suddenly "psychotic" behavior is not explainable on the basis of toxic reactions, drugs, or organic brain disease. The behavior cleared up within a few days when sensory input (social, visual, auditory) increased (Leiderman, 1958; Jackson, Pollard, and Kansky, 1962). The largest body of literature regarding clinical sensory deprivation deals with "eye-patched patients"—people, generally with cataracts or detached retinas, whose eyes are patched and who are relatively immobilized after eye surgery (summarized in Jackson, 1969). They are thus temporarily or partially blind. These studies point to a high incidence of temporary mental impairment in patient-clients with this major sensory deficit. Almost all the people with detached retinas and 30 to 50 percent of those with cataracts experience restlessness or anxiety, or become involuntarily noncompliant with medical therapy (get out of bed or tear off bandages). Some become confused, have hallucinations, or experience "dreamlike" visual images.

The nursing literature contains a few reports of patients in institutions (a perceptually monotonous environment) who became better oriented, less apathetic, more aware of self, and more socially active after one- to eight-week periods of sensory and social stimulation (Cockburn, 1967; Carlson, 1968; Moody et al., 1970). These reports cannot be taken together to "prove" that sensory-perceptual deprivation occurs clinically. The reports do not compare similar situations, nor similar groups with and without the "therapeutic" stimulation. However, they point to a hypothesis to be tested—that institutionalized people and people whose acute condition restricts their social and perceptual field experience at least some of the subjective effects of sensory deprivation.

The general concept of sensory-perceptual restriction and overload has several implications for nurses. These include the management of the sensory-perceptual environment for the developing infant and child and the prevention and management of sensory-perceptual restriction and overload in the susceptible patient-client.

Sensory-Perceptual Restriction in Development

There is growing evidence that the environment during infancy of animals and human beings affects their subsequent perceptual, motor, and social abilities. The nervous system of human beings and of many animals is not completely developed at birth. Therefore, many investigators postulate that early sensory and perceptual experiences influence the anatomic development of the neural networks by which general arousal of the brain is translated into specific perception (Sackett, 1970).

Studies of the early behavior of many kinds of animals, birds, and other organisms suggest that there is a critical stage during infancy after which the effects of sensory, perceptual, and social deprivation become at least partially irreversible (Beach and Jaynes, 1954). Riesen's (1961) studies of primates and cats demonstrate that visual deprivation in infancy resulted in

irreversible visual-perceptual defects when the animals were subsequently placed in a normal visual environment. Primates deprived of normal social and sensory environment during a critical period of infancy are never able to achieve certain normal social and perceptual abilities. For example, female rhesus monkeys raised without mothers are brutally aggressive toward their first offspring and do not learn mothering behavior. Socially isolated monkeys tend to be sexually inept, less gregarious, and more easily frightened than those raised in social contact (Reisen; Sackett, 1970).

Evidence of the critical nature of early perceptual and social environment in human beings comes primarily from observations of children raised from infancy in institutions and anecdotal reports of feral children, or those raised in the wilds. Feral children are those raised in isolation from human beings, either locked away by their parents or supposedly raised by animals. Such children are often quite retarded, mentally as well as socially.

The classic observations of Spitz (1945) and Goldfarb (1955) of children institutionalized in their first and second to third years of life emphasize the critical nature of early experiences on the development and socialization of children.

Spitz observed the motor, perceptual, and social development of 130 children in two institutions and compared them with 30 children raised in their own homes. The children raised at home and those raised by their mothers in the prison nursery (one of the institutions) maintained a normal developmental level during the year. The infants in a "foundling home" began at a normal developmental level but dropped markedly below that level and below that of all the other children by the end of the year. The major difference between the two institutions was the kind of maternal and sensory environments.

The children in the foundling home, after

weaning, had contact with a nurse for only brief periods at feedings, could not see out of their cribs, and had few toys or objects to look at. They spent the majority of the day on their backs, ultimately wearing such hollows in the crib mattresses that they could not turn over when physically mature enough to do so.

In contrast, the children in the prison nursery could see one another and see activity in the corridors. They had many toys and, most important, had frequent and consistent contact with their own mothers or with mother substitutes. Spitz emphasized that the presence of a mother or mother substitute was more important than the mere presence of sensory-stimulating objects. He felt that the emotional attachment to the mother was the "bait" which induced the child to explore the sensory environment.

Goldfarb observed children institutionalized from the first to third years. He found these children to be less gregarious, of lower intelligence, more impulsive, and more asocial than children of similar background raised in foster homes (a more normal environment). The major emphasis in both these works is the influence of maternal deprivation. However, sensory contact is an integral part of mothering—all the more so if an institutional environment offers little variety and sensory stimulation.

More recently, the effects of increasing sensory stimulation for children have been investigated. A group of infants exposed to increased handling and to objects hanging overhead spent more time looking at objects and were able purposefully to grasp objects sooner than a group who spent their time in cribs with nothing to look at but their hands (White, 1967). The abundance of "educational" toys for infants attests to public interest in these observations.

It is hard to demonstrate unequivocally that early stimulation, and thus earlier motor development, increases intelligence or socialization. However, it is clear that the converse is true. A marked decrease in normal levels of social and

sensory stimulation may lead to later emotional and learning problems.

Nursing Management Nursing management of the sensory environment of adults is primarily necessary in health crises, in institutions, and when there are specific sensory defects. However, when infants and children are concerned, the nurse's role encompasses management of the normal environment, as well as the environment during illness. The nurse may teach and support the parents in maintaining an adequately stimulating environment, or he may directly manage the sensory-perceptual-social environment.

Guiding Parents in Environmental Management Many people "automatically" raise their children in an adequately stimulating environment. Others, however, because of custom, lack of knowledge, or lack of materials, raise their infants in a sensorily impoverished environment.

Mrs. W. S. was a 32-year-old mother of six, ages 12 years to 3 months. Mr. S. worked on a corn-seed farm, receiving $40 to $60 per week, plus the use of a decaying house owned by his employer. Two of the school-age children were in special classes for children with learning difficulties. A public health nurse visited the family for a variety of reasons. One of her concerns was for George, the 14-month-old. George spent most of his time in his crib, out of the traffic of the other children. He was slow in motor development—did not stand, rarely crawled in his crib, seemed apathetic, and was increasingly likely to lie in his bed staring at the ceiling.

Mrs. S. had noticed this "slowness" and agreed that it might help to expand George's horizons, but felt he could not be put on the floor, as it was so cold. Her concern was valid, for the only source of heat was not adequate to keep the house warm. She had no money for toys to put in the crib, and had not thought of using household items. Together, she and the nurse made "cradle gyms" of measuring cups, bright plastic lids, and cloth. They used washed plastic bottles, scraps of cloth and wooden spoons to create a variety of objects which George

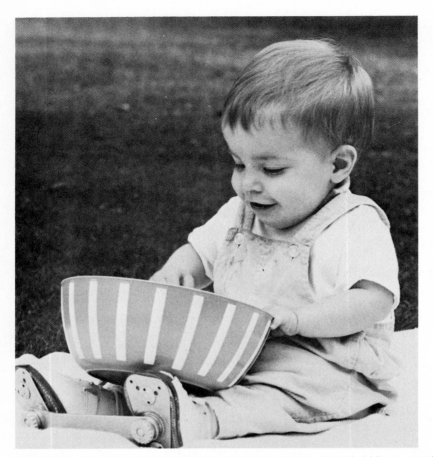

Figure 11-2 Helping a baby explore the world. Inexpensive household items may be used as toys to feel, grasp, and chew upon.

could feel, see, and chew on (see Fig. 11-2). His crib was moved to the center of activity, except for nap time.

Gradually, he became more interested in his environment and interested in the other children. On her own, Mrs. S. constructed similar items for Bonnie, the 3-month-old.

Mrs. S. is an example of a person whose lack of knowledge and materials led to an impoverished sensory-perceptual and social environment for her infants. Once the nurse had helped her with both, her own motivation led her to apply the knowledge to her younger baby.

More difficult problems arise when culture or custom dictate minimal handling and quiet surroundings for babies beyond the first month or two. Out of concern for "spoiling" a child, some mothers hold them only for feedings, and provide little in the way of stimulation when the infant is in its crib. Citing scientific evidence for increased stimulation will probably get the nurse nowhere, when culture and custom dictate otherwise. However, if the nurse can demonstrate the practical value of bright objects and variety in amusing a fussy baby, he may be on the way to helping a family increase the environmental stimulation. Several references at the end of this chapter give practical and inexpensive ideas for stimulation appropriate to the child's developmental level.

It is possible to provide too *much* stimulation for a young infant, thereby producing sensory overload. White and his associates (1967) demonstrated that massive enrichment of the environment actually slowed the onset of sustained attention to the baby's own hand, and seemed to produce more crying during the first five weeks of life. After two to three months, however, this group of infants achieved purposeful, directed grasp much earlier than those in a nonenriched environment.

Thus, the same set of stimuli produced opposite effects in the same children. This supports the idea that the sensory environment must be tailored to fit the individual child's motor and sensory abilities at any one level.

Direct Environmental Management Nurses are most likely to manage the sensory environment directly when caring for infants and children in institutions. These institutions may be general hospitals or specialized hospitals, such as those for the retarded or for rehabilitation. In institutions or social agencies, such as orphanages or agencies dealing with foster homes, a nurse may serve the same consultative role that he serves with the child's own parents.

One of the major goals of care of any hospitalized child is to support his level of development and his developmental potential. In terms of the sensory-perceptual development, this means providing an environment which will support the natural drive for sensory stimulation and which will encourage development of perceptual-motor skills.

In practical terms, this includes hanging mobiles over an infant's crib (visual stimulation) and alternating bright toys and objects which he can touch and feel (variety, tactile sensation). If the infant has begun to reach for things, hanging toys provide reinforcement for reaching and grasping—they move, make noise, or bounce. Reaching leads to normal eye-hand coordination.

Variety of sensory-perceptual environment is essential for infants and children of all ages. The attention span increases as a child grows, but all children become bored rather quickly with an unchanging environment, i.e., they experience perceptual monotony. During nap time, a monotonous, relatively nonstimulating environment may help a child get to sleep, but continuation of the same environment all day leads to apathy and fussiness. Infants may be set in special infant seats and moved to other rooms for a change of scene. Bedfast children can be gotten into wheelchairs or onto stretchers or carts for socializing and change of scenery (see Fig. 11-3). Even infants benefit from being able to see and to make noises at other infants and children. Older children certainly need the opportunity for group contact.

The child who is isolated from others either to prevent him from transmitting pathogens or to protect him from potential pathogens is in a particularly vulnerable situation. He is vulnerable both in terms of the general effects of sensory-perceptual-social restriction and in terms of potential retardation of perceptual motor and social development. Since he cannot be moved to join other children or to see new areas, his own room must be made as stimulating and full of variety as possible. Nursing personnel and his parents need to try to spend time socializing with him. He will need more toys, games, or whatever amusements are appropriate to his age. However, only a few should be available at one time, and they need to be changed frequently to prevent boredom. Television, used judiciously, may be a help. However, indiscriminate use of television will eventually lead to perceptual monotony.

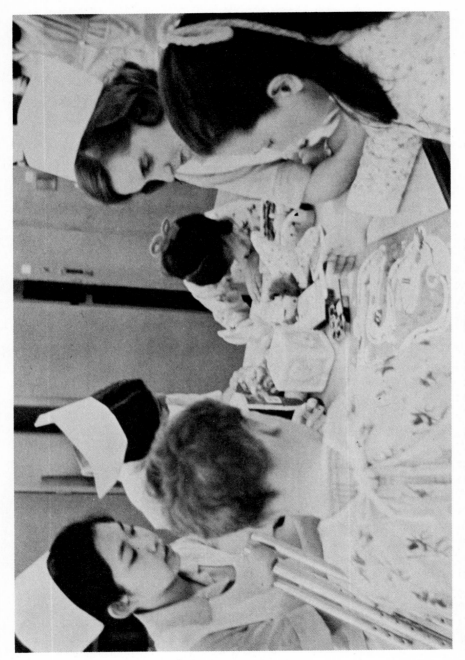

Figure 11-3 Providing social stimulation for hospitalized children. Wheelchairs, stretchers, and carts could be used to help otherwise isolated children join a group such as this. *(Photograph, courtesy of University of Washington Medical Photography, Health Sciences Division.)*

Prevention and Management of Sensory-Perceptual Restriction and Overload

Most of the medical and nursing literature related to clinical sensory-perceptual-social restriction deals with measures used to reduce actual manifestations of deprivation, rather than with preventing these manifestations altogether. There have been almost no reports of controlled studies to measure the effect of ways to prevent these manifestations. Thus, we do not know at this time if it is possible to prevent these effects in susceptible persons, or if there are differences in the preventability of acute and long-term variations of the syndrome. Many clinicians are just beginning to feel that sensory-perceptual-social restriction is a common denominator in some "psychotic" or inexplicable behavior of some groups of patient-clients.

In order to determine how common this syndrome is and if it is indeed related to restricted environments, practitioners must first develop a high "index of suspicion" in relating restricted environments to aberrant behavior. "Index of suspicion" is a term referring to the degree to which a specific entity is considered as related to a symptom or group of symptoms. Patient-clients are too often labeled "disoriented," "confused," "difficult," "hostile," "apathetic," without looking at potential sources of their behavior or symptoms. The case of Mr. L. illustrates this observation:

Mr. A. L. was a 65-year-old man in a body cast (midchest to ankle). The student nurse caring for him was told that he was "confused." On her initial assessment, she found that he called her by anyone's name, did not know where he was, and spent much time sleeping or talking to himself. During his morning care, she found some eyeglasses in his drawer and put them on him. He looked rather surprised and asked who she was. He was considerably more animated and alert for the next hour in which she was there. After a week of wearing his glasses and daily three-hour contacts with student nurses, he was no longer confused, recognized

nursing personnel by name, and slept only at night and for an hour in the afternoon.

The influence of sensory-perceptual and social deprivation on Mr. L.'s behavior was hypothesized in retrospect, and only because of the serendipitous use of his eyeglasses. If assessment for potential situations of sensory restriction becomes a part of nursing practice, we may begin to gather enough evidence to confirm or refute the existence of a clinical sensory-perceptual restriction syndrome and to determine if it is preventable.

There are several groups of people who seem to be in potentially restricted situations. They include persons whose environment, sensory deficit, or personality in a restricted environment could be expected to lead to actual or potential sensory-perceptual restriction (Fig. 11-4).

Therapeutically Restricted Environment One general class of susceptible people includes those whose therapeutic environment is restrictive. Certainly, patient-clients who are socially isolated for therapeutic reasons (to protect them or others from pathogenic organisms) are in a highly susceptible position. They are socially isolated, except for contacts with gowned, and often masked, staff members. The environment is usually devoid of pictures and is unchanging. In addition, this patient-client is often acutely ill. The effect of the attendant anxieties and drug therapy on the level of awareness may intensify any general effects of social isolation and perceptual monotony.

A variation of this group includes patient-clients whose therapeutic environment is sensorily overloaded and thus perceptually restricted, i.e., so overloaded as to be without meaningful patterns. Intensive-care and coronary-care units may be overloaded environments. The acutely ill person is attached to a variety of tubes and machines and is in a constant hubbub of activity, with little variation from night to day. There is little to help orient him to the limits of himself

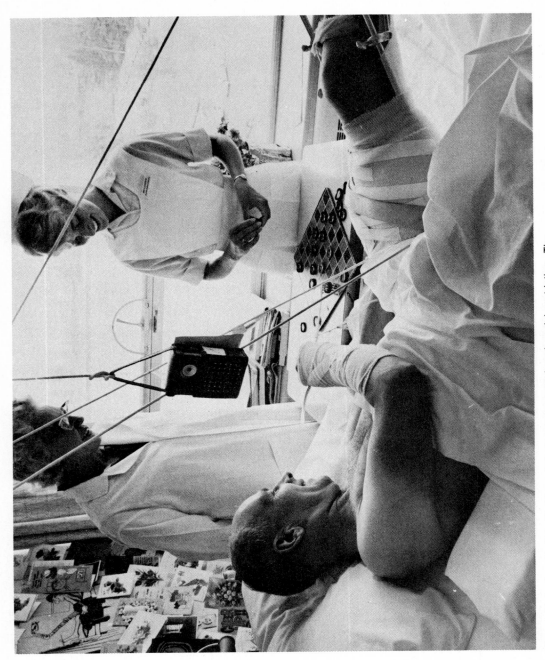

Figure 11-4 A potential situation of sensory-perceptual and social restriction. The nurses are helping to provide social stimulation to an immobilized man. *(Photograph, courtesy of University of Washington Information Services.)*

and his day. The perceptual restriction (meaningless pattern) of the intensive-care unit may be one factor which precipitates the many instances of post-cardiac-surgery "delirium."

Patient-clients on Stryker frames, in traction, in body casts, and simply confined to bed are also in a therapeutically restricted environment. Their tactile stimuli are restricted to the bed, sheets, and covers. Depending upon how much immobilized they are, their visual field may be limited to the ceiling or the floor (with the Stryker frame). At best, the field may encompass the ceiling and whatever is at eye level. Because the hospital environment is unfamiliar, sounds may be perceptually useless stimuli, since they have no known meaning.

Socially Restricted Environment Another group of susceptible persons includes those whose environment is deprived by reason of living circumstances. This group would include infants raised in nonstimulating institutions or by families who do not provide normal levels of stimulation. People of any age who live in institutions where the social and perceptual scene is relatively static would be in this group.

Many people who live in their own homes but are physically or emotionally unable to get out may be in a socially restricted or perceptually monotonous environment. The elderly are probably the largest single group of such people. Retarded children "hidden away" by their parents, depressed or psychotic people who avoid contact with others, or people with chronic illness who are physically unable to leave the house would also be in this group.

Sensory-Perceptual Deficits The last major classification of people susceptible to sensory, perceptual, or social restriction or overload consists of those whose sensory or perceptual deficits restrict their total sensory input.

People who have sensory deficits may have them in only one modality or in many modalities. Certainly, the modality affected and the number of senses affected will influence the total amount of sensory input and the susceptibility to effects of sensory-perceptual restriction.

When only one modality is affected, the others tend to become more sensitive to stimuli. Experimentally, temporary blocking of only visual stimuli in human beings results in an increase in tactile acuity, pain sensitivity, auditory discrimination, and appreciation of taste and odor (Zubek, 1969). Temporary deprivation of auditory and tactile stimulation resulted in increased sensitivity in these modalities after the deprivation ceased.

These observations support the theory of sensoristasis—organismic attempts to maintain a level of sensory stimulation.

People who are blind tend after a time to compensate for this deficit by increasing auditory acuity, tactile acuity, sense of smell, and kinesthetic awareness. People who are deaf tend to become keen observers. However, people who are suddenly or temporarily blinded or deafened experience a period in which the loss of a major sensory modality is not compensated by increased acuity of the other senses and by development of alternative sensory cues. It is reasonable to hypothesize that they are most susceptible to the effects of sensory-perceptual deprivation during this initial period.

The reactions of eye-patched patients (described earlier) are markedly similar to those of some subjects in sensory-deprivation experiments, leading many investigators to hypothesize that these reactions are the effects of sensory-perceptual restriction. Certainly, the eye-patched patient is in a restricted environment. A major sensory modality is lost; he is in an unfamiliar environment, and thus has few cues by which to order the perceptions which he does receive.

The extremely limited clinical research with eye-patched patients suggests that preventive measures may not preclude the incidence of unpleasant reactions to sensory deprivation. Theoretically, an increase of input from the other senses and increased structuring of the environment should prevent this syndrome. Only one investigator reports attempting to do this, and he was unable to reduce the incidence (Ziskind, 1965). However, it is not clear from his statements whether the measures taken were intended to prevent the occurrence of these effects or to reduce them after they occurred.

Because the visual sensation is so essential to perception and orientation, it is possible that sudden underload in the modality is too disorganizing to be compensated by increasing input in other areas. In view of this, Ellis et al. (1969) suggest that approaches for these patients center upon determining if the patient is having disturbing experiences and then helping him cope with these experiences. Specific measures related to this attempt are discussed under "Nursing Intervention in Clinical Sensory-Perceptual Restriction," later on in this chapter.

Many neurologic illnesses decrease perception and reception in one or more of the sensory modalities. For example, loss of kinesthetic and tactile perception often occurs together with paralysis or weakness after a stroke. People so afflicted may not be able to tell the nature of an object by feeling (stereognosis), or may have no idea where an arm or leg is without looking at it. Many people with cerebral infarcts of the nondominant hemisphere lose perception of one-half of their body and act as if it did not exist. They must consciously remember to dress that half as well. Children with brain lesions which impair stereognosis have considerably more difficulty in learning about the world by touch and feel.

Some inflammatory diseases of the nervous system seem to disorder the normal inhibition of "background" stimuli to the extent that a normal sensory environment becomes an overloaded one. People with meningitis and encephalitis often are agitated and disturbed by normal daylight, bright colors, or voices at normal levels.

Esther Frankel (1969) describes her subjective reactions to the normal level of activity during the acute phase of her encephalitis:

> The yellow wall opposite me seemed to come at me and engulf me. . . . The multi-colored flowers whose shapes were blurred were so painful to my eyes. I had to hide my face in the pillow to avoid the agony. It was somewhat like keeping one's eyes open to a blinding sun. I would like to make the humble suggestion that patients in the acute stage of encephalitis be placed in a room where there are no bright colors, just neutral gray.

Personality and Developmental Factors   Most persons can tolerate some degree of sensory-perceptual restriction and monotony without untoward behavioral and perceptual effects. However, individual tolerance for experimental sensory deprivation varies considerably. Empirical observations suggest that the amount of clinical sensory-perceptual restriction tolerated varies a great deal also.

How do we apply these findings and impressions from experimental studies (see "Individual Tolerance for Sensory-Perceptual Deprivation," earlier in this chapter) in predicting which patient-clients might have more difficulty in tolerating therapeutically imposed restrictive conditions? The evidence of specific personality factors is so scanty that they can be suggested only as hypotheses which have not been adequately tested. They may, however, serve as hunches concerning which the clinician may gather substantiating or refuting data.

First, we may propose that people whose developmental level or personality is characterized by short attention spans, a need for physical activity, and dependence upon others to provide entertainment or amusement might have more difficulty in restricted situations than more contemplative, self-reliant persons. Most children exhibit these kinds of behavior as a normal part of their personality; many adults have never gone beyond this reliance upon external stimulation.

People of any age who are anxious might also be expected to have more difficulty in coping with a restricted environment. Anxiety, by definition, narrows focus and perception; therefore, the restriction of pattern and level of sensory-perceptual stimuli might intensify this reaction. Certainly, many health crises and health problems which result in decreased sensory ability are in themselves anxiety provoking. Therefore, a normal, mature person who might tolerate experimental sensory deprivation well might have much difficulty in a clinical sensory restriction.

A final factor affecting individual susceptibility and tolerance to sensory restriction is the use of drugs. Central nervous system depressants, such as narcotics and alcohol, decrease awareness of the environment. If this decreased awareness is coupled with a monotonous or restricted environment, behavioral aberrations may occur.

Consciousness-expanding drugs, such as LSD, and central nervous system stimulants, such as the amphetamines, alter and distort perception of the environment. Some of the behavioral reactions to these drugs may be related to a drug-induced sensory overload (Brawley and Pos, 1967).

In summary, we may hypothesize four major factors which could predispose an individual to manifest a clinical sensory-perceptual-deprivation syndrome:

1 An environment which is monotonous, meaningless in terms of sensory patterns, or characterized by decreased sensory input in one or more modalities. This restriction may be a characteristic of the usual living environment or may be therapeutically imposed.

2 Deficits or distortions in a major sensory modality, or in multiple modalities, coupled with an environment which has few meaningful sensory cues.

3 Developmental level or personality which leads to dependency upon activity and external stimulation.

4 Drugs or level of anxiety sufficient to decrease or distort the level of awareness.

Nursing Intervention in Clinical Sensory-Perceptual Restriction

These hypotheses about which patient-clients might be likely to develop manifestations of sensory-perceptual restriction suggest the emphasis in assessment of sensory status for these groups of people.

Such an assessment should include the person's sensory status, i.e., intactness of the sensory systems and degree and nature of deficits. The sensory, perceptual, and social environment must be assessed not only in terms of the current environment but also in relation to its appropriateness to developmental stage and its relation to the normal environment for that person. An elderly person who lives alone may be accustomed to a very quiet environment; thus, the noises and bustle of a hospital may be a relative overload for him. Spalding's (1969) report on infant care among low-income women discusses the need to assess social as well as physical environment before concluding that an infant from a "poor" home is socially deprived. She utilizes an example of the large amount of social handling and contact which lower-class Negro babies get, despite the impoverished material environment.

Last, one makes some estimate of the individual's need for structure and his resources for coping with monotony. This may be done partly through observation, but also by asking the patient-client or his family the kind of activities he enjoys when alone, what bores him, how he reacts when alone in the dark.

We can attempt to prevent sensory-perceptual and social restriction by using whatever measures will increase input and make the pattern meaningful for the individual person. Input cannot be solely through passive means such as a television set or a radio. These do not require a person to interact with the environment, and therefore soon become monotonous in themselves. Television and radio are of value but cannot be relied upon as the sole means to reduce perceptual monotony and restriction.

Toys of different textures and shapes, objects hung overhead to encourage reaching, and objects which make noises help children and infants to explore the sensory-tactile environment. Modeling clay, knitting, leather tooling, and other crafts serve a similar purpose for adolescents and adults. Volunteers and occupational therapists can be utilized by the nurse and physician to provide such preventive activities.

The environment can be made more structured by use of clocks and calendars, fairly fixed time schedules, a regular television or radio program. Interests outside the institution or home can be stimulated with newspapers, news broadcasts, and magazines.

Structure and pattern can be introduced into the world of the acutely ill, less aware person by careful brief explanations of everything which the nurse is doing, by describing the surroundings, and by interpreting the various sounds and activities. Try standing in a busy hospital ward with your eyes shut to appreciate some of the confusion the restricted patient-client may feel.

Management of manifestations of restriction and overload is based upon a high level of suspicion that this restriction is the source of aberrant behavior. It is common to sedate and isolate or restrict a patient-client who becomes disoriented and combative. If the cause of his behavior is a relative sensory restriction, these measures can only increase his restricted state. Conversely, if we use increased sensory stimulation in an attempt to decrease agitation of someone who is reacting to sensory overload or distortion, we only increase the problem.

What are the cues which differentiate sensory restriction or overload? There has been so little medical or nursing investigation of the clinical syndrome that we cannot offer a clear-cut listing of differentiating symptoms. Moreover, anxiety, agitation, confusion, slow thinking, and other manifestations of sensory-perceptual restriction are also manifestations of a number of other behavioral and physiologic reactions. At this point, one has to proceed rather empirically: suspect sensory restriction or overload as the source of the behavior, then increase or decrease the input and compare pre- and postintervention behavior. "If it works, use it."

There are, however, a few general guideposts which may help determine if sensory restriction or overload is a reasonable possibility in a particular situation. Clinical reports seem to define two general syndromes—acute and chronic.

Acute Syndrome   Acute manifestations of restriction generally include the rather sudden onset of psychotic-like behavior: acute anxiety, delusions, hallucinations, confusion, disorientation, and noncompliance with treatment. These symptoms usually occur within a few hours to many days after the environment becomes restricted. This reaction occurs more often in older people (whose general sensory input is often altered) and appears unrelated to toxic effects of illness or drugs. It seems to occur in perfectly "normal" people, as well as in those who had previous emotional instabilities.

This acute syndrome often clears up spontaneously or with an increase in social and sensory input. Television is of short-term value here, as is getting the patient-client into the company of others. Other methods of increasing the patterning of the environment include leaving a night light on, occupational-therapy projects, and encouraging auto-stimulation—singing or reciting to oneself.

Increased social contact is a consistent feature of successful attempts to reverse the acute syndrome. Sometimes a relative or friend is asked to stay with and talk to the patient-client. In other cases, nursing personnel increase their conversational and physical contacts.

Dealing with Hallucinations   The people who experience hallucinations sometimes act as if they are real. Other patient-clients are aware that the objects they "see" are not really there. In either case, the experiences may be frightening.

Nurses frequently wonder how to help the hallucinating person. Often they do not want to agitate the person further, and so "go along" with the hallucination. The nurse may be uncomfortable about doing this, feeling foolish and concerned that the patient will lose trust if his sensorium suddenly becomes clear. Certainly, this approach does not help the patient find reality or reassure him that he is not mad.

There are several ways in which the nurse can help without going along with the content of the hallucination. Some of these experiences are more appropriately called delusions—misinterpretations of the environment. Simply clarifying the nature of the misinterpreted object or event is often enough to reassure the person that he is sane.

> Mrs. B. T. was a 26-year-old woman who had had a baby six weeks before developing a neurologic disorder characterized by rapidly ascending loss of sensory and motor function. She was confined to a tank respirator to aid her breathing. She became very much agitated the second day after being placed in the tank, shouting, "They're killing the babies." The nurse realized that Mrs. T. was hearing the commotion of the linen carts and seeing, via the mirror on the respirator, people throw laundry into bags. When the nurse explained what was happening and adjusted the mirror, Mrs. T. looked markedly relieved and said she had thought she was losing her mind. She had a number of other delusions which quickly ended when the environment was interpreted to her.

Some patient-clients have experiences which they know are unreal—yet they have experienced them. "I know there is no one there, but he frightens me!" The important action in these situations is to let the person know that you appreciate his fear and that he can talk about the experiences. Ellis et al. (1969) emphasize that this kind of experience is frequent among patients who have their eyes patched after surgery; therefore, it is useful to assure them that this experience is not abnormal. Explaining these experiences on the basis of misinterpretation of

the environment is a mistake, for the patient-client knows that he had unreal experiences, and may simply stop mentioning them if the staff minimizes his concern.

It may or may not be effective to tell the patient who thinks his hallucinated scenes are real that this is a common occurrence. He may feel that he is being belittled, since he feels they *are* real. In these situations, it is probably best to avoid discussing the content of the hallucination. Therefore, the focus might be on the feelings of the patient-client; e.g., "It must be frightening to feel that people are watching you; I will stay with you until you feel more comfortable." Simply holding the person, if he is frightened, may be of help.

Acute sensory-perceptual overload may cause the same symptoms as restriction. One clue to the existence of overload may be the patient's medical diagnosis. Inflammatory disease of the brain and spinal cord, or toxic and feverish reactions often lead to delirious, agitated behavior. This may be the result of overload of internally generated stimuli to the reticular activating system. Another clue to the existence of overload is the patient-client's response to sensory stimuli applied. If increasing social contact and sensory input only increases the symptoms, it is worthwhile to try subduing or decreasing them.

Chronic Syndromes We are only recently beginning to suspect the long-term effects of sensory-perceptual and social restriction in adults. The nursing literature has begun to publish accounts which relate the "apathetic," "difficult," or "senile" behavior of institutionalized adults to chronic social and perceptual monotony. The description by Judith Morris (1969) of the perceptual environment of an institution for retarded children is similar to that experienced by many institutionalized persons:

> Here there is little, if any, change from day to day. The routine is always the same. The sounds are the same. If you were to *feel* this environment, as

Duncan must, you would find that most things are hard: the floors, the beds, the walls, the sinks, the chairs. Everything is of the same temperature and texture. Conversation does not vary much; the same sounds are heard over and over. The same bland foods are served again and again. There is little reason to respond to this world. There is little hope for learning in it either, for it is only through what our senses tell us of our world that we may progress and develop to anything approaching our full potential.[2]

Cockburn (1967) and Moody, Barron, and Monk (1970) describe group sessions with chronically institutionalized adults which led to rather startling increases in motivation, awareness of self and environment, and general enjoyment of life.

Cockburn divided chronic schizophrenic patients (average hospitalization, twenty to twenty-three years) into experimental and control groups. Those in the experimental groups were given objects designed to stimulate specific senses. They handled the objects and discussed them, went for walks, and discussed these experiences. The control group were presented with the same objects, but did not discuss them. Both groups were tested before and after the eight-week stimulation period in terms of interpersonal communication, self-care, work and recreation activity, and hospital adjustment. Final scores of the experimental group were significantly higher in all areas than those of the control group, and significantly improved over their prestimulation scores. Since both groups were presented with stimulating objects, these findings would suggest that the social interpretation and structuring of the stimulation were more important than the presentation of sensory objects alone. Unfortunately, the author did not report whether these effects were long-lasting.

Moody, Barron, and Monk used similar group meetings to stimulate elderly people in a nursing home. All the patients in their group experienced brief periods of confusion which the authors hypothesized were due to sensory deprivation. The patients were typically depressed, tired, and despairing. The group met for forty-five minutes a day for one week and discussed topics related to a specific object—strawberries, fishing poles, doughnuts. At the end of the week, the patients were considerably more animated and alert. Their scores on a measure of life satisfaction were considerably higher.

This study was not controlled and does not report systematic evaluation of any measure other than subjective satisfaction. Therefore, it does not substantiate any assumption about sensory restriction as the cause of the patients' behavior. However, it again suggests that social contact and variety are important in subjective reactions and the level of alertness in chronically institutionalized people.

Carlson (1968) used flower arrangements, pictures, mobiles, exercises, music, and physical nursing care (such as back rubs) to increase the sensory input for a small group of elderly immobilized women. She compared their subjective satisfaction with that of a group of women in the usual monotonous ward environment and with those whose beds were in a solarium, a natural gathering place for patients and staff. She found that the group which was stimulated changed from six women who "spent a great deal of time staring at the ceiling—apathetic, expressionless" to women who ". . . were now a cohesive group—active physically as well as emotionally."[3] Even more interesting is her finding that those in the solarium group, who had constant, naturally occurring social and perceptual stimulation, were more satisfied and alert than those in either the experimental or the control group. This again suggests that social stimulation is a key part of the sensory-perceptual environment.

The emphasis in decreasing the manifestations

---

[2] Judith Morris, The Senses and the Environment, *1967 ANA Regional Clinical Conferences*, Appleton-Century-Crofts, Inc., New York, 1969, pp. 170-171.

[3] Sylvia Carlson, Selected Sensory Input and Life Satisfaction of Immobilized Geriatric Female Patients, *ANA Clinical Sessions*, Appleton-Century-Crofts, Inc., New York, 1968, pp. 117-123.

of a chronic restrictive syndrome includes keeping social interaction high and providing a varied input of sensory-perceptual stimuli. Cockburn's work suggests that structuring and interpreting the meaning of the stimuli are more important than simply making them available. Moving a person's stretcher to a place where other patients are gathered does not ensure that he will interact with them. An apathetic, withdrawn person needs some props to being interactive, such as the group discussions described.

Busy institutional nurses cannot necessarily provide these stimulating experiences by themselves. However, they can arrange for volunteer groups, friends, and families to help decorate a ward, to conduct discussion groups, or to move patient-clients about. The professional nurse uses his knowledge to assess sensory-social environment and to plan the structure of the environment. Many other hands can rearrange it.

Summary of Common Problems, with Approaches

Problems	Approach
Acute sensory-perceptual restriction	Pattern and clarify environment
	Increase light-dark contrast
	Explain activities
	Television-radio
	Clock-calendars
	Increase social contact
	Help patient-client cope with "unreal" experiences
Acute sensory-perceptual overload	Reduce intensity and quantity of input
	Increase pattern or meaning of input
	Explain environment
	Introduce change slowly (e.g., from light to dark, hard to soft)
Chronic sensory-perception restriction	Provide activity requiring exploration of sensory environment
	Exercise
	Smelling
	Feeling
	Tasting
	Moving
	Increase purposeful social contact
	Discuss sensory experiences
	Group games, exercises (adults or older children)
	Play time
	Increase tactile contact
	Handling, cuddling (babies, children, regressed adults)
	Back rubs
	Increase visual and auditory input
	Music, mobiles, variety of pictures
	Limited radio and television

REFERENCES

Books

Bennett, A., Sensory Deprivation in Aviation, in P. Solomon et al. (eds.), "Sensory Deprivation," Harvard University Press, Cambridge, Mass., 1961.

Cannon, Walter B., "The Wisdom of the Body," rev. ed., W. W. Norton Company, New York, 1939.

Goldberger, Leo, and Robert Holt, Experimental Interference with Reality Contact: Individual Differences, in P. Solomon et al. (eds.), "Sensory Deprivation," Harvard University Press, Cambridge, Mass., 1961, pp. 130–141.

Jackson, C. W., Clinical Sensory Deprivation: A Review of Hospitalized Eye-surgery Patients, in J. Zubek (ed.), "Sensory Deprivation: 15 Years of

Research," Appleton-Century-Crofts, Inc., New York, 1969, pp. 332-373.

Lindsley, Donald, Common Factors in Sensory Deprivation, Sensory Distortion and Sensory Overload, in P. Solomon et al. (eds.), "Sensory Deprivation," Harvard University Press, Cambridge, Mass., 1961, pp. 174-194.

Meyers, Thomas, Tolerance for Sensory and Perceptual Deprivation, in J. Zubek (ed.), "Sensory Deprivation: 15 Years of Research," Appleton-Century-Crofts, Inc., New York, 1969, pp. 289-331.

Riesen, Austin, Excessive Arousal Effects of Stimulation after Early Sensory Deprivation, in P. Solomon et al. (eds.), "Sensory Deprivation," Harvard University Press, Cambridge, Mass., 1961, pp. 37-40.

Sackett, Gene, Innate Mechanisms, Rearing Condition, and a Theory of Early Experience Effects in Primates, in M. Jones (ed.), "Miami Symposium on the Prediction of Behavior, 1968: Effects of Early Experience," University of Miami Press, Coral Gables, Fla., 1970, pp. 11-53.

Schultz, Duane, "Sensory Restriction," Academic Press, Inc., New York, 1965.

Solomon, P., et al. (eds.), "Sensory Deprivation," Harvard University Press, Cambridge, Mass., 1961.

Suedfeld, Peter, Changes in Intellectual Performance and Susceptibility to Influence, in J. Zubek (ed.), "Sensory Deprivation: 15 Years of Research," Appleton-Century-Crofts, Inc., New York, 1969, p. 165.

Zubek, J. (ed.), "Sensory Deprivation: 15 Years of Research," Appleton-Century-Crofts, Inc., New York, 1969.

Zuckerman, Marvin, Hallucinations, Reported Sensations and Images, in J. Zubek (ed.), "Sensory Deprivation: 15 Years of Research," Appleton-Century-Crofts, Inc., New York, 1969, pp. 85-125.

Periodicals

Beach, Frank, and Julian Jaynes: Effects of Early Experiences upon the Behavior of Animals, *Psychological Bulletin,* **51**:239-263 (1954).

Brawley, Peter, and Robert Pos: The Informational Underload (Sensory Deprivation) Model in Contemporary Psychiatry, *Canadian Psychiatric Association Journal,* **12**:105-124 (1967).

Carlson, Sylvia: Selected Sensory Input and Life Satisfaction of Immobilized Geriatric Female Pa-

tients, *ANA Clinical Sessions,* Appleton-Century-Crofts, Inc., New York, 1968, pp. 117-123.

Cockburn, Kathleen: Sensory Stimulation in the Nursing Care of Chronic Schizophrenic Patients, *1965 ANA Regional Clinical Conferences,* Appleton-Century-Crofts, Inc., New York, 1967, pp. 261-267.

Ellis, Rosemary, et al.: Suggestions for the Care of Eye Surgery Patients Who Experience Reduced Sensory Input, *1967 ANA Regional Clinical Conferences,* Appleton-Century-Crofts, Inc., New York, 1969, pp. 131-137.

Frankel, Esther: I Spoke with the Dead, *American Journal of Nursing,* **69**:105-107 (1969).

Goldfarb, William: Emotional and Intellectual Consequences of Psychological Deprivation in Infancy: A Revaluation [sic], *Psychopathology of Childhood,* Proceedings of American Psychopathological Association, 1954, Grune & Stratton, Inc., New York, 1955, pp. 115-119.

Heron, Woodburn: The Pathology of Boredom, *Scientific American,* **196**:52-56 (January, 1957).

Jackson, C. W., J. Pollard, and E. W. Kansky: The Application of Findings from Experimental Sensory Deprivation to Cases of Clinical Sensory Deprivation, *American Journal of the Medical Sciences,* **243**:558-563 (1962).

Leiderman, Herbert, et al.: Sensory Deprivation: Clinical Aspects, *Archives of Internal Medicine,* **101**:389-396 (1958).

Lilly, John: Mental Effects of Reduction of Ordinary Levels of Physical Stimuli in Intact, Healthy Persons, *Psychological Research Reports,* **5**:1-9 (1956).

Moody, L., V. Barron, and G. Monk: Moving the Past into the Present, *American Journal of Nursing,* **70**:2353-2356 (1970).

Morris, Judith: The Senses and the Environment, *1967 ANA Regional Clinical Conferences,* Appleton-Century-Crofts, Inc., New York, 1969, pp. 170-171.

Spalding, Margaret: Adapting Post-partum Teaching to Mothers' Low Income Life Styles, in B. Bergerson et al. (eds.), *Current Concepts in Clinical Nursing,* **2**:280-291 (1969).

Spitz, Rene: Hospitalism, *Psychoanalytic Study of the Child,* **1**:53-74 (1945).

Studies in Sensory Overload; Parts 1 to 4, *Tohoku Psychologica Folia,* **28**(3-4):69-103 (1970).

Suedfeld, Peter, R. J. Grissom, and J. Vernon: The Effects of Sensory Deprivation and Social Isolation on the Performance of an Unstructured Cognitive Task, *American Journal of Psychiatry,* **77**:111–116 (1964).

White, Burton: An Experimental Approach to the Effects of Experience in Early Human Behavior, *Minnesota Symposia on Child Psychology,* **1**:201–226 (1967).

Ziskind, Eugene: An Explanation of Mental Symptoms Found in Acute Sensory Deprivation Researches, 1958–1963, *American Journal of Psychiatry,* **121**:939–946 (1965).

Zubek, John, and L. Wilgosh: Prolonged Immobilization of the Body: Changes in Performance and in the Electroencephalogram, *Science,* **140**:306–308 (Feb. 25, 1963).

ADDITIONAL READINGS

General

Chodil, Judith, and Barbara Williams: The Concept of Sensory Deprivation, *Nursing Clinics of North America,* **5**:453–465 (1970).

Jackson, C. W., and Rosemary Ellis: Sensory Deprivation as a Field of Study, *Nursing Research,* **20**:46–54 (1971).

Ohno, Mary: The Eye Patched Patient, *American Journal of Nursing,* **71**:271–274 (1971).

Sensory Restriction in Children

Cohen, Sidney: Contact Deprivation in Infants, *Psychosomatics,* **7**:85–88 (1966).

Fleming, Juanita: Sensory Losses in Children, in B. Bergerson et al. (eds.), *Current Concepts in Clinical Nursing,* **1**:339–352 (1967).

Sensory Stimulation for Children

Boston Children's Medical Society and Elizabeth Greg, "What to Do When There's Nothing to Do," Delacorte Press, New York, 1967. (Also in Dell paperback.)

Dodson, Fitzhugh, "How to Parent," Nash Publishing, Los Angeles, 1970. (Also in Signet paperback.)

Williams, Karin, and Constance Bain, "Just in Case," Ryther Child Center, 2400 Northeast 95th Street, Seattle, Washington 98115. (Available only from the Center.)

Motor Status

Pamela Mitchell

MOBILITY

Mobility, the ability to move about freely, is one of the central attributes by which men define and express themselves and by which they measure their health and physical fitness. Because mobility is so central to one's daily life, the problems associated with changes in mobility and the adaptation to these changes are among the most important problems with which nurses deal.

To appreciate the importance of mobility in defining self, consider your reactions if you were suddenly paralyzed from the neck down, able to move only your head. How would you think of yourself? What do you think others would think of you? What changes would this event make in your aspirations and in your relationships with others? Indeed, what changes would it make in your whole life? Throughout your life, you have learned about the world and made your place in it through movement. Suddenly, your ability to carry on as usual is gone, and a tremendous adjustment in self-concept must be made.

Movement is a means by which we express ourselves. Gestures, mannerisms, and facial expressions are all forms of nonverbal communica-

Data to Be Assessed

Medical restrictions on activity
Musculoskeletal status
  General movement
  Muscle strength, tone, mass
  Range of joint motion
  Posture
  Handedness
  Deformities
  Abnormal innervation to muscles
Mobility
  Method of ambulation
  Gait
  Endurance

tion and are dependent upon movement. Motor activity is a primary means of discharging emotion, particularly in children. Small children show their anger and frustration by hitting, crying, or running away. Later, they learn to sublimate anger, sexual desire, and anxiety by vigorous exercise. We punch a pillow rather than the other fellow, or take a walk to "simmer down." Adults have generally learned to control verbal expression of emotion, but they often express it through movements—the tense drumming of fingers, fiddling with hair or buttons.

Many people define physical fitness or health in terms of mobility. Loss of mobility becomes "proof" of illness. Schwartz et al. studied a group of elderly persons who were patients in a hospital clinic. She reported:

> Despite clinic attendance and current medical diagnosis of illness, 44 percent of the group [studied] did not think of themselves as having been "sick" during the last month.[1]

However, some of those who thought they had been sick mentioned loss of mobility as "proof" of sickness: "I couldn't get to the park for two days"; "I can't get out . . . I've slowed down."

Bauman (1961) surveyed conceptions of health among 100 medical students and 100 clinic patients with chronic diseases. One of the three major classes of response was in terms of "performance orientation"—what a healthy person should be able to do. Sixty-four percent of the patients mentioned performance as a criterion of health—"they're able to work, do household chores, shopping, washing, ironing."[2] Obviously, what a person is able to do depends upon his mobility.

[1] Reprinted by permission of The Macmillan Company, from "The Elderly Ambulatory Patient," by Doris Schwartz, Barbara Henley, and Leonard Zeitz, copyright The Macmillan Company, New York, 1964, p. 102.

[2] Barbara Bauman, Diversities in Conceptions of Health and Physical Fitness, *Journal of Health and Human Behavior*, **2**:39–46 (1961).

FACTORS ALTERING MOBILITY

What events or situations alter a person's mobility? Motor function or mobility is changed in three basic ways: (1) it is lost or becomes quiescent, through disease or trauma; (2) it is externally restricted, through a prescription for bed rest, or by means of mechanical devices; and (3) it is voluntarily curtailed to conserve energy or to maintain equilibrium.

Motor Function Is Lost or Quiescent

The most obvious situations in which motor ability changes are those involving disease or trauma. Disease occurs when internal pathological processes alter function; trauma is externally induced alteration of function through accident or design (e.g., surgically induced trauma).

Motor function is dependent upon the intact functions of the central nervous system, the muscles, and the bones. Pathologic change or injury to any of these components may cause a loss of motor ability or a change in it. For example, the contraction of a muscle is mediated by the central nervous system. If a hemorrhage in the brain (cerebrovascular accident, stroke) interrupts transmission of motor impulses to muscles on one side of the body, partial paralysis results (hemiplegia), even though the bones and muscles of that side of the body are perfectly normal. Nervous transmission can also be interrupted by severing a nerve or by degeneration secondary to toxins.

Nerve and muscle may be normal, but there may be a defect at the juncture between them, at the motor endplate. This produces a disorder called *myasthenia gravis*. In this disorder, the muscles are overstimulated and become rapidly fatigued, thereby decreasing the person's mobility.

Changes in a muscle itself may contribute to loss of mobility. The muscle may be atrophied through disuse or through loss of innervation. Its fibers may have been cut, either therapeutically (surgical incision) or through accidental trauma. Or the muscle may have been sprained or bruised, rendering its movement too painful.

Finally, the skeletal framework may be diseased or injured, preventing effective use of an intact nervous and muscular component. The bones may be too weak, whether through congenital malformation, osteoporosis, or fracture, to support the person's weight. The joints may be fibrosed and unable to move freely. Arthritis is an example of a disease which causes joints to become painful. These painful joints are thus not moved freely and become fibrosed because of lack of movement, as well as because of the disease process itself. (The effects of disuse on muscles and joints are discussed later in this chapter.)

Loss of consciousness or heavy sedation are examples of situations in which motor activity is quiescent, rather than truly lost. The central nervous system may initiate little voluntary activity, but the peripheral nerves, muscles, and bony structures are intact. Unless motor nerve tracts are disrupted, motor ability will return when consciousness does, provided that complications due to disuse have not occurred during the period of heavy sedation or unconsciousness.

Certain psychological states also may cause loss or quiescence of motor activity. These are usually temporary states, but they may become progressive or permanent.

Most of us have been "frozen with fear" at one time or another. Fortunately, this is usually a transient phenomenon, particularly if one must move in order to avoid the feared object! More long-term loss of motor ability may occur in such psychological conditions as catatonia and conversion reaction.

A catatonic state occurs in some people who are psychotic. The person thus affected is so much out of contact with reality that he makes no overt reaction to his environment or to other persons. He initiates little voluntary activity, although physiological disease can not be demonstrated. It is almost as if the only way in which he can cope with the anxieties which interaction

arouses is to withdraw totally from any motor or verbal interaction with his environment.

Conversion reaction refers to physical symptoms (often limb paralysis) for which no abnormal physiologic cause can be found. The person generally has had a tremendous emotional conflict which he cannot resolve and which is "converted" into a physical symptom. Physical illness is more acceptable than emotional illness in our society, and the unconscious mind chooses this means to cope with the conflict. The psychophysiologic dynamics of catatonic states and conversion reactions are beyond the scope of this textbook but may be found in psychiatric and psychosomatic readings.

Motor Function Is Externally Curtailed

The second group of situations in which motor ability is altered is that in which external limits are placed on movement. A physician's prescription for bed rest is the most common external limitation. Obviously, it will be a limitation on movement only to the extent to which the patient-client follows the prescription.

Bed Rest   A great deal of attention has been focused on the dangers of bed rest, and health professionals have begun to realize that indiscriminate use of rest in bed may harm more than it helps. There are, however, some legitimate occasions in which bed rest is used as therapy.

The primary reason for rest is to prevent further damage to the body, or a part of the body, when the normal demands of use exceed the ability to respond. For example, in an acute myocardial infarction (called a "heart attack" or "coronary" by lay persons), a portion of the cardiac muscle is dead. The heart's efficiency as a pump is impaired, and it cannot provide the volume or force of blood necessary for the body to carry out its usual activities. Therefore, the whole person is put to rest to decrease the demands on the heart. Similarly, in acute pneumonia, the alveoli cannot diffuse sufficient oxygen to meet the normal demands of the body cells. If the person decreases his activity, the damaged organ (the lungs) can meet the metabolic demands. Rest in bed has been shown to decrease the basal metabolic rate (Deitrick, 1948), an index of the metabolic demands of the body.

A second purpose of rest is to allow an injured or diseased part to heal. This is certainly inherent in resting the whole body in the examples above. Further damage to the heart or lung is prevented, and they are given time to heal. If a bone is broken, it cannot heal properly if subjected to continued use; the same is true of a sprained muscle. When the injured or diseased part is a limb, it is possible to limit use of that part only, rather than impose bed rest on the whole body. Sometimes the whole person must be put to bed even for a limb injury; for example, when a broken leg must be immobilized in traction. Unfortunately, when the whole person is put to bed, the normal parts of the body will begin to deteriorate because they are not used. The harmful effects of loss of mobility will be discussed later in this chapter under "Consequences of Immobility."

Mechanical Limitations on Movement External limitations on movement may also be mechanical. Such therapeutic devices as casts and traction are designed to immobilize an injured part and rest it. Unfortunately, these devices effectively immobilize, or at least limit the mobility of, the rest of the body as well. Respirators, intravenous tubing, and cardiac monitors are other examples of therapeutic devices which mechanically limit a person's motion and interaction with his environment.

Institutional Limitations on Movement Institutional restrictions may also place limits on a person's mobility. These limits are primarily in terms of scope and variety of the world in which he exists. If a person is in an institution such as a hospital, mental hospital, nursing home, or alcoholic treatment center, he will have certain limitations on his movement. In terms of space,

his environment may be as small as the bed to which he is confined or as wide as several acres of land in a state institution. Rules and regulations may limit his mobility; he may not be allowed to leave his ward, his room, or his building. He may have limitations on his visitors, which decreases his social mobility. Finally, the drabness and monotony of most institutions may limit his intellectual mobility, leading to boredom or even mental deterioration.

Motor Function Is Voluntarily Curtailed

The third class of limitation on mobility is voluntary limitation of movement. The primary psychophysiologic purpose of this decrease in activity is to maintain physical or emotional equilibrium. The person himself may be totally unaware of this purpose; he knows only that he "doesn't feel well," doesn't "feel like" meeting new people, or "can't get around like I used to."

Many kinds of situations precipitate voluntary limitation of activity. Generally, they involve (1) a response to temporary illness, or (2) a response to an environment which makes demands greater than the person's ability to respond.

Response to Temporary Illness The response to temporary illness is familiar to us all. We "just don't feel well," and want to "take it easy" for awhile. The demands of normal activity are greater than the ill body can handle, and fatigue results. This fatigue usually induces us to decrease our demands upon the body until equilibrium has been restored. Often we take to our beds with no need to have anyone "prescribe" bed rest.

Temporary emotional or social instability (conflict) may also lead to voluntary limitation of activity or mobility. "Getting away from it all," meditating, and sitting quietly and thinking are all ways of restoring emotional equilibrium which involve decreased physical activity.

Response to Environmental Demands Other conditions may reduce the capacity of a person to respond to the normal demands of his environment. Pregnancy is an example of a nondis-eased state which does this. The pregnant woman, particularly in the last months, may drive to the grocery store rather than walk, or need to have help with housework, because her physical bulk prevents her from carrying out this previously normal activity. This is a temporary limitation in activity.

Progressive and permanent illness or disability also affects a person's ability to respond to the normal demands of his environment. If the person cannot change the environment, he must limit his activity to live within it. For example, Mr. B., a man with congestive heart failure, cannot climb a flight of stairs without becoming severely dyspneic (short of breath). He lives in a third-floor walk-up apartment and cannot afford to move. Therefore, he rarely leaves his apart-ment and has been severely limited by his environment. Similarly, a person who is de-pressed may find the demands of social interac-tion more than he can cope with and may withdraw to his home. There he spends much of his time alone, thinking of his unworthiness. He is physically capable of activity but cannot respond emotionally to the interpersonal de-mands of such activity.

THE CONCEPT OF IMMOBILITY

When one or more of the three factors altering mobility is in operation, some degree of *immobil-ity* results. Often we think of immobility as an *absolute* lack of movement. However, immobility is a relative term, encompassing a variety of situations in which mobility is restricted or decreased. As Carnevali and Brueckner (1970) point out, this restriction of movement may be in any area of life—physical, emotional, intellec-tual, or social.

Spencer et al. define the following four quali-tative aspects of immobility which help deter-mine the degree of immobility present:

1 *Physical inactivity.* This inactivity consists of a decrease in body movement, with concomitant decrease in energy needs.

2 *Physical restriction or limitation of movement.* This may occur with extreme physical inactivity, motor paralysis, a physically restricting environ-ment (such as a space capsule or "iron lung" respirator), or with mechanical devices such as casts, traction, or restraints.

3 *Constancy of body posture in relation to gravity.* Prolonged maintenance of *any* position (recumbent, sitting, or standing) leads to a loss of the normal range of adjustment to change in position. This loss of normal adjustment is one of the basic conse-quences of immobility.

4 *Sensory deprivation of stimuli.* This deprivation leads to a decrease in stimulation to movement and response, which in turn leads to physical inactivity.[3]

Any or all of these aspects of immobility may be present in a given patient-client. The more aspects which are present, the more complete the immobilized state. The presence of one aspect may lead to the development of all, as shown in the following example (Fig. 12-1).

Mr. X. has had a cerebral thrombosis (stroke) which causes paralysis of the left side of his body, thus inducing physical restriction of movement. In addi-tion, the damage to his nervous system decreases sensation in his left side and has caused aphasia (a disturbance in speaking and understanding). These defects create a relative sensory deprivation. He is put to bed in a hospital, which adds physical inactivity to his restricted motion. Because he is always recumbent, his body posture is constant in relation to gravity. The hospital environment de-creases his usual social and intellectual input (per-ceptual stimuli). Thus, Mr. X. has a high degree of immobility, as he is affected in all four aspects. Immobility is not total, however, for he has the ability to move one side of his body, to see, and to hear.

The Consequences of Immobility

When immobility occurs, certain predictable consequences follow. The extent and number of physiological and psychological changes depend

[3] W. A. Spencer, C. Vallbona, and R. E. Carter, Jr., Physiologic Concepts of Immobilization, *Journal of Physical Medicine and Reha-bilitation,* **46**:89–100 (1965).

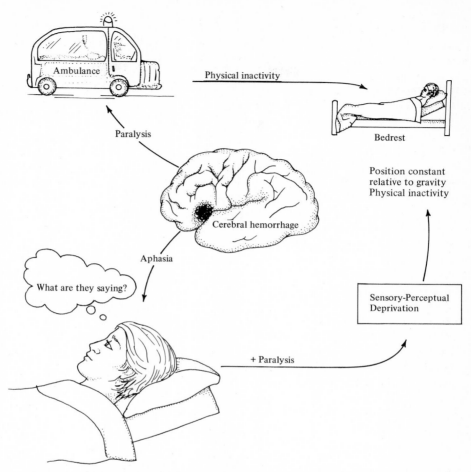

Figure 12-1 Interrelation of the four aspects of immobility. The cerebral hemorrhage (stroke) created restricted movement and partial sensory deprivation. These aspects led to constancy of body position and physical inactivity.

upon the degree and duration of immobility. The greater the extent and duration of immobility, the greater is the chance that pathological consequences will occur.

The classic study documenting the effects of immobilization upon the body was conducted in 1948 by Deitrick, Whedon, and Schorr. Prior to World War II, physicians generally felt that the weakness, fatigue, and complications (such as pneumonia and thrombophlebitis) seen in surgical and other hospitalized patients were the result of their various disease processes. Long periods of rest in bed were commonly prescribed

after surgery, childbirth, and for most illness. During the war, there simply were not enough beds to allow wounded soldiers these long periods of bed rest; they were rapidly gotten up and out of the hospital.

Physicians began to notice that the "inevitable" complications were not occurring so frequently in these soldiers, and began to wonder if bed rest itself were not the cause of these problems. Prompted by these questions, Deitrick, Whedon, and Schorr conducted an experiment to demonstrate the effect of immobility itself on the body.

Four healthy young men had both legs immobilized in plaster casts for a period of six to seven weeks. Heart rate, muscle size and strength, response to position change, and by-products of metabolic activity were measured and compared to pre- and postexperimental recordings for the same factors. The investigators documented decreased basal metabolism, decreased muscle size and strength in all limbs, decreased exercise tolerance, decreased ability to tolerate the head-up position, decreased blood volume, increased pulse rate, and increased nitrogen, calcium, and phosphorus excretion. In addition, the young men showed signs of anxiety, hostility, and changes in mental activity, physical activity, and sleep patterns. The men required four to six weeks after immobilization ended to regain their preexperimental levels of function.

The investigators concluded that immobility per se was a greater factor in the metabolic and functional changes noted secondary to trauma and surgery than had been previously realized. Their study has been replicated and the results verified by other investigators. These studies, and more current work by the Air Force and the National Aerospace Administration, form the basis of theoretical and factual knowledge of the consequences of immobility.

The functional and metabolic changes seen in immobility are the result of *deconditioning*—a loss of physiologic condition, or functional capacity, secondary only to lack of use (Spencer et al., 1965; Kottke, 1966). Spencer defines deconditioning in terms of (1) diminished maximum range of response usually evoked in physiologic activity, (2) decreased endurance for activity, and (3) changes in the regular adjustments during transient states, such as position change. Anyone who has spent any length of time in bed knows what this means in everyday English. You feel weak (diminished range of response to muscular activity); you cannot walk across the room without tiring (decreased endurance); and you are dizzy, or even faint, upon arising (loss in regulatory adjustment to position change). You

are simply "out of shape" (deconditioned). These phenomena are common simply with physical inactivity. Consider how they are compounded when other aspects of immobility are present: joints are stiff after a cast is removed; muscles are too weak for walking after recovery from paralysis; tempers are short because aggression could not be expended through activity.

Physiologic deconditioning occurs simply because a part, or all of the body, is not used. Kottke and Blanchard summarize the principle of disuse:

> The physiological basis of the development of functional ability by any tissue or organ of the body is use. . . . Inactivity or non-use results in regression of the organ with loss of ability to function.[4]

Kottke and Spencer do not discuss disuse and deconditioning in other than physiologic terms. However, these concepts can be easily applied to the effects of immobilization on psychosocial response as well. For example, confinement to bed restricts a person's social environment and the range of response which he may normally have to conflict and to frustration. Blake (1969) points out the social and emotional problems encountered by school-age and adolescent children, for whom activity is an important means of communication. Hospitalized children are socially confined, and often physically immobilized as well. Aggressive feelings cannot be so easily discharged by activity and may be expressed outwardly through tears and temper tantrums. Or these feelings may be kept inward, leading to withdrawal and depression.

If a defective motor system or imposed immobility leads to disuse of normal social-motor function in a child, his psychosocial development may be hampered. Disuse of the usual psychosocial responses in an adult may make it difficult for him to interact normally when the

---

[4] F. J. Kottke and R. B. Blanchard, Bedrest Begets Bedrest, *Nursing Forum*, **3**(3):56–73 (1964).

period of immobilization ends. An extreme example of this is the person who has spent many years in a state mental institution, which induces restrictions of physical and social mobility. When he is no longer in need of psychiatric care, he may be unable to take care of himself "on the outside." His ability to make decisions and care for himself has atrophied from disuse.

THE DISUSE PHENOMENA

Disuse phenomena occur in all the systems of the body during immobilization. The functional consequences of many of the phenomena depend upon the duration and degree of immobilization. For example, postural hypotension (drop in blood pressure upon arising) does not occur after only a few days of bed rest, but may be a real problem after three weeks.

Many of the disuse phenomena are reversed when the system is used after immobilization ends. However, loss or decrease in function from disuse can lead to pathological consequences (damaged function). For example, the decrease in muscle tone and strength which is a physiologic consequence of disuse can lead to poor function of the "muscle pump" in the legs, which normally aids venous return to the heart. This situation may contribute to pooling of blood in the veins, which may, in turn, lead to thrombus formation (blood clot) in the vein. These thrombi are loosely attached to the vein and may break loose. This loose thrombus, called an *embolus,* may occlude a major vessel when it reaches the pulmonary circulation. Interruption of circulation to a portion of the lung for an extended period may cause cell death (infarction) in the affected area. Consequently, pulmonary embolism can be a very serious pathological consequence.

Many of the functional and pathological consequences of disuse can be avoided if a body part or system can be used while other portions of the body are rested. The consequences of disuse and the means for their prevention are given in the following pages. Disuse phenomena involve all the systems of the body; therefore, all the phenomena will be discussed in this chapter to avoid fragmentation of the concept.

Musculoskeletal, Neurosensory Effects

The musculoskeletal and neurosensory systems are primary in maintaining mobility, as was discussed earlier in this chapter. Therefore, disuse effects in these systems will ultimately affect all body systems. Figures 12-2 and 12-3 illustrate the cyclical nature of disuse effects.

Loss of Muscle Strength and Mass   One of the most obvious and dramatic changes attributed to immobility occurs in the muscles. Deitrick, Whedon, and Schorr (1948) reported a 13 to 20 percent decrease in the strength of their subjects' immobilized limbs and a 6 percent loss in the nonimmobilized arms. Four to six weeks were required to regain former strength. Mass loss was documented by a decrease in girth, by decreased mass as seen in cross-sectional roentgenograms, and by decreased creatinine tolerance. Creatinine tolerance measures the ability of muscles to retain injected creatinine; the less muscle mass, the less creatinine retained.

Muscle strength is an extremely important aspect of mobility. When strength decreases, so does endurance or tolerance for exercise. When a person's endurance is impaired, he generally limits his activity to match his capacity. Thus, a cycle begins which leads to further loss of strength and endurance.

Muscle strength decreases during immobility simply because the muscle is not used. The more completely the muscle is immobilized, the less it is used and the greater the loss of mass, strength, and endurance.

A muscle maintains or increases strength through frequent contractions. Maximal tension is the greatest contraction a muscle can sustain,

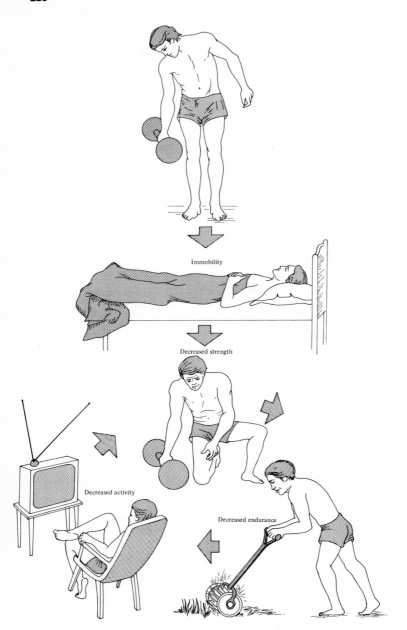

Immobility

Decreased strength

Decreased activity

Decreased endurance

Figure 12-2 The effect of muscular atrophy on strength and endurance. The ability to tolerate exercise (endurance) decreases as muscular atrophy impairs strength. Decreased endurance leads to decreased activity, which initiates further loss of strength secondary to disuse of muscles.

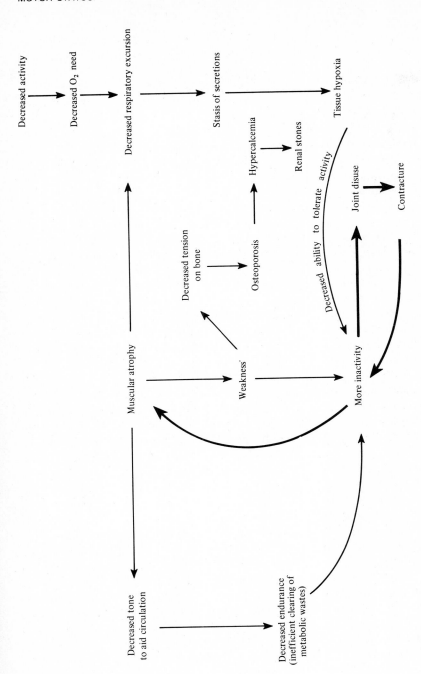

Figure 12-3 The cyclic nature of disuse effects. Disuse atrophy of muscles affects more than muscular strength. Loss of strength from disuse may eventually lead to pathologic consequences in the respiratory, skeletal, and renal systems.

and strength is increased when maximal tension is produced regularly. Strength is maintained with a contraction of 20 to 30 percent maximal tension (Kottke, 1966). Therefore, disuse atrophy and loss of strength can be prevented if muscles can exert at least 20 percent of their maximal tension. Isometric bed exercises are one way in which this can be accomplished. Indications and contraindications for isometric exercises are discussed under "Nursing Management in Immobility," further on in this chapter.

Loss of Joint Mobility   Through a process of fibrosis, muscle and joint mobility is decreased or lost when these structures are not used. Normal mobility is dependent upon the free movement of the joints and their muscular attachments. When the joints and muscles are not used, the normal metabolic activity within joints and muscles is altered and this leads to a loss of mobility.

Connective tissue fibers are continually being laid down in the subcutaneous tissue, muscle planes, and joint capsules. The normal range of motion of joints and muscles keeps this fibrous network loose, or areolar. It stretches to accommodate the maximum range of movement of any one joint. When motion is limited, the normal stretching forces are absent, and the collagen meshwork becomes less pliable. Eventually, this meshwork becomes quite dense, a process called *fibrosis.* Recent experimental work suggests that the amount of connective tissue does not increase, but that the connective tissue simply becomes more fixed (Akeson et al., 1968).

A dense collagen network may form in as few as five days of immobilization, and motion may be restricted within a week (Kottke, 1966). If allowed to progress to a dense scar, fibrosis can lead to a permanent loss of joint mobility. The process of fibrosis may be hastened in any situation in which circulation to the immobilized joint is impaired. Such situations include the presence of edema, fracture, and inflammation.

Fibrosis within a muscle plane leads to progressive shortening of the muscle in a contracted shape. Contracted muscles will pull the joint to

which they attach into an abnormal position, creating a *contracture* (Fig. 12-4). Contractures may become permanent deformities if the fibrosis is severe enough. They are more apt to occur when disuse is secondary to paralysis or other conditions resulting in loss of motor power than when the disuse is due to bed rest alone. However, fibrosis and contractures may occur in any extremity which is not used, regardless of the cause of disuse. Poor position in bed during prolonged bed rest may lead to deformed posture through atrophy of muscles, fibrosis, and contractures of postural muscles. Figure 12-5 shows such an example. This deformity of posture is important not only because it is unattractive but because it requires more of the person's energy to remain erect when he cannot maintain good posture. If the back or weight-bearing joints cannot assume their normal position because of contractures, more effort must be exerted to stand than normally. This increased effort may lead to easy fatigue, which may lead the person right back to his bed!

Preventive Measures   The obvious preventive measure against fibrosis is to maintain the full range of motion for the joint. This may be done by the patient-client himself (active range of motion) or may be done for him by the nurse (passive range of motion). Details of range-of-motion activities are included under "Nursing Management in Immobility," further on in this chapter.

Changes in Bone   A second factor in maintaining mobility is the condition of the bones. Disuse of normal muscular tension on bones leads to *osteoporosis,* literally, "porous bone."

When bones are subjected to the normal muscular stresses of weight bearing and moving, bone formation (osteoblastic activity) and bone resorption (osteoclastic activity) are balanced. The pull of muscle on the bone creates these normal stresses. When these pulls are absent, osteoclastic activity appears to increase and shift the normal balance toward bone resorption. The normally dense matrix of the bone becomes thinned and porous. The collagen fibrils become

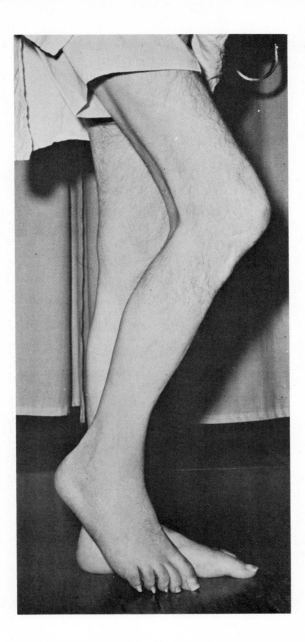

Figure 12-4 Contracture of the leg with foot drop (inability to flex the foot). This partially paralyzed limb has been pulled into a permanently flexed position by fibrosis of the collagen tissue around the joint and in the muscles. Both hip and knee are flexed because of prolonged sitting without range-of-motion exercise. The patient also has foot drop, because of contracture of the calf muscle. *(Courtesy of Jane Jones, Stroke Nurse with the Washington-Alaska Regional Medical Program.)*

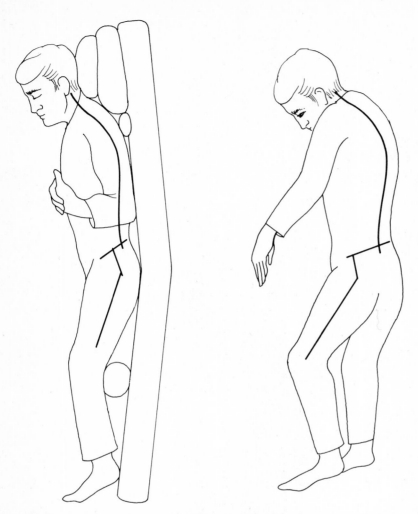

Figure 12-5 Poor position during prolonged bed rest. The contractures in the standing posture on the right closely resemble the body angles in the poor bed position on the left. Note the misalignment of spine and hip girdle. *(Adapted from Frank Krusen and Frederick Kottke, in F. H. Krusen, et al., "Handbook of Physical Medicine and Rehabilitation," 2d ed., W. B. Saunders Company, 1971. By permission of authors and publisher.)*

degraded, apparently by a chemical liberated by the osteocytes (bone-resorbing cells). Because the collagen substrate normally holds the mineral components in the matrix, its degradation and resorption release the mineral constituents, primarily calcium and phosphorus (Little, 1963). These minerals are dissolved into the general circulation and excreted. Contrary to older theories, osteoblastic (bone-forming) activity does not decrease during immobility; rather, it ap-

pears to increase but not sufficiently to compensate for increased resorption. In a man with one paralyzed wrist and one which was weak but used for muscular activity, Heaney (1962) demonstrated increased mineral uptake and thus increased bone formation in the flaccid (paralyzed) wrist, as compared with the stronger wrist.

Osteoporosis, which is a physiologic response to immobilization, begins soon after muscular activity ceases. In the Deitrick study (1948), urinary levels of calcium (which reflect that mobilized from bone) rose in the second to third day and reached a peak in the fourth to sixth week. No roentgenographic changes suggestive of osteoporosis were found. However, the subjects excreted only about 2 percent of normal body calcium, whereas 25 to 30 percent of the body mineral must be lost before conventional roentgenographic changes are seen (Vogt, 1969). Using specialized x-ray densitometric technique, Mack and LaChance (1967) demonstrated measurable loss of calcium in two weeks of bed rest in healthy young men. Similar findings were made during the Gemini earth orbital flights. Significantly, this loss of density was reduced both in the astronauts and in controlled laboratory conditions by daily isometric and isotonic muscular exercises which produced muscular stress on the bones. An increase in dietary calcium simply caused more calcium to be excreted.

Osteoporosis is reversible in normal people once immobilization ends. However, osteoporosis may become pathologic if enough bone and mineral are lost. The bone which becomes too porous through disuse may break when again subjected to weight bearing. This is known as a *pathologic fracture;* the bone breaks because of abnormality within it, rather than because of external trauma. Pathologic fractures are more apt to be the result of osteoporosis when the process is caused or accentuated by factors such as disease, medication, or aging. Osteoporosis is concomitant with aging, particularly in women. It also occurs as a side effect of steroid therapy and in such diseases as multiple myeloma.

Preventive Measures The basic preventive measure is to maintain muscular stress upon the bones. This can be done either through active weight bearing or through isometric exercise (q.v., under "Nursing Management in Immobility," further on in this chapter). Passive weight bearing (e.g., on a tilting table) is not effective unless the person is able to contract his muscles in response to the weight; it does not prevent osteoporosis in people with paralyzed legs. Increasing the calcium in the diet does not prevent osteoporosis. The calcium mobilization is a result of bone resorption, rather than the cause of it; therefore, adding dietary calcium simply adds to the amount in the bloodstream.

Neurosensory Effects

The third principal factor in mobility is the state of the nervous system. The central nervous system is the primary regulator of movement. Because the peripheral sensory nerve endings are so numerous and respond to such a variety of stimuli, there is no such thing as disuse of the intact adult nervous system. Portions of the nervous system which are severed from their central connections through trauma or pathologic change do die. However, this is the result of the disease or trauma, rather than of disuse per se. Disuse of portions of the developing nervous system in animals can lead to permanent impairment (Reisen, 1950).

Loss of Innervation Loss of innervation to a part of the body can lead to disuse phenomena in that part of the body, however. For example, paralysis is loss of innervation to a muscle or group of muscles. Thus, these muscles will atrophy and lose strength rapidly, for there is no stimulus to move. Even the tone of the resting muscle is lost. Similarly, a loss of peripheral sensory innervation reduces the sensory stimulation to move, even though motor power is intact. This may occur in such conditions as multiple sclerosis.

Improper body positioning or improper use of restraints can lead, in turn, to nerve damage. Superficial nerves, particularly those which course around bony prominences, may become compressed and then ischemic (i.e., their blood supply is decreased); they will then die if pressure is not relieved. The damage to the nerve is more properly called a *misuse* phenomenon; the resultant muscle atrophy in the area innervated is called a *disuse* phenomenon.

One example of the loss of nerve function from

misuse occurs when a plaster cast used to immobilize a fractured leg compresses the peroneal nerve as it courses around the head of the fibula. Portions of this nerve serve the ability to flex the foot and toes. Prolonged compression can result in foot drop, or inability to flex the foot at the ankle (Fig. 12-4). Sleeping positions which compress the ulnar nerve may result in wrist drop, if body weight compressing the nerve is not removed. All of us have experienced the "pins-and-needles" sensation which occurs in a portion of the body served by the temporarily ischemic nerve. Normally, a person moves and relieves the compression of the nerve or of the blood vessel supplying the nerve, and no damage results. The unconscious, weak, or paralyzed person cannot do this. The nurse is responsible in these situations for preventing nerve damage from misuse.

Sensory and Perceptual Restriction In addition to being subject to potential nerve damage, the immobilized person is subject to a decrease in environmental sensory and perceptual input. This decreased stimulation produces both physiologic and psychosocial effects.

The normal erect sitting or walking position produces a great variety of stimuli from which we learn to determine the position of body parts; this is called *proprioception*. We know whether we are on a hard or soft surface and whether we are sitting, standing, or lying. People in experiments where the sensory and motor stimuli are reduced or made monotonous often report strange, disembodied feelings. They become physically inactive, even though they are not externally restrained. This inactivity is secondary to the loss of tactile stimulation to movement (Freedman, 1961; Zubek and Wilgosh, 1963).

The decrease in sensory and tactile stimulation inherent in the more complete degrees of immobilization tends to produce certain changes in a person's behavior, such as anxiety, boredom, ego-centeredness, difficulty in problem solving,

and changes in body image. Any changes in behavior seen in an immobilized person will be affected by the immobilization per se, by the immobilizing condition, and by the person's own personality structure.

When a person is put to bed or must remain in a confined space, his role changes from independence to dependence. His perceptual axis changes if he is supine. He now looks up at people, rather than being eye to eye with them. This tends to reinforce the dependency, as well as decrease the amount of visual input.

Certainly there are changes in sensory perception and input, in addition to the changed axis. The environment may be new; consequently, many of the noises and smells cannot be identified by the immobilized person. This increase in the area of the unknown may lead to anxiety. Monotony and boredom frequently accompany immobilization, for a person is dependent upon others to introduce variety. If the immobilizing condition changes or decreases motor or tactile input, the person may have little information about where the parts of his body are. Indeed, there is evidence that immobility in itself may decrease proprioceptive and tactile information of this nature (Freedman, 1961; Zubek and Wilgosh, 1963). This decreased tactile information, plus the dependent status, may lead to changes in body image and sensations of being detached from oneself. Research in sensory and perceptual deprivation gives some clues to the behavioral changes which might be related to the decreased sensory and motor stimuli associated with immobility and many immobilizing conditions.

Behavioral changes have been consistently reported in experiments in which sensory and perceptual stimuli are reduced to a minimum (see Part 3, Chapter 11, for a discussion of these experiments). These behavioral changes include anxiety, exaggeration of usual psychological defense mechanisms, decreased ability to concentrate and to solve problems, dreamlike quality of thoughts, loss of orientation to time and place, sensation of floating, and auditory and visual hallucinations (Freedman, 1961; Heron, 1957). Investigators have postulated that variety in perceptual stimulation is necessary to maintain one's orientation and alertness (Zubek and Wilgosh, 1963). Immobilization usually does not produce the extreme deprivation achieved in these experiments, but does decrease the variety and familiarity of the environment for the immobilized person. Zubek and Wilgosh (1963) conducted an experiment in which young men were allowed normal sensory and perceptual stimuli but were immobilized for a week in a special box. Using the same tests of intellectual and motor function given to subjects in sensory-deprivation experiments, they found that the immobilized condition alone accounted for some of the decreased efficiency in verbal recall, abstract reasoning, and verbal fluency previously attributed to sensory and perceptual deprivation. When they added perceptual deprivation to the immobilized condition, more than half of the subjects quit before the week was up! The remaining men showed greater impairment of intellectual function than did the control group or the group which was immobilized only. In addition, depth perception of the experimental subjects was impaired (Zubek et al., 1969). More recently, Ryback and his associates (1971) demonstrated that prolonged bed rest alone resulted in a number of changes in psychomotor and intellectual abilities which are usually seen in sensory-deprivation experiments. The subjects were all supine for five weeks but were allowed to read, watch television, and interact with the other subjects. Nevertheless, in addition to the expected decrease in muscle strength, the men were significantly more anxious, hostile, and depressed than they were prior to bed rest. They were interacting more superficially and felt more sluggish mentally. The authors hypothesize that the condition of sensory deprivation was present because of decreased kinesthetic muscle input and environmental monotony.

Preventive Measures Nurses must recognize that immobilized persons may suffer from sensory, perceptual, and tactile deprivation. The behavioral effects may be reduced through an increase in social and sensory stimulation. Frequent visits from staff, family, or friends help maintain social contact; newspapers and television help maintain contact with the outside world. Clocks and calendars, rarely evident in hospital rooms, can help orient the person to time. Moving the person from room to room or to the outdoors can help change the environment. A person who must remain in his bed can be moved in the bed or on a stretcher.

Children who are bored may introduce variety by "naughty" behavior, which brings some attention, albeit negative. Others may withdraw and isolate themselves further. An important part of a child's development is socialization with others and learning about the world. Unless opportunities for this are provided for the immobilized child, his development will suffer.

Respiratory Effects

Recumbent immobility in itself has no effect on pulmonary function in healthy people. The work of breathing is increased, however, in the supine position; intraesophageal pressure increases and tidal volume decreases slightly, thereby requiring more effort to expand the lungs and exchange gas (Browse, 1965). Deitrick (1948) carried out several tests of pulmonary function and found no changes from the preimmobilization base lines. He did note, however, that the subjects exerted more muscular effort to perform the maximum ventilatory capacity test. This was because of the decreased strength of the muscles of respiration.

Although recumbency does not pose ventilatory problems in healthy young men, it may lead to hypostatic pneumonia in ill or debilitated persons. Pneumonia is an inflammatory process in the alveoli which interferes with the exchange of oxygen and carbon dioxide. Hypostatic pneumonia is pneumonia resulting from the stasis of secretions; it is caused by several factors.

The decreased strength of muscles of respiration may lead to decreased chest expansion. The pressure of the bed against the chest also decreases expansion, predisposing the person to shallow breathing. Lack of activity decreases the usual stimulus to deep breathing. All these factors lead to stasis of the normal secretions of the lungs. If these mucous secretions become static, they form a good medium for bacterial growth. In addition, when a person is supine, the effects of gravity tend to draw the mucus in a bronchiole toward the bottom of the tube, leaving a dry upper epithelium, as shown in Fig.

12-6. This epithelium is more vulnerable to bacterial invasion. Bacterial growth, if unchecked, may cause pneumonia. Atelectasis, or collapse of a portion of the lung, may occur if static secretions become thick and block a bronchiole. Normally, if excess mucus is present, we cough it out, and pneumonia does not occur. If, however, a person is too weak to cough well, if it is painful to cough, or if he is unconscious, stasis of secretions may occur and lead to pneumonia.

Because this type of pneumonia is caused by *stasis* of secretions, the best preventive measure is to *move* the secretions. This can be accomplished by deep breathing, coughing, and changing position. Frequent change of position from side to side, to sitting, to standing, or walking will allow more complete ventilation of all areas of the lungs and will stimulate deep breaths.

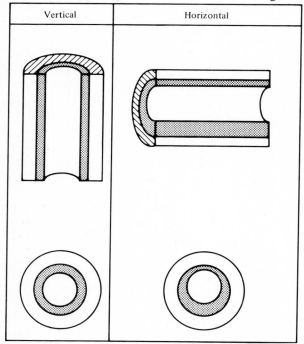

Figure 12-6   The effect of gravity on the distribution of mucus within a bronchus. Any excess mucus pools on the dependent side of a horizontal tube, and the upper surface may dry out. *(From Norman L. Browse, "The Physiology and Pathology of Bedrest," Charles C Thomas, Publisher, Springfield, Ill., 1965. By permission of the author and publisher.)*

Circulatory Effects

The major circulatory effects of immobility are increased work of the heart, decreased exercise tolerance, postural hypotension, and dependent edema. Pulmonary embolism from venous thrombosis is a pathological effect which may occur in certain circumstances.

Immobility leads to circulatory changes only when it involves long periods of recumbent inactivity. Immobilization of one limb has no effect on the heart and circulation as long as the person is able to change his position in relation to gravity.

Increased Work of the Heart Deitrick (1948) and Taylor (1949) both document an increase in heart rate during several weeks of recumbent bed rest and immobilization. Six weeks were required for the rate to return to normal after immobilization ended. This increase in heart rate may occur in compensation for the greater work load imposed by the supine position. Cardiac output increases when we change from standing to supine. This increase reflects the volume of blood "dumped" into the general circulation from the legs. Normally, about 1 liter of blood is in the legs; lying down adds this volume to the venous return. Therefore, the heart has to work harder to put out this extra blood in each stroke.

Decreased Exercise Tolerance A decrease in exercise tolerance during and after physical inactivity is a function of both the cardiovascular effects and the muscle strength. In the Deitrick and Taylor studies, immobilized experimental subjects show a marked increase in pulse rate during exercise testing, and required twice as long to return to resting-level heart rates as they had during a preliminary control period. Men in both studies required several weeks to recover preimmobility exercise tolerance levels. These findings are reflections of the deconditioned state of the cardiac and skeletal muscles. The fact that six to eight weeks were required to recondition the men helps explain why it takes so long for people to feel "really themselves" after a period of bed rest or inactivity.

Postural Hypotension Anyone who on getting up after several days in bed has become dizzy or has fainted has experienced postural hypotension—a fall in blood pressure upon rising. This phenomenon is an example of the loss of normal regulatory adjustment to transient states which occurs because of disuse of these adjustments.

Normally, a change from lying to standing produces vasoconstriction of splanchnic and peripheral vessels, so that central blood pressure is maintained. During immobility in any one position relative to gravity (lying, sitting, or standing), these regulatory adjustments are not used and somehow become dormant. When the person changes position, the central neurovascular response to position change seems intact; but the peripheral vessels fail to respond, blood pools in the legs, central blood pressure drops, and fainting may occur. After one week of bed rest with plaster immobilization of the legs, Deitrick's subjects began to faint regularly when passively raised on a tilt table to the upright position. Browse (1965) points out that passive tilting is more apt to result in fainting because there is no muscular contraction of the legs, as there is in active standing. This muscular contraction tends to compress leg veins and offset their lack of response to nervous stimulation to constrict. If the leg muscles have been considerably weakened by disease, this "muscle pump" effect will be lost. Spencer (1965) and Taylor (1949) both document postural hypotension, but without fainting, in subjects whose legs were not immobilized.

Preventive Measures Changing position in relation to gravity during the period of immobility is the most obvious measure to prevent postural hypotension (Fig. 12-7). This change of

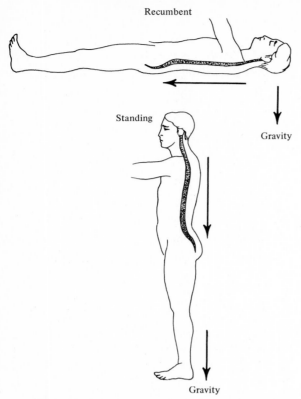

Recumbent

Gravity

Standing

Gravity

Figure 12-7 Position in relation to gravity. The supine, or recumbent, position places the spinal axis at right angles to the force of gravity, whereas the standing spine is in direct line with gravity.

position can be accomplished by seating the patient-client in a chair if he is most often in bed, or by having him sit on the edge of the bed periodically. His feet need to be supported if he is on the edge of the bed, so that the edge does not exert pressure on the popliteal vessels and impair venous return (see "Dependent Edema" and "Thrombus Formation," further on in this chapter). If the patient-client must remain in bed, a Circolectric bed, which has a revolving frame, will allow position change. These beds are expensive and are usually available only for patients who will be immobilized a long time.

There are many situations in which the patient-client's position relative to gravity cannot be changed during the period of immobility. In these situations, several measures will help to reduce the effects of postural hypotension when he gets up. The simplest measure is to make the postural changes gradually—slowly moving from lying, to sitting, to standing. It may take a few attempts before the person can stand without dizziness or faintness. A second measure is to apply elastic bandages or stockings. These supply an even, external compression of the vessels and complement the muscular activity of the legs in constricting the blood vessels. The stockings are easier to apply than the bandages, and do not require frequent rewrapping.

Dependent Edema Edema is swelling of tissues when fluid is held intercellularly. The general subject of edema is discussed in Part 3, Chapter 15. We are concerned here only with edema caused by circulatory stasis in dependent parts.

Most of us are familiar with the foot and leg swelling which occurs during long periods of sitting, as in a car or airplane. This swelling occurs in a dependent (lower-than-the-heart) part of the body because of circulatory stasis—hence the term *dependent edema*. The circulatory stasis is the result of two factors: vasodilatation, and impairment of venous return to the heart.

The veins in the legs or other dependent parts tend to dilate during muscular inactivity. Normally, venous return is aided by a pumping mechanism: the contraction of leg muscles exerts pressure on the veins and acts as a pump to return blood from the periphery to the heart. If there is no muscular activity, as in prolonged sitting, veins dilate, and the blood pools in the dilated veins. Here it exerts pressure greater than tissue pressure, and some of the fluid portion of the blood "leaks" into the interstitial space.

The second factor leading to stasis is impairment of venous return. The sitting position puts pressure on the popliteal vessels, particularly if the bend of the knee hits the surface of the chair. The pressure tends to impede the venous return, resulting in more backing up and pooling of venous blood. This adds to the increased venous pressure in the legs, and forces more fluid into the tissues.

Dependent edema can occur in any part of the body which is lower than the heart, if this part remains dependent for any length of time and if venous return is slowed. This edema is most apt to occur in the legs if the person is sitting; in the sacrum, if the person is lying in bed. If the patient-client has any loss of muscular function, dependent edema may occur in the affected limbs whenever they are dependent. The loss of the muscle pump is the prime factor in these situations.

Dependent edema may be a problem in many ways: (1) it may be uncomfortable if the swelling is great enough; (2) it may impede resumption of mobility if severe enough to prevent the person from putting on his shoes; (3) edematous tissues are more susceptible to injury and breakdown of tissues. This occurs because the accumulation of interstitial fluid, in effect, pushes the cells further from the capillaries and, thus, from their means of nutrition and waste removal. Adequate blood supply is one factor which promotes healing of injured cells. If prolonged pressure on an edematous area such as the sacrum, heels, and ankles further compromises circulation, a pressure sore may result. Pressure sores are discussed later in this chapter and in Part 3, Chapter 18.

Preventive Measures Circulatory stasis may be prevented by active contraction of muscles, which activates the muscle pump. Elastic stockings may be used to supplement the muscle pump in persons who are in bed more than a week, or in postoperative patients. McLachlin (1960) showed that elevation of the legs produced less venous stasis than either muscular contraction or elastic stockings. Thus, elevation of the dependent part is indicated when edema is not easily managed by other means. Obviously, elevating his legs reduces the mobility of the patient-client during that time.

Impairment of venous return may be prevented by avoiding positions which compromise flow in the veins. Sitting with pillows under the knees, crossing the legs at the knee, and sitting on chairs which compress the popliteal space are all situations in which position exerts pressure on veins and impedes flow.

Thrombus and Embolus Formation A thrombus is a blood clot loosely attached to the wall of a vein. If the thrombus breaks loose from the vein and enters the general circulation, it becomes an *embolus*. Emboli may pose problems when they enter the pulmonary circulation. Emboli which are large enough may block off vessels supplying a large portion of the lung; very small emboli (microemboli) lodge in pulmonary capillaries. Microemboli interfere with lung function

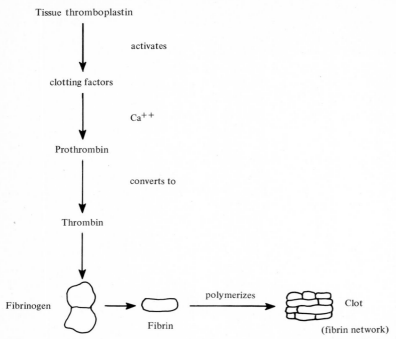

Tissue thromboplastin

activates

clotting factors

Ca^{++}

Prothrombin

converts to

Thrombin

Fibrinogen

Fibrin

polymerizes

Clot

(fibrin network)

Figure 12-8 A simplified diagram of the clotting reaction. Tissue thromboplastin activates a number of other coagulation factors, which, in the presence of the calcium ion, convert prothrombin to thrombin. Thrombin, in turn, converts fibrinogen to fibrin by proteolysis. The fibrin polymerizes into a fibrin network, or clot.

by causing reflex bronchoconstriction or vasoconstriction (Hume et al., 1970). Large emboli or multiple microemboli may cause death of a portion of the lung if they completely interrupt circulation for any length of time. This dead or necrosed area is termed an *infarct.* If the infarcted area is extensive enough, function of the organ is compromised, and death or disability may result. Obviously, a major nursing and medical responsibility is the prevention of thrombi and, thus, of emboli.

Three factors may combine to cause thromboembolism in immobilized persons: hypercoagulability of the blood, trauma or infection of the vessel walls, and circulatory stasis. Immobility per se contributes only circulatory stasis. Browse (1965) surveyed the literature and found no convincing evidence that stasis by itself causes

thrombosis. However, stasis in the presence of the other two factors can potentiate thrombus formation. Hypercoagulable blood will clot rapidly if flow is stopped. If the intima of the vessel is damaged or inflamed, a "rough spot" forms, over which pooled blood may deposit platelets and form a clot. In addition, damaged vascular tissue initiates the clotting process by releasing tissue thromboplastin. Thromboplastin, along with plasma clotting factors, converts prothrombin to thrombin. Thrombin activates the formation of a fibrin clot, as illustrated in Fig. 12-8.

Simply lying in bed does not produce generalized venous stasis, as measured by venous velocity and circulation time in experiments with normal immobilized men (Browse, p. 27). However, McLachlin (1960) demonstrated "pockets" of stasis in the venous valves in clinically immo bilized people. This tendency of blood to pool in the valve pockets was more pronounced in older people. Earlier studies with postoperative patients on bed rest also document a decrease in venous velocity in the legs (Wright, 1951).

Hypercoagulability has been demonstrated following surgery, accidental trauma, and childbirth. No such changes have been demonstrated in immobility in healthy persons (Browse).

The intima of vessels may be damaged during surgical procedures, or possibly by prolonged heavy pressure such as that produced when an unconscious person lies on his side with one leg atop the other. However, there is no good evidence that such positional vessel damage actually contributes to deep-vein thrombosis (Hume et al., 1970, p. 86).

Preventive Measures Preventive measures are aimed at eliminating or attenuating the factors predisposing to thrombus formation. Independent nursing action is aimed at preventing circulatory stasis and preventing damage to vessels. Decreasing coagulability is accomplished through drugs and is thus the physician's responsibility. Nursing measures are secondary to the drug therapy and consist of observing the patient-client for signs of increased bleeding secondary to drug therapy.

The measures described to decrease stasis and promote venous return in dependent edema are equally applicable in the prevention of thrombi.

Certain positions in bed and chair may contribute to circulatory stasis and possibly to vessel damage. Side-lying positions in which one leg rests atop the other and sitting positions with the knees crossed are two such positions. No bed patient should be positioned with one leg on top of the other. A proper side-lying position is illustrated in Fig. 12-15 in the section on nursing management, further on in this chapter. People who are susceptible to thrombi should be cautioned against crossing their legs at the knees and should be reminded about this. Susceptible people are those who are aged, who have had previous thrombi or recent trauma (surgical or accidental), who have delivered a baby, or who have a disease which increases the coagulability of the blood.

Physicians have attempted to prevent thrombus formation in persons at risk of such formation by anticoagulant drug therapy. These drugs interfere with various clotting factors and thereby slow blood clotting. Anticoagulant drugs have been effective in preventing thromboembolism in patients immobilized following surgery for fractured hips (Salzman, 1966). They are also used to prevent systemic emboli after cardiac valve surgery and to prevent further emboli in pulmonary embolism and myocardial infarction (Hume et al., 1970). Nursing responsibilities with patients taking anticoagulants involve observing them for signs of overdosage and encouraging them to remain under medical supervision. Since the drugs interfere with the normal clotting mechanisms, a fine line exists between adequate dosage to prevent intravascular clots and a dosage low enough to prevent bleeding into the tissues. Signs of overdosage include bleeding of the gums, epistaxis (nosebleed), and blood in the urine or stool. Blood in the urine may not be bright red but may give the urine a smoky or dark red color. Blood in the stool may make the stool appear tarry, or it may be detectable only by a simple laboratory test—the guaiac test. People receiving anticoagulant therapy must be under medical supervision. Periodic blood samples are taken to determine the clotting ability of the blood. The physician regulates the dosage on the basis of these tests.

Effects on Metabolism, Nutrition, and Elimination

Metabolism, nutrition, and elimination are considered together, for they are closely related. The metabolic requirements are partially supplied by nutritional intake, and the metabolic by-products are excreted in body wastes.

Metabolic Changes   The metabolic effects induced by immobility which are important to nurses are decreased basal metabolic rate, negative nitrogen balance, and negative calcium balance.

Deitrick documented an average of 6.9 percent decrease in basal metabolic rate and oxygen consumption induced by immobility. These decreases reflect a decreased energy requirement of the body—one of the aims of immobility as therapy.

Negative Nitrogen Balance   Normally, protein synthesis is in balance with protein breakdown (anabolism balances catabolism). Nitrogen, which reflects protein degradation, is lost through the urine and stool. This loss is usually balanced by dietary intake of amino acids in protein, which are used to synthesize new protein. During immobilization of healthy persons, a marked increase in urinary nitrogen excretion occurs (Deitrick, 1948; Lynch et al., 1967) about the fifth to sixth day. This large excretion of nitrogen occurs earlier in persons immobilized after surgery or accidental trauma.

The marked urinary excretion of nitrogen results in a negative nitrogen balance—more nitrogen is excreted than is taken in. Deitrick theorized that the source of the excreted nitrogen is muscle tissue, suggesting that negative nitrogen balance is a factor in atrophy. The evidence for this theory is the unchanged sulfur/nitrogen ratio in the urine; e.g., the sulfur excreted rose proportionately to the nitrogen excreted. This phenomenon suggests that the nitrogen came from a source also rich in sulfur; this source is presumably skeletal muscle.

Negative nitrogen balance is important, because it represents a depletion of stores for protein synthesis. Protein synthesis is essential in tissue healing after trauma or surgery. Increasing the protein in oral feeding has not been effective in restoring nitrogen balance. However, current work in hyperalimentation (intravenous feeding of amino acids and fats) has resulted in reversal of negative nitrogen balance (Peaston, 1969; Morgan et al., 1970).

Nursing responsibility consists primarily of keeping the negative balance at a minimum. Although diet alone cannot reverse negative balance, a balanced, protein-rich diet can prevent further imbalance. *Anorexia,* or loss of appetite, is common in people who are immobilized for a time. This anorexia is probably secondary to inactivity, boredom, and unpalatable institutional diets. If pronounced, it can contribute to negative nitrogen balance by decreasing protein intake. Protein-rich foods are filling and may be tolerated better if provided in several small meals, rather than in three large ones.

Negative Calcium Balance   Negative calcium balance also occurs solely as a result of immobility. Calcium is mobilized from the bone in the process of bone resorption (see "Changes in Bone," earlier in this chapter), and is excreted in excess of dietary intake.

The urinary loss of calcium is important for two reasons: (1) the developing osteoporosis reflected in the mobilized calcium, and (2) the physical presence of calcium in the kidneys and urine, which potentiates the formation of urinary tract stones.

Calcium is normally present in the urine and is dissolved if the urinary volume, pH, and citric acid concentration are normal. If the increase in calcium excretion during immobility were accompanied by proportionate changes in the other three factors, there would be no problem with calcium precipitation. However, only the calcium output changes. Citric acid concentration remains the same, thus altering the important ratio between calcium and citric acid. Urinary pH rises slightly rather than falling, as would be necessary to retain an acid urine. The volume rises slightly, but not in proportion to the calcium increase. These factors combine to make precipitation of calcium and formation of stones quite likely. Coupled with these chemical factors is the fact that urine is more apt to pool and remain stagnant in the recumbent kidney, as illustrated in Fig. 12-9. Browse estimates that 15 to 30 percent of patients who have had prolonged bed rest have recumbency stones (1965, p. 185).

Nursing measures to prevent stones consist of encouraging a large fluid intake (sometimes called "forcing fluids") to increase urine volume,

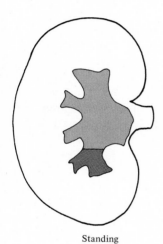

Standing

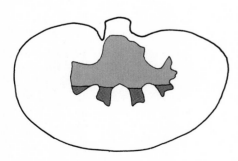

Supine

Figure 12-9 Pooling of urine in the recumbent kidney. Renal stones are more apt to form in stagnant urine. The supine position allows urine to pool in a greater number of calyces than the standing position.

encouraging an upright position part of the day to aid in emptying the kidney, and encouraging foods with an acid residue. The latter helps lower urine pH. Foods with an acid residue include cereals, meat, poultry, and fish. Exercises which produce stress on the bones will decrease bone resorption and thus decrease the amount of calcium mobilized into the circulation. If any of these measures is contraindicated by the medical problem or by the medical plan of care, alternatives will have to be coordinated with the physician.

Elimination Changes The only eliminatory effects attributable to supine immobility are an increase in renal blood flow, an increase in urine volume, and the increased urinary excretion of calcium and nitrogen discussed earlier. The increase in urine volume is secondary to the increase in renal blood flow. This change occurs normally upon lying down.

Among the several pathologic changes which often occur in ill people who are immobilized are renal stones, urinary retention, and constipation.

Renal Stones Gravity plays an important role in the normal emptying of the kidney and bladder. The kidney actively moves urine into the bladder by contractions of the calyces, renal pelvis, and ureters. If the person is supine, gravity impedes this process, for the urine must be pushed upward from the calyces to the renal pelvis. Stagnant pools of urine may form readily in the prolonged supine position. In an immobilized person, these pools are ideal places for the increased mineral content of the urine to precipitate and form renal stones.

Urinary Retention The upright position somehow facilitates the emptying of the bladder. Past the age of two or three, voiding is a voluntary process, controlled by relaxation of perineal muscles controlling the external sphincter and contraction of the detrusor muscle (the muscle around the bladder). A full bladder initiates a stretch reflex in the detrusor muscle. This muscle contracts, raising intrabladder pressure. This increase in pressure automatically opens the internal urethral sphincter. If the external sphincter is relaxed, urine will leave the body. The external sphincter is under voluntary control and can be contracted to prevent urination. Many people who try to void in bed, using either a bedpan or urinal, find it extremely difficult, if not impossible, to relax the perineal muscles sufficiently to initiate voiding. These same people may have no difficulty if allowed to sit on a commode or stand to void. If a person must remain in bed and cannot initiate voiding, he will develop *urinary retention,* and the bladder will distend. A distended bladder may develop small tears in the mucosa which form a focus for infection. In addition, the person with a distended bladder is acutely uncomfortable. Occasionally in urinary retention just enough urine will dribble out to relieve intrabladder pressure. This does not allow complete emptying of the bladder, and stagnant urine remains. This is called *retention with overflow.* A palpable bladder "bulge" with frequent voiding of small amounts (less than 100 ml) are signs of retention with overflow.

Preventive Measures Prevention of renal stones is discussed under "Negative Calcium Balance," earlier in this chapter.

The most obvious means of trying to prevent urinary retention is to help the immobilized person void in a normal position: standing for men, sitting for women. Women who are immobilized in long leg casts (which preclude sitting) can void with a special female urinal.

If the person must remain in bed, he or she needs to be helped to as close to the sitting position as is possible. A woman should have the backrest of the bed as nearly 90° as possible, with the bedpan well under her hips. A man may be able to void lying on his side or sitting with the urinal between his knees. If relaxation is difficult, running water in a sink or pouring warm water over the perineum may help relax muscles. Privacy is essential to help a person relax. Past the age of toilet training, few of us are accustomed to having others around when we are using the toilet.

Children who have just mastered voluntary control of urination may regress under the stress of illness or hospitalization. This may be distressing to them and/or their parents. The child may be assured that he will be able to control his urine (or stool) when he is better and that it is not bad to be wet. His parents need the same reassurance, particularly if toilet training has been a source of contention with their child.

Constipation Constipation is not a sequela of immobility per se, but is so common in ill persons who are immobilized that it will be briefly discussed here. A more detailed discussion of constipation is given in Part 3, Chapter 14.

Normal frequency of bowel movement depends upon the softness of the stool, muscular ability to defecate, and the heeding of the urge to defecate. Changes in any or all of these factors may lead to constipation.

The consistency of the stool depends upon the roughage content of the diet and the amount of fluid absorbed from it in the intestine. If the person is anorexic, his solid intake may be decreased, thus providing little roughage to increase the bulk of the stool. If his fluid intake is low or he is dehydrated, the body may try to compensate by increasing fluid absorption in the colon. This results in a hard, dry stool.

Many people have experienced the "summer-camp syndrome"—simply being too busy to take time to defecate and, subsequently, becoming constipated. When stool remains too long in the colon, more fluid is reabsorbed, and the stool becomes progressively dryer and harder to pass.

People in bed, particularly in a hospital, may succumb to this same kind of constipation because they are reluctant to try to defecate in a bedpan in a room with other persons. Thin curtains around a bed create only visual privacy, but do not hide the sounds and smells of having a bowel movement. Consequently, many bedfast patients suppress or ignore the urge to defecate. Eventually the sensation passes, and the stool mass remains in the colon, becoming drier and drier.

In addition to suppressing the desire to defecate, some immobilized people have not the muscle strength to pass stool, particularly if it is hard and they must strain. Perineal and abdominal muscles used in defecating are weakened by bed rest. In addition, the position one must assume on a bedpan does not favor effective use of whatever muscle strength remains. The physiologic position for defecating is a squatting one. Western man has altered this somewhat with a toilet, but the position is still upright. In contrast, the position in which bed patients are usually put forces them to lean backward and does not favor effective pushing (Fig. 12-10). A bedside commode is preferable to a bedpan, whenever the person's medical condition allows sitting. The commode allows the patient-client to be in an upright position. Getting on the commode requires less effort than getting on and off a bedpan.

If constipation is allowed to continue, fecal impaction may result. This is a situation in which stool has become so bulky or so hard that the person cannot defecate. In such situations, the stool must be removed manually. This is a most painful process.

Preventive Measures Constipation should be anticipated and prevented in anyone who is immobile. A daily glass of prune juice or an increased fluid intake may be sufficient to maintain regular stools in some persons. Others may require a daily laxative or stool softener. Whenever possible, the patient-client should be helped to an upright position and privacy should be provided. Knowledge of the person's usual bowel habits, any tendency to constipation, and any changes in bowel habits during immobility

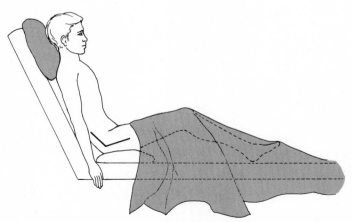

Figure 12-10 Bed position which interferes with normal position for defecation. Nursing personnel frequently leave patients in this position, or in one with the back even more reclined. Note the backward angle of the spine, which does not favor effective leverage and use of the muscles involved in defecation.

are important in predicting that a person may develop constipation.

Skin and Integumentary Effects

Reports of studies of immobility in healthy persons do not discuss any problems pertaining to the skin and subcutaneous tissues which result from immobility alone. However, the clinical situations which necessitate immobility lead to two problems which merit nursing attention: maintenance of personal hygiene and prevention of pressure sores.

Maintenance of Personal Hygiene A person who is bedfast is dependent upon others to help him keep clean. This is particularly true if he must void and defecate in bed. It is nearly impossible to clean oneself adequately after defecating on a bedpan. Women have the additional problem of drying after urination. The normal perineal odors of a woman are compounded when she must use a bedpan and has no facilities for washing her hands and perineum. These are subjective problems for the patient-client but are important to his comfort. Therefore, the nurse who is sensitive to the patient's need in this area will make washing materials available and will aid the patient-client in cleaning after elimination.

Prevention of Pressure Sores The problem of preventing pressure sores is a major one in the immobilized person, if he cannot change his position frequently by himself. Pressure sores will be discussed here very briefly; a complete discussion of etiology, prevention, and treatment will be presented in Part 3, Chapter 18.

Pressure sores are also called "bedsores" or "decubitus ulcers"; they are cutaneous and sub-cutaneous ulcers which occur in areas of the body subjected to unrelieved pressure. Skin and subcutaneous tissues die, slough away, and leave ulcerated areas. Cells in these tissues die because

sufficient nutrients cannot diffuse from the capillaries to them, and their waste products cannot be carried away. This lack of diffusion to and from the capillaries occurs because pressure on the tissues is greater than the hydrostatic pressure in the capillary. This pressure difference effectively opposes diffusion from the capillaries. Thus, *unrelieved pressure* in skin and subcutaneous tissues is the major factor in the development of pressure sores.

This unrelieved pressure must occur over a period of time. Anytime you cross your legs, pressure at the place where the legs touch is greater than capillary pressure, and diffusion cannot occur there. The blood flow increases, producing a red spot. This effect is called *hyperemia*. You uncross your legs after a bit because they are uncomfortable, thereby relieving the pressure before any cell damage has occurred. The person who is unconscious, paralyzed, or encumbered by mechanical equipment cannot change position for himself. Or perhaps he is unwilling to move. Prolonged pressure from the bed or chair may prevent nourishment of some of his tissues. Tissues which are compressed between bony prominences and external surfaces are particularly apt to be deprived of circulation. When cells are deprived of nutrients long enough, they die. If enough cells die, a bluish area forms. This area inevitably breaks down and forms an ulcer, or pressure sore. Pictures of such ulcers are shown in Part 3, Chapter 18.

Once a pressure sore forms, it is extremely difficult to bring about healing. Healing replaces normal tissue with scar tissue. Scar tissue is less well supplied with blood than normal tissue, and this lack of vascularity makes scar tissue more liable to further formation of pressure sores. In addition, a pressure sore becomes easily infected, then drains serous or purulent fluid. This fluid contains protein, further depleting the immobilized person's nitrogen reserve (Fig. 12-11).

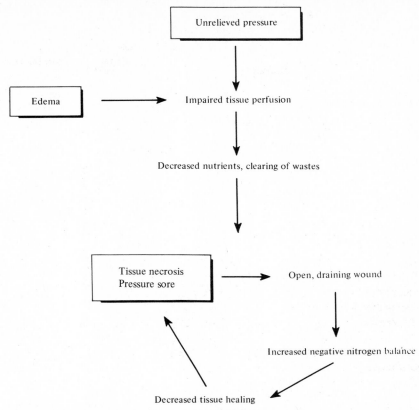

Figure 12-11 Factors contributing to the formation of pressure sores. Once a pressure sore has begun, it may become a draining, infected wound. Loss of protein in this drainage contributes to negative nitrogen balance and makes tissue repair more difficult.

Prevention of pressure sores is an extremely important and difficult nursing responsibility. The basic objectives in prevention are to relieve pressure periodically and to distribute pressure over as wide an area as possible. Specific measures to accomplish these objectives are given in Part 3, Chapter 18.

People who are particularly subject to developing pressure sores must be identified and given priority in the use of mechanical preventive equipment. People at risk are those with edema of subcutaneous tissues, those who cannot move themselves, those who are malnourished or debilitated, and those who are obese or very thin. Families need to be taught how to prevent pressure sores in persons immobilized at home; patient-clients who are permanently immobilized (such as those with paralysis) need to learn to change position frequently, since they cannot rely upon sensations of discomfort to tell them that pressure is prolonged.

NURSING MANAGEMENT IN IMMOBILITY

The preceding pages of this chapter are devoted to specific problems which occur with disuse of parts of the body. The overall nursing problem associated with immobility is the *prevention* of the outcomes of disuse. Specific preventive measures have been included in each section of the preceding discussion. Some general aspects of nursing management are included here. These general principles are discussed here, rather than at the beginning of the chapter, so that the student can better relate them to the concept of immobility and problems of disuse.

In order to help any individual patient-client who is immobilized, the nurse must diagnose the potential disuse problems, determine which problems require nursing intervention, select appropriate preventive actions, assist the patient-client to apply these measures or act for him, and evaluate the efficacy of the actions.

Diagnosis of potential disuse problems involves determining the degree of immobility or potential immobility and the patient-client's abilities to help himself. Mr. X., the man with hemiplegia discussed earlier in this chapter, is an example of a person with a high degree of immobility, and we may expect that this man will develop all the effects of disuse unless preventive measures are taken. He is able to use his left side, so he can help with some exercises and position changes. An example of a person with a low degree of immobility is a person wearing a long leg walking cast. He can get around by himself, although the weight and clumsiness of the cast slow him somewhat. The only disuse changes which he is likely to experience involve the casted leg. He will probably have muscle atrophy, knee and ankle stiffness, and some degree of bone resorption.

In order to determine which problems require nursing help, the nurse must determine the abilities of the patient-client to help himself, and must know the scope of action within nursing practice.

The Scope of Independent Nursing Action

In general, people are immobilized because of some pathological process. Prevention or treatment of disuse phenomena and pathological consequences of immobility which occur in the diseased system or part of the body are primarily the physician's responsibility and prerogative. Nursing measures in these situations are assis-

tive; they require delegation or direction from the physician, and they assist him in the medical treatment. Independent nursing measures are those which aim at preventing or dealing with the disuse phenomena in parts or systems not directly affected by the pathologic process.

A clear-cut example of independent and assistive intervention occurs in a person immobilized in traction for a fractured femur. Clearly, his whole body is immobilized by the treatment, but only one leg is injured. Any exercises or positioning of that leg must be done under supervision of the orthopedist. However, a nurse may independently institute measures to meet such goals as maintaining muscle strength and joint mobility in all other limbs, and preventing pressure sores.

In some conditions the whole body must be put to rest in order to heal one part. Myocardial infarction and rheumatic fever are two such conditions. In these situations, the whole body is considered the affected "part," and nursing preventive measures which involve physical activity on the part of the patient-client must be discussed with the physician before they are used.

Obviously, if the nurse is to use good judgment in determining the scope of independent action, he must understand medical science well enough to know what systems or body parts are affected by the disease. Beginning students possess a minimum of such knowledge and must rely upon the judgment of more experienced nurses in order to determine which actions are independent and which require consultation with the physician. Increased knowledge and experience will aid the student in exercising sound judgment in this area.

Preventive Nursing Intervention

Four general kinds of nursing actions are helpful in preventing most of the disuse phenomena: (1) body positioning, (2) muscle conditioning exercises, (3) joint mobility exercises, and (4) environmental structuring.

Body Positioning   Natural body positions can be used to help prevent contractures, renal stones, postural hypotension, hypostatic pneumonia, pressure sores, circulatory stasis, elimination problems, and sensory-perceptual deprivation. The aims of body positioning are to (1) prevent nerve damage from pressure on superficial nerves, (2) prevent nonfunctional positions which may contract into permanent deformities, (3) distribute body weight over as large an area as possible, (4) prevent prolonged pressure on any body prominence, and (5) provide stimulation to postural adjustment mechanisms. These aims will be met if position is changed regularly and frequently and if every position in bed or chair approximates normal sitting or standing alignment.

Position Change Patient-clients who can move themselves will automatically shift position when pressure on any one part becomes uncomfortable. People who cannot move themselves depend upon the nurse to do this for them. Animal studies have shown that normal tissues begin to degenerate in two hours of unrelieved pressure, and much faster in paralyzed tissues (Krusen et al., 1971). In practice, helpless patients are often helped to change positions only

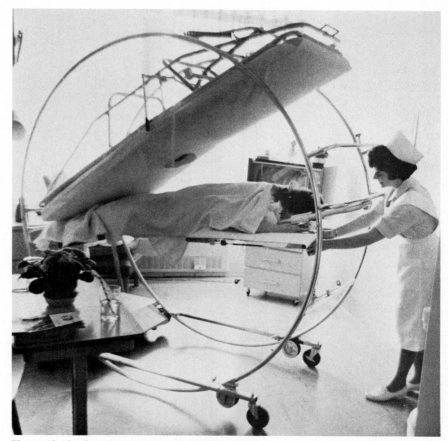

Figure 12-12 Rotating electric bed. This is one of the types of beds and frames used for people who must be immobilized for long periods. It allows one or two persons to move the patient easily and provides for change of position relative to gravity. *(Photograph, courtesy of University of Washington Information Services.)*

every three to four hours. Paralysis does not necessarily include loss of sensation, and these people are miserably uncomfortable after even one to two hours in any one position. Air cell mattresses and special turning frames (Stryker, Foster and Circolectric frames) (Fig. 12-12) help vary the pressure on various parts of the body and allow longer intervals between turnings. The frames make turning a person much easier, which may allow him to be moved more frequently.

Changing position not only relieves pressure on any one part of the body, but "stirs up" secretions and may promote muscular and joint movement.

Position must be changed in relation to gravity in order to prevent postural hypotension, stones, and, to some extent, pneumonia. This is not possible in some pathologic states (e.g., a fractured back or neck), but should be done when possible. Even unconscious people can be moved to a chair once or twice a day with the aid of mechanical lifting devices, as shown in Fig. 12-13.

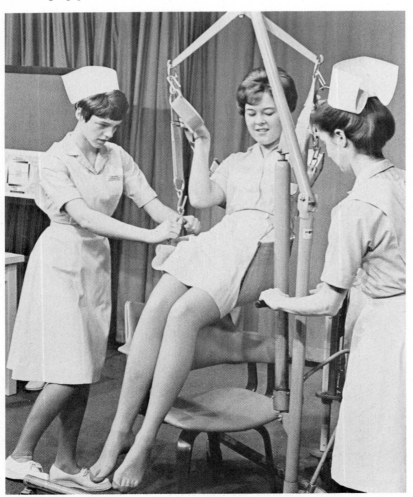

Figure 12-13 Mechanical lift. Device used to move helpless or immobilized people. *(Photograph, courtesy of University of Washington Information Services.)*

Proper Alignment of the Body The normal standing alignment is described as follows: the center of gravity is just over the instep, and the knees are lightly flexed. Natural hollows occur at the lumbar portion of the back and at the bends of the knees. Natural hollows exist at the side of the head and at the waist, when a person is viewed from the front. Hands are relaxed, fingers are slightly flexed, and feet are at nearly right angles to the tibia. Normal standing posture maintains the planes of the shoulders and hips at right angles to the axis of the spine.

When a person is in bed or in a chair, this same general alignment must be maintained, both for comfort and to prevent deformity. Natural hollows must be filled in or supported to maintain the axes of the hips and shoulders in relation to the spine. Figures 12-14 to 12-16 illustrate the application of this principle in several bed positions. The solid lines overlying some of the photographs demonstrate the way in which hip and shoulder girdles are kept at right angles to the spine.

These photographs illustrate supportive devices used to maintain functional position for a helpless person. A person who can move about by himself should not be encumbered with many pillows and bolsters. Pillows on which to rest his arm and leg when he is lying for a long time on his side will provide comfort and proper alignment. However, he should not be surrounded by pillows to the extent that he cannot easily change position.

Joint Mobility Exercises Each joint has a maximum range in which it can move; this is referred to as *full range of motion* for that joint. Figure 12-17 illustrates the range of motion of major joints. Joint mobility is maintained through frequent motions which move the joint through its full range of motion and thus keep the fibrous network in the muscles and joint loose. Normally, activities such as stretching, brushing hair, walking, and reaching accomplish this movement. In bed, the activities stimulating full joint motion are decreased.

If the patient-client is able to move his own joints in the portions of his body not affected by the pathologic process, the nurse's task is to teach him the necessity of keeping these joints mobile while he is immobilized. Exercises which the patient-client can do by himself are called *active range-of-motion exercises;* they consist of merely moving the joint through its full range of motion. Patient-clients who have chronic joint disease, such as arthritis, or who have some degree of contracture may not be able to accomplish the full range of motion. These people should move the joint only to the point of resistance or pain.

A person who is weak or partly paralyzed may be able to move a limb only partially through its range. He needs *assisted range-of-motion exercises;* the nurse assists him in finishing the full range. For example, he may be able to raise his arm only to shoulder level; the nurse helps him to raise it straight overhead. Both active and assisted exercise require muscle contraction, and thereby also help maintain muscle tone.

Sometimes the patient-client cannot perform range-of-motion exercise, either because he is too weak, paralyzed, or unconscious, or because muscular activity might be detrimental to his recovery. In these situations, the nurse performs *passive range-of-motion exercises* for the patient-client. The nurse supports the limb at the joints and moves the joint for the patient. This does not help maintain muscle tone, as no active contraction of the patient-client's muscle is involved. Passive range-of-motion exercises are used most often in parts of the body where disease exists, or they are performed for patients whose whole body must rest. Therefore, the nurse must use some judgment in deciding when to institute passive range-of-motion exercises independently and when to consult the physician before doing so.

The nurse cannot assume that activities of daily living will automatically accomplish full range of motion for all joints in a person who is in bed. The joints most liable to contractures are those to which large muscles attach—the hip and

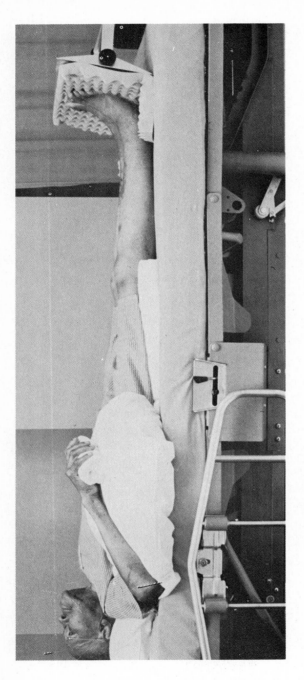

Figure 12-14 Good supine alignment. A small, flat pillow is well under the shoulders as well as the head; this prevents forward flexion of the neck. This patient's paralyzed arm is supported by pillows; finger and wrist flexion are maintained by a hand roll. The trochanter roll is placed hip-to-knee to prevent external rotation of the hip. A footboard maintains dorsiflexion of the feet. *(Photographs, courtesy of Jane Jones, Stroke Nurse with Washington-Alaska Regional Medical Program.)*

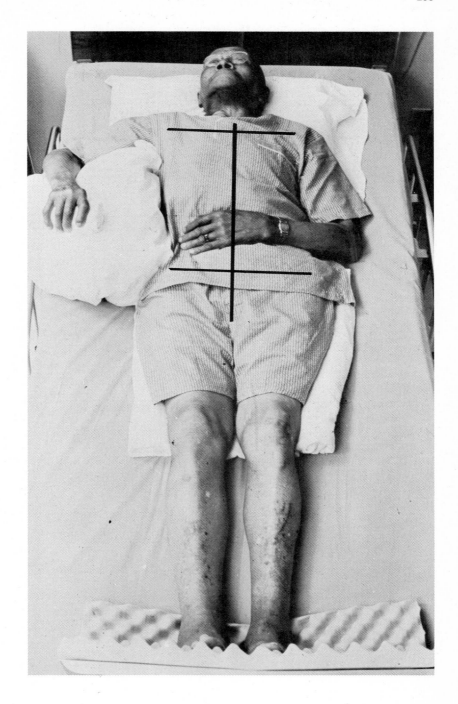

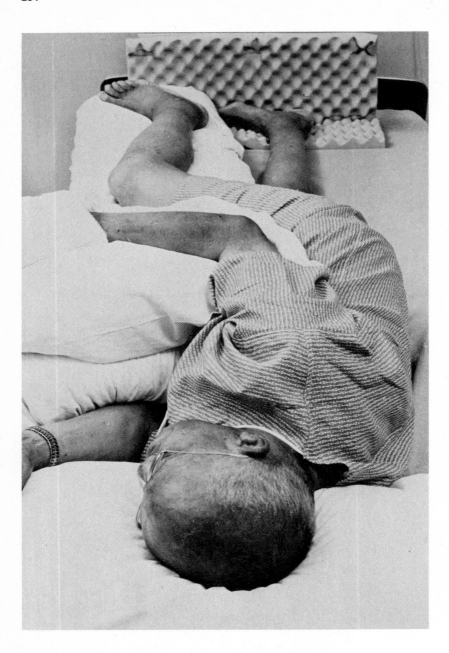

Figure 12-15 Side-lying position. Ordinary pillows are used to support the upper leg and to prevent internal rotation at the hip. Another pillow maintains the axis of the shoulder girdle by elevating the forearm. A large handroll is used to maintain the natural flexion of wrist and fingers. Note the straight back and absence of a pillow at the back. These supports might be used for a hemiplegic person. Note the difference in posture of hip and shoulders in the poorly positioned example on the right. *(Photographs, courtesy of Jane Jones, Stroke Nurse with the Washington-Alaska Regional Medical Program.)*

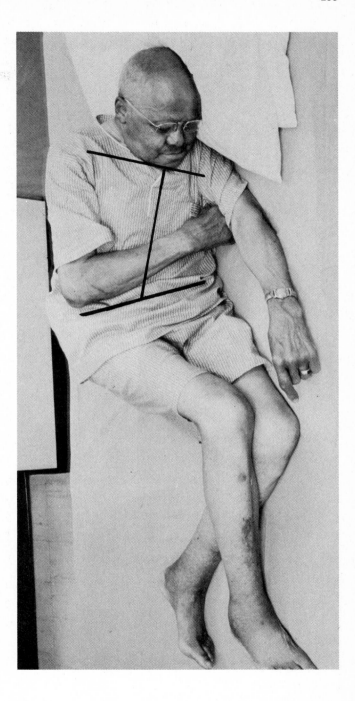

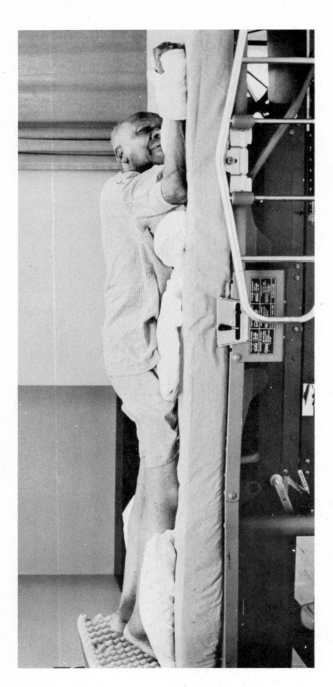

Figure 12-16 Prone position. The normal standing alignment is maintained by dispensing with almost all pillows and supports. The head is turned to one side, and small pads may be used to prevent the shoulders from dropping forward (see detail in picture on the right). The natural position of the feet is maintained either by allowing them to extend

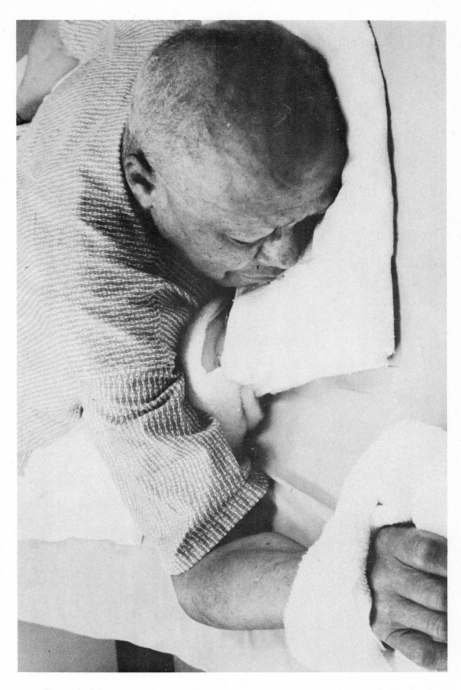

over the end of the mattress, or by placing a pillow from knee to ankle and allowing the feet to hang over the pillow. This patient had a "barrel" chest, so padding was placed to fill in the hollow at his waist. *(Photographs, courtesy of Jane Jones, Stroke Nurse with the Washington-Alaska Regional Medical Program.)*

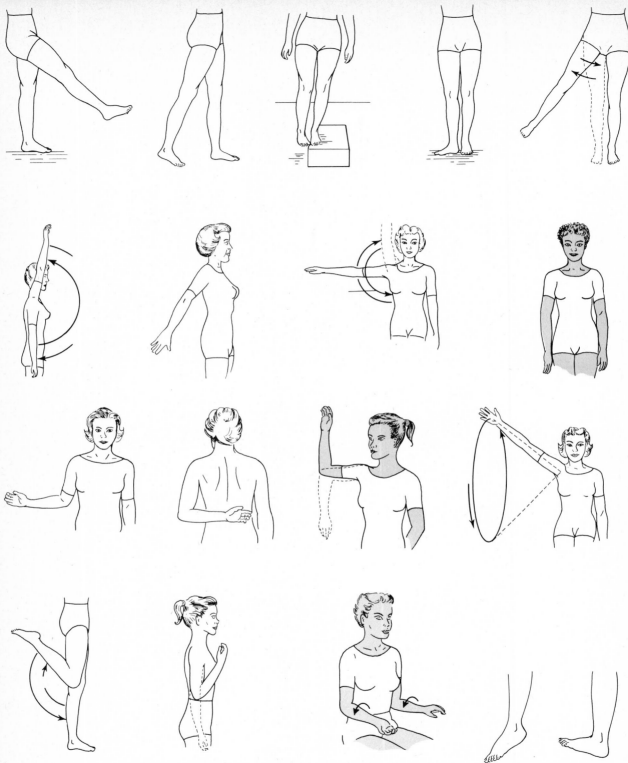

Figure 12-17 Range of motion of joints. *(From H. Moidel et al., eds.), Nursing Care of Patients with Medical-Surgical Disorders, Copyright McGraw-Hill Book Company, New York, 1971. Used with permission of McGraw-Hill Book Company. Exercises after M. Winters, Protective Body Mechanics in Daily Life and Nursing, W. B. Saunders Company, 1952.*

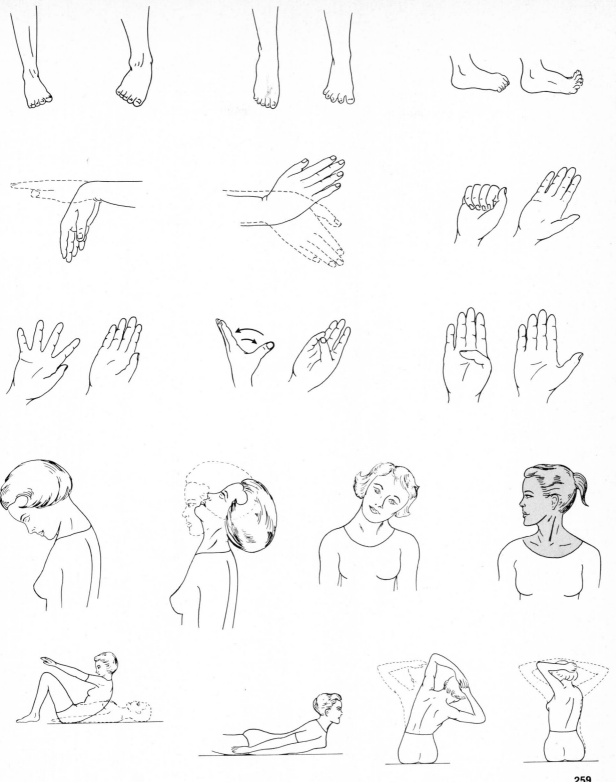

knee joints. The legs are the limbs least likely to be exercised when a person is in bed. Patients in hospitals commonly sit hunched in bed, a large pillow behind their neck, with hips and knees bent (Fig. 12-5). This position puts the neck, hips, and knees into flexion and may lead to postural deformity. Even if a person lies prone and flat in bed, his hip joint cannot extend the full 175° to which it normally extends upon standing (Krusen et al., 1971). Consequently, people who must remain in bed or who otherwise cannot maintain full range of motion themselves need a planned program of exercise. The nurse must assess which joints get full range of motion in the patient-client's normal activities and which do not. Not every patient needs to have nursing help to maintain joint mobility. However, each patient-client should be assessed on the basis of his ability to move his joints, rather than on the basis of his medical diagnosis. Nurses commonly assume that any patient with a stroke or paralysis will need range-of-motion exercise, but neglect to assess the joint mobility needs of the elderly patient with pneumonia or the person with arthritis who is hospitalized for some other illness. Consequently, many patient-clients may become stiff without anyone having noticed it. Such a situation is exemplified by Mr. J. M.:

Mr. J. M. was a 66-year-old man hospitalized for acute pneumonia. He was frequently out of contact with the environment, sleeping, or rambling incoherently. This latter behavior may have been due to organic brain disease. A student nurse cared for him on his fifth hospital day, by which time the pneumonia was clearing up. While giving him a bath, the nurse realized that she could not raise Mr. M.'s arm above shoulder level. She then tested his other joints and found decreased range of motion in all, particularly shoulders, hips, and knees. She began passive range-of-motion exercises to all joints, because he was unable to follow directions for active exercise and because of his general weakness. She prescribed this routine three times daily in the nursing Kardex.

After three days of this regimen, Mr. M. had regained full range of motion of all joints.

There seems to be no consensus as to how often range-of-motion exercises should be performed. Authorities recommend anywhere from one to three times daily (Kelly, 1966; Krusen, 1971). Empirically, the exercises should be done as often as needed to keep the joints easily movable.

Muscle-conditioning Exercises Muscle strength is maintained by frequent isometric contractions of 20 to 30 percent maximal tension. Therefore, isometric contraction of muscles is one way to maintain muscle strength. Several kinds of exercises are recommended for selected bedfast or immobilized patient-clients. These exercises involve both isometric and isotonic contractions. Isometric contractions are those in which force is exerted without change in the length of the muscle. Isotonic contractions occur when the muscle shortens, as when it is used to lift a load.

Setting exercises are truly isometric. The muscle is simply contracted as hard as possible for ten seconds and then released. Muscles commonly involved in setting exercises are the abdominal, gluteal, and quadriceps. *Resistive* exercises are those in which the muscle contracts in pushing or pulling against a stationary object. For example, pushing the feet against a footboard accomplishes resistive contraction of the gastrocnemius and quadriceps muscles. This exercise is useful in maintaining strength and in aiding in venous return. Another useful resistive exercise is to push against the bed with the hands and simultaneously lift the hips off the bed. This exercises the triceps, important muscles in walking with crutches. Pulling oneself up to a sitting position with the aid of a rope attached to the end of the bed exercises arm and shoulder muscles, and enables a person to help himself up when his abdominal muscles are weak. Figure

12-18 shows a series of graded exercises used by one medical center with patients who have had myocardial infarctions. These exercises are not begun until the cardiac rhythm is stable.

Isometric exercises raise the blood pressure in normal people (Bartels et al., 1968; Nutter, Schlant, and Hurst, 1972). This elevation is transient and of no consequence in people with a healthy cardiovascular system. However, this brief elevation of blood pressure may compromise cardiac blood flow in people with vascular or cardiac disease. The heart must pump harder to maintain adequate output against an increased arterial pressure. If the heart cannot meet this sudden increased work demand, the amount of blood pumped to the coronary arteries will be inadequate to meet the oxygen needs of the heart muscle itself, and myocardial ischemia may result. This, in turn, may precipitate a myocardial infarction or heart failure. The decision to avoid isometric exercises in patient-clients who are hospitalized for treatment of acute unstable cardiac disease is obvious. However, a great many people who have controlled heart failure, valvular disease, or arteriosclerotic heart disease are hospitalized for reasons unrelated to their cardiac condition. For example, the woman immobilized with a broken leg may have mitral stenosis as a consequence of rheumatic fever in her childhood. Isometric exercise should not be initiated in such situations without consultation with the physician. When it is used, the patient-client must be instructed to exhale during the muscular contraction, so that he does not hold his breath. A phenomenon called the *Valsalva maneuver* occurs when a person holds his breath during isometric exercise or certain straining activities, such as pushing oneself up in bed or having a bowel movement. The Valsalva maneuver is defined as an increased intrathoracic pressure produced by forced expiration against the closed glottis. Holding one's breath while straining produces this entrapment of air by the glottis. The increased intrathoracic pressure decreases venous return and filling pressure to the heart and thereby decreases cardiac output and coronary blood flow. Again, this decreased coronary blood flow may be sufficient to precipitate a myocardial infarction in a person whose coronary vessels are relatively clogged by atherosclerosis, or whose heart muscle is diseased. More than one "heart attack" has occurred while someone was straining to pass a hard stool on the toilet or bedpan.

An inadvertent Valsalva maneuver can be avoided by preventing constipation and by teaching patient-clients to exhale through the mouth while moving themselves in bed or while performing isometric exercise. The glottis cannot be closed while the person is exhaling through the mouth.

Environmental Structuring The last general class of nursing measures involves introducing variety into the environment in order to decrease sensory and perceptual restriction. Introducing variety also helps prevent simple boredom. Methods of producing variety may vary from such simple measures as providing a clock and calendar to arranging for special dinners or entertainments. Moody, Barron, and Monk (1970) describe the dramatic effect of forty-five minutes a day spent in talking and sharing food and experiences with a group of elderly people in a nursing home. Many of these people had previously had little interaction with others, were sloppy in their personal habits, and were felt to be senile. After only a week of this social stimulation, they "blossomed." Structuring the environment is an area in which nurses may need to call upon others to provide the direct services to the patient-client. Institutions often use volunteer groups to visit and provide entertainment. A nurse in the community may recruit friends and volunteers to visit a person who must be immobilized at home, or to take him for a ride regularly.

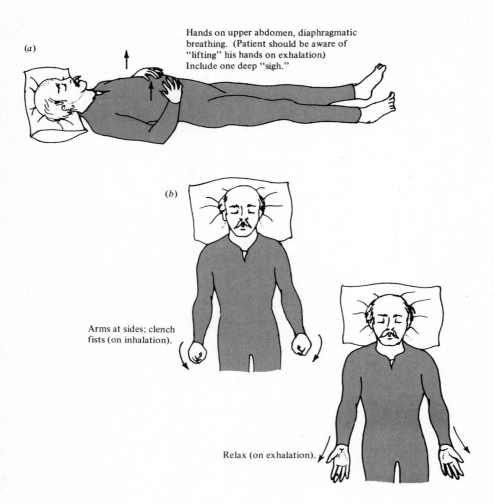

(a)

Hands on upper abdomen, diaphragmatic
breathing. (Patient should be aware of
"lifting" his hands on exhalation)
Include one deep "sigh."

(b)

Arms at sides; clench
fists (on inhalation).

Relax (on exhalation).

Figure 12-18 Exercises to prevent deconditioning and pathological consequences of
bed rest (a and b). Exercises c, d, and e are for reconditioning. These are from a series
of exercises designed for coronary-care patients; they are begun at the discretion of the
physician when heart rhythm and general condition are stable. *(By permission of
Stanford University Hospital—Coronary Care Activities Program.)*

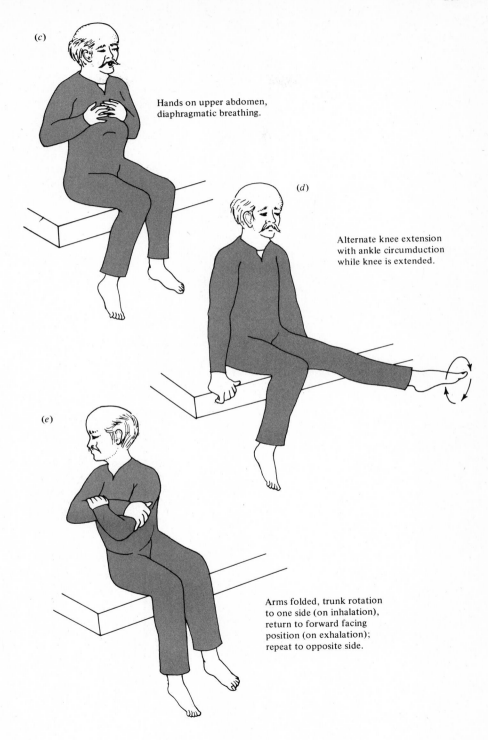

(c) Hands on upper abdomen, diaphragmatic breathing.

(d) Alternate knee extension with ankle circumduction while knee is extended.

(e) Arms folded, trunk rotation to one side (on inhalation), return to forward facing position (on exhalation); repeat to opposite side.

THE CONCEPT OF REHABILITATION

Rehabilitation is the process of restoring a person to his previous capabilities, or helping him make the most of his existing capabilities. The term often connotes a process of helping a person to become a contributing or relatively independent member of society. For example, we speak of the rehabilitation of convicts, as well as the rehabilitation of handicapped people. Rehabilitation is considered in this chapter, because a large proportion of people requiring this service have impaired mobility. Examples of such persons are someone whose lung disease prevents him from working, a person who is paralyzed in one or more limbs, a homemaker whose cardiac disease limits her ability to do household tasks, and a child with long-term immobilizing treatment of such deformities as scoliosis (curvature of the spine).

Rehabilitation is not a static something which is done to a person; it is a process in which the person himself must participate if he is to make the most use of his abilities after disabling injury or illness.

Formal rehabilitation involves a team which is most often composed of a physician (often a physiatrist, i.e., a specialist in rehabilitation medicine), nurse, physical and occupational therapist, vocational rehabilitation worker, social worker, and psychiatrist. These professionals and the patient-client plan a program designed to capitalize on his remaining capabilities in returning him to as productive and fulfilling a life as possible. Wright points out the importance of this "co-management" attitude in rehabilitation:

Barring special circumstances, this support on the part of the client in the long run is enhanced when he takes an active part in decision-making; it is often weakened when he feels his life is being manipulated behind the scenes, even when it is by the experts, who know best "where he is to go and how he is to get there."[5]

[5] Beatrice Wright, "Physical Disability—A Psychological Approach," Harper & Row, Publishers, Inc., New York, 1960, p. 345.

She further clarifies active participation, not as a "cooperative" attitude, but as asking questions as well as answering them, evaluating data as to his ability and disability, and having the right to veto decisions.

Because formal rehabilitation usually occurs in a separate hospital unit or in a special institution, many nurses assume that rehabilitation is a "specialty" and that the nurse in the hospital for acute conditions, or in the home or industry, has no rehabilitative skills to offer. This is simply not true. Nursing in the process of rehabilitation is based upon exactly the same premises as all nursing; namely, that a person is assisted in using his abilities to cope with whatever changes in daily life his disabilities have created. The primary goal of the rehabilitation process is to achieve maximum physiologic and psychosocial function within the limitations of the person's disability. Broadly speaking, this is accomplished by protecting remaining abilities, preventing further disability, and helping the person incorporate his changed self-image and abilities into his life. The way in which the particular nurse and patient-client work together toward this goal depends upon where they meet, in time, during the rehabilitation process. For example, a young man who is paraplegic (paralyzed from the waist down) will need a great deal of physical preventive nursing care in the hospital period immediately following the accident. In order to preserve ability, disuse phenomena must be prevented in his nonparalyzed parts, such as his arms, neck, and trunk. Disuse atrophy and osteoporosis cannot be prevented in his paralyzed legs, but the nurse can prevent further disability by preventing contractures and pressure sores. The major means of mobility for this person will be a wheelchair. If he has marked contractures of his legs or pressure sores, he cannot use a wheelchair and will be more immobile than is necessary. Thus, the nurse who cares for the patient-client early in the process may focus primarily on preserving ability and preventing further disability; the nurse who meets this person after the disability is stable may work more with him in incorporating his new self-image and abilities into his life. The process of adjusting to disability is a long, often slow one. Nurses in acute-care systems may not be with the patient-client long enough to see more than the initial stages of shock and denial; therefore, they cannot expect the person to accept the situation while under their care.

Adapting to Disability

People who have suffered a physical disability which they view as causing a major change in their self-image commonly experience a form of grief reaction—a grief and mourning for the lost self (Crate, 1965). A facial scar may alter a young woman's self-image sufficiently to cause this reaction; paralysis, blindness, or amputation is likely to cause it in almost anyone.

The initial reaction to disability is one of shock and disbelief. This reaction is often manifested in denial of the disability or anger directed toward medical and nursing staff. When the person can no longer avoid the reality of the situation, denial may be replaced by regression and depression. The person may make no attempt to do even what he is capable of, and may be so depressed as to contemplate suicide. This is an extremely trying time for both the patient-client and the professionals trying to help him. He feels that life is not worth living, and rebuffs any attempts to help. Health professionals support their self-images by being helpful, and these rebuffs make them feel helpless. Helplessness may turn to anger, if the professional does not recognize and accept the patient-client's depression as a common, and perhaps necessary, stage of psychosocial recovery. Eventually, most patient-clients find some meaning in their new lives and beings to work toward making the most of their abilities. Some "get stuck" in one of the earlier stages of psychological recovery and need more intensive help from a psychiatrist, psychiatric nurse therapist, or psychiatric social worker. This is more often true in persons whose

psychosocial coping was tenuous before their disability occurred.

The work of resolving the loss of a person takes a year or more (Lindemann, 1944; Engel, 1964); similarly, the mourning of the lost self may take this long. This psychological work involves as much effort as physical labor. Consequently, people involved in the rehabilitation process need to be sensitive to signs that the patient-client is being "overworked." He may not be able to handle a vigorous program of physical rehabilitation measures and his "grief work" at the same time. Or he may be able to avoid thinking of his plight during the day while he is busy with occupational therapy, physical therapy, and other appointments, only to have his thoughts overwhelm him once evening comes and this activity ceases. This is a time when a nurse can be of real help by simply listening, letting him cry, or encouraging whatever releases tension. The rehabilitation unit is "home" for a time, and the nurse is the only member of the team who is home with the patient-client. Consequently, the nurse has one of the best opportunities to help the person with his grief work.

George Perrine (1971) has written poignantly of his personal experiences during the rehabilitation process. He describes the changes in his assessment of himself and his abilities in three periods: (1) protest, (2) despair, and (3) detachment. After these periods he felt he had worked through his grief and felt "good" about himself. He felt that nurses and other professionals·could have helped him during each stage by listening to his protests, being "compassionate waiters" until he was ready for help, being honest but supportive when he asked questions about his future, and helping him understand the grieving process which he was experiencing. The ways in which nurses can help a person grieve are discussed in Part 3, Chapter 9, and will not be repeated here.

Grief work may well extend beyond institutionalization; in fact, the necessity of coping with the attitudes of people "on the outside" may precipitate another period of mourning. The community nurse (in the home, school, or job) may help the patient-client at this point. This nurse's role is primarily one of consultation to both patient-client and his family. Presumably, the person and his family have learned physical measures to prevent deformity and preserve abilities. Therefore, the nurse in the community helps them adapt these measures to the home or work. For example, the nurse may show a woman's husband how to fix a safe shower stool for his partially paralyzed wife; he may ask the patient-client to demonstrate the exercise which he has been taught; or he may help parents give moral support to their child when schoolmates taunt her about her braces.

Psychosocially, this nurse may be an important help to the patient-client in the final stages of his grief work. He may help the person vent his feelings and cope with his anxiety and anger over the stares of friends or strangers. He may help him focus on his accomplishments at work, rather than on his deformity. Society tends to regard a physical handicap as undesirably deviant or inferior, with the implication that the whole person is inferior and must be hidden away (Wright, 1960; Friedson, 1965). If the disabled person accepts this judgment, he will try to hide himself physically or psychologically. One of the tasks of rehabilitation is to accept one's disability and focus on what one *can* do, rather than on what one *cannot* do. The achievement of this goal is essentially the patient-client's job, but the nurse who works with him along the way can help him accept himself as he is.

Summary of Common Problems, with Approaches, in Prevention of Disuse and Misuse Phenomena

Problem	Approach
Muscular atrophy	Isometric/isotonic exercise (see precautions)
Contractures	Range-of-motion exercise
	Position
Osteoporosis—negative calcium balance	Isometric/isotonic exercise
Peripheral nerve ischemia	Position
Sensory restriction	Environmental structure—variety, social contact, exercise, social mobility
Hypostatic pneumonia/ atelectasis	Deep breathing
	Position change, posture
	Exercise
Postural hypotension	Position change (relative to gravity)
	Elastic stockings
Increased work of heart	Avoid prolonged supine position
Valsalva maneuver	Avoid straining while moving or defecating
	Exhale through mouth during bed exercises
Dependent edema	Elevate limb
	Avoid compression of veins
	Elastic stockings
	Exercise (muscle pump action)
Thromboembolism	Elevate limb
	Avoid compression of veins
	Elastic stockings
	Exercise (muscle pump action)
	Anticoagulants (medical prophylaxis)
Negative nitrogen balance	Encourage protein foods (cannot be prevented by this)
	Hyperalimentation (medical management)

Anorexia	Frequent small feedings
	Variety food from home, if possible
	Attractive eating place
Constipation	Privacy
	Roughage, adequate fluids
	Upright position for defecation
	Laxatives
Urinary retention	Maintain as close to normal voiding position as possible
	Privacy
Renal stones	High fluid intake
	Acid-ash foods
	Upright trunk position whenever possible
	Muscular exercise (to decrease calcium mobilization secondary to bone resorption)
Pressure sores	Relieve and vary pressure on any part, particularly bony prominences
	Turn; use positions with large body surface
	Air-cell mattress, water bed, polyurethane foam, synthetic-fat mattresses

REFERENCES

Books

Browse, Norman, "The Physiology and Pathology of Bedrest," Charles C. Thomas, Publisher, Springfield, Ill., 1965.

Freedman, S. J., H. U. Greenebaum, and M. Greenblatt, Perceptual and Cognitive Changes in Sensory Deprivation, in P. Solomon et al. (eds.), "Sensory Deprivation," Harvard University Press, Cambridge, Mass., 1961, pp. 59-71.

Friedson, Eliot, Disability as Social Deviance, in Marvin Susman (ed.), "Sociology and Rehabilitation," American Sociological Society and Vocational Rehabilitation Administration, U.S. Department of Health, Education, and Welfare, 1965, pp. 71-99.

Hume, M., S. Sevitt, and D. P. Thomas, "Venous Thrombosis and Pulmonary Embolism," Harvard University Press, Cambridge, Mass., 1970.

Krusen, F. H., F. J. Kottke, and P. M. Ellwood, "Handbook of Physical Medicine and Rehabilitation," 2d ed., W. B. Saunders Company, Philadelphia, 1971.

Schwartz, Doris, Barbara Henley, and Leonard Zeitz, "The Elderly Ambulatory Patient," The Macmillan Company, New York, 1964, p. 102.

Wright, Beatrice, "Physical Disability—A Psychological Approach," Harper & Row, Publishers, Inc., New York, 1960, p. 345.

Periodicals

Akeson, W. H., D. Amick, D. LaViolette, and D. Secrist: Connective Tissue Response to Immobility: An Accelerated Aging Response? *Experimental Gerontology,* **3**:289-301 (1968).

Bartels, R. L., E. L. Fox, R. W. Bowers, and E. P. Hiatt: Effects of Isometric Work on Heart Rate, Blood Pressure, and Net Oxygen Cost, *The Research Quarterly,* **39**:437-442 (1968).

Bauman, Barbara: Diversities in Conceptions of Health and Physical Fitness, *Journal of Health and Human Behavior,* **2**:39-46 (1961).

Birkhead, N. C., G. J. Haupt, R. N. Meyers, and J. W. Daly: Circulatory and Metabolic Effects of Prolonged Bedrest in Healthy Subjects, *Federation Proceedings,* **22**:520 (1963).

Blake, Florence: Immobilized Youth: A Rationale for Supportive Nursing Intervention, *American Journal of Nursing,* **69**:2364-2369 (1969).

Carnevali, Doris, and Susan Brueckner: Immobilization: Reassessment of a Concept, *American Journal of Nursing,* **70**:1502-1507 (1970).

Crate, Marjorie: Nursing Functions in Adaptation to Chronic Illness, *American Journal of Nursing*, **65**:72–76 (1965).

Deitrick, John, G. D. Whedon, and G. Schorr: Effects of Immobilization upon Various Metabolic and Physiologic Functions of Normal Men, *American Journal of Medicine*, **4**:3–36 (1948).

Engel, George: Grief and Grieving, *American Journal of Nursing*, **64**:93–98 (1964); also in M. Meyers (ed.), "Nursing Fundamentals," Wm. C. Brown Company Publishers, Dubuque, Iowa, pp. 88–100.

Heaney, Robert: Radiocalcium Metabolism in Disuse Osteoporosis in Man, *American Journal of Medicine*, **33**:188–200 (1962).

Heron, Woodburn: The Pathology of Boredom, *Scientific American*, **196**:52–56 (January, 1957).

Jackson, C. W., J. C. Polland, and E. W. Kansky: The Application of Findings from Experimental Sensory Deprivation to Cases of Clinical Sensory Deprivation, *American Journal of the Medical Sciences*, **243**:558–563 (1962).

Kelly, M.: Exercises for Bedfast Patients, *American Journal of Nursing*, **66**:2209–2213 (1966).

Kottke, F. J.: The Effects of Limitation of Activity upon the Human Body, *Journal of The American Medical Association*, **196**:117–122 (June 6, 1966).

——— and R. B. Blanchard: Bedrest Begets Bedrest, *Nursing Forum*, **3**(3):56–73 (1964).

Lindemann, Erich: Symptomatology and Management of Acute Grief, *American Journal of Psychiatry*, **101**:141 (1944).

Little, K.: Bone Resorption and Osteoporosis, *The Lancet*, **2**:752–756 (Oct. 12, 1963).

Lynch, T., et al.: Metabolic Effects of Prolonged Bedrest: Their Modification by Simulated Altitude, *Aerospace Medicine*, **38**:10–20 (1967).

McLachlin, Angus, J. A. McLachlin, T. A. Jory, and E. G. Rawling: Venous Stasis in the Lower Extremities, *Annals of Surgery*, **152**:678–685 (1960).

Mack, Pauline, and Paul LaChance: Effects of Recumbency and Space Flight on Bone Density, *American Journal of Clinical Nutrition*, **20**:1194–1205 (1967).

Meyer, Ovid: Treatment with Anticoagulants, *Cardiovascular Nursing*, **4**:11–15 (1968).

Moody, Linda, V. Barron, and G. Monk: Moving the Past into the Present, *American Journal of Nursing*, **70**:2353–2356 (1970).

Morgan, Alfred, R. M. Filler, and F. D. Moore: Surgical Nutrition, *Medical Clinics of North America*, **54**:1367–1381 (1970).

Nutter, Donald O., Robert C. Schlant, and J. Willis Hurst: Isometric Exercise and the Cardiovascular System, *Modern Concepts of Cardiovascular Disease*, **41**:11–15 (1972).

Peaston, M. J. T.: Modification of the Early Metabolic Response to Trauma by Adaptive Calorie-Nitrogen Feeding, *British Journal of Medical Practice*, **23**:11–14 (1969).

Perrine, George: Needs Met and Unmet, *American Journal of Nursing*, **71**:2128–2133 (1971).

Reisen, A. H.: Arrested Vision, *Scientific American*, **183**:16–19 (1950).

Ryback, Ralph, Oliver F. Lewis, and Charles S. Lessard: Psychobiologic Effects of Prolonged Bedrest (Weightless) in Young, Healthy Volunteers (Study II), *Aerospace Medicine*, **42**:529–535 (1971).

Salzman, E. W., W. H. Harris, and R. W. DeSanctis: Anticoagulation for Prevention of Thromboembolism Following Fracture of the Hip, *New England Journal of Medicine*, **275**:122ff. (1966).

Spencer, W. A., C. Vallbona, and R. E. Carter, Jr.: Physiologic Concepts of Immobilization, *Journal of Physical Medicine and Rehabilitation*, **46**:89–100 (1965).

Taylor, H. L., A. Henschel, J. Brozek, and A. Keys: Effects of Bedrest on Cardiovascular Function and Work Performance, *Journal of Applied Physiology*, **11**:223–239 (1949).

Vogt, F. G., L. S. Meharg, and P. B. Mack: Use of a Digital Computer in the Measurement of Roentgenographic Bone Density, *American Journal of Roentgenography, Radiotherapy, and Nuclear Medicine*, **185**:870–876 (1969).

Wright, A. P.: Effect of Post-operative Bedrest and Early Ambulation on the rate of Venous Blood Flow, *Lancet*, **1**:22 (1951).

Zubek, John, and L. Wilgosh: Prolonged Immobilization of the Body: Changes in Performance and in the Electroencephalogram, *Science*, **143**:306–308 (1963).

———, L. Bayer, S. Mitstein, and J. Shepard: Behavioral and Physiological Changes during Prolonged Immobilization Plus Perceptual Deprivation, *Journal of Abnormal Psychology*, **74**:230–236 (1969).

ADDITIONAL READINGS

Christopherson, Victor: Role Modifications of the Disabled Male, *American Journal of Nursing*, **68**:290–293 (1968).

Madden, Barbara, and John Affeldt: To Prevent Helplessness and Deformity, *American Journal of Nursing*, **62**:59–61 (1962); also in M. Meyers (ed.), "Nursing Fundamentals," Wm. C. Brown Company Publishers, Dubuque, Iowa, 1967.

Rehabilitative Aspects of Nursing, Part I: Physical Therapeutic Nursing Measures—Units 1 and 2, National League for Nursing, Research and Studies Service, New York, 1966, 1967. (A programmed instruction series.)

Rusk, Howard: Rehabilitation Belongs in the General Hospital, *American Journal of Nursing*, **62**:62–63 (1962); also in M. Meyer (ed.), "Nursing Fundamentals," Wm. C. Brown Company Publishers, Dubuque, Iowa, 1967, pp. 274–277.

Chapter 13

Nutritional Status

Pamela Mitchell

"Tell me what you eat, and I shall tell you what you are," said the gourmet Brillat-Savarin. His statement is true in many more ways than he may have realized. Most basically, what we eat is physically converted to what we are—our cells.

Beyond this, what we eat defines and is defined by nearly every aspect of our social, psychological, and spiritual being. By and large, we can tell a man's culture, socioeconomic position, and often religion by examining his food habits. In

Data to Be Assessed

Dietary habits	Factors in food ingestion
Usual eating habits	State of teeth, mouth, consciousness
Appetite	Swallowing ability
Changes related to health problem	Gastrointestinal motility
Person responsible for food preparation at home	Digestion
Adequacy of diet	Nausea, vomiting
Height, weight; gain-loss pattern	Eructation
General appearance	Medication affecting
Attitudes toward eating	Non-oral means of feeding
Importance of food	Parenteral fluids' hyperalimentation
Religious restrictions	Naso-gastric tube, gastrostomy
Symbolic meaning	

all cultures, eating and food are integral parts of human social and emotional relationships from birth onward. Whether a man is a primitive hunter, who spends his life finding enough food just to keep alive, or a member of a wealthy industrial society, food and eating are central to his social and physical existence.

Nutritional status reflects the adequacy or inadequacy of a person's diet in supplying nutrients essential to life and well-being. Adequate nutrition requires a balance between body needs and available nutrients, and is associated with a subjective feeling of well-being and health. Extremes of under- and oversupply of food can lead to illness and death, as shown in Fig. 13-1. The ultimate measure of nutritional status is the

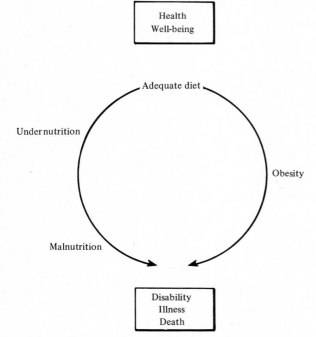

Figure 13-1 Relation of nutritional status to health. Both under- and oversupply of food can lead to illness and death. Malnutrition can directly cause debilitation and death. Overeating to the point of obesity can contribute to disability in any number of diseases, and appears to be associated with the manifestation of some diseases, such as diabetes and coronary artery disease.

ability of the foods eaten to meet the body's need for nutrients—calories, carbohydrates, fats, proteins, vitamins, and minerals. However, many factors influence the foods we eat. Such factors include the availability of food, cost, attitudes toward food, cultural, social, and religious prescriptions, and physical states altering ability to eat.

Nutrition is essentially a scientific concept, implying knowledge of cellular metabolism, quality of diets, and the effects of nutrition in health and disease. The average layman has a rudimentary knowledge of nutrition; his concept is food and eating. Some foods are "good for you"; vitamins come in a bottle. Even when the layman has some knowledge of nutritional food concepts, taste and food habits will ultimately determine his choice of foods. A nurse who is to help people with nutritional problems must combine his scientific knowledge of nutrition with knowledge of his patient-client's basis for food choice. In addition, he must understand the forces which inhibit or promote change of food habits.

The purpose of this chapter is to help the nurse to recognize the central nature of food to our physical, social, and cultural being; to analyze the factors which affect the choice of foods we eat; to determine when a nutritional problem exists; and to use knowledge of food habits to define nursing help with these problems. Specific nutritional needs, metabolism of nutrients, and specific nutritional disorders and attendant diet therapy are not discussed in this chapter. Information related to these topics is more appropriately found in formal nutrition courses and in textbooks of nutrition. The supplementary readings at the end of this chapter include such references.

FOOD AND NUTRITION

We often speak of eating foods which provide adequate nutrition; yet the concept of "adequate" nutrition is not quite so simple as it may seem. We must ask, "Adequate for what?" Medical dictionaries define an adequate diet as one which meets the body's needs for normal growth and health. Herein lies the difficulty in defining adequate nutrition. Norms, or definitions of what is normal, vary from culture to culture and within a culture. In addition, individual requirements for nutrients vary according to activity, age, and growth needs. Much of the variation in defining norms of adequate nutrition among cultures stems from differences in health goals. These differences in goals arise partly from differences in available resources. For example, the recommended daily protein intake in India is lower than that recommended in the United States for a person doing the same amount of work (*Recommended Dietary Allowances*, 1968). This is not because the Indian needs fewer amino acids, but because there is insufficient protein supply available in India for authorities to recommend the large margin over minimal requirements which is feasible in the United States. A person in an underdeveloped country who has never known a plentiful food supply may consider himself adequately fed on a diet which we might consider barely sufficient to keep one alive. Similarly, some people may consider their diet adequate because they are not hungry. A nutritionist, however, may find their diet inadequate in essential nutrients. The layman tends to define adequate nutrition in terms of satiation (lack of hunger) and his standards of well-being; the professional defines it in terms of consumed nutrients, body needs, and objective measures of health, as health is defined by his culture.

The nurse must recognize these cultural and individual differences in defining adequate nutrition for two reasons. First, more and more nurses eventually participate in health programs involving other cultures. If upgrading nutrition is a goal in these programs, participating professionals must be aware that their own concept of adequate nutrition may be far in excess of the resources or goals of the people with whom they work. The Food and Agriculture Organization (FAO) of the United Nations World Health Organization (WHO) has compiled resources to help health professionals work with the available foods and concepts of nutrition of several cultures around the world.[1]

The second reason for recognizing differing concepts of adequate nutrition is more immediately applicable to the beginning practitioner. In order to help people change their eating habits and nutritional status, the health worker must recognize that his definition of adequate nutrition may or may not be the same as that of his clients. In the United States the professional's definition of optimum health and nutritional status is most apt to coincide with the definition of upper-middle- and middle-class people, and least apt to match that of lower-class, less-educated citizens. Therefore, the nurse can expect to find a poor "fit" of nutritional concepts when working with people from these groups, and must ascertain where and how their concepts differ. Until nurse and client find a common ground, the motivation of the client to change his food habits may be low.

Standards of Adequate Nutrition in the United States

Recommended Dietary Allowances   In 1940, the National Research Council of the National Academy of Sciences appointed a Food and Nutrition Board to review available research and establish human requirements for specific nutrients. They formulated a set of recommended dietary allowances (RDA), which were first published in 1943. These recommendations have been revised every few years as more research data have become available. Each revision is published by the National Research

---

[1] A table with comparative standards of the United States and several other countries is published in the *Recommended Dietary Allowances* (see bibliography). Other resources are available from the Food and Agriculture Organization, WHO, Rome, Italy.

Council with documentation of the research supporting the recommendations. Tables of the recommendations are available in all nutrition textbooks and in journals of nutrition, dietetics, and public health. The recommended dietary allowances are different from the minimum daily requirements (MDR) published by the Federal Food and Drug Administration (FDA). The MDR are believed to be the minimum required to prevent deficiency symptoms. The recommended levels are lower than those of the RDA, which provide a wide margin above minimum requirements. Commercial food processers who provide nutrient analysis of their products usually refer to the MDR figures.

The National Research Council definition of adequate nutrition reflects the prevalent professional philosophy of health in the United States. The Council's recommended dietary allowances provide a wide margin above minimal physiologic needs sufficient to "allow for greatest dividends in health and disease prevention."[2] Thus good nutrition is defined in terms of realization of potentials, not merely in terms of avoiding illness secondary to deficient diet. The Board further states that the allowances should "*maintain* good nutrition in practically all *healthy* persons in the United States" (italics mine).[2] Thus these recommendations are not meant to be standards of nutrition for ill or malnourished people. Because the RDA are based on research regarding nutrition of groups of people, they can be only a rough guide in assessing the nutritional status of any particular person. Individual nutritional status depends upon the balance between the nutrients which each person needs and those which he actually eats, absorbs, and utilizes. The RDA nevertheless represent a professional standard in considering optimum nutrition, and they

provide practitioners with a means of communicating among themselves about good nutrition.

The average person cannot easily translate the RDA into terms of what foods he should eat to maintain health. Therefore, nutritionists have prepared guides such as the Daily Food Guide (U. S. Department of Agriculture) to help people choose from a variety of foods. This is commonly referred to as the "basic four." Figure 13-2 shows these basic food groups. The examples of foods in each group are based on the eating patterns of the majority of Americans. However, other ethnic or regional foods can supply adequate nutrition. Examples used in the basic four groups should be modified when a nurse is working with people whose ethnic foods differ from those shown.

Recommended Dietary Allowances provide only one guide in assessing the nutritional status of a group or of individuals. History of food intake may be compared with the RDA to see if there are patterns of over- or underconsumption. However, this evidence in itself says little about the true status of the group or individual. To give a complete picture, it must be combined with clinical observation (e.g., signs of nutritional deficiency disease), the person's feeling of health or well-being, and laboratory analysis of excreted metabolic by-products. The biochemical studies are used primarily in surveys of the nutrition of groups, or by physicians who suspect that a disease may have been caused by a nutritional deficiency.

The terms commonly used in connection with deviation from good nutritional status are malnutrition, undernutrition, and overnutrition.

Malnutrition Malnutrition occurs when the diet is inadequate in quality (essential nutrients) and often in quantity (calories) as well. Overt malnutrition manifests itself by deficiency disease; disorders caused by deficiency states are rickets (vitamin D), scurvy (vitamin C), pellagra (niacin), and the protein-calorie deficiencies—

[2] "Recommended Dietary Allowances," 7th rev. ed., Report of the Food and Nutrition Board, National Research Council, National Academy of Sciences Publication 1694, Washington, D.C., 1968.

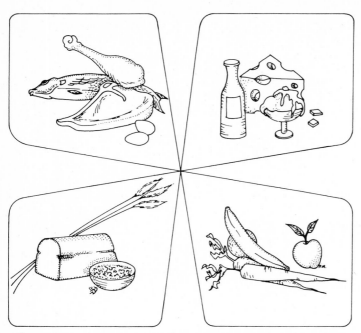

Figure 13-2 The "basic four" food groups. The suggested number of servings from each of these groups will provide the recommended dietary allowances. The *meat group* consists of meat, poultry, fish, and eggs. Two or more 2- to 3-oz servings daily are recommended. The *milk group* is composed of milk and dairy products (cheese, yogurt, ice cream). Adults should have two glasses or more daily, children two to three glasses. Four or more daily servings are recommended in the *bread and cereal group*. Enriched or whole-grain items should be used. Four or more daily servings are also recommended for the *fruit and vegetable group*. A source of vitamin C should be served daily (citrus fruit or juice, tomatoes); a dark-green or deep-yellow vegetable should be included three to four times a week. *(Recommendations from the Institute of Home Economics, U.S. Department of Agriculture.)*

kwashiorkor and marasmus. Marginal malnutrition exists when laboratory analysis of nutrient breakdown products in blood and excretions show deficiencies but signs of overt deficiency disease are not present. People who are marginally malnourished seem to be more susceptible to infectious disease and less productive than those who are adequately nourished (Eichenwald and Fry, 1969; Spengler, 1968).

Undernutrition Spengler differentiates undernutrition from malnutrition, describing undernutrition as a deficiency in quantity (calories) and malnutrition as a deficiency in quality (spe-

cific nutrients). Thus, a person who is undernourished might not show signs of deficiency disease but would have less energy for his daily work. Large numbers of people in nonindustrialized and developing countries are undernourished and malnourished. The National Nutrition Survey is revealing that the extent of undernutrition and outright malnutrition in the United States is greater than many people would like to think (Schaefer, 1969).

Overnutrition Overnutrition is a national problem in relatively wealthy, industrialized countries such as the United States and in some countries where carbohydrate forms a large part of the diet. We use the term to mean an excess of calories, not of essential nutrients. Many people who are overnourished, e.g., overweight or obese, actually may be deficient in some basic nutrients. The problem of obesity is discussed later in the chapter.

The Relationship of Nutrition to Health

Nearly every culture and civilization throughout history has had specific ideas about the relationship of food to general and spiritual well-being. Gout was long thought to be caused by gluttonous eating and drinking. Special herbs or foods are thought to be curative in nearly all cultures. Several religions prescribe vegetarian food habits for their members, believing that killing for food is wrong and that blood and flesh contribute to ungovernable passions in people. Spanish-Americans in the Southwestern United States believe that "hot" and "cold" foods, as defined by inherent quality rather than by temperature, must be kept in balance to keep man's temperament in harmony. Similar beliefs were held by ancient medical practitioners, who felt that a balanced diet kept the internal humors in proper balance.

The science of nutrition is considerably younger than many of these beliefs about the relationship of food to well-being. Scientists from many disciplines, interested in how the foods we eat affect our health and well-being, have documented and explained a number of relationships between health and food. Many of the essential nutrients have been isolated and identified, and the mechanisms of their action in the body are at least partially understood. Scientific study is "proving" what the many folk and primitive beliefs about food have long indicated: that poor diet can cause disease, impair growth, impair mental development, affect temperament, and reduce productivity. In short, what we eat affects every aspect of our well-being.

Nutrition and Disease   Prolonged lack of specific nutrients can cause nutritional deficiency diseases such as scurvy and rickets, as well as more general conditions such as the disorders of peripheral nerve function related to vitamin deficiency. Captain Cook was able to prevent scurvy in 1768 by adding sauerkraut and greens to his sailors' soup (Villiers, 1971). However, understanding of vitamin C and its role in preventing scurvy was not attained until this century.

Not only does poor nutrition cause actual disease, but it contributes to a person's susceptibility to nonnutritional disease and seems to impede recovery. We know that calories, proteins, and vitamins are essential for tissue building and repair, and that requirements for them are often increased during physiologic stress. People who are malnourished or chronically undernourished seem more likely than the well-nourished to develop infectious disease. Protein deficiency in particular seems to lead to a decreased inflammatory response to infection and decreased ability of the cells to resist bacterial and viral invasion (Eichenwald and Fry, 1969).

Nutrition and Growth   Nutritional status also affects physical and mental growth. The increasing average stature of people in the United States is often attributed to increasingly better nutrition during the past two centuries. Animals which are malnourished during early life and then fed adequately tend to grow rapidly during the period of adequate nutrition, but they never catch up with their litter mates who were fed well all the time. This same pattern has been documented in malnourished children.

The effects of nutrition on mental development are not so well documented. Investigators have long noted the apathy, irritability, and general dullness of malnourished children. However, it is difficult to separate the effects of nutrition from the general environment of poverty and disease which usually accompanies malnutrition. Both disease and a chronically impoverished environment may contribute to slow mental development.

Eichenwald and Fry review a number of recent investigations which strongly suggest that malnutrition itself is an important factor in retarded mental growth. The most rapid neural growth occurs during the early part of life, and animals which have been fed diets inadequate in calories and protein during this period have smaller, less functional brains at maturity. If the underfeeding occurs during a critical period of brain growth, subsequent adequate nutrition does not reverse the slow growth. If a restriction occurs during cell multiplication, maturation is slowed. If the deprivation occurs during the increase in cell size, growth is slowed. In experimental animals, protein deprivation in early life reduced the capacity to learn. Rats born of malnourished mothers also had decreased learning ability. The implications of this research for human malnutrition are obvious, even though we cannot separate the effects of malnutrition from social and emotional factors in intellectual performance in human beings.

Nutrition and Behavior   The link between the level of nutrition and such factors as temperament and productivity is not clear-cut. However, there is considerable evidence that a poor diet is a factor in the listlessness and decreased productivity of undernourished and malnourished people. Apathy is a characteristic sign of kwashiorkor, one of the protein-calorie deficiency states (Cravioto, 1966). This apathy could be due to a number of social and environmental factors as well. However, the dramatic increase in alertness and vitality of the child with this disorder when he is adequately nourished suggests a rather direct link between the state of his nutrition and his behavior.

Anemia (a decrease in the number of red blood cells) also causes listlessness, as well as fatigue and inability to function optimally. Al-though many circumstances other than poor nutrition cause anemia, an iron-deficient diet is one of the major causative factors. Preliminary results from the National Nutrition Survey showed that 15 percent of the population sampled (predominately low-income people) were anemic according to laboratory analysis. Thirty percent of the surveyed children from birth to five years of age had inadequate hemoglobin levels. Although infestation with parasites (hookworm) and genetically abnormal red blood cells (sickle-cell trait) also contribute to this incidence of anemia, the investigators believe that iron-deficient diet is the major factor (Schaefer, 1969).

Inadequate caloric intake is another factor in decreased productivity or decreased physical performance. The undernourished person simply has not enough fuel available for the energy output necessary for optimum performance.

This impaired capacity is reflected in the sluggish performance of the school child who routinely goes to school without breakfast and carries an inadequate lunch, or in the diminished productivity of the adult worker, here or abroad. If undernutrition is coupled with malnutrition, even more severe reduction in potential occurs. Although people of any socioeconomic level may be malnourished through ignorance of what constitutes a good diet, malnutrition is most commonly associated with poverty. The effects of poor nutrition on learning and productivity, in turn, tend to hinder people in these situations from improving their lot. The inadequate diet appears to have severe effects on the development and productivity of many children and adults in the United States. Doctor Schaefer, in testifying before the Senate Select Committee on Nutrition and Human Needs in January 1969, stated that in the first subsample of the National Nutrition Survey:

. . . we found every kind of malnutrition that any of us has seen in similar studies in Central America,

Africa, and Asia. It is just as prevalent in these areas [surveyed in the United States] as it is in many of the remote countries.[3]

The surveyors found not only biochemical evidence of deficiency but also overt signs in many people of rickets, scurvy, goiter, and vitamin A deficiency. Children with kwashiorkor and marasmus (the severe protein-calorie deficiencies of infancy and early childhood) were found, thus refuting the notion that these conditions are seen only in very poor, underdeveloped countries. The investigators themselves had not expected to find these conditions in the United States.

FACTORS AFFECTING NUTRITIONAL STATUS

Several factors affect a person's nutritional status, including the body's requirements for nutrients and energy, the actual intake of foods and fluids, and the efficiency of the mechanisms for absorption, storage, utilization, and excretion of nutrients. We will consider only the first two factors in this chapter. Textbooks of nutrition, advanced nursing, and medicine should be consulted for information regarding problems related to alterations of absorption, storage, and excretion.

Nutritional Requirements

Requirements for calories (available energy) vary with growth, needs, amount of activity, and unusual metabolic needs (e.g., needs for tissue repair after surgery). Thus, the rapidly growing infant needs more calories per pound than the adult. The pregnant woman needs more calories, to support the growth of the baby, than the nonpregnant woman of the same age and activity. The manual laborer needs more calories than the sedentary executive.

Requirements for the essential nutrients increase steadily during the growing years of childhood and then remain steady during adult-

[3] A. E. Schaefer, Are We Well Fed? *Nutrition Today*, 4:7 (1969).

hood when growth is attained. Requirements for calories and other nutrients increase during pregnancy and lactation (nursing the baby) to provide for the growth needs of the fetus and baby. Traumatic stress, such as surgery, and illness also increase requirements for nutrients to compensate for the increased metabolic rate and needs for tissue healing.

Intake of Food—Eating

Nutritional imbalance may occur when the calories and other nutrients eaten in food exceed or fall below the requirements of the body. People particularly at risk of nutritional imbalance are infants, children, adolescents, pregnant women, and the aged. Adolescents' diets may be inadequate in both quality and quantity to meet their increased growth needs. Lowered income, loss of health, or lowered living standards may decrease the quality of the diet in the aged. In addition, many older people continue to eat the quantity of food which they ate in their younger years. Since their caloric requirements are usually decreased, this may result in overweight and obesity. The poor of any age group are also at risk, for their diet is apt to be deficient in essential nutrients at any age, and in both calories and other nutrients during the periods of increased growth.

Very few people eat because they are consciously aware of specific body requirements. They eat because they are hungry, because it is time to eat, because they are at a party, because they are lonely, or because there is nothing else to do. Although there are physiological, psychosocial, and physical factors which determine what and when we eat, the social and psychological aspects of eating will ultimately determine what a person eats and what changes he will make in his dietary habits. Before examining the psychosocial and physical factors, we must look at the physiological determinants of eating behavior.

Physiological Factors:
The Regulation of Food Intake

One reason why we eat is that we are hungry, but what makes us feel hungry, what tells our body that it needs more food or drink? The fact that animals and man, for the most part, maintain weight and eat a relatively balanced diet when the food supply is adequate point to a homeostatic mechanism regulating food intake. In both man and experimental animals, aberrations of intake—i.e., eating more or less than the body requires—may occur, both because of changes in the physiological mechanisms and because of conditioning or selective reinforcement of certain eating behavior. In man, this conditioning is the result of complex social, cultural, and emotional events associated with eating. In animals, it is usually due to deliberate laboratory manipulation. The conditioned aspect of eating will be discussed later in this chapter.

Most of the evidence about the nature of physiologic regulation comes from studies with rats and other laboratory animals. Therefore we must use caution in applying the findings to human beings. However, there are corollary types of eating behavior in human beings who have disease in certain areas of the brain believed to regulate eating, or who have had surgery in such areas.

The brain is the ultimate regulator of eating, although the alimentary canal, the peripheral nervous system, and the bloodstream all appear to play a part in regulating food intake. Research with rats and other animals has demonstrated that certain areas of the midbrain and forebrain are critical in initiating and terminating eating. Areas in the hypothalamus have been termed feeding, satiety, and drinking "centers." However, these so-called centers are only one part of a regulatory network comprising an anatomic circuit, which ascends toward and descends from the cerebral cortex (Morgane and Jacobs, 1969). Because the most dramatic aberrations in eating

behavior occur when discrete areas in the hypothalamus are stimulated or destroyed, there are many references in the literature to the hypothalamic "center."

Morgane and Jacobs review current thinking about the major pathways to the regulatory circuits in the brain. These connections include a metabolic pathway via the metabolites in the bloodstream which circulate to the brain, and a sensory pathway via the peripheral and central nervous systems. The relationship of these mechanisms is diagrammed in Fig. 13-3.

Metabolic Pathway   The various nutrients ingested are broken down into glucose, amino acids, fatty acids, and various other metabolites. There are apparently receptors in the brain specific for one or more of these chemicals. When circulatory levels decline below a set point these chemoreceptors somehow initiate the cycle which results in a search for food and eating. When the circulating metabolites rise to a certain level, the "stat" turns off, so to speak, and eating ceases.

The metabolic pathway is fairly slow, however, for food must be absorbed and broken into its component nutrients before metabolites enter the circulation. A more immediate feedback system appears to be mediated via the peripheral nervous system and cortical neural pathways. The cortical pathways (from the "thinking" portion of the brain) mediate the conditioned responses. These conditioned influences on eating will be considered later in the chapter.

Sensory Pathways   There appears to be an immediate feedback system regarding hunger and satiety via stretch receptors and chemoreceptors in the stomach, liver, and intestines. Distension of the stomach creates the sensation of satiety or fullness, thus providing an immediate feedback regarding the quantity of food ingested. In addition, specific nutrients seem to stimulate receptors in the stomach, and intes-

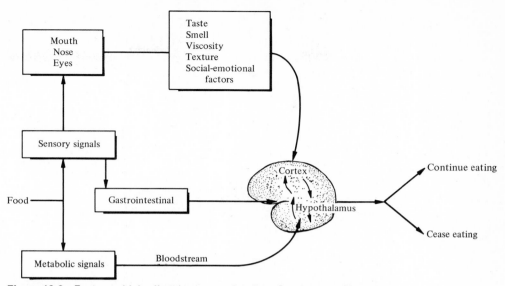

Figure 13-3 Factors which affect hunger and satiety. See text for discussion.

tines, which relay this immediate information about quality of food to the central nervous system. The connections of this pathway with the regulatory areas in the central nervous system are not understood as yet. Rats will tend to "eat for calories"; once they have established a base-line caloric intake, they will continue to eat the same number of calories regardless of whether these calories are in concentrated form or whether cellulose has been added to the diet to increase bulk but add no calories. When cellulose is added, the rats simply eat more food until they have consumed their usual number of calories. Presumably there is some immediate feedback system which enables them to ignore the signals from the stretch receptors and eat until caloric intake is normal.

This immediate feedback regarding caloric content does not appear to operate so accurately in human beings, however. Walike et al. (1969) had volunteers rapidly ingest a liquid formula a short time before a regularly scheduled "meal" of the same formula. Although these people could not see the amount of formula taken, they had all established a constant intake over several days. Rapid "preloading" with formula before the meal caused all the subjects to decrease their normal amount of formula at the meal. However, the decrease was not sufficient to compensate for the extra calories in the preload.

Taste, smell, viscosity, and texture of food generate sensory signals in the mouth and nose which influence eating in human beings. Peripheral nerves relay this sensory information to the brain, where it is interpreted by the cortex on the basis of previous experiences with food. Somehow this information is relayed through the hunger/satiety network and influences the regulation of intake. Input from these sensory pathways may influence the regulatory circuit to "instruct" the cortex to continue or cease eating even though sufficient nutrients have been consumed or hunger is still present. For example, a person may eat a piece of chocolate cake even though he is quite full. Conversely, he may be quite hungry but will not eat a strange food with an unpleasant texture.

The anatomical and physiological relationships between cortical and midbrain influences in the regulation of eating are not at all clear.

However, it is evident that both animals and people develop preferences for certain tastes and are influenced by textures, smells, and conditioned experiences with foods.

Psychosocial Factors—Food Habits

The food habits of men are as much a product of selective reinforcement or conditioning as those of experimentally conditioned laboratory animals. However, man learns his food habits in a much more complex social, cultural, and emotional environment. Animals in the wild generally select a diet adequate in nutrients for that species. They are rarely obese or undernourished, except in illness or time of food scarcity.

Similarly, primitive man was apparently able to select from natural foods a diet sufficient for survival of the species. Long before nutrition was a science, folk practitioners knew which kinds of foods and herbs prevented deficiency diseases. Central American Indians used limestone and lime water in preparing tortillas; American Indians used rose hips as food. These provide calcium and vitamin C, respectively. Even the alcoholic drinks of some cultures (pulque in Mexico and kaffir beer in South Africa) are important sources of necessary vitamins (Le Gros Clark, 1968).

However, as society became more civilized and complex, each person was more dependent on imported food and could rely less upon his appetites and the natural foods about him to supply his nutrient needs. LeGros Clark suggests that once primitive cities began to develop and to depend upon farmers for food, the stage was set for the beginning of ritual and symbolism connected with food. He states:

> Though the origins of food beliefs and prohibitions are obscure, they would usually have occurred where a community was stable in its habitat and reasonably prosperous over a long period of years. The beliefs would have arisen from chance observations, imagined analogies or the conflicting claims that different age groups were able to establish for foods in relatively short supply. For instance, the "elders" of a tribe have often managed to enforce priority rights over such foods. . . . Since the beliefs thus held are normally left unchallenged for many generations, they tend to harden into elements of the total patterns of the dietary habits of a people.[4]

Animals in the laboratory can be taught to prefer an unbalanced or nonnutritive diet. Thus conditioned habits can alter the natural tendency of animals as well as of man to select an adequate diet.

In man, food habits and feelings about food are probably the major determinants of diet. Even when he is starving, taboos or feelings about certain kinds of food may prevent a person from eating. From earliest infancy we learn what foods are and are not considered appropriate for people, what foods different age groups eat, what taste, texture, and viscosity each food "should" have. These notions are a product of social and cultural learning (conditioning). For example, Puerto Rican children from San Juan would not eat the sweetened rice prepared by a United States mainland school cook. The cooks knew "Puerto Ricans like rice" but did not realize that rice to these children was a dish made of short-grain rice and lard, not the sweetened long-grain rice which was served to them (DeZayas, 1962).

Food habits begin in the eating experiences in one's family. These in turn, are affected by the cultural and subcultural groups (regional, ethnic, religious, and socioeconomic) with which the family identifies.

The broadest cultural difference in eating is the distinction between the Western and the cereal diets of the world. The Western diet contains 30 percent or more animal protein, while the cereal diet contains less than 10 percent animal protein (Ohlson, 1969). Large amounts of cereal grains and legumes are used to fulfill caloric and protein needs. The Western diets

---

[4] F. Le Gros Clark, Food Habits as a Practical Nutrition Problem, *World Review of Nutrition and Dietetics,* **9**:56–84 (1968).

vary considerably with ethnic and regional preferences but are more like what we in the United States consider a "good" diet than are the cereal diets. People in the Oriental countries and in industrially undeveloped countries are more apt to be cereal eaters than those in the Western and developed countries. Different cultures use different grains as their staple cereal—rice for the Orientals, maize (corn) for Western Hemisphere Indians and Spanish-speaking people, wheat for India. Either type of diet can provide minimum nutrition provided enough calories are eaten. However, the cereal diet may be deficient in riboflavin and protein, the Western diet lower in iron and thiamine. The typical United States diet is particularly high in meat, fat, and sugar, but tends to be low in the valuable nutrients in cereal carbohydrates (Ohlson, 1969).

Regional and Ethnic Influences Within these broad cultural dietary patterns are regional and ethnic patterns as well. The spaghetti of the Italian-American, the cornbread of the Southern American, and the tortilla of the Mexican-American are foods familiar to us all. Very early in life we learn to associate certain foods and styles of eating with home and family, and later with a social group. These patterns become an integral part of the idea of self. They provide part of the feeling of identity with a regional or ethnic group. The "typical American" meal of meat, potatoes, and vegetable is as ethnic as any of the "foreign" foods we eat.

Religious Influences Religion is another factor within a culture which affects food habits. Feasting and fasting form a large part of any religion. Certain foods are reserved for certain religious observances—hot cross buns are associated with Easter in Anglo-Saxon countries, matzos with Passover. Several religions have laws about daily eating, such as the Orthodox Jewish proscription against pork. Vegetarianism is a part of the Seventh-Day Adventist and Hindu practices.

Socioeconomic Influences Social and economic status is a third factor which affects food habits within a culture. Most directly, income affects how much money can be spent for food. Social factors (the prestige value of food, or ethnic eating patterns) and knowledge of nutrient value will affect how the available money will be spent. Certain kinds of foods have social prestige value. For example, steak is a prestigious cut of meat, hot dogs and stew meat are not. "Soul food" (typical Southern black food) had its origins in the socioeconomics of the Old South. The slaves and tenant farmers ate the scraps—the fatback, chitterlings (hog intestines), and greens, while the landowners ate "high off the hog," with pork chops, roasts, and sweet potatoes.

Low income, lack of education, and poor nutrition often go hand in hand. However, simply raising a person's income, or teaching him about which foods are both cheap and nutritious, will not automatically result in better nutrition. The social status factors in food choices are powerful determinants of food buying. Children, poor or not, who see advertisements for carbonated soft drinks, candy, and sugar-coated cereal on television will want to snack on these empty-calorie prestige items rather than on fruits, vegetables, and cheese. Parents may take money from the food budget for more conspicuous, socially prestigious items such as cars and television.

Symbolic Influences A final factor influencing food habits is the symbolic aspect of food. These symbolic meanings apply not only to the foods themselves but also to the setting and manner of eating. For example, the Thais teach their children to take only a small portion of the protein dish which is served with the rice. This is designed as a lesson in frugality (Burgess and Dean, 1962, p. 83). The stereotype of the Jewish mother who berates her family for lack of love if they do not eat heavily is based on the symbolism of love in the giving and taking of food. Eating certain foods may create fond memories of home and love; consequently, many people eat when lonely and tense. Eating together symbolizes acceptance, friendship, and kinship. Most of our social gatherings include some kind of food or drink.

Specific foods may be symbolic. For example, meat is considered masculine; salads are feminine. Some vegetarians see meat and blood as purveyors of aggression and undesirable passions; others feel that killing for food betrays their reverence for life.

There is symbolism in foods, in eating, and in feeding. Because nurses often engage in feeding people, these symbolic aspects are particularly relevant. Feeding often symbolizes loving; the majority of an infant's waking time is occupied with being fed. Food then becomes associated with the loving acts of his mother. If his mother is unloving, feeding may come to symbolize anxiety or hostility to that child. Being fed frequently symbolizes helplessness and dependency. These symbols are derived from the helpless dependency of the infant. Feeding also symbolizes femininity, since feeding is generally a woman's task. A more detailed discussion of the symbolism of feeding and being fed is given in Reva Rubin's excellent article, "Food and Feeding" (1967).

Influence of Habits on Hunger and Satiety Hunger, satiety, and appetite are terms frequently used in connection with eating. Food habits can affect all three, although hunger and satiety are more physiologically based than appetite. Hunger is the unpleasant physical sensation which compels a person or organism to seek food. Gastric contractions often accompany this

sensation. The brain areas mediating hunger initiate the signal which results in stimulation of the stomach. Lowered blood levels of key nutrients probably form the strongest stimulus to hunger, but certain conditioned stimuli, such as smell, can also stimulate hunger sensations if the organism has been without food long enough. Appetite is the desire for and anticipation of food or specific foods. Appetite may or may not be accompanied by hunger; it is more directly affected by learned cues than hunger is.

Satiety is the sensation accompanying the end of the desire for further food. Circulatory levels of the key nutrients influence the nervous system signals to cease eating; however, the sense of satiety is also dependent upon learned cues. Some people do not feel satiated until they are "stuffed" or until all the food before them is gone; others can be replete with far less intake. Much of this variation reflects early learning about the sensation which accompanies a child's parents' estimations as to whether he has eaten "enough." Small children generally gauge their own needs pretty well if left alone and provided with a variety of foods.

Changing Food Habits

Food habits provide a part of the stabilizing force of a culture and of a person's sense of identity. Because of this, they are of primary importance in determining a person's nutritional intake. Some food customs stabilize and perpetuate nutritionally sound practice. Witness the limestone and lime water used to prepare tortillas in Old Mexico as a source of vitamin C. Other customs or beliefs may deprive a group of important nutrients. A Zulu taboo which prohibited pregnant women from drinking the milk of their own cows or those of kindred tribes prevented these women from getting any milk at all (Cassel, 1957). Because food habits are so much a part of self, attempts to change them in adult life may be highly unsuccessful. Immigrants to a new country may alter all their outwardly visible customs (dress, speech, even religion), but often do not change their food customs unless such customs are highly visible signs of being different (Stoetzel, 1962). People often do not adhere to diets prescribed for medical problems because these diets require them to alter their food habits. The teen-age diabetic may be denied the snack food which "everybody" eats; the person with hypertension may be denied the salt which he sees as essential to decent-tasting food; the hospitalized person used to a specific ethnic diet may be served typical American food, which he finds repulsive.

There are occasions, however, when eating patterns of individuals or of groups must be changed in the best interests of their health. Shortage of basic food supply, diet modification essential to therapy, travel to another country, and outright malnutrition are some of the reasons why change must occur if the person or group is to maintain or regain health. Following are some general observations about changing habits. The application of these generalizations to nursing practice is discussed here and toward the end of this chapter.

Change within the Cultural Context Most basically, food habits and nutritional practices must be examined and altered within the context of the culture of which the person or group is a part. This seems an obvious approach, but prior to World War II and the formation of the World Health Organization, little attention had been paid to culturally based difficulties in changing food habits. The cultural basis of food habits is important in practice in the United States as well as abroad. The community health nurse or dietitian who expects to convert a poorly nourished Spanish-American family in New Mexico to the "basic four" patterns of eating may get a polite nod from the family but is not apt to see much change in eating habits. Only if he can put the customary foods of the family into the four basic food groups can he hope to make any real changes.

Obviously, translating culturally available food into a basically sound food pattern requires knowledge of the nutrient values of the foods, the food habits, and the symbolism of foods for that culture or subculture. Government nutrition projects often employ anthropologists to study the food habits and meanings within the cultural context, and nutritionists to analyze the nutrient values of the common foods. The nurse practitioner may be able to consult such professionals directly or may need to turn to the literature for a better understanding of the culture, food habits, and nutritional composition of common foods. Most nutrition textbooks have some information on food patterns of various ethnic subgroups in the United States. Resources for further cultural information are listed in the additional readings at the end of this chapter.

Food habits cannot be analyzed out of context of the whole society. Groups attempting to improve the nutritional status in underdeveloped countries soon realized that changing food habits may have ramifications far beyond eating. In addition, changes in other aspects of the culture may affect eating as well. For example, the use of eggs as a "cash crop" deprived a Malawi village of a previously plentiful source of protein. Yet encouraging the villagers to eat the eggs would have left them without money in a country rapidly changing from a barter economy to a cash economy (LeGros Clark, 1968). Similarly, when a physician prescribes a very low-sodium diet for a man, either the entire family must eat an altered diet, since salt cannot be used for cooking, or the patient must have his foods cooked separately. In either case, the wife must alter long-established methods of cooking if her husband is to adhere to the diet.

Change Involving Symbols A second generalization is that habits and practices which are the most symbolically invested are the hardest to change. If possible, these should be left alone and more peripheral changes made. If this is not possible, we should try to follow Mead's advice: ". . . if we must make a substitution, this should also substitute adequately for the symbol." [5] This type of symbolic investment probably explains why attempts to reestablish use of brown (unpolished) rice in the Orient failed. Polished, white rice lacks the B vitamins lost in the milling process, but it is a status symbol as it is more expensive than brown rice. Similarly, in the United States white bread came to be considered more desirable than the coarse dark bread of the "old country." Since the symbol was not easily replaced, the nutritional content of many such refined or processed foods has been increased by fortifying them with some of the nutrients lost in processing.

Duration of Habits Food habits which have existed for a short length of time are easier to change than those which are deeply ingrained. For example, habits acquired in adulthood can be altered more easily than those acquired during formative years. The person who became obese as an adult is more apt to be able to decrease his caloric intake than the person who established excessive eating as a child.

Availability of Substitutes Food substitutions or changes must be economical and easily available if the change is to endure. This means that health workers seeking to help people change dietary practices must know what foods are readily available, which are seasonal, and which are economical. Economical foods are not necessarily the cheapest in terms of retail price. Spare ribs, a common food in some diets, are relatively

---

[5] M. Mead (ed.), "Cultural Patterns and Technical Change." World Federation for Mental Health. UNESCO, Paris, 1953, pp. 214–215.

cheap in terms of price per pound. However, because of the large proportion of bone and fat, the price per pound of edible meat is high.

Motivation As in any kind of change, the motivation of an individual or group to change is the key to success. The person who is motivated to change for his own reasons, whatever they may be, is more apt to alter his eating habits successfully than the person who is pressured to do so. The immigrants to the United States whose "different" eating patterns were highly visible, such as workers who took lunch to their jobs, changed to American diets more readily than those who took all their meals at home (Stoetzel, 1962). The obese child whose personal desire to look like his peers overrides his comfort from eating is more apt to lose weight than the one whose parents' nagging represents external pressure to reduce. The institutionalized person who has retained his ethnic eating patterns may be forced to change them. He may find the food uninteresting but nevertheless eat it, or he may lose all appetite, thus adding inadequate diet to other stressors. Even though the institution has no overt policies related to changing food habits, this lack of adaptation to ethnic diets amounts to coercion of the patient-client to change, albeit temporarily.

Age, education, and socioeconomic level all influence individual motivation to change diets. The differences are particularly important when an outside person or group is trying to motivate people to change. Infants are motivated to eat by hunger. Their natural desire to pop anything into their mouths can be used to encourage them to try new foods. Teen-aged boys are also motivated by hunger, as well as by what their peers eat. Teen-aged girls are interested in good figures, but are also strongly influenced by the food fads of their friends. Adults for whom optimum health is an important value can be motivated to change by appealing to their desire for health for themselves and for their families. Adults to whom health is simply the absence of incapacitating illness may not respond to this same approach. The aged generally are not motivated by claims for better health as they are aware that they are already in the years of declining health.

Peer or group pressure is a strong factor in motivation. Lewin (1952) compared lecture, individual instruction, and group methods of teaching new food habits. The method which required the housewife to state before the group that she would use the new foods proved to be the most effective in actually altering food practices. Similar effects are evident in the success of weight-reducing groups which require their members to state publicly their intent to lose weight, and to weigh in at each meeting. The evidence for the motivating effect of group decision is from work within middle-class Western culture. Little evidence is available as to the efficacy of peer pressure across cultural and socioeconomic lines.

Learning   Change in food habits is essentially a process of learning. Hence one who attempts to help others change must facilitate that learning. The concept of learning is presented in Part 3, Chapter 9. Certain general aspects related to nutrition education will be discussed here.

Some learning about food changes is informal, as when an immigrant observes indigenous food habits and patterns his own after them. Few mothers consciously teach their children about foods, but the experiences children have with food and the attitudes of others toward food teach them a great deal.

Deliberate teaching about foods is intended to alter or change the food habits of the target group or person. The teaching methods may range from an informal discussion of the merits of whole milk versus powdered skim milk with a housewife, to a formal class in nutrition for nursing students. If the learner is highly motivated, just about any learning resource will produce some changes in his behavior. He will pick up and use the tidbits of information from a lecture which the uninterested listener ignores. If the learner is not particularly motivated to learn about or change his eating habits, the didactic (telling) method is a waste of time and breath.

Packard and VanEss (1969) report a significant increase in selection of three nutritious foods by postpartum patients (women who had just had babies) when they were taught about some aspects of nutrition by a nurse. The greatest changes occurred when the nurse explicitly identified the roles of nurse and patient as those of teacher and learner. Ankenbrandt and Tanner (1971) were unable to replicate these results with a group of elderly hospitalized patients. They found no improvement in selection of nutritious foods for groups taught either with or without specific definition of student-teacher roles. They postulate that the difference in motivation was a major reason for their lack of success in changing behavior. Women who have just had babies are usually highly motivated to eat well for their babies' well-being, whereas the older person may see no point in eating for better health.

Another factor which may have led to the lack of success in the second study was the teaching method itself. In both studies the teaching was essentially didactic. Even though there was some opportunity for discussion of the facts, there was no real participation by the student with the teacher, nor any immediate feedback as to the student's progress. Since the learners were not even aware that their selection of foods on the menu constituted a measure of learning (i.e., a "test"), they certainly were not concerned with how well they did. As pointed out earlier, if the learner is highly motivated, as the mothers were, this may not deter learning. If motivation is low, simply presenting information to someone does not ensure that he will use it.

Lewin's work with group discussion and decision and current educational research about the efficacy of participant, active learning suggest that active participation is a more effective method for learning about nutrition, particularly for those who are not highly interested. Participation does not guarantee learning, but it has a better chance than the "talking *at*" method.

Howell and Loeb (1969, pp. 66–73) describe a project in which the nutritional status and food choices of elderly, low-income people were improved as a result of active learning experiences. The people cooked together, taking turns, planned menus, and discussed foods under the supervision of nutritionists and local community nutrition workers. The learning resources incorporated the following factors which learning theory postulates as important to changing behavior:

1 Practice, i.e., the opportunity to try new methods with immediate feedback from the "teacher."

2 Active, as opposed to passive, learning. In the project this meant actually preparing new foods, rather than watching the nutritionist do it, and actually planning menus, rather than using a prepared menu.

3 Overlearning—the opportunity to practice enough so that the skill or method of thinking is comfortable and natural. Cooking meals several times provided overlearning.

4 Spaced rather than massed practice, i.e., practice in small amounts over a period of time. This method seems to be particularly important for some elderly people, whose ability to assimilate information has slowed. It allows a person to proceed at his own pace.

5 Feedback of progress. Feedback helps the learner gauge his progress and know if he is "catching on." Immediate feedback helps encourage the learner and prevent him from incorporating errors into his learning. In the project, other learners provided feedback about the taste of the food or the cooking methods.

6 Success: each woman saw success in the praise which others gave her meals.

7 Replacement of old habits with new ones. Since one of the aims of the project was to improve nutrition, attempts were made to replace inappropriate responses to food cues with more appropriate ones. For example, the word "hunger" initially elicited responses of "sweet roll" and "coffee" in many of the women. Through discussion and preparation of snack food, this response was gradually changed (in words and in what they ate) to "milk," "fruit."

Physical Factors in Food Intake

Along with physiological factors and food habits, several physical states may affect food intake. We do not refer here to disease states affecting digestion and absorption, but to states affecting actual ingestion. Debilitating illness may produce anorexia (loss of appetite), which will decrease intake. Similarly, decreased level or loss of consciousness will affect one's voluntary eating. If such situations are prolonged, parenteral (intravenous) nutrition may be necessary, or feeding may be accomplished via a tube into the stomach.

The state of the teeth and oral mucosa are also factors in ingestion. The edentulous person (one without teeth) may have developed gums tough enough for chewing meat. In all likelihood, however, he will have to avoid foods requiring much chewing. Inflamed or diseased gums and teeth also make eating difficult.

The state of a person's gums, teeth, and oral mucosa both affect and are affected by his nutritional and fluid status. Inadequate calcium and phosphorus in the diet of a pregnant woman and her infant are reflected in the poor quality of the baby's teeth. A diet high in refined sugars is often reflected in a high incidence of caries (cavities). The development of dental caries is dependent upon the pH of the saliva, the bacterial flora of the mouth, and the quality of the tooth enamel. Some people rarely develop caries despite a high intake of sugar; others readily develop them. Differences in oral bacteria, saliva, and quality of the teeth account for differing susceptibility to caries. The fact that primitive people often develop caries for the first time after refined sugars are introduced to them suggests that sugar intake is an important factor in tooth decay.

Fluoridation of the water supply appears to decrease caries in children who drink that supply during their early years. In addition, brushing teeth and using dental floss between the teeth are effective preventive measures. These techniques help remove the debris available for action by the bacteria in the mouth. The acids which this bacterial action release are the real culprits in the creation of decay. Finally, a decrease in refined sugar intake helps decrease the type of food most apt to interact with oral bacteria to produce caries.

Nurses share with other health professionals an obligation to educate the public in methods and goals of oral hygiene, as well as in the purpose of fluoridation of water supplies. Many people can benefit from a simple demonstration of correct brushing technique. Two nurses recently demonstrated the effectiveness of a single demonstration in improving the oral hygiene of a group of hospitalized men (Klocke and Suddith, 1969).

DIAGNOSIS AND MANAGEMENT OF NUTRITIONAL PROBLEMS

A nurse and patient-client may diagnose far more nutritional problems than the nurse can help with directly. He may need to refer the person to a physician or dietitian, or he may need to obtain advice from professionals in the field of nutrition. Nutrition is an area in which roles of professionals are particularly blurred and in which much collaboration and consultation are needed in the best interests of the client.

Initially we will look at some of the kinds of problems a nurse and patient-client might be involved in, and then at some of the roles commonly assumed by the nurse in managing these problems.

Client-recognized Problems

Nutrition problems may include both those for which the patient-client seeks help and those which are recognized by health professionals but not necessarily by the client. The patient-client may come directly to the nurse for help or may encounter a nurse secondary to seeking medical care for a problem in eating. Examples of people who seek nursing help directly might include the obese child who seeks help from the school nurse, the mother who asks the community health nurse for advice about foods, or the man who asks a nurse to help him understand the diet prescribed by his physician. An example of a secondary contact with a nurse might include the hospitalized patient who needs help to eat. Other examples include physician referrals to the hospital or community nurse to aid patients in learning and adapting therapeutic diets.

Problems Recognized by the Health Professionals

Many times people are not aware that they have a nutritional problem. Often their belief system or level of knowledge is such that they do not attribute their lack of well-being or actual illness to poor nutrition. Hunger for many people in the world is a way of life, which may or may not be amenable to change. In other people, situational stress may physiologically or psychologically decrease the desire to eat. Over a long period of time this may impair nutrition. Nurses in institutions often see this kind of anorexia, and view it as a possible nutritional problem. The anorexic person may see his lack of appetite as unimportant.

Although nutritional status should be evaluated as part of the health assessment of any patient-client, certain groups of people are more likely to have inadequate or imbalanced intake, or are more susceptible to the problems arising from poor intake. These people should be evaluated quite specifically for nutritional status as it relates to their health. Such groups are those with increased growth needs—infants, children, adolescents, pregnant and lactating women—and those with decreased resources (monetary, food supply, knowledge), most particularly the many aged persons and those who are poor. Obviously one must be alert for signs of overt malnutrition, e.g., symptoms of the deficiency diseases. However, most signs of undernutrition are more vague and elusive. Apathy, fatigue, listlessness, and lack of motivation in persons at risk can be a sign of undernutrition. Obesity is an obvious sign of overnutrition in terms of calories. However, the obese person may have a grossly unbalanced diet; its components also need to be assessed.

Nursing Roles in Managing Nutritional Problems

Whether the patient-client or the nurse has initiated contact for help with nutritional problems, there are several basic kinds of help which the nurse may offer him.

Coping for the Patient Most fundamentally, the nurse may cope for the person to some degree when he is physically or emotionally unable to solve or recognize his own nutritional problems. The nurse may feed him, help him feed himself, or motivate him to eat. These activities range from coping for him to motivating him to cope for himself.

Feeding Feeding is one of the most basic and symbolic of all caring activities. Feeding is often a symbol of maternal caring, and being fed is a symbol of dependence and helplessness. The two-year-old who is unsure of his place with a rival baby may wish to be dependent, and ask his mother to feed him. The twenty-two-year-old who is quadriplegic (paralyzed in all limbs) or the sixty-two-year-old with a severe heart attack may fight their imposed dependence and resist being fed. Most people, once they have mastered feeding themselves, resent being fed, unless they are too ill and tired to help themselves. Whenever possible, a nurse should allow a patient-client to feed himself as much as he can or wants to, rather than feeding him in the interests of speed or tidiness.

There are many ways in which a nurse can help a patient maintain some degree of independence while still helping him get enough food. These ways must be geared to his habits, his nutritional needs, and the level of his ability. If a person tires easily, the nurse can cut the food in order to spare him that effort, or feed him the last part of his meal. If he is untidy, the nurse can allow privacy, spread the dishes out enough to prevent spilling, or use weighted dishes for increased stability.

Usually the patient who must be fed is in an institution, but community nurses may need to help families feed a person at home as well. Whenever you feed a person, you must realize that he may find being fed a distressing experience. It is better to acknowledge that you appreciate this ("It *is* hard to have to be fed"; "It's a helpless feeling, isn't it?"), rather than shutting off his concern by such comments as, "That's all right, it's part of my job."

The patient-client has certain patterns or habits of eating which, if followed, may make being fed a less distressing experience. Some people eat a little bit of each item, in a circular fashion around the plate. Others eat all of one food before going on to the next. Some drink beverages with their meals, some after the meal. A few minutes used to ask the patient-client how he likes to eat may pay dividends in a good appetite.

Most middle-class people, at least, are accustomed to washing their hands before meals and their teeth afterward. Yet, how many institutions provide opportunity to do this? Many people say grace before a meal. If this is the patient's practice, a sensitive nurse will ask him, before beginning to feed him, if he would like a moment to say grace.

Motivating the Person to Eat *Anorexia* refers to lack of appetite or desire to eat. It may be secondary to many conditions—physical illness, unpalatability or unfamiliarity of foods, or unconscious psychological motivation to stop eating. Beginning students are most apt to encounter people with anorexia secondary to illness, to the quality of the food itself, or to stresses surrounding eating. When patient-clients mention loss of appetite, or when a nurse in an institution notices that a person is not eating, the nurse needs first to ascertain the patterns of food intake to determine if anorexia is truly present. When a person feels that he has lost his appetite, a problem exists, at least subjectively. If his food and fluid intake has decreased significantly and is reflected in weight loss, an objective problem exists as well. A small food intake in one or two days of hospitalization does not necessarily indicate a nutritional problem; however, a regular pattern of low intake does. Low food intake is often coupled with low fluid intake. This can add problems of fluid balance to problems of nutrient intake. Part 3, Chapter 15, discusses fluid problems in detail.

When a person in the community seeks nursing advice about anorexia, he should be referred to a physician, to determine if there are physiologic or psychologic reasons for it. The anorexia of the hospitalized person should also be brought to the attention of his physician. However, unless his illness is directly causing the decrease in appetite, environmental factors may play an important part.

How does the nurse help someone increase his appetite? First, he must try to find the source of the problem. If physical illness is ruled out as a basic cause, perhaps the food is unfamiliar, unpalatable, or served in too-large quantities. A measure as simple as decreasing the size of

portions or having the family bring a familiar dish from home may solve this kind of problem. If the person is on a therapeutic diet, it is still possible to bring in familiar food from home if the specific foods to be brought are compatible with the restrictions of the diet. A dietitian should be consulted for this kind of information. In some institutions, the physician's approval must be obtained before any food is brought in from home.

Often, anorexia in the hospital is due to a combination of the effects of illness, stress of hospitalization, and fears about the prognosis of the illness. Here the nurse needs to be a detective. He needs to observe what the person does eat, find out from him what he dislikes, see that the room environment is conducive to eating (e.g., remove bedpans and smelly dressings before meals). The institutional dietitian may be able to take a diet history and find food which the patient likes. However, the nursing staff are the ones who must observe what he actually eats.

Assisting the Person to Cope for Himself

The majority of nursing help in the area of nutrition involves assisting people to cope with their problems, or helping them recognize that a problem exists. The patient-client may need help in understanding and adapting a therapeutic diet to his life, or he may need to alter a great many of his food habits. The need for an obese person to change his whole pattern of eating is an example of major change.

Obesity is often defined in terms of degree of weight over the standard for age and height (greater than 20 percent overweight). A more precise definition involves the measurement of subcutaneous fat in certain areas of the body. When a piece of skin is pinched between the examiner's fingers, the distance between the two fingers is measured with a special instrument and computed for amount of fat (Mayer, 1966). This technique is called measurement of skin-fold thickness. In general it is not too hard to look at a person and roughly estimate if he is obese or not. Treatment of true obesity is notably unsuccessful. The reports of large groups of obese people treated with any of a number of methods indicate that only about 2 percent lose enough weight to get into the normal weight range and then maintain that weight for at least a year. All the others either lose small amounts and quit or fail to maintain a desirable weight for any length of time (Miller, 1964; Stunkard, 1968).

The origins of obesity are not at all well understood. Fundamentally, a person or animal becomes obese because he takes in more calories than he expends, and the excess calories are converted to fat and stored. This fact has led to some oversimplified approaches to the problem of excess weight, however. Many people feel that all the obese person has to do is to "stop eating so much" and he will lose weight. This overlooks some of the complex interactions of physiological and psychological factors in obesity.

For some time, scientists have realized that destroying the hypothalamic area related to satiety causes rats to overeat and become obese. As they become fatter, their activity decreases, and fewer calories are necessary to maintain their obesity. In addition, rats so affected will eat to excess if food is freely available, but eat very little if some barrier is put in the way of the food. Scientists interpret this as an actual decrease in hunger drive, or apparent lack of hunger, but inability to be satiated (Miller, 1964; Stunkard, 1968).

These observations may have direct corollaries in the eating behavior of obese human beings. To date, there is no evidence that gross abnormalities exist in the hypothalamus of obese human beings. However, some observations of their eating behavior are similar to those made about the experimental rats.

Some obese people report that they never feel hungry but cannot stop eating once they start. Their eating appears to be motivated by availability of food cues rather than by hunger. However, some people of normal weight do not respond to hunger, either. Some prominent investigators hypothesize that external cues, such as the time of day, availability of food, odors of food, and anxiety-producing situations are paramount in regulating the eating of obese people (Schachter, 1968; Stunkard, 1968).

Lack of activity apparently is important in maintaining obesity with a relatively low caloric intake in human beings, just as it is in rats. Obese teen-aged girls are more sedentary than their normal-weight counterparts (Monello and Mayer, 1963). The same appears to be true in obese women (Stunkard, 1958). Such people thus remain obese with a lower caloric intake than many people of normal weight.

Finally, obesity is directly related to socioeconomic class. Data regarding weight were collected as a part of a large study in New York City regarding the epidemiology of mental illness. The prevalence of obesity was considerably greater among people of the lowest class than among people of the uppermost class. This difference apparently reflects social values and fashions, as well as other as yet undetermined social and environmental influences. There were also ethnic associations with obesity, but the origins or significance of these associations are not clear (Stunkard, 1968).

These observations and ongoing trials of behavioral modification as therapy suggest that the old approach of giving an obese person a low-calorie diet and sending him to an exercise class did not succeed because it was not based on the eating behavior of obese people. Some current attempts to modify eating behavior hold some promise for weight control. Stuart (1967) initially helps the person master techniques to control eating behavior. These techniques included counting mouthfuls of food or putting down utensils in the middle of a meal and sitting quietly from two to five minutes. This helps the person learn to stop eating before consuming everything in sight. Once the person can control his eating, he starts trying to cut down the number of calories and increase energy expenditure in order actually to lose weight.

The success of group efforts such as Weight-Watchers, Incorporated, and TOPS (Take Off Pounds Sensibly) is probably related to group pressure and group support through difficult times. One technique of such groups is to have a member call another member when he is tempted to overeat. This substitutes some other behavior for eating, and may help him gain some control over his eating behavior.

Nursing Roles in Assisting People to Cope Nurses are only one group of professionals who may help people in coping with their nutritional problems. The primary functions of many such health workers include supervising, facilitating learning, counseling, and assisting the person to adapt recommendations to his life situation. These functions are shared with physicians, nutritionists, dietitians, or community workers trained to help with nutritional problems. The professional's formal title should not determine who helps the patient-client; the person who can best meet the client at his level of understanding ought to be the one to help him.

Adapting Therapeutic Diets Physicians prescribe modified diets in the treatment of a number of diseases. Examples of these modifications include high- or low-calorie, low-sodium, diabetic, and high- or low-protein diets and diets altered for people with food allergies. The physician may refer the client to a dietitian or provide him with written material about the food allowed in the diet. However, simply receiving information about a diet is a far cry from

actually incorporating it into one's life. This is clearly evident in the lack of success of low-calorie diets in helping obese people to lose weight.

In some instances, a nurse may be asked to help the client learn a new diet. The ability of a particular nurse to understand the dietary prescription and facilitate the client's use of it depends upon his background in nutritional principles and his knowledge of consultative resources in the community. Each nurse should become familiar with these resources for his particular area.

When helping a person adapt a therapeutic diet, the nurse must determine several factors: the "fit" of the diet to the patient-client's food habits, the patient-client's level of understanding of the purpose and methods of the diet, and his motivation to use it.

The closeness of fit of the prescribed diet to the person's food patterns will determine the extent to which he will need to alter his usual habits. Cultural patterns, economic factors, and individual preferences will all enter into this. In other words: Are the foods familiar to him, can he afford to buy them, will he eat them?

Most printed materials regarding modified dietary patterns are based upon typical middle-class Anglo-American eating patterns. The menus contain few of the foods familiar to the Chinese-American or Orthodox Jewish patient-client, for example. If the client's family and peer group eat an ethnic diet, chances are that this person will not completely alter his habits to conform to the printed diet, no matter what his motivations for better health may be.

Therapeutic diets can be formulated for ethnic food patterns as well as for the Anglo-American patterns. There are, however, few printed materials available regarding these adaptations. The New York City Health and Hospital Corporation recently compiled diet guides for basic modified diets for people whose food patterns are predominantly Spanish, Chinese, Southern American, Orthodox Jewish, Italian, and Anglo-American ("Hospital Food Notes," 1971). Nutritionists and dietitians employed by institutions and community health agencies can help nurses adapt therapeutic diets to specific cultural patterns by analyzing the patient's normal foods for the restricted or increased nutrients. Readings regarding cultural food patterns are given at the end of this chapter.

Economics is an important determinant of food habits and of the person's ability to afford a prescribed diet. Again, the nurse, in consultation with the dietitian and the patient-client, can often find more economical substitutes for recommended foods. Diet prescriptions given to patients often contain specific menus. If the nurse understands the principles behind the menu, he can help the client alter these menus to his own situation. Examples of such principles are those which govern diabetic exchange diets. Certain groups of foods have roughly equivalent proportions of fat, carbohydrate, or protein. The foods in these groups are thus interchangeable in a diabetic diet. The diabetic person can then be given a prescription for a certain number of meat, or carbohydrate, exchanges per day, rather than rigid menus.

The patient-client's level of understanding and motivation are vital factors in the success of a therapeutic diet. If the client does not understand that the diet is intended to help him feel and function better, or if he does not believe that these changes will occur, he is not apt to make any major alterations in his eating.

Conversely, he may be willing to stop using table salt on a low-sodium diet, but he may not understand that many common foods also contain sodium. He may continue to eat such foods as milk and cheese, which contain sodium, in sufficient quantities to negate the intent of the diet.

The patient-client's level of understanding will determine the level of language which the nurse uses—whether the nurse speaks of "nutrients" or "foods," whether he interprets the diet in terms of groups of interchangeable foods (an abstract concept) or in terms of specific menus (a more concrete approach).

Counseling about General Nutrition

Nurses in the community, by virtue of their position as health professionals, are often asked advice about food and eating by neighbors, clients, and community groups. Nurses may be asked for advice about current food fads, feeding problems in children, weight loss, or they may be asked to teach formal classes for pregnant women, school children, or civic groups. The nurse's ability to give sound advice will obviously depend upon his own background in nutrition and ability to apply it to practical problems.

Harrison et al. (1969) tested the level of general nutrition knowledge among public health nurses in seven agencies. The test measured knowledge of tools used to plan and evaluate diets, psychological and physiological factors affecting intake, and facts about nutrients in foods. There was a wide range of scores, particularly in the segments related to physiological and psychological factors affecting eating. Nurses with baccalaureate education scored higher than those with technical education. These differences tended to even out with years of experience in the agencies which had ample written resources about nutrition and a full-time nutrition consultant. Experience did not affect the scores in agencies without these resources. These findings emphasize the importance of supplementing the nurse's formal education with consultation and reading facilities. The nutrition textbooks and other works listed in the additional readings in this chapter are sources of reliable nutrition information.

Nurses in the community tend to be seen by the public as sources of nutrition information. In contrast, nurses in hospitals are not often regarded by patients as nutritional information sources. One recent study suggests that although nurses in hospitals do a significant amount of informal nutrition education, the lay public sees the physician as the only reliable source in hospitals of nutrition information.

This would imply that a nurse who is attempting to do any teaching about nutrition to a hospitalized person needs to establish clearly the purpose of the teaching and, if need be, his credentials as an informed source. Nurses in the institution surveyed had a generally negative attitude toward nutrition and attached a low priority to the patients' nutritional needs. In contrast, the patients viewed food as an important part of their hospital life, and focused on the food in voicing their complaints or praise about care (Newton et al., 1967). To the hospitalized patient, food and eating often become the high points of an otherwise monotonous day. Nurses in hospitals need to remember this and appreciate the importance of food to the person who does not have a nutritional "problem" but has little else to look forward to in the day.

REFERENCES

Books

Burgess, A., and R. Dean (eds.), "Malnutrition and Food Habits," The Macmillan Company, New York, 1962.

DeZayas, E., in A. Burgess and R. Dean (eds.), "Malnutrition and Food Habits," The Macmillan Company, New York, 1962, p. 81.

Lewin, K., Group Decision and Social Change, in G. Swanson (ed.), "Readings in Social Psychology," Holt, Rinehart and Winston, Inc., New York, 1952, pp. 459-475.

Mead, M. (ed.), "Cultural Patterns and Technical Change," World Federation for Mental Health, UNESCO, Paris, 1953.

"Recommended Dietary Allowances," 7th rev. ed., Report of the Food and Nutrition Board, National Research Council, National Academy of Sciences Publication 1694, Washington, D.C., 1968.

Stoetzel, J., The Social Psychology of Food Habits, in A. Burgess and R. Dean (eds.), "Malnutrition and Food Habits," The Macmillan Company, New York, 1962, pp. 76-84.

Periodicals

Ankenbrandt, M. D., and L. K. Tanner: Role-delineated and Informal Nurse-teaching and Food Selection Behavior of Geriatric Patients, *Nursing Research,* **20**:61-64 (1971).

Cassel, J.: Social and Cultural Implications of Food and Food Habits, *American Journal of Public Health,* **47**:733-740 (1957).

Cravioto, J., in: *Pre-School Child Malnutrition,* National Academy of Sciences–National Research Council Publication 1282 (1966).

Eichenwald, H. F., and P. C. Fry: Nutrition and Learning, *Science,* **163**:644-648 (Feb. 14, 1969).

Harrison, G. G., A. M. Sanchez, and C. M. Young: Public Health Nurses' Knowledge of Nutrition, *Journal of the American Dietetic Association,* **55**: 133-139 (1969).

Hospital Food Notes: Outpatient Diets Match Cultural Background, *Journal of the American Hospital Association,* **45**:70-71 (June 16, 1971).

Howell, S., and M. Loeb (eds.): Nutrition and Aging: A Monograph for Practitioners, *The Gerontologist,* **3**:1-122, Part 3 (Autumn, 1969).

Klocke, J., and A. G. Suddith: Oral Hygiene Instruction and Plaque Formation during Hospitalization, *Nursing Research,* **18**:124-130 (1969).

LeGros Clark, F.: Food Habits as a Practical Nutrition Problem, *World Review of Nutrition and Dietetics,* **9**:56-84 (1968).

Mayer, J.: Some Aspects of the Problem of Regulation of Food Intake and Obesity, *New England Journal of Medicine,* **274**:610-731 (Part 1) (Mar. 17, 1966).

Miller, C. H.: Current Understanding of Eating and Dieting, *Psychosomatics,* **5**:119-126 (1964).

Monello, L. F., and J. Mayer: Obese Adolescent Girls, an Unrecognized "Minority" Group? *American Journal of Clinical Nutrition,* **13**:35-39 (1963).

Morgane, P. J., and H. L. Jacobs: Hunger and Satiety, *World Review of Nutrition and Dietetics,* **10**:100-213 (1969).

Newton, M., M. E. Beal, and A. L. Strauss: Nutritional Aspects of Nursing Care, *Nursing Research,* **16**:46–49 (1967).

Ohlson, M. A.: Dietary Patterns in Nutrient Intake, *World Review of Nutrition and Dietetics,* **10**:13–43 (1969).

Packard, R. B., and H. VanEss: A Comparison of Informal and Role-delineated Patient-teaching Situation, *Nursing Research,* **18**:443–446 (1969).

Rubin, R.: Food and Feeding: A Matrix of Relationships, *Nursing Forum,* **7**:195–205 (1967).

Schachter, S.: Obesity and Eating, *Science,* **161**:751–756 (Aug. 23, 1968).

Schaefer, A. E.: Are We Well Fed? *Nutrition Today,* **4**:3–11 (1969).

Spengler, S. S.: World Hunger: Past, Present, and Prospective, *World Review of Nutrition and Dietetics,* **9**:1–31 (1968).

Stuart, R. C.: Behavioral Control of Overeating, *Behavior Research and Therapy,* **5**:357–365 (1967).

Stunkard, A. J.: Physical Activity, Emotions and Human Obesity, *Psychosomatic Medicine,* **20**:366 (1958).

———: Environment and Obesity: Recent Advances in Our Understanding of Regulation of Food Intake in Man, *Federation Proceedings,* **27**:1367–1373 (1968).

Villiers, A.: The Voyages and Historic Discoveries of Captain Jas. Cook, *National Geographic,* **140**:328 (September, 1971).

Walike, B., H. Jordan, and E. Stellar: Studies of Eating Behavior, *Nursing Research,* **18**:108–113 (1969).

ADDITIONAL READINGS

Brennan, R., et al.: A Bookshelf on Foods and Nutrition (1st rev.), *American Journal of Public Health,* **58**:621–637 (1968). (An annotated bibliography of books and pamphlets of importance to health professionals.)

Cornelison, S.: Guidelines to Feeding a Helpless Patient, *Journal of Psychiatric Nursing,* **2**:184–187 (1964).

Leininger, Madeleine, Some Cross-cultural Universal and Non-universal Functions, Beliefs, and Practices of Food, in J. Dupont (ed.), "Dimensions of Nutrition: Proceedings of the Colorado Dietetic Association Conference," Fort Collins, Col., 1969, Colorado Associated University Press, 1970, pp. 153–173.

Mitchell, H., H. Rynbergen, L. Anderson, and M. Dribble (eds.), "Cooper's Nutrition in Health and Disease," 15th ed., J. B. Lippincott Company, Philadelphia, 1968.

Morris, Ena: How Does a Nurse Teach Nutrition to Patients? *American Journal of Nursing,* **60**:67–70 (1960).

Newton, M., and J. Folta: Hospital Food Can Help or Hinder Care, *American Journal of Nursing,* **67**:112–113 (1967).

Trillin, C.: U.S. Journal: Manhattan; The Ordeal of Fats Goldberg, *The New Yorker,* **47**:57–63 (July 3, 1971).

Elimination Status

Margaret E. Auld

In order to make a thorough nursing assessment and diagnosis of a patient-client's elimination status, the nurse must have a complete under- standing of normal human excretory function and patterns. Knowledge of the common devi- ations and alterations that he may encounter is

Data to Be Assessed

I Bladder
   A Bladder habits
     1 Frequency of micturition
     2 Characteristics of urine
       a Quantity
       b Color
       c Odor
       d Sedimentation
       e Unusual constituents
     3 Aids to elimination
   B Special problems
     1 Abnormal sensation
     2 Diversion of urine
     3 Care of special problems
II Bowel
   A Bowel habits

     1 Time of defecation
     2 Frequency
     3 Changes in response to stress, illness, trips
     4 Character of stool
       a Amount
       b Color
       c Odor
       d Consistency
       e Unusual constituents
     5 Aids to elimination
   B Special problems
     1 Abnormal sensation
     2 Artificial orifices
       a Colostomy
       b Ileostomy
     3 Caring for special problems

also necessary. This chapter focuses on the normal patterns of elimination from the bladder and bowel, factors that help maintain normal patterns, common deviations from the normal, and means by which the nurse can assist the patient to live within the limitations of the alterations.

Americans have been characterized as a bladder- and bowel-conscious nation. Sociologists have made light of it. Miner (1956), in his classic article, "Body Ritual among the Nacirema," has labeled the bathroom the "shrine" in American homes, and relates a number of practices occurring here. Americans traveling in Europe and the Far East are appalled by and annoyed with the available toilet facilities, as well as the lack of privacy and cleanliness in the communal toilets found in many of the hostels.

We are accused of yearly spending millions of dollars for laxatives which would be unnecessary were we to "eat a correct diet," "answer the call of nature," and "exercise more." The ideal of having one bowel movement a day may be considered the "national goal," but it is neither physiologically correct nor essential for proper body functioning. There is less consensus on the "correct" number of times a day to void (urinate), but abnormalities from the person's "normal" are easily recognized.

Maintenance of privacy is paramount for elimination from either the urinary bladder or the colon. We expect to lock doors in public toilets; of even greater status is the "pay toilet." Cleanliness is considered essential.

The sights and smells of the normal bowel movement are considered repugnant. Frequently, joking behavior is associated with the bowel and its function. The flush toilet is our way of dealing with the immediate reality of human waste and its disposal. The quiet flush toilet has high social value.

In the American middle class, discussion of bowel and bladder function is generally not acceptable socially. Such discussions may be held between good friends or between an acknowledged health worker (physician or nurse) and the person seeking help. The most acceptable open discussion of elimination patterns occurs when attempts are made to "toilet-train" children.

In light of the above reservations and hesitation to discuss elimination patterns and normalcy, it may be difficult for the nurse to gather data essential to guide nursing action. Ease in gathering data about elimination may be achieved by matter-of-factness, knowing why information is wanted, and setting the patient at ease by sharing with him the reasons why such information is necessary for nursing care.

Normal patterns of excretory function are variable, although well-defined limits to normalcy exist. In one study, 99 percent of the persons studied had a bowel movement frequency within the range of three bowel movements a week to three a day. Only 1 percent had more than three movements (stools) a day or only one a week. The authors do suggest that three stools daily may be regarded as unusual and more than three a day as abnormal (Connell et al., 1965). The desire to empty the urinary bladder (void) occurs when the bladder has reached a capacity of 250 to 450 ml urine. The desire to void is dependent upon the integrity of the stretch receptors. Voiding is dependent upon fluid intake, an intact neuromuscular system, and the ability of the kidneys to produce urine. Also affecting voiding is the opportunity to urinate at a socially acceptable time.

Emotionally charged and stressful situations, illness, and hospitalization may interfere with normal habits of elimination. During limitation of usual activity alteration in bowel or bladder functioning may occur. Examples of limited mobility include long trips in confined spaces, such as cars or airplanes; confinement in body casts or skeletal traction for the treatment of fractured bones; or an illness in which the person does not have the strength to get out of bed.

Social situations not conducive to meeting one's needs to empty the bladder or colon interfere with normal functioning. Examples of such social situations include holiday dinners or cocktail parties. Similarly, in large hospital wards where the noises and smells of defecation are cause for embarrassment, a person may attempt to ignore the defecation reflex; the reflex then is diminished, eventually weakened, and lost. Other factors contributory to alteration in "normal" bowel and bladder patterns are major changes in diet and use of medications such as morphine sulfate, barbiturates, and atropine (Bisgard, 1959; Goodman and Gilman, 1970); anticipation of an important date or examination; and mental depression.

BLADDER FUNCTION

The urinary bladder serves as a reservoir for the urine constantly being produced by the kidneys at a rate of 30 to 50 ml per hour. This urine is transported down the ureters by peristaltic activity and is deposited for storage in the bladder. Normally, this storage continues slowly and without our knowledge until sufficient urine is present to make us aware of it (Kropp, 1967). Then evacuation may be started at will and is usually complete without hesitation within one minute. The process of emptying the urinary bladder is known as *micturition;* the terms *voiding* and *urination* are also used. This process allows us to be independent in our daily activities and to choose when and where we will urinate. Effective functioning of this system is dependent upon the coordination of bladder-wall smooth muscle and the external sphincter.

Children are toilet-trained to meet cultural demands. They must substitute voluntary control for what is initially an involuntary reflex process. When the child's bladder is physiologically able to hold urine for a two-hour period, it is thought that he is ready to begin bladder training. This may be expected to occur at fifteen

to eighteen months of age (Blake et al., 1970).

If the physiology, innervation, and muscles are normal and a person has once learned the control of his bladder functions, a loss of bladder functioning is significant. When urinary abnormalities exist, intervention must be considered a critical aspect of the person's care. Unlike bowel derangement, which is more annoying than critical, dysfunction of the lower part of the urinary tract can lead to subsequent loss of renal function, uremia, and, ultimately, death if intervention does not occur.

Micturition

Micturition is the process in which the urinary bladder empties itself of urine when it becomes filled. Voluntary micturition is characterized by the sensation of fullness of the bladder (need to void) and contraction of the detrusor muscle, followed by relaxation of the sphincters (Delehanty, 1970). Any pain or difficulty in voiding is abnormal and needs immediate attention. Involuntary micturition occurs when only the spinal reflex mechanism operates, as in those who are not toilet-trained or have some spinal cord injuries. The normal innervation is diagrammed in Fig. 14-1.

The steps in micturition follow a normal course. The bladder is slowly filled with urine until from 150 to 500 ml is collected. This amount then stimulates the stretch receptors in the detrusor muscle to send impulses to the voiding reflex center located in the spinal cord at the level of the second to fourth sacral segments. The impulses are carried to the higher voluntary cortical micturition control centers. If the time for voiding is appropriate, the brain sends impulses to motor neurons in the sacral area of the spinal cord, causing parasympathetic efferent fibers of the pelvic nerve to stimulate the contraction of the detrusor muscle, relaxation of the sphincters, and voiding. The exact mechanism of

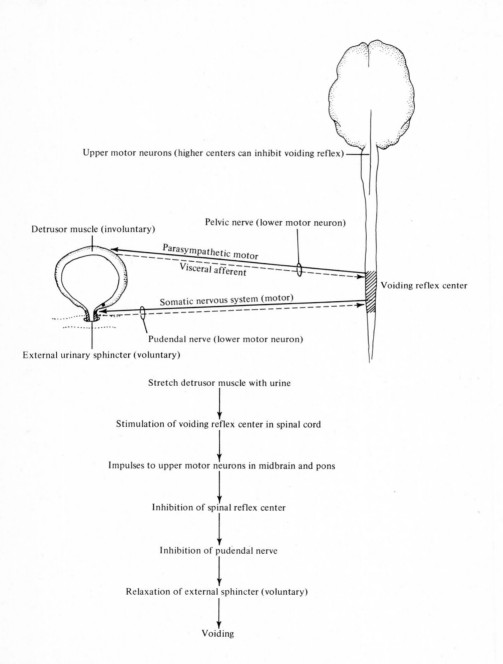

Figure 14-1 Normal innervation and the mechanism of micturition.

the micturition initiation is unknown. The conscious desire to void probably occurs when the bladder has already begun to contract and closure of the external urethral sphincter still persists (Kropp, 1967). The identification of a "continence reflex" has been made on observations of increased activity of the urethral sphincter as the bladder is filling; it is thought to develop through teaching and constant conditioning.

Normal and Abnormal Urine Characteristics

In the normal person, the kidneys form urine by a complex process of filtration, reabsorption, and secretion of the blood plasma which passes through the 2 million nephrons in the kidneys. Urine is a waste product, formed by the excretion of the by-products of body metabolism and the concentration of most of the constituents of the body fluids. Review of urine formation in a physiology textbook is recommended. Some characteristics of normal urine are depicted in Table 14-1.

Table 14-1   Characteristics of Normal Urine

Color	Straw, amber, or transparent
pH	4.5–7.5
Specific gravity	1.010–1.025
Amount	1,200–1,500 ml/day
Frequency of voiding	Varies with bladder capacity, sensations, acceptability, and availability of toilet facilities
Odor	Specific aromatic

The urine volume is variable and depends on normal kidney functioning, amount of fluids ingested, environmental temperature, fluid requirements of other organs, diuretic drugs, and presence or absence of open wounds (such as burns). Urine output of 30 to 50 ml per hour indicates adequate kidney function. Less than 25 ml per hour or 500 ml urine in a 24-hour period should be brought to the physician's attention.

The amount of urine voided varies with the above factors as well as with the person's bladder capacity and ability to control micturition until a socially acceptable time. Normally, the response to void is felt when the bladder contains between 200 to 500 ml urine, but it is not uncommon for a bladder to have a capacity of up to 1,500 ml in cases of obstruction.

Voiding five to ten times a day is common. Most common times of voiding are upon arising and before retiring. Other times vary with individual habits and correspond to coffee breaks for some and availability of a toilet for others.

The normal color of urine is described as pale, straw, amber, or golden yellow. The coloration of normal urine is due to the pigment urochrome. Pale urine may be due to temporary diuresis due to an excessively large fluid intake, sudden absorption of edema fluid, diabetes insipidus, or diabetes mellitus. Dark urine usually represents a dehydrated state but may also indicate the presence of urobilin and small amounts of bilirubin. Consumption of large amounts of carotene-containing foods (e.g., carrots) will result in a urine of brighter yellow color.

Red urine may be due to the presence of blood in the excretory system from injury, from a urinary tract infection, or from diseases which hemolyze (disintegrate) red blood cells. Red urine (described as smoky) has also been noted after ingestion of beets, rhubarb, senna, blackberries, and red dyes used in confectionery products (McLagen, 1967). Persons with the disease porphyria note that their urine turns red if left standing. The antituberculosis drug rifampin colors urine red-orange, as does Pyridium.

In the disease alkaptonuria, urine turns dark brown or black on exposure to light and air. Dark brown urine is also seen in extensive burn and crush injuries (Cone, 1968).

Normal urine is transparent in the freshly voided state. Upon standing, however, it may become cloudy because of deposits or sediment.

Freshly voided urine which is not transparent needs to be accurately described, as it may well herald an inflammatory process. Mucous shreds are not common in urine but are seen frequently in persons with indwelling urinary catheters or other urinary diversion methods.

Urine odor may be described as aromatic and specific. If allowed to stand, urine products decompose and the characteristic ammonia odor is detected. Food, such as asparagus, can alter the urine odor, as can inflammatory processes.

Special Problems

Urinary Incontinence Urinary incontinence is the inability of the urinary sphincters to control the movement of urine from the bladder. Incontinence among the elderly is thought to be a natural process of aging. Putting up with the uncomfortable situation of constantly smelling like urine, fearing another "accident," and living with the inability to reach a bathroom in time to void contribute to fewer social contacts for the elderly.

Elderly women may have some relaxation of the perineal musculature which interferes with complete emptying of the bladder, or they may have some loss of muscle strength because of multiparity (i.e., because of having borne several children). Any stress or increase in the intra-abdominal pressure, as in laughing, sneezing, or crying, may cause them to be incontinent. One frequently finds that the elderly woman rolls up toilet paper to wear in her underpants, begins to wear perineal (Kotex) pads in an attempt to catch the incontinent urine, and stays home most of the time rather than seek medical assistance. She is highly conscious of her odor.

Elderly men who have enlarged prostates urinate with difficulty and have a tendency to "dribble" because of retention (inability to empty the bladder completely). Like elderly women, they are highly conscious of their apparent inability to control their urinary function, and of concomitant odors.

Heavy intake of sedative and barbiturate drugs (Hillman, 1969), as well as the ingestion of large amounts of alcohol, reduces the sensation of having to void and the ability to control the external sphincter. Reduction or discontinuation of the use of sedative drugs frequently removes the cause for incontinence. Fecal impaction, urinary infection, many kinds of neurologic conditions, and physical limitations such as hip fractures also contribute to the incontinence problem (d'Entrecasteaux, 1971; Hardy, 1971).

Nursing care of the incontinent patient is aimed at enlisting his active participation in a bladder-retraining program (Saxon, 1962; Tudor, 1970). It is essential for the nurse to know the physician's diagnosis and how it may affect the training program, the pattern of incontinence, the person's ability to perform activities of daily living, and the mechanics of normal micturition.

One of the most successful methods of reducing incontinence found by Saxon was restoration of a person's hope that he could once again become continent. Adjusting the fluid schedule (Schofield, 1970), increasing physical activity, surgical intervention, positioning for elimination, wearing street clothes, placing toilets or bedpans within reach, and the simple removal of underpads secured as diapers were all of benefit (Saxon, 1962).

It is usually the geriatric person who is thought of as being incontinent. However, children may also be incontinent as the result of disease or birth defects. One of the most common defects is meningomyelocele, in which the spinal cord is spread out in the lumbar region and the nerve supply is deranged, resulting in both fecal and urinary incontinence (Woodward, 1970). Spinal cord injuries or transections in adults or children will result in incontinence. Special bladder- and bowel-retraining programs are essential in these circumstances. Information about such programs may be found in textbooks of rehabilitation.

Urinary Retention Urinary retention occurs as the production of urine continues to distend the bladder and the urine is not excreted from the bladder. Retention of urine may occur with prostatic enlargement, after gynecologic or bowel surgery, after childbirth (due to meatal swelling), and in supine immobility (see Part 3, Chapter 12).

Urinary retention is potentially dangerous. If the bladder is allowed to collect an excessive volume of urine, the transitional epithelium of the bladder wall will be stretched thin and will become hypoxic because of the increased pressure on the arterial vessels. The discomfort is acute, and the person seeks assistance in a very distressed manner.

There are characteristic signs of the distended bladder. The abdomen appears swollen as the level of the bladder rises above the symphysis pubis. Palpation with a light pressure on the abdomen reveals a tense, highly sensitive area, and percussion over the swollen area results in a "kettle-drum" sound. Discrepancies in intake and output exist, and great lengths of time since last voiding are noted. Men with hypertrophied prostates who continue to put off elective surgery may be victims of distended bladder.

Removal of the urine and pressure reduction are important. Any nursing measures to assist the patient to void should be attempted in an effort to avoid catheterization. Early ambulation after surgery, warming the bedpan, placing the hands in warm water, providing privacy, reducing anxiety-producing situations, pouring warm water over the vulva of females, suggestion, or running water from the tap are all reputed to help. A sitting position for females and a standing one for males are physiologically ideal.

If nursing measures do not aid the patient, the physician may order Urecholine in an attempt to empty the bladder. Catheterization is the last resort. The dangers of catheterization are well spelled out later in this chapter. The additional danger in decompression of the greatly distended bladder must also be considered. The bladder may well lose tone, and with the rush of blood back into the pelvic area, the person may experience lightheadedness, fainting, or even shock if more than 700 to 1,000 ml urine is removed at one time. The exact mechanisms of lightheadedness and shock are unknown. Perhaps they may be due to the reflex dilatation of previously effaced pelvic arteries and veins. No clinical studies are available at this time. Mr. W. suffered mild clinical shock thought to be related to removal of a large volume of urine:

Mr. W. is a 72-year-old retired accountant who arrived in the Emergency Room early one Saturday morning. His complaint was of bladder distension due to prostatic enlargement. Through the previous day and night, he had forced fluids upon himself in an attempt to "make himself go," since this technique had been successful previously.

Physical examination revealed a hard, tender abdomen, enlarged to a size comparable to that of a pregnancy of four months. He was acutely uncomfortable, unable to assume any comfortable position, and short of breath.

Relief by catheterization was attempted. Removal of 1,000 ml clear yellow urine produced great relief without any change in vital signs. The decision to remove the remaining urine was made. After the removal of another 400 ml the patient was ashen and complained of being lightheaded; a drop in blood pressure was recorded, as well as an increase in heart rate.

Further removal of urine was discontinued; the catheter was clamped and left in place. An intravenous fluid line was established, and the patient given fluids intravenously to aid in restoration of his blood pressure.

Removal of a hypertrophied prostate afforded clinical relief from further episodes of bladder distension.

Retention with Overflow Retention with overflow is exactly what the name implies; the overfull bladder "dribbles" because the increased pressure overcomes the sphincter control. In addition, the person may void frequently in small amounts, his condition mimicking that of a person with an acute urinary infection, but upon observation it is obvious that the bladder is still distended. Detection is somewhat more difficult than detection of simple retention, as the feeling of a need to void is diminished, but the treatment is aimed at the same objective: removing the urine from the bladder while maintaining the bladder-wall tone and preventing shock. Medical or surgical intervention must then be instituted.

Alteration in the Method of Eliminating Urine Because dysfunction of the lower part of the urinary tract can lead to serious loss of renal function if allowed to progress or to proceed untreated, methods of urinary diversion are necessary adjuncts to care. Any diversion of the urinary stream must be compatible with continued good function of the kidneys and should provide the patient with a method of collecting his urine which will not impair him socially to any degree. An ideal method is yet to be available, and the dangers of using a catheter are extreme. In 1883, Clarke stated that "the entrance upon catheter life occasionally gives rise to a pernicious fever which destroys life and is sufficient to cause death." It has been well documented that the presence of an indwelling catheter has a direct relation to infection. A catheter left in the bladder from twenty-four to forty-eight hours inevitably results in bacteriuria (microbiologic evidence of organisms in the urine) (Ansell, 1962).

Shackman (1954) clinically investigated the relation of an indwelling urinary catheter to the bacterial status of the urine and presented evidence that organisms gain entrance to the bladder by way of the catheter. Dutton (1957) and Gillespie (1960) carried out similar investigations, concluding that bacteria enter through the catheter. Kass (1959) used *Serratia marcescens* swabbed on the perineum to demonstrate how

gram-negative organisms can enter the bladder around the catheter in the fluid-filled space between the catheter and the urethral mucosa twelve to twenty-four hours after insertion. Significant bacteriuria is then induced by bacterial multiplication in the bladder and/or in the collecting device (Ansell, 1962; Kass and Sossen, 1959; Petersdorf, 1965).

Fecal and skin bacterial action has been inhibited by a variety of methods. Martin and Bookrajain (1962) suggest abandoning the indwelling catheter. Two general methods to minimize frequency of bladder contamination have been suggested: meticulous asepsis and use of continuous or intermittent irrigation with antibacterial solutions. The use of Neosporin Gu Irrigant in conjunction with a three-way catheter after five, ten, and fifteen days of indwelling catheterization has shown an incidence of bacteriuria of 4, 6, and 10 percent (Meyers et al., 1965), in contrast to 95 to 100 percent with an indwelling straight catheter (Martin et al., 1964). The drug was shown to have a high degree of bactericidal activity and safety (Hodari, 1966).

Desautels (1959) investigated daily cleaning of the urethral meatus with aqueous benzalkonium chloride followed by application of a wet benzalkonium chloride dressing around the glans penis and adjacent catheter. He found that of 82 patients, only 14 had positive cultures (bacteria in the urine) after fifteen days of using a closed system. Routine irrigation of indwelling catheters almost always leads to contamination. If the system must be broken, he found that use of 70 percent alcohol before disconnecting the catheter junction permitted irrigations to be done more safely. The only criterion for instituting bladder irrigation is the presence of mucous shreds or unclear urine. McLeod (1963) found that a paraplegic whose catheter was changed daily and whose perineum was sprayed with Neosporin remained free of urinary tract infection.

Nursing care should be aimed at maintenance of a closed system with a bacteriostatic catheter to prevent entry of bacteria about the meatus, and an air break at the end of the drainage tube to prevent retrograde invasion of bacteria. Provision for maintenance of continuous free drainage by gravity into the collecting container is essential, as is sufficient fluid intake so that the kidneys produce urine at the rate of at least 50 ml per hour. Such a rate prevents motile bacteria from migrating upward. The tubing should be circled on the bed and taped to provide for gravitational drainage, as shown in Fig. 14-2 (Ansell, 1962).

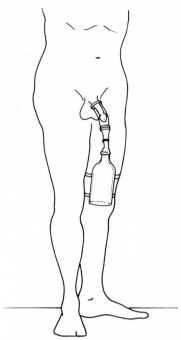

Figure 14-3 Condom appliance for external urinary collection.

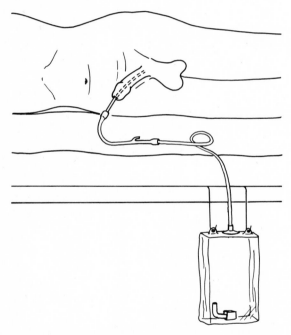

Figure 14-2 Provision for gravitational drainage with indwelling catheter. In males, the penis is directed headward to prevent erosion of the urethra by the catheter.

Instead of an indwelling catheter, a "condom catheter" is sometimes used to collect urine from males (see Fig. 14-3). It is not a catheter at all, but rather an apparatus affixed to the external genitalia, connected to tubing which may be attached to a leg bag or a larger collecting bag, and used when the person is unable to control elimination from the bladder. It has the decided advantage of entailing a great deal less risk of bladder infection than catheters. There is, unfortunately, no such device for women. The goal of nursing care is to prevent skin breakdown at the site of attachment. Frequent removal of the condom and cleaning of the penis and scrotum are necessary.

Permanent methods of urinary diversion are varied. A *cystostomy* is used primarily as a temporary measure after prostatectomy and in surgery of the urethra or perineum. It consists of placing a tube directly into the bladder through the abdominal wall. Permanent cystostomies are used for persons with severe urethral strictures, periurethral abscesses, or multiple perineal abscesses, as well as for paraplegic or quadriplegic persons. Nursing care is aimed at maintaining cleanliness of the skin, preventing infection, and helping the person with socialization if he wishes.

Ureterosigmoidostomy (Fig. 14-4) procedures are appealing as a means of maintaining urinary continence because of the convenience of not having to wear an appliance. The ureters are transplanted into the sigmoid colon as low as possible. The person experiences an increase in the number of "stools," as the stools are, of course, more watery. The number of "stools" is related to the amount of fluid intake. Drawbacks to this artificial means of eliminating urine are that the person may have nocturnal bowel movements because of the increased fluidity of the stool, bacterial contamination of the ureters and kidneys is a constant threat, and sometimes stricture forms at the transplant location.

A more frequently performed procedure is the *ileal conduit.* (Fig. 14-5). A short segment of terminal ileum is isolated with its intact mesentery, intestinal continuity is reestablished by anastomosis (suturing together), the proximal end of the isolated segment is closed, the ureters

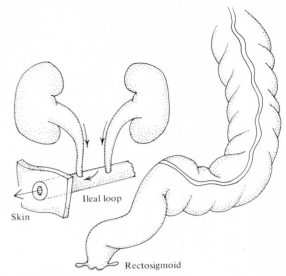

Figure 14-5   Ileal conduit.

are implanted in the ileum, and the distal end is brought out to the abdominal wall. Peristalsis is maintained. Continence is lost, so the person must wear an ileostomy appliance on the skin stoma (Fig. 14-11). The rate of infection is less than with an indwelling catheter or with the ureterosigmoidostomy, as the peristalsis in the ileal loop prevents pooling and there is no cross-contamination from the fecal stream. As with an ileostomy, the aim of nursing care is to assist the person to maintain an intact skin, prevent odor formation, prevent infection, and remain clean and socially acceptable.

BOWEL FUNCTION

Efficiency of body function requires that food residue in the gastrointestinal tract be eliminated and that toxic substances produced or ingested be rendered harmless. The function of the colon is to receive liquid chyme from the terminal small intestine and transport it to the anus. While the liquid chyme is in the colon, most of the water is absorbed from the colonic contents, and the contents become firm. Sodium and chloride ions are absorbed, and potassium and

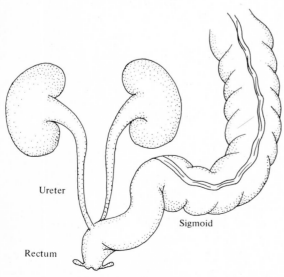

Figure 14-4   Ureterosigmoidostomy.

bicarbonate ions are excreted. The colon absorbs about 2 liters of water in twenty-four hours. Although the colonic products represent a blend of meals eaten over the preceding several days, 80 percent of food residue from any one meal is excreted by the end of the fourth day (Truelove, 1966). Transit of the colonic contents through the gastrointestinal tract is affected by the quantity of residue in the diet, the motility rate, and presence or absence of chemicals or infections within the gut.

Muscle of the large intestine exhibits automaticity and can be stimulated by a number of factors. The intrinsic nervous supply—the mesenteric plexuses—is essential to normal bowel functioning. Motility of the gastrointestinal tract depends to a lesser degree on the extrinsic nervous system and the ability of the muscle fibers to respond to stimuli (Bennett, 1966). Disruption of the integrity of the intrinsic nervous supply results in grave alterations in colonic functioning. Any alteration in neuromuscular

control of the intestine will require a special bowel program to maintain continence or provide for effective elimination of fecal waste.

Reflex activity is common in the human intestinal system. Three commonly identified reflexes are the gastrocolic, duodenocolic, and the defecation reflex. Essentially they are activated by distension of a portion of the gastrointestinal tract, which initiates another action. The gastrocolic reflex is a response to distension of the stomach, which initiates contraction of the rectum and frequently a desire to defecate (Ganong, 1967). The duodenocolic reflex is similar, but the original stimulus is initiated by distension of the duodenum.

Defecation

In healthy subjects, the rectum is usually empty. The desire to defecate is initiated by distension of the sigmoid colon and rectum by the presence of feces. Normal defecation is a complex voluntary and involuntary act. As distension occurs in

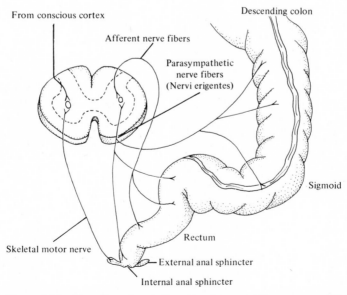

Figure 14-6 The afferent and efferent pathways of the parasympathetic mechanism for enhancing the defecation reflex. *(From Arthur C. Guyton, "Textbook of Medical Physiology," 5th ed., W. B. Saunders Company, Philadelphia, 1971. By permission of the publisher and author.)*

the sigmoid and rectum, sensory nerves are stimulated, which in turn stimulate reflex activity in the sacral nerves. Simultaneously, impulses travel up the spinothalamic tract to the brain. Figure 14-6 depicts this mechanism. Once the fecal mass in the rectum has initiated the reflex activity, the fecal mass is driven from the rectum by a sustained mass contraction of the lower part of the colon, assisted by characteristic straining movements of contracting the abdominal muscles and setting the diaphragm, which markedly increase the intra-abdominal pressure. However, unless the urge to defecate is responded to, the urge will disappear.

Movements which assist defecation are fixing the diaphragm, contracting the abdominal and chest muscles, and voluntarily relaxing the anal sphincter while raising the pelvic floor muscles. Straining is also assisted by forced expiration against a closed glottis, which markedly raises the intra-abdominal pressure. Without a glottis (as in persons with laryngectomies) this additional assistance is unavailable.

Aids to defecation that are commonly used include beverages, positioning, medications, laxatives, enemas, smoking cigarettes, and establishing a regular time for defecation. People use a variety of beverages to stimulate bowel action, including hot coffee, warm water with a squeeze of lemon juice, or prune juice. The habit of drinking a warm fluid upon arising to stimulate defecation is common. Although they may not know it, people who do this are utilizing the gastrocolic reflex. Adequate fluid intake has long been recognized as an essential adjunct to the prevention and treatment of constipation (Bockus, 1964). Authors do not agree on the amount of fluid which is "adequate."

The squatting position is the most physiologically correct position for defecation. Leaning forward from the hips raises the intra-abdominal pressure; this is sometimes necessary to assist the fecal mass from the colon. If a person must use a bedpan for defecation, the nurse may approximate the physiologically correct leaning-forward position by rolling the head of the bed up to a high Fowler's position, if this position is not contraindicated.

Providing a footstool to aid in flexion at the hips will assist the short person using the commode or toilet to raise his intra-abdominal pressure. Pregnant women notoriously have difficulty in defecating. This is thought to be due to their altered shape, which prevents them from easily assuming the leaning-forward position, as well as to the loss of abdominal muscle strength, which prevents effective straining.

Defecation requires the assistive contraction of the muscles of the abdomen and the pelvic floor. Bockus (1964) advocates abdominal strengthening exercises for better bowel elimination. Persons who would benefit from such exercises include those who are immobilized or debilitated, pregnant women, and people whose muscles are without tone because they have gained or lost a great amount of weight.

Enemas stimulate peristalsis by distension or by chemical irritation and lubrication. Laxatives are effective because of their bulk-forming properties, lubrication, chemical irritation, or their ability to soften the stool in the colon.

The enema requires introduction of a substance into the rectum to produce evacuation. Essentially, three kinds of enema are now in use: the volume enema, the electrolyte enema, and the oil enema. The volume enema requires that a large quantity of fluid (from 500 to 1,000 ml) be introduced into the colon, causing distension and, it is hoped, evacuation. Tap water (hypotonic) and saline (isotonic) solutions are used most frequently, sometimes with the addition of soapsuds to provide chemical irritation of the rectal mucosa. The electrolyte enemas are usually dispensed in disposable plastic containers. The active ingredients are either sodium phosphate or sodium biphosphate solutions, which act because they are hypertonic, causing slight distension and mild chemical irritation. Oil enemas are small-volume enemas which are given to soften hard feces.

Laxatives and enemas are abused (Tillery, 1966). Correctly used, they can be a real assistance to the person in need, providing him with profound relief. Chronic users of harsh laxatives and enemas disrupt their normal functioning, empty the intestinal tract of fecal material for one or two days while sufficient fecal material accumulates to stimulate again the desire for bowel action, and generally repeat the purgative when a "normal" bowel movement is not achieved every day. Once the cycle is established, it becomes difficult to disrupt. The person expects a bowel movement every day. Without it, his anxiety increases about its absence, little else can be thought of until bowel action takes place, and so assistive means are sought. The intestines soon lose their ability to act without aids; the normal reflexes diminish and are soon lost. The person then has become enema- or laxative-dependent. The decreased expulsive power as a result of the disuse atrophy of the muscles of the abdominal wall, pelvic floor, and intestine only contributes to the patient-client's further need for aids.

Enemas may be hazardous. The irritation of the rectal mucosa by the chemical irritant can be severe. Pike (1971) reported a single case of fetal death following a soapsuds enema given to the mother in preparation for delivery. Following administration of a soapsuds enema, the mother became pale and had no discernible pulse or blood pressure. After restoration of her pulse and blood pressure, she delivered a stillborn infant. Study of the nurses' preparation of soapsuds enemas revealed that the enema had contained an excessive amount of soap (more than 5 ml in 1 liter of water). The hazards of multiple tap-water enemas in the elderly and in infants are discussed in Part 3, Chapter 15.

Color and Characteristics, Normal and Abnormal Stools

Some characteristics of normal feces are outlined in Tables 14-2 and 14-3.

Table 14-2 Characteristics of Normal Stool

Color	Brown
Form	Shaped to rectum; cylindrical
Consistency	Soft
Odor	Varies with diet, medications, person
pH	6.8–7.3
Amount	150 gm/day
Frequency	3 times/day to once a week

Table 14-3 Composition of Normal Feces

	Percent
Water	75
Solid matter	25
Dead bacteria	30
Fat and fat derivatives	10–20
Inorganic matter	10–20
(calcium and phosphates)	
Proteins	2–3
Undigested roughage varies, bile	
pigment, sloughed epithelial cells,	
cellulose	30

Source: (Adapted from Guyton, 1971).

Guyton (1971) states that fecal composition is relatively unaffected by variations in diet because a large fraction of the fecal mass is of nondietary origin. This knowledge assists the nurse in understanding that appreciable amounts of feces continue to be passed even during prolonged starvation. Thus the patient-client who has not taken anything by mouth (n.p.o.) for surgical or medical reasons may still be expected to pass fecal material. The movement of the bowel cannot be expected to be "normal" for that person until the normal or near-normal preillness condition is achieved, or food restrictions are removed, normal functioning of the body is restored, or the alteration in functioning is corrected or living is adjusted to it. Examples of persons who could be expected to have altered stools because of diminished food intake would be those who maintain strict diets for weight loss, political activists who refuse anything but liquids to dramatize and support their claim that injustice is being done, and, historically, prisoners in concentration camps such as Dachau and in the United States Civil War camp at Andersonville.

In Truelove's studies (1966) of the human intestine, he found that the colon normally retains food residues from meals taken during the preceding week, or before, and that ordinarily 80 percent of any one meal is extruded by the fourth day. We may then expect that any stool passed represents a mixture of the residues of what has been eaten over the previous days.

The characteristic brown color of normal fecal matter is caused by the bilirubin derivatives, stercobilin and urobilin, and the action of the normal intestinal flora. Abnormal stools may be important diagnostically to the physician, as well as in planning nursing actions. Absence of bile entering the bowel, as seen in persons with biliary obstruction, results in a characteristic white or putty-colored stool—an *acholic* stool. Blood in stools is usually present in one of two forms: occult (hidden) or frank (observable). A fecal mass which has occult blood is dark, sticky, has a pungent odor, and is termed *tarry*. It is the result of digestive action on the red blood cells in the gastrointestinal tract. Frank bleeding may first be noted by the presence of bright red blood in the stools. The guaiac test for occult blood is an easy, inexpensive, and reliable index that the nurse can do with the proper reagents. It is important for the nurse to determine if bright red blood is mixed within the stool or is on the surface of the stool. Blood on the surface of the formed stool may be from hemorrhoids; blood mixed in the stool must come from a more distal bleeding site.

Watery stools have a larger percentage of water than the "normal" 75 percent. The stool has had a shorter transit time in the intestine, with resultant decrease in absorption of important ions and water. Glistening, pale stools mixed with considerable mucus and observable fat are *steatorrheic*. Steatorrheic stools are seen in patient-clients with defects in fat absorption.

Large, mushy stools with *undigested food particles* may indicate a lack of hydrochloric acid in the stomach. Undigested food in the stools is common in infants and small children. Large, pale gray or green, semiliquid stools with a *putrid odor* are seen in the digestive disorder of sprue. A great deal of mucus surrounding the stool may indicate constipation, as the body has attempted to lubricate the hardened stool in order to pass it from the body. The stool in this case is frequently described as "rock hard." A stool surrounded by mucus is different from one in which a large amount of mucus is intermixed, and needs to be observed and accurately recorded. "Rice-water" stools are characteristic of prolonged periods of diarrhea, as in cholera.

Medications as well as food may alter the normal color of stool. Oral hematinics (agents such as iron which tend to increase the hemoglobin content of the blood) result in a stool which resembles the "tarry"-colored stool seen in gastrointestinal bleeding. Some observers have described such stools as "coal-like." Chlorophyll and red beets also color the stool green or red.

The odor of the fecal matter is derived principally from the products of bacterial action, and therefore varies from person to person, depending upon the individual intestinal bacterial flora and the foods ingested.

The normal consistency of stool is soft, but the stool is formed, assuming the shape of the rectum; it is important to observe alterations in the shape of the normal stool. Narrowed, or pencil-like, stools indicate obstruction in the bowel. More critical than the exact size and shape is a change from what the person considers normal. In "apple-core" carcinoma, the stool might resemble a pencil or shoestring (see Fig. 14-7).

Special Problems

Flatulence Gas (flatus) in the gastrointestinal system is normal, being present in the stomach

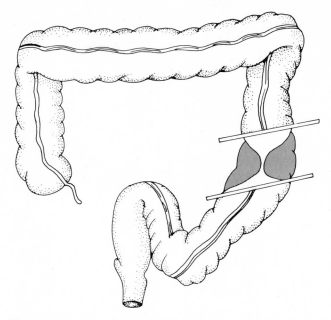

Figure 14-7 Cutaway view of carcinoma resembling "apple core" attached to wall of the descending intestine. Stools passing by this obstruction are pencil or shoestring size.

and in the small and large intestines. Abnormalities and potential problems arise when flatus cannot pass or when an abnormally large amount of flatus is passed.

Gases can enter the gastrointestinal tract from three different sources:

70 percent from swallowed air
20 percent from diffusion of gases from the bloodstream into the gastrointestinal tract
10 percent from bacterial decomposition of food residue (Roth, 1968; Roth and Bockus, 1957)

Excessive swallowing of air may occur in nausea, postnasal drip, emotionally upsetting situations, and with the use of drinking straws. The habit of swallowing to relieve discomfort from peptic ulcer, gallbladder disease, and angina is common. Persons who eat rapidly, consume vast amounts of carbonated beverages ("pop," beer), or hypersalivate through the frequent chewing of

gum, candy sucking, or excessive smoking are liable to excessive air swallowing.

Although the incidence of gas formation from food residue is small, many persons are able to identify particular foods which increase the amount of intestinal gas. Foods which are widely acclaimed as contributing to gas formation are beans, cabbage, onions, cauliflower, radishes, cucumbers, and highly irritant foods such as pizza and hot peppers. Highly irritant foods are suspected of causing a faster transit time, thus reducing the amount of time for gases to be absorbed, rather than actually being gas formers.

Flatus is normally without odor. Odoriferous flatus is the result of putrefaction of certain proteins, inadequately cooked starches, and cellulose.

Motility inhibition and obstruction in the gastrointestinal tract caused by a number of factors will increase the amount of intestinal gas, as reabsorption is diminished and removal per rectum becomes difficult. Common causes of diminished reabsorption of gas are constipation, the administration of certain medications decreasing intestinal motility [e.g., morphine sulfate, codeine, and barbiturates (Bisgard, 1959)], anesthetic agents, and lack of activity. The inevitability of postoperative ileus (halt in gastrointestinal movement) is disputed (Baker, 1964), as gastrointestinal sounds do not disappear completely following abdominal or chest surgery, but are diminished; many persons, however, experience postoperative distension. The person with distension is acutely uncomfortable and seeks relief (Fig. 14-8).

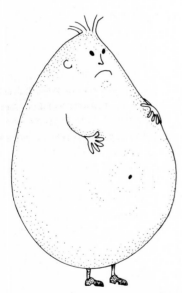

Figure 14-8 Caricature of a person who states that he has "gas."

Belching may bring temporary relief from the pressure of the gases within the stomach; however, attempts to relieve a "bloated stomach" by conscious belching will only increase the discomfort. Greater discomfort occurs because more swallowed air is retained than is belched back (Roth, 1957).

Small amounts of gas are usually present in the small intestine, and greater amounts are

present in the large. Transit of the gas through the gastrointestinal tract is an indication of peristaltic activity. If there is little peristaltic activity, accumulation of gases causes distension. Distension, in turn, can cause extreme discomfort, relieved by belching or by passing flatus per rectum. Distension may contribute to respiratory difficulty, by impinging upon the diaphragm, and may contribute to further inhibition of gastrointestinal motility (Farrar, 1955).

Distension and flatulence are treated according to the suspected cause. Decreasing the amount of swallowed air may be the greatest help, since air swallowing ranks as the highest source of intestinal gas. Identifying the means of decreasing swallowed air and interrupting the air-swallowing behavior should lead to diminished air in the gastrointestinal tract. Observing the person's ingestion habits, not letting him use straws, reducing ingestion of carbonated beverages, reducing gum chewing, and stopping postnasal drips with medications may reduce the amount of swallowed air. Decreasing or removing known or suspected gas-forming foods from the diet is another means of prevention and intervention. If reduced or diminished activity is suspected as the cause of gaseous distension, an increase in activity is essential. Walking about while gently massaging the abdomen is suggested to relieve distension; assuming the knee-chest position with a backward-and-forward rocking movement sometimes helps (Roth and Bockus, 1957). Medically, nasogastric tubes may be inserted to remove gas. Food and fluids may be withheld; an enema using a pint of lukewarm tap water may be given, or a rectal tube may be ordered.

Nursing care is aimed at minimizing air swallowing, educating the patient-client about foods, beverages, and condiments that contribute to distension, and increasing peristalsis.

Constipation Constipation is one of the oldest and most common physical disorders. Interpretation of the concept of constipation varies, and the condition of being constipated is relative. Simply, constipation is the defecation, after an abnormally long period, of a stool which is abnormally dry and which requires excessive use of voluntary muscles (Giblin, 1971). Connell (1965) surveyed 1,000 normal factory workers regarding their normal bowel habits. He found that the passage of three stools daily may be regarded as unusual, and that passage of more than three stools daily is probably abnormal. It is not the number of stools passed in a certain length of time that differentiates between a nonconstipated and a constipated state, but rather the consistency and the difficulty in passage.

Causes of constipation vary. The patient-client describes himself as being "all bound up" (Fig. 14-9). Gastroenterologists have identified many factors that contribute to constipation. Probably the single greatest factor contributing to constipation is the failure to establish or maintain habituation, thereby allowing reflexes which assist defecation to diminish. A variety of systemic diseases (cancer, peptic ulcer, heart failure), lack of sufficient bulky food, excessive

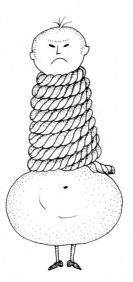

Figure 14-9 Caricature of a person who states that he is "all bound up" (constipated).

use of laxatives and enemas, and weakened abdominal, perineal, and intestinal muscles are contributory. Also contributory are intrinsic lesions of the ileum and colon (hemorrhoids and anal fissures), severe dehydration, prolonged confinement and immobility, and medications which slow intestinal motility (codeine, barbiturates, and morphine sulfate) (Coombs, 1969; Geigy, 1966; Giblin, 1971; MacBryde, 1970).

Children are not immune to the development of constipation. In addition to the above causes of constipation, a child may actively withhold the bowel movement in rebellion against toilet-training efforts of the mother.

Medical and nursing care is aimed at identifying factors contributing to the constipation, and intervening on the basis of information gathered in the assessment. Primarily, the nurse's role is to intervene, help the patient identify contributing factors, and guide him to substitutive behavior, at the same time using his skills as a health teacher to meet these objectives.

Fecal Impaction Fecal impaction is the sequela of prolonged retention and accumulation of fecal material in the sigmoid and rectum. The fecal mass that remains in the intestine progressively becomes harder as the moisture in the stool continues to be absorbed, and serves as an obstruction and irritant.

The person who has a fecal impaction is unable to pass a normal stool. Rather, fecal seepage is noted as small amounts of feces bypass the hardened mass, leaking through the anus. Bacterial action upon the fecal mass may produce an enormous soft or liquid stool which is passed in incontinent flashes through the anus. Not all of the hardened mass is expelled in this way, leaving a core of feces that is still hard.

The desire to defecate is felt, but the person is unable to do so. Severe rectal pain, abdominal fullness, an everted anus, and a rock-hard mass in the sigmoid flexure on digital exam are all present.

Prevention of fecal impaction is important. If

constipation is allowed to progress to impaction, the patient-client suffers unnecessary discomfort, and may thereafter be liable to further formation of fecal impactions.

Treatment consists of the administration of an oil enema to soften the hardened stool, followed by a mild cleansing enema in two to three hours. Digital manipulation and removal of the hardened stool are frequently necessary. This is an uncomfortable and embarrassing procedure. Impactions are easier to prevent than to treat.

Diarrhea   Diarrhea is the frequent passage of unformed or liquid stool. This reflection of abnormal intestinal motility and function has wide ramifications. Diarrhea may be merely a transient, uncomfortable, and inconvenient state, or it can create major physiological problems.

With increased intestinal motility, there may be less absorption in the small intestine of essential nutrients for optimum body functioning and reduced ability of the body to form critical substances such as vitamin B_{12}, thiamine, riboflavin, and vitamin K. Severe, major physiological problems may occur in diarrhea, with the loss of water, sodium, and potassium which are not reabsorbed from the chyme passing through the ileocecal valve (Guyton, 1971; Bortoff, 1969). The potential danger from the excessive fluid loss is great. Children and people with massive infectious dysentery (cholera) are affected the most. The reader is referred to Part 3, Chapter 15, for further discussion of fluid-loss problems.

If diarrhea goes unchecked and untreated, the body continues to lose amino acids; carbohydrate and fat absorption is diminished; and with the diminished fat absorption, fat-soluble vitamins are lost. Saline loss is critical. This loss, then, may become a vicious circle; the person feels less and less like ingesting nutrients, so that further depletion occurs. Hypoproteinemia leads to edema, as described in Part 3, Chapter 15.

After great famines and diseases following typhoons in southeast Asia and India, we see and work with the terribly emaciated, pot-bellied, spindly-legged children who have fallen victim to this syndrome. Figure 14-10 diagrams loss in untreated diarrhea.

There are many causes of the increased peristalsis of the intestinal column which produces diarrhea. As with constipation, stressful situations may interfere with normal habits of elimination. Emotions may affect visceral activity. Symptoms presented may reflect inability to handle a stressful situation (Sherbaniuk, 1964). Contaminated foods may be an offender. Local and national health agencies investigate reports of "food poisoning" (gastroenteritis) from canned and other foods. Infectious organisms may be present also in unrefrigerated foods, particularly mayonnaise, whipped cream, and meats. The organisms that most commonly cause gastroenteritis are *Staphylococcus* and *Streptococcus*. Travelers frequently report being victims of "Montezuma's revenge" while traveling in Mexico. The primary cause of this ailment is not the drinking water, which is often blamed, but the organisms carried in the water which are foreign to the person's intestinal flora.

Irritating foods, or dietary indiscretions such as eating a high preponderance of fried, greasy, or carbohydrate foods, may also be the primary cause of diarrhea. High-protein, high-carbohydrate tube feedings and certain antacids (those with more magnesium salts) may also cause diarrhea. The body's defense mechanism for removing irritating chemical irritants (highly spiced foods) is remarkable.

Nursing responsibilities in diarrhea depend upon the severity of the symptoms and the contributing factors. A primary nursing responsibility is to assist in maintaining or replacing fluid loss in severe or prolonged diarrhea. Replacement should be aimed at known electrolyte loss (potassium and sodium) and increasing the number of bacterial flora (e.g., by giving the

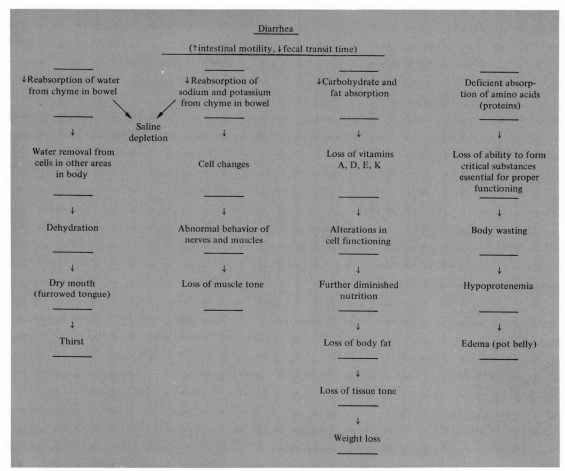

Figure 14-10 Losses in untreated severe diarrhea and physical symptoms present.

patient yogurt). The nurse also should note any abnormal constituents of stool, provide a well-ventilated room with privacy and a commode, bedpan, or bathroom in proximity, and prevent secondary complications. Most frequently seen physical complications are anal irritation and excoriation, and alterations in the body chemistry. Anal irritation may be reduced by providing a means of gently removing the liquid stool from the perianal region (either soft tissue or gentle washing after each stool). Diarrhea that produces alterations in body chemistry requires medical attention.

Anal Incontinence Anal incontinence is the inability of the anal sphincter to control the discharge of fecal and gaseous material voluntarily. It is a most distressing problem. Alert persons who are plagued by it characteristically have a limited environment, as they tend to stay where they will suffer the least embarrassment from an incontinent stool. Hospitalized persons tend to stay within the confines of their room, and persons at home stay home. Socialization is minimal, if at all, and usually limited to the professional staff or to family. The desire to dress in "street clothes" is lost, as the person chooses not to soil his clothing. Characteristically, one who is incontinent of stool dresses in easily washable night clothes and absorbent and waterproof underpants, so that if he cannot reach the toilet to complete the bowel movement, the soiling will be minimal.

This inability of the anal sphincter voluntarily to control the discharge of fecal and gaseous material occurs in patient-clients with neuromuscular disturbances. A case history is presented:

Mr. H. L., a 48-year-old laborer, was admitted to a large city medical center hospital with complaints of increasing "hemorrhoids," and difficulty, pain, and bleeding when trying to defecate. On examination it was found that Mr. H. L. had a cystic growth in the muscles of the external anal sphincter. Because of its location and disturbance to the patient, an attempt to remove the cyst with minimal disturbance to the muscle itself was made. Postoperatively, he was incontinent of feces because of the loss of muscle control and because the sensory and motor nerves had been severed.

A bowel training program was initiated. It consisted of utilizing the known physiological principles of the gastrocolic reflex and defecation. With the cooperation of the patient and staff, Mr. H. L. was given two cups of hot coffee each day at 6 A.M., followed by a bisacodyl suppository; he was assisted to the bathroom (if necessary) 20 minutes after the initiation of these actions. Oral stool softeners were also administered daily. He was instructed in positioning on the toilet to achieve the best possible results (leaning forward from the hips while applying external pressure over abdomen with the hands) and was provided with maximal privacy.

During the hospital stay of five days after his operation, Mr. H. L. had but two small "accidents"; he felt confident that he could continue his regimen in his boarding house without difficulty.

The physicians felt that much of Mr. L.'s neuromuscular control would be regained as innervation

returned to the operative site. The nursing goal of assisting the patient, through bowel training, to prevent accidents because of anal incontinence was successful.

Other examples of persons who have anal incontinence are those who have explosive diarrhea, those who have had an excessive number of enemas in preparation for bowel studies and whose liquid stool seeps through the sphincters, and some elderly persons who have lost the ability to sense that the rectum is full.

Surgical treatment for fecal incontinence has included electrical stimulation of incompetent or denervated muscles (Hopkinson, 1966) and substitution of muscle flaps or fascia for incompetent sphincter control (McGregor, 1965). Stanley created an artificial anus-occluding prosthesis encircling the bowel with an inflatable balloon to control incontinence in sheep; he proposes to use a similar device in man (1970).

Skin care of the anal region is critical and focuses upon removal of harmful agents and protection of the integrity of the skin. Skin moist with fecal matter has a greater potential for decubitus formation because of the acid nature of feces and bacterial multiplication. Without fail, the anal region must be washed with a gentle soap after *each* episode, gently and thoroughly dried, and protected either with a protective agent (petroleum jelly) or a material to reduce potential friction between the buttocks (talcum powder).

Artificial Orifices for Elimination Obstructive lesions of the colon caused by cancer and ulcerative colitis which are not amenable to treatment by medical or dietary regimens are treated surgically by the creation of an artificial opening bypassing the lesion. A surgically created opening in the small intestine is termed an *ileostomy;* a surgically created opening in the large intestine is called a *colostomy.* The fecal stream, or move-

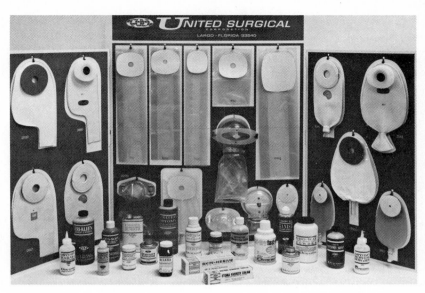

Figure 14-11 Variety of appliances used for the collection of fecal and urinary excretions. *(Photo courtesy of United Surgical Corporation.)*

ment, is diverted to an opening (stoma) created by the surgeon on the abdominal wall.

Preparation of the patient-client for extensive surgical alteration in normal bowel function requires that the nurse review the normal functioning of the intestinal tract, understand the past functioning of the bowel, assess the patient-client's emotional state, and introduce him to the postoperative appliances he might be using. Preparation for a new set of habits is critical (Katona, 1967). Secor (1970) presents some very detailed care and planning for rehabilitation of the person with a colostomy.

Appliances for the collection of fecal excretions of the body vary. The goals in the use of ileostomy appliances are to provide the patient with security that his clothes will not be stained by leakage of the fecal contents, to maintain cleanliness, to prevent irritation of surrounding skin by the digestive enzymes, and to maintain privacy, modesty, and freedom from embarrass-

ment. The goal with colostomy control is not to rely upon an appliance but to regulate fecal movement with irrigations (Katona, 1967). Some of the appliances used are shown in Fig. 14-11.

Katona has spent a great deal of time studying persons with colostomies, and has suggestions for care of postsurgical problems, irrigations, diet modification, personal adjustment, and care of the stoma (Katona, 1967). The student is referred to other articles of note (Devlin, 1968; Shaw, 1969; Seargeant, 1968; Devlin and Plant, 1969) for further study. If a person has an ileostomy or colostomy and must enter the hospital, it is of utmost importance that the nurse gather data about prehospital care and effectiveness so that care may continue without interruption of established habits.

Common bladder and bowel problems and appropriate nursing care are summarized in the accompanying table.

Summary of Common Problems, with Approaches

Problem	Approach
Bladder	
Urinary incontinence	Discontinue large amounts of barbiturates, alcohol
	Prevent fecal impaction and urinary infections
	Retrain bladder
Urinary retention	Encourage early ambulation; upright sitting position for females, standing for males
	Remove urine by catheters
	Remove cause (e.g., enlarged prostate), by physician
Retention with overflow	Determine cause
	Provide skin care
Urinary diversion	Use meticulous aseptic technique
Indwelling catheter	Provide for adequate drainage
Condom	Provide skin care of anus, abdominal wall
Cystostomy	
Ureterosigmoidostomy	
Ileal conduit	
Intestinal tract	
Flatulence	Identify and remove causes of excessive air swallowing, gas formation, or inability to release formed gas
	Increase activity, exercise, withhold food and fluids
	Use enema or rectal tube
Constipation	Establish or maintain bowel habituation
	Provide bulk-forming foods, water
	Remove causes
	Assist in treating systemic disease
Fecal impaction	Encourage abdominal exercise
	Teach correct positioning
	Prevent constipation
	Administer oil enema, followed by cleansing enema
	Remove digitally
	Prevent recurrence
Diarrhea	Assist in maintaining or replacing fluid and electrolyte loss
	Provide for cleanliness
	Prevent anal excoriation
	Identify and remove cause (food, medicine, organize data on causes)
Anal incontinence	Institute bowel-training program
	Provide skin care
Artificial orifices, colostomy, ileostomy	Prepare for surgery
	If there is an "old" artificial orifice, gather data about prehospital care and effectiveness of continuing such treatment in hospital

REFERENCES

General

Kropp, Kenneth A., and Vincent J. O'Conor: Normal Human Excretory Functions, *American Journal of Physical Medicine,* **46**:648–652 (1967).

Miner, Horace: Body Ritual among the Nacirema, *The American Anthropologist,* **58**(3):503–508 (1956).

Urinary Problems

Ansell, Julian: Some Observations on Catheter Care, *Journal of Chronic Diseases,* **15**:675–682 (1962).

Blake, Florence G., F. Howell Wright, and Eugenia H. Waechter, "Nursing Care of Children," 8th ed., J. B. Lippincott Company, Philadelphia, 1970.

Clark, Sir Andrew: Remarks on Catheter Fever, *Lancet,* **2**:1075–1077 (1883).

Cone, Thomas E., Jr.: Diagnosis and Treatment: Some Syndromes, Diseases and Conditions Associated with Abnormal Coloration of the Urine or Diaper, *Pediatrics,* **41**(3):654–658 (1968).

Delehanty, Lorraine, and Vincent Stravino: Achieving Bladder Control, *American Journal of Nursing,* **70**:312–316 (1970).

d'Entrecasteaux, J. S.: Electronic Control of Urinary Incontinence, *Nursing Mirror,* **132**:43 (1971).

Desautels, Robert E., and J. Hartwell Harrison: The Mismanagement of the Urethral Catheter, *Medical Clinics of North America,* **43**:1573–1584 (1959).

Dutton, A. C., and M. Ralston: Urinary Tract Infection in a Male Urologic Ward, *Lancet,* **1**:115–127 (1957).

Gillespie, W. A., et al.: The Diagnosis, Epidemiology and Control of Urinary Infection in Urology and Gynecology, *Journal of Clinical Pathology,* **12**:187–200 (1960).

Hardy, Shirley: Incontinence in the Elderly, *Nursing Mirror,* **132**:12 (1971).

Hillman, Iris E. O.: Practical Problems in the Care of the Elderly, *Nursing Times,* **65**:207–212 (1969).

Hodari, A. A., and C. P. Hodgkinson: Iatrogenic Bacteriuria and Gynecological Surgery, *Journal of Obstetrics and Gynecology,* **95**:153–162 (1966).

Kass, Edward H., and Lawrence J. Schneiderman: Entry of Bacteria into the Urinary Tracts of Patients with Inlying Catheters, *New England Journal of Medicine,* **256**:556–557 (1957).

——— and Harold S. Sossen: Prevention of Infections of Urinary Tract in Presence of Indwelling Catheters, *Journal of the American Medical Association,* **169**:1181–1183 (1959).

McLagen, N. F.: Urine, Abnormal Coloration, in A. H. Douthwaite (ed.), "French's Index of Differential Diagnosis," 9th ed., The Williams & Wilkins Company, Baltimore, 1967.

McLeod, J. W., and J. M. Mason: Prophylactic Control of Infections of the Urinary Tract Consequent on Catheterization, *Lancet,* **1**:292–295 (1963).

Martin, Christopher M., et al., Prevention of Gram-negative Rod Bacteremia Associated with Indwelling Urinary Tract Catheterization, in J. C. Sylvester (ed.), "Antimicrobial Agents and Chemotherapy," American Society for Microbiology, Ann Arbor, 1964.

——— and Edward N. Bookrajain: Bacteriuria Prevention after Indwelling Urinary Catheterization, *Archives of Internal Medicine,* **110**:703–711 (1962).

Meyers, M. S., et al., Controlled Trial of Nitrofurazine and Neomycin-Polymyxin as Constant Bladder Rinses for Prevention of Post-indwelling Catheterization Bacteriuria, in J. C. Sylvester (ed.), "Antimicrobial Agents and Chemotherapy," American Society for Microbiology, Ann Arbor, 1965.

Petersdorf, Robert G., and M. Turck: Urinary Tract Infections, *General Practitioner,* **32**:131–134 (1965).

Saxon, Jean: Techniques for Bowel and Bladder Training, *American Journal of Nursing,* **62**:69–71 (1962).

Schofield, Derek: Management of Urinary Incontinence, *Nursing Mirror,* **131**:39–46 (1970).

Shackman, Ralph, and David Messent: The Effect of an Indwelling Catheter on the Bacteriology of the Male Urethra and Bladder, *British Medical Journal,* **2**:1009–1012 (1954).

Tudor, Lea L.: Bladder and Bowel Retraining, *American Journal of Nursing,* **70**:2391–2393 (1970).

Woodward, Sister M. Hiliary: Urinary Incontinence in the Physically Handicapped Child, *Nursing Times,* **66**:1098–1100 (1970).

Bowel Problems

Baker, W. L., et al.: Intestinal Activity after Operation, *Proceedings of the Royal Society of Medicine,* London, **57**:391–394 (1964).

Bennett, Alan, and Brian Whitney: A Pharmacologic Study of the Motility of the Human Gastrointestinal Tract, *Gut,* **7**:307-316 (1966).

Bisgard, J. Dewey, and E. K. Johnson: The Influence of Certain Drugs and Anesthetics upon Gastrointestinal Tone and Motility, *Annals of Surgery,* **110**:802-822 (1959).

Bockus, H. L., "Gastroenterology," 2d ed., vol. 2, W. B. Saunders Company, Philadelphia, 1964.

Bortoff, Alex: Intestinal Motility, *New England Journal of Medicine,* **280**(24):1335-1337 (1969).

Connell, A. M., Claire Hilton, G. Irvine, J. E. Lennard-Jones, and J. J. Misiewicz: Variations of Bowel Habit in Two Population Samples, *British Medical Journal,* **2**:1095-1099 (1965).

Coombs, Harrison S., et al.: When Your Patient Says, "Doctor, I'm Constipated," *Patient Care,* **111**:90-102 (1969).

Devlin, H. B.: Abdominoperineal Resection of the Rectum, *Nursing Times,* **64**:1364-1368 (1968).

——— and J. A. Plant: Colostomy and Its Management, *Nursing Times,* **65**:231-234 (1969).

Farrar, John T., and Franz J. Inglefinger: Gastrointestinal Motility as Revealed by Study of Abdominal Sounds, *Gastroenterology,* **29**:791-800 (1955).

Ganong, William F., "Review of Medical Physiology," 3d ed., Lange Medical Publications, Los Altos, Calif., 1967.

Geigy Chemical Corporation: "Bowel Evacuation: A Teaching and Reference Manual," Ardsley, New York, 1966.

Giblin, Elizabeth C., Abnormalities in Gastrointestinal and Urinary Output, in Harriet C. Moidel et al., "Nursing Care of the Patient with Medical-Surgical Disorders," McGraw-Hill Book Company, New York, 1971.

Goodman, Louis S., and Alfred Gilman, "The Pharmacological Basis of Therapeutics," 4th ed., The Macmillan Company, New York, 1970.

Guyton, A. C.: "Textbook of Medical Physiology," 5th ed., W. B. Saunders Company, Philadelphia, 1971.

Hopkinson, B. R., and L. Lightwood: Electrical Treatment of Anal Incontinence, *Lancet,* **1**:297-304 (1966).

Katona, Elizabeth A.: Learning Colostomy Control, *American Journal of Nursing,* **67**:534-541 (1967).

MacBryde, Cecil M., and Robert S. Blacklow (eds.), "Signs and Symptoms," 5th ed., J. B. Lippincott Company, Philadelphia, 1970.

McGregor, R. A.: Graulis Muscle Transplant in Anal Incontinence, *Disease of the Colon and Rectum,* **8**:141-143 (1965).

Pike, Benjamin F., et al.: Soap Colitis, *New England Journal of Medicine,* **285**:217-218 (1971).

Roth, James L.: The Symptom Patterns of Gaseousness, *Annals of New York Academy of Science,* **150**:109-126 (1968).

——— and Henry Bockus: Aerophagia: Its Etiology, Syndrome and Management, *Medical Clinics of North America,* **41**:1673-1696 (1957).

Seargeant, P. W.: Management of a Colostomy, *Nursing Times,* **64**:36-42 (1968).

Secor, Sophia M.: Colostomy Rehabilitation, *American Journal of Nursing,* **70**:2400-2401 (1970).

Shaw, B. L.: Current Concepts of Stoma Care, *RN,* **32**:52 (1969).

Sherbaniuk, Richard W.: The Physiology of Diarrhea, *Canadian Medical Association Journal,* **91**:1-6 (1964).

Stanley, Theodore H.: Artificial Control of Fecal Incontinence, *Surgery,* **68**:852-856 (1970).

Tillery, Betty, and Barbara Bates: Enemas, *American Journal of Nursing,* **66**:534-537 (1966).

Truelove, Sydney C.: Movements of the Large Intestine, *Physiological Reviews,* **46**:457-512 (1966).

ADDITIONAL READINGS

Andriole, Vincent T., et al.: Preventing Catheter-induced Urinary Tract Infections, *Hospital Practice,* **3**:61-68 (1968).

Cleland, Virginia, et al.: Prevention of Bacteriuria in Female Patients with Indwelling Catheters, *Nursing Research,* **20**(4):309-318 (1971).

Curtis, C.: A Child with Sigmoid Colonic Urinary Conduit, *Nursing Times,* **64**:1370-1374 (1968).

Desautels, Robert E., et al.: Technical Advances in the Prevention of Urinary Tract Infection, *Journal of Urology,* **87**:487-490 (1962).

Flocks, R. H., and David A. Culp, "Surgical Urology," 3d ed., Year Book Medical Publishers, Inc., Chicago, 1967.

Frohman, I. Phillips: Constipation, *American Journal of Nursing,* **55**:65-67 (1955).

Gallo, David, and David Presman: Urinary Retention Due to Fecal Impaction in Children, *Pediatrics,* **45**:292–294 (1970).

Given, Barbara A., and Sandra J. Simmons, "Nursing Care of the Patient with Gastrointestinal Disorders," The C. V. Mosby Company, St. Louis, 1971.

Gutowski, Frances: Ostomy Procedures: Nursing Care Before and After, *American Journal of Nursing,* **72**:262–267 (1972).

King, J. M.: Ileo-cutaneous Ureterostomy, *Nursing Times,* **57**:1531–1533 (1961).

Kunin, C. M., and R. O. McCormack: Prevention of catheter-induced urinary tract infections by sterile closed drainage, *New England Journal of Medicine,* **274**:1151–1161 (May 26, 1966).

Mohammed, Mary: Urinalysis, *American Journal of Nursing,* **64**:87–89 (1964).

Murphy, B. M.: Principles of Management of the Neurogenic Bladder, *Hospital Medicine,* **3**:88–91 (1967).

Scharli, A. F.: Defecation and Continence: Some New Concepts, *Disease of the Colon and Rectum,* **13**:81–107 (1970).

Wells, Charles, et al.: Postoperative Gastrointestinal Motility, *Lancet,* **1**:4–10 (1964).

Weyrauch. H. M., and J. B. Bassett: Ascending Infection in Artificial Urinary Tract: An Experiment Study, *Stanford Medical Bulletin,* **9**:25–30 (1961).

Circulatory and Fluid-Electrolyte Status

Pamela Mitchell

Data to Be Assessed

Circulatory status		Fluid and electrolyte status
Pulse	*Blood pressure*	*Normal patterns of intake and output*
Rate	Systolic/diastolic	Pattern and type of food and fluid
Volume	Pulse pressure	Pattern of output—stool, urine,
Rhythm	Lying and standing	perspiration
Pulse deficit	Postural changes	Change in pattern due to health problem
Response to activity, stress	Discrepancy between arms	
Medications affecting heart rate	Factors altering accuracy	*Measurements*
	(obesity, cuff size)	Oral and parenteral intake
		Output, all routes
General appearance		
Color—skin, nails, lips		*Indirect data*
Signs of saline/water excess or depletion		Weight trends—rapid gain, loss
Urine output/fluid intake balance		Skin turgor
Warmth and color of extremities		Condition of mouth, mucous membranes
Data from electronic monitoring devices		Visible edema
Quality of respiration (see Part 3, Chap. 16, for		Thirst
respiratory assessment)		Venous filling, distension
		Level of consciousness
		Muscular weakness, irritability
		Laboratory values
		Medical therapy directed toward fluid,
		electrolyte imbalances

Concepts which relate to circulatory status and fluid equilibrium cannot be easily separated. Adequate circulation depends partially upon the volume and distribution of the fluid circulated; conversely, the volume and distribution of the fluid depend upon how well it is pumped and upon the vascular resistance which it meets. Because of the close relationship of these two components of body function, they will be considered together in this chapter. Disease of the heart and blood vessels will not be dealt with here, except to illustrate points, nor will the disorders which create fluid and electrolyte imbalances.[1] Rather, the focus of this chapter is on basic measures by which the nurse can assess circulatory-fluid status and upon concepts basic to the patient's problems in connection with many circulatory or fluid dynamic disorders. Thirst, edema, and shock are examples of such problems.

CIRCULATORY STATUS

The basic function of the circulatory system is to provide adequate oxygen and nutrition to the cells, and to remove wastes from them. This basic movement of fluid, nutrients, and metabolic by-products is accomplished via the capillaries which surround the cells. Circulation through tissues is called *perfusion,* i.e., a pouring through. Adequate perfusion depends upon three factors: the pump, the pipes, and the fluid. Figure 15-1 shows this relationship.

The pump is the heart; the pipes are the blood vessels. The fluid consists of the blood, the fluid around the cells, and the fluid within the cells. Because these fluids readily flow from one compartment to another, all portions may be considered as potential circulating fluid. The dynamics of intercompartmental fluid movement is discussed under "Fluid and Electrolyte Status," further on in this chapter.

[1] Information about these disorders and attendant nursing care can be found in Beland (1970) and Moidel et al. (1971).

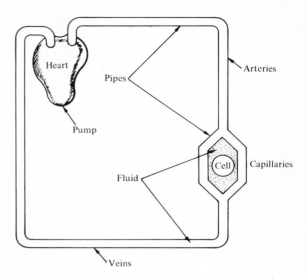

Figure 15-1 The relations between the pump, pipes, and fluid in the circulatory system. The circulatory system is relatively closed; therefore, alterations in composition or function of any of the components affect the other parts. See the text for further discussion.

The pipes, or blood vessels, become progressively smaller as they move from the heart to the capillary bed. In accordance with the laws of physics, this progressive decrease in diameter creates increasingly more resistance to the flow of fluid (blood) through the vessels. Therefore, the heart must actively pump blood to overcome this resistance and perfuse the cells. If vascular resistance decreases when, for example, capillaries and peripheral vessels dilate, blood pools; and cardiac force will not be sufficient to perfuse the organs unless cardiac output increases. Conversely, increased vascular resistance, such as that found in arteriosclerosis (hardening of the arteries) or induced by certain drugs may be too great for the pump to overcome. Poor peripheral circulation will result.

The sympathetic nervous system is the primary regulator of vascular resistance. Normally, increases or decreases in fluid volume, cardiac output, or metabolic needs of specific organs are met with appropriately increased or decreased peripheral resistance, and appropriate shunting of blood to needed areas. Pathological alterations in circulation occur when these sympathetic impulses are altered, when transmission of them is interrupted via anesthesia, drugs, or nervous system injury, or when vessels do not respond to the signals. Often, circulation to the periphery is more severely interrupted than circulation to vital organs. For example, people with generalized arteriosclerosis may first notice difficulty with cold hands or feet, delayed healing of feet, or pain when walking.

Assessment of Circulatory Status

Functional status of the heart and blood vessels may be assessed both directly and indirectly. Function may be assessed directly by using cardiac catheterization (placement of small cannulas directly into the chambers of the heart) to measure oxygen and carbon dioxide content and blood pressure in the various chambers. This type of data is gathered by the physician to assist him in diagnosing specific disorders of the heart and great vessels. Indirect data may be gathered by both nurse and physician. The electrocardiogram indirectly measures electrical activity of the heart, which in turn gives some information about the pump action (but not the force of pumping). Laboratory analysis of gases and electrolytes in the blood can reflect a variety of circulatory, pulmonary, and electrolyte imbalances.

Observations of the patient-client's general appearance and of his vital signs are indirect measures frequently used by nurses in assessing circulatory status. Color and temperature of skin, weight gain or loss, and the response of pulse, blood pressure, and respiration to activity are examples of such indirect data. These observations offer clues as to the adequacy of vital organ perfusion essential to normal everyday activity. These data may be of help to the physician in estimating the severity of disease.

They are of great help to the nurse in determining how much help the person needs in meeting the demands of ordinary life. They also help the nurse to plan with the patient-client to avoid overtaxing his functional capabilities.

For example, a man who says he has "heart trouble" may come to a physician because of increasing dyspnea (difficult breathing during activity); he can walk only a few yards without labored respiration. The physician may want to hospitalize the man and perform specific tests of cardiac and lung function before establishing the cause of the disorder underlying this symptom. The nurse can use the data about his dyspnea upon exertion to help the patient-client adapt to hospital life within his physical limitations. If bathrooms are not in each patient's room, the man would need to be in a room close to a common bathroom. In addition, he might need planned and uninterrupted rest periods in each day.

Vital Signs

Measurements of the pulse, blood pressure, and respirations are often called "vital signs," for they indirectly reflect the function of vital organs—heart, blood vessels, and lungs. Pulse and blood pressure will be discussed in this chapter. Part 3, Chapter 16, is devoted to respiratory function.

Pulse   Each time the heart ejects blood from the left ventricle (systole), a pulse wave is generated. The rate, strength, and rhythm of these waves are palpable in arteries located in several superficial areas of the body. The most commonly used points are illustrated in Fig. 15-2. Rate and rhythm can be more accurately measured by the electrocardiograph, and this electronic monitoring is used for patients in whom small changes in rhythm may have immediate serious consequences. Such patients include those with myocardial infarction.

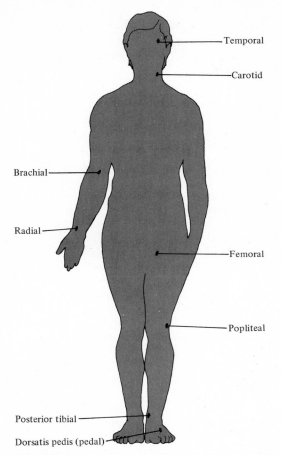

- Temporal
- Carotid
- Brachial
- Radial
- Femoral
- Popliteal
- Posterior tibial
- Dorsatis pedis (pedal)

Figure 15-2 Common points for palpating pulses. The artery most commonly used to palpate the pulse is the radial. However, this artery does not provide information about the circulation to the legs and feet, nor is it always easily palpable in severe illness. Therefore, the nurse should also be able to locate other points.

Pulse rate is expressed in beats per minute. However, most practitioners count the beats for fifteen or thirty seconds and multiply accordingly to obtain the rate. There has been controversy regarding the accuracy of this practice. Jones (1967) compared the accuracy of fifteen-, thirty-, and sixty-second counts with a simultaneously obtained electrocardiograph recording. The fifteen-second count was significantly more accurate than the sixty-second count for the

normal pulse. However, even the most accurate count was significantly less accurate than the actual rate taken from the cardiograph. When the rate was rapid, after exercise, all the counting intervals gave grossly inaccurate rates compared with the electronic measure.

There are several relevant implications of this study. First, pulse rates obtained by palpation should probably be considered as estimates. In general, the trend of readings—e.g., stable, steady increase, increase with activity, steady decrease—is more important than any one absolute figure. Consequently, this estimation by palpation is acceptable for both nursing and medical data. When accuracy is necessary, electronic monitoring should be used.

The second implication relates to the counting interval; fifteen seconds is the recommended interval for normal pulses. Jones states that there is no advantage to counting the normal pulse for sixty seconds; in fact, inaccuracy increases with the long interval. When the pulse is markedly irregular, or when marked deviations from normal are present, a longer interval may be indicated. There are at present no studies similar to Jones's involving abnormal rates.

The rate detected in a peripheral artery may not be the same as the actual number of ventricular contractions. These ventricular beats can be heard, however, through a stethoscope placed over the apex of the heart (at midclavicular level, between the third and fifth ribs). The magnitude of the discrepancy between apical and radial pulse readings is called a *pulse deficit*. It occurs in atrial fibrillation when ventricular contractions are too weak to open the semilunar valves and expel enough blood to produce a palpable pulse wave. The pulse deficit reflects inefficient ventricular contraction, since blood is not circulated with each beat.

Alterations in rate reflect cardiac compensation for increased or decreased metabolic demands, cardiac disease which alters the transmission of impulses generated in the sinoatrial node to the ventricles, or dysfunction of cerebral centers regulating heart rate. Since cardiac output is a product of the heart rate and the volume ejected with each beat,[2] an increase in rate increases the output to meet body demands during exercise, febrile illness, or the normally increased metabolism of children. The increased heart rate seen with decreased blood volume represents a compensatory attempt to maintain normal cardiac output. The supine position, if prolonged, adds the blood from the legs to the central circulation and will slowly increase heart rate by increasing stroke volume (see Part 3, Chapter 12). A marked increase in rate is called *tachycardia.*

The nurse can use the rate response as one means to gauge the patient's response to normal activity, particularly in a patient-client recovering from an illness. Rate normally increases about 20 to 30 beats per minute with mild-to-moderate activity (equivalent of 10 knee bends or 50 hops on one foot), and returns to normal within two minutes (Friedburg, 1966, p. 334). If the patient has marked tachycardia, or if the pulse rate does not return to resting levels for several minutes, he may need to resume activity more slowly. Pulse rate as a measure of tolerance to exercise is a particularly important observation in people with cardiac and pulmonary disease.

A slow pulse, generally below 60 beats per minute, is called *bradycardia.* Bradycardia occurs when metabolic demands decrease, as in hypothermia, when hypoxia or mechanical pressure alters regulatory centers in the brain, or when some of the sinoatrial impulses to the ventricle are blocked. Obviously, when rate falls, cardiac output will fall unless stroke volume is increased. Increase in stroke volume is exactly what occurs in the bradycardia commonly seen

in athletes; each beat is stronger and ejects more blood. In ill people, bradycardia usually suggests some condition which is compromising cardiac output or central nervous system regulation of heart rate.

The clinical significance of the discovery of bradycardia during a routine hospital assessment is illustrated in the following example:

Mr. T. M., a 52-year-old accountant, was hospitalized for evaluation of dizziness and fainting episodes. There seemed to be no pattern to these attacks. Neurologic examination and an electrocardiogram revealed no abnormalities, and the physician wondered if these episodes were not a psychological reaction to emotional stress.

One day, while taking routine afternoon temperature, pulse, and respiration readings, a nursing student noted Mr. M.'s pulse to be 32 beats per minute. Certain that he had miscounted, the student took the pulse for a full minute and got the same rate. He asked the assistant head nurse to confirm his finding. Until this point, Mr. M. had been fully alert and appeared to be in no distress. However, he now complained of dizziness and looked pale.

The nurse immediately called the intern, who took an electrocardiogram, which documented a 2:1 heart block: for every two beats initiated by the sinoatrial node, only one reached the ventricle. Mr. M. had been having transient attacks of heart block, which had decreased cardiac output and caused the dizziness and fainting. This current attack persisted, however. Treatment was rapidly instituted to counteract the heart block and increase cardiac output before irreparable tissue hypoxia occurred. In Mr. M.'s case, this treatment included drug therapy and electrical stimulation, or "pacing," of the ventricle to ensure a heart rate of 60.

The rhythm of the pulse is probably of more diagnostic significance than the rate. Small variations in rhythm are within normal limits but are rarely palpable. Frequent, palpable irregularities should be brought to the attention of the physi-

---

[2] $CO = HR/\text{min} \times SV$, ml/min, where CO = cardiac output, HR = heart rate, and SV = stroke volume.

cian if this is a change from the person's usual status. If he is being treated for arrhythmias, careful observation of irregularity is extremely important.

The character of the irregularity is as important as its presence. Irregular beats may be completely random, or they may follow a regular pattern. For example, *bigeminal rhythm* consists of two beats followed by a pause. These coupled beats may occur quite regularly, or they may be interspersed among regular single beats. This rhythm represents an ectopic (out-of-place) beat which originates elsewhere than the sinoatrial node. The ectopic focus is usually in the ventricle. This bigeminal rhythm may indicate, among other conditions, digitalis[3] toxicity. In order to assist in drug therapy, it is important that a nurse note and report the characteristics of this arrhythmia.

The quality or strength of each beat can be only roughly assessed by palpation. A forceful pulse may be described as "full" or "bounding," a weak one as "thready."

Palpation of peripheral pulses (arms and legs) gives information about the patency of the vessels. Figure 15-2 shows the location of some peripheral pulse points. Weak or absent pulses in the palpable arteries of the ankle and foot indicate that circulation to that area is greatly diminished. Evaluation of pedal and popliteal pulses gives some clues to the severity of peripheral vascular disease and the efficacy of vascular surgery.

Blood Pressure Measurement of blood pressure is a better indicator of the force of the cardiac beat than is the estimation of the strength of the pulse. Intra-arterial measurements are, of course, the most accurate, but they are used clinically only in specialized acute-care

---

[3] Digitalis is a drug often used to slow and strengthen ventricular contraction.

units. Arterial pressure is most commonly measured indirectly by use of the stethoscope and sphygmomanometer (blood pressure cuff). Properly used, measurements by this technique are within 10 mm Hg of intra-arterial pressure values. This is accurate enough for most situations. As is true for all vital-sign determinations, trends are usually more important than single absolute figures.

Blood pressure is essentially a reflection of the cardiac output (stroke volume multiplied by the heart rate) and the vascular resistance which it meets. Thus:

$$BP = CO \times R \quad or \quad BP = SV \times HR \times R$$
$$\text{where } BP = \text{blood pressure}$$
$$CO = \text{cardiac output}$$
$$R = \text{vascular resistance}$$
$$SV = \text{stroke volume}$$
$$HR = \text{heart rate}$$

The mechanisms which maintain systemic blood pressure exemplify the interacting relationship of pump force, condition of the pipes, and quantity and location of fluid. Figure 15-3 illustrates the relationship of these factors.

The force with which blood is ejected against the arterial wall during systole is called *systolic pressure.* This represents the height of the pressure wave. The lowest force, occurring when the heart is in diastole, is called the *diastolic pressure.* The difference between the two figures is the *pulse pressure.* An increase or decrease in pulse pressure gives important diagnostic information in such states as increased intracranial pressure, shock, and hypertension.

Blood pressure is normally measured in millimeters of mercury, i.e., the number of millimeters a column of mercury would rise if subjected to the force exerted in the artery. The inflatable bladder of the sphygmomanometer is pumped to a pressure somewhat exceeding the person's systolic pressure. As the pressure is

Blood Pressure

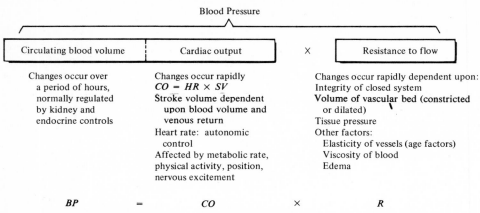

Circulating blood volume	Cardiac output	X	Resistance to flow
Changes occur over a period of hours, normally regulated by kidney and endocrine controls	Changes occur rapidly $CO = HR \times SV$ Stroke volume dependent upon blood volume and venous return Heart rate: autonomic control Affected by metabolic rate, physical activity, position, nervous excitement		Changes occur rapidly dependent upon: Integrity of closed system **Volume of vascular bed (constricted or dilated)** Tissue pressure Other factors: Elasticity of vessels (age factors) Viscosity of blood Edema

$$BP \qquad = \qquad CO \qquad \times \qquad R$$

Figure 15-3 Relationship of factors which maintain blood pressure. Alterations in any one factor will stimulate compensatory measures in the others in order to keep blood pressure constant. For example, if circulating blood volume decreases, thereby decreasing stroke volume, heart rate must increase to maintain the cardiac output. If the cardiac output decreases, resistance to flow must increase to maintain blood pressure. *(Modified, with permission from Louise Mansfield, in H. Moidel, et al. (eds.), "Nursing Care of the Patient with Medical-Surgical Disorders, McGraw-Hill Book Company, New York, 1971.)*

slowly released, tapping or beating noises are heard. The point at which two consecutive tapping sounds are heard is considered the systolic pressure. The point at which the sounds are *muffled* is now considered to be the diastolic pressure (Kirkendall et al., 1967). At one time, the disappearance of sound was recorded as diastolic pressure; however, recent studies show that muffling of sound is consistently closer to intra-arterial pressure (7 to 10 mm Hg higher) than is the disappearance. The American Heart Association recommends recording the pressures as follows to avoid confusion: systolic/muffling/disappearance; e.g., 122/68/60 or 142/-78/78. This is particularly important when several persons, trained at different times, may be measuring blood pressures.

Measurements of blood pressure, pulse, and respiration frequently become routine observations made on the basis of a time schedule rather than on the basis of cues from the patient indicating the need to evaluate circulatory, fluid,

and respiratory status. If the nurse sees these measurements as valuable data in assessing the patient-client's ability to oxygenate his tissues in response to normal or abnormal living demands, he will be better able to help the patient meet these demands, as well as aid the physician in diagnosing disorders involving these systems.

FLUID AND ELECTROLYTE STATUS

In the course of evolution, as living things became more complex and emerged from the sea, they carried some of the sea with them in the fluids which bathe the cells. The fluids which surround each of man's cells still are quite similar to that ancient sea. Even though man enclosed his sea within his skin, he is just as dependent upon it for life as was his most primitive sea-living ancestor. This solution carries oxygen, nutrients, and other essential chemicals into the cells, removes the wastes from them, and provides the chemical environment necessary for cells to do their specific jobs.

The composition and volume of fluid may vary only within a narrow range, if the cells are to perform their functions optimally. Despite wide fluctuations in the amount of fluid drunk, quantity of electrolytes eaten in food, and amount of fluid and dissolved substances excreted, this narrow range is maintained. Various mechanisms help the body compensate for these variations and maintain homeostasis. Although many illness or environmental situations may dangerously alter the normal balance, the ability of the body to compensate for most alterations is remarkable.

In this section of this chapter, we will review some of the basic concepts related to fluid-electrolyte homeostasis in order to apply them to nursing responsibilities. The last part of the chapter will be devoted to problems common to alterations in both circulatory and fluid status.

BASIC ELEMENTS OF FLUID HOMEOSTASIS

Three elements of the fluid system are of importance in this discussion: (1) distribution of fluids, (2) volume of fluid, and (3) concentration of dissolved substances. The interrelationship among these elements is complex indeed. However, fluid and electrolyte balance need not be the mysterious subject which nurses so often feel it to be, if we look at these components systematically. It is also helpful to keep in mind the uses to which the nurse will put the information, namely: (1) to design plans to maintain normal fluid balance, (2) to support the physician in therapy of fluid and electrolyte disorders, and (3) to help the patient-client cope with problems induced by therapy, such as thirst.

This discussion is not intended to be an encyclopedic review of the normal physiology of fluid balance. Rather it is meant to highlight those points which the student will find helpful in application to the problems of patient-clients. Nurses usually study the basic sciences when they have no exposure to clinical situations, and the essential points are often only half-remembered. Therefore, some individual review of the physiology may be in order while studying this chapter.

Distribution of Fluid and Solute

The fluids and all that is dissolved in them comprise about 60 percent of an adult's weight and about 70 percent of the infant's total body weight. They are distributed everywhere in the body, but for simplicity are considered to be in three major "compartments," or spaces—*intracellular* (in the cells), *interstitial* (around the cells), and *intravascular* (in the blood vessels). Because there is so little difference in composition of the fluid portion of the intravascular and interstitial compartments, they are frequently classified as one *extracellular* space. The proportionate distribution of fluid in each of the compartments in the adult and infant is shown in Fig. 15-4.

The fluid within these compartments is a solution of water, protein, cells, and dissolved organic and inorganic chemicals. The dissolved chemicals (such as $NaCl$, KCl, H_2CO_3) dissociate into positively and negatively charged particles called *electrolytes*. Extracellular fluid is a mildly alkaline (pH 7.35), saline solution. The composition of intravascular fluid and that of interstitial fluid are almost identical, except for the presence of red blood cells and other protein molecules in the vascular compartment. Intracellular fluid is primarily a potassium solution. The significance of these differences will be discussed further on under "Concentration of Electrolytes."

The fluid compartments are not rigidly separated from each other. The semipermeable membrane of the vascular capillary walls, lymphatic

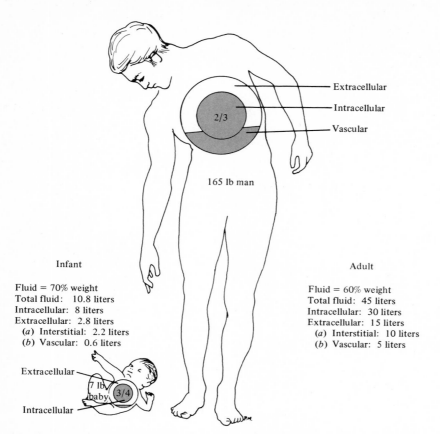

Extracellular

Intracellular

Vascular

2/3

165 lb man

Infant

Fluid = 70% weight
Total fluid: 10.8 liters
Intracellular: 8 liters
Extracellular: 2.8 liters
   (a) Interstitial: 2.2 liters
   (b) Vascular: 0.6 liters

Adult

Fluid = 60% weight
Total fluid: 45 liters
Intracellular: 30 liters
Extracellular: 15 liters
   (a) Interstitial: 10 liters
   (b) Vascular: 5 liters

Extracellular

7 lb
baby

3/4

Intracellular

Figure 15-4 Proportionate amount of fluid in each compartment. Fluid comprises about 60 percent of an average adult man's body weight, and approximately 70 percent of an average infant's weight. Two-thirds of the fluid is inside the cells of an adult; three-quarters is intracellular in an infant. *(Based upon B. H. Scribner (ed.), "A Teaching Syllabus for the Course on Fluid and Electrolyte Balance," 7th rev., University of Washington School of Medicine, Seattle, 1969.)*

capillary walls, and tissue cells permits free flow of fluid and dissolved electrolytes, as well as some exchanges of larger particles such as protein. Alterations in intravascular volume generally affect distribution in all the compartments: the body attempts to protect this compartment first, in order to maintain sufficient volume for effective circulation. Fluid is first drawn to the vascular compartment from the interstitial space and then from the cells themselves if necessary.

Distribution of fluid is dependent upon vol-ume (particularly intravascular volume, as noted above) and concentration of electrolytes and protein, as will be shown later in this chapter. Movement between compartments is constant—in fact is necessary, if cellular nutrients and wastes are to be exchanged between the blood and the cells. The mechanisms for this fluid movement are (1) diffusion, (2) osmosis, and (3) filtration.

Diffusion Diffusion is the simple dispersion

of the dissolved substances throughout a fluid until the concentration (proportion of dissolved particles) is equal in all parts of the container. Mixing a drop of food color or a teaspoon of salt in a glass of water is an example of diffusion. Since cell membranes are freely permeable to the small-particle (nonprotein) electrolytes in body fluid, these substances can diffuse between compartments whenever concentrations are unequal. The protein molecules cannot diffuse freely, because the membrane is normally almost impermeable to them.

Diffusion is important in maintaining *electrochemical neutrality,* the state in which the number of anions (negative charge) and cations (positive charge) is equal within each fluid compartment. If this neutrality is disturbed, some substance must combine with the excess ion to neutralize the charge, or appropriate ions must diffuse into the compartment to balance the charge.

Osmosis Osmosis is the movement of water from an area of lesser solute concentration to an area of greater solute concentration through a membrane permeable to the water but not to the solute. In other words, the *water* moves to dilute the more concentrated solution. Whereas diffusion involves the movement of solute (dissolved particles), osmosis involves the movement of the water or other solvent.

Osmotic force is the attraction of particles in solution for water, shown in Fig. 15-5. These particles may be ions or noncharged molecules (such as glucose). Since plasma proteins diffuse very little, they tend to exert their osmotic force within the blood vessels. This force is termed *oncotic* force, to distinguish it from the osmotic force exerted by diffusible ions.

The total concentration of dissolved substances is termed the osmolarity (or osmolality) of the solution. Concentration refers to the

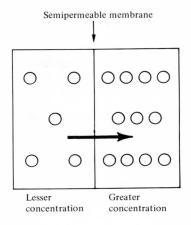

Semipermeable membrane

Lesser concentration   Greater concentration

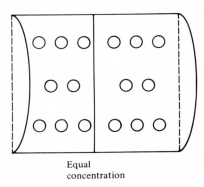

Equal concentration

Figure 15-5 Osmosis. In the first figure, concentrations of solute (circles) are unequal on either side of the semipermeable membrane. Water then moves to "dilute" the side of greater concentration. The arrow indicates the direction of water movement. The second figure shows the concentration equilibrium which has resulted from osmosis. The curved surfaces indicate the volume changes which have occurred with water movement.

number of dissolved particles per unit of solution. The conventional unit of concentration is Osmols (number of particles) per liter. Because of the relatively small numbers of particles in the body, milliOsmols per liter (mOsm/L) are the units used clinically.

Osmolarity is controlled by the movement of

the body water, rather than of solutes. Even though most of the electrolytes are freely diffusible through the cell membranes, they tend to stay in their compartments, whatever their concentration, and let the water come to them.

Filtration   Hydrostatic pressure, or filtration force, is the third factor affecting the distribution of fluid between compartments. The laws of physics require that fluids flow from an area of greater pressure to an area of lesser pressure. Hydrostatic pressure (the force exerted by a column of water) in the arterial end of the capillary bed is greater than total tissue pressure (interstitial fluid plus solid tissue). This fluid, plus whatever solute is permeable to the membrane, is literally pushed from the capillary into the interstitial space. The cell probably transports specific solutes in and out by means of "carrier systems" (Guyton, 1971). This involves an active mechanism, rather than purely mechanical filtration force.

At the venous end of the capillary, net tissue pressure is greater than hydrostatic pressure in the capillary. Fluid and solute (including products of cellular metabolism) are forced back into the vascular compartment. Normally, the flow in and out of the capillary is balanced so that the net interstitial pressure is negative (Guyton, p. 246). If, for any number of reasons, fluid and protein begin to accumulate in the interstitial spaces, net positive pressure will result. This increasing pressure interferes with normal fluid movement and further increases the *edema,* or fluid accumulation. Problems related to edema are discussed near the end of this chapter, under "Problems Related to Both Circulatory and Fluid-Electrolyte Status."

In summary, the distribution of fluids within the body compartments is affected by vascular volume, concentration of solutes, and hydrostatic pressures in the vascular and interstitial compartments.

Volume of Fluid

The volume of fluid in a 165-lb man is about 45 liters. The largest proportion in both adults and infants is intracellular. Figure 15-4 shows the proportionate volumes for each.

Regulation of Volume   The volume of each fluid compartment is determined primarily by the relative amount of solute, or its osmolarity. The vascular volume (about 4 to 5 liters in the adult, 0.6 liter in the infant) is the most crucial, for it must be maintained within a narrow range to prevent circulatory underload or overload. Concentrations of sodium ion and plasma proteins are the most important factors in maintaining blood volume in an intact system, by virtue of the osmotic force which they exert. Water continually moves in and out of the three compartments, and by this small shifting maintains a dynamic volume equilibrium.

The total volume of body fluid is regulated by balancing fluid gains against fluid losses. Since body fluid is a solution of water and the various chemicals dissolved in the water, the intake and excretion of water and these chemicals are also balanced. The components of body fluid are ingested daily, in food and drink, and are formed during the metabolic activity of cells. Despite rather large variations in amount and composition of food and fluid, we still maintain the internal fluids within the narrow ranges compatible with optimum function.

Fluid and electrolytes are lost from the body via the lungs, skin, feces, and urine. Average adult gains and losses from these routes are shown in Table 15-1. It is extremely important for nurses to realize that fluid is gained from food and oxidation, as well as in free (liquid) forms. Thus, if a patient-client eats less than usual or ceases eating, it is necessary to increase the amount of free fluid taken in order to maintain the same balance.

Table 15-1 Average Daily Fluid Intake and Output of a Normal Adult*

Intake, ml		Output, ml	
Free fluid	1,650	Urine	1,700
Preformed		Feces	150
(in food)	750	Insensible (skin)	500
Oxidation	350	Respiration	400
Total	2,750	Total	2,750

*These figures vary widely from person to person. However, the fluid intake from all sources equals the output via all routes in a normal person. Note that a significant portion of fluid intake is preformed, in food. Oxidative fluid is that formed during metabolic processes within the body.
  Source: Values from Wolf, 1958.

The body has several means of selecting necessary amounts of fluid and solute, and then excreting or storing the rest. In general, the body regulates intake through thirst, and regulates output by increasing or decreasing urinary output of fluid and electrolytes, increasing absorption of gastrointestinal fluids, and increasing or decreasing the amount of expired carbon dioxide and water. The insensible (unobservable) loss of water through the skin is obligatory; it does not change regardless of internal fluid balance. The amount lost in perspiration varies with activity and environmental temperature. This amount is regulated more by temperature-regulating mechanisms than by those varying fluid output.

Volume Imbalance Volume imbalances may occur at the entry or exit from the fluid system or within the system itself. The diagram in Fig. 15-6 indicates the sources of volume imbalance. Intake may be decreased in the face of normal output, or output may be markedly increased with a normal intake. In such situations, specific volume and concentration receptors (osmoreceptors), located in the brain, will activate compensatory mechanisms. Antidiuretic hormone (ADH), secreted by the posterior pituitary gland, and aldosterone, secreted by the adrenals, promote retention of fluid and electrolytes in the kidney. The midbrain and forebrain circuit regulating thirst and eating will stimulate thirst. If fluid is freely available, the person or animal will drink an amount sufficient to restore volume and concentration. There is some experimental evidence that an organism may selectively eat foods

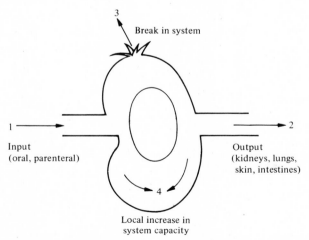

Figure 15-6 Major causes of volume imbalance. (1) Input exceeds output: net volume gain; (2) output exceeds intake: net volume loss; (3) output through a break in the system exceeds replacement input: net volume loss; and (4) system capacity increases locally—fluid pools in dilated capillaries or body space and is essentially lost to the general circulation: net volume loss.

high in the specific electrolytes missing, e.g., salty foods after excessive sweating. This specific appetite is not so well documented, nor is it evident, in more highly developed species such as man (LeGros Clark, 1968).

Volume imbalance may also occur because of gain or losses within the fluid system itself. Gain within the total system can occur only if the exit is altered or blocked, e.g., in renal failure or renal retention of fluid. If the intake of either water or sodium continues normally and the output of either is decreased, fluid volume will continue to build up in the system, creating edema. This excess fluid will accumulate primarily in the interstitial spaces, with perhaps a slight increase in intravascular volume.

Intravascular loss occurs when there is a break in the integrity of the system, which allows fluid to escape either to the outside of the body, as in hemorrhage from a blood vessel, or to a body space which is not part of the vascular system, such as the abdominal cavity. This may occur either through actual hemorrhage or by the loss of large amounts of the plasma (noncellular) portion of the blood. Intrasystem volume loss may also occur if a localized portion of the vascular system expands through vasodilatation and blood pools in the dilated portion. The pooled blood is essentially lost to the circulating volume.

Intrasystem imbalances are usually the result of pathologic change or disturbed functioning of mechanisms which regulate fluid and electrolyte balance. Because of this, the mechanisms which compensate for simple intake-output imbalances are often not adequate to remedy intrasystem imbalances.

Sodium as the Chief Volume Regulator Sodium ion is the principal determinant of the volume of extracellular fluid. Sodium comprises approximately 98 percent of the extracellular cation. Thus, the sodium ion and its corresponding anion account for almost all the extracellular osmotic activity. The regulatory mechanisms of the body attempt to maintain the concentration within the range of 130 to 145 mEq per liter or mOsm per liter. A milliequivalent of sodium equals a milliOsmol, since each available charge also represents one particle in solution. Therefore, any increase or decrease in the total number of sodium ions will be matched by an increase or decrease in amount of water in that compartment.

If sodium ion increases in any compartment, water increases to maintain the concentration. This extra water may be ingested, as a transient serum sodium rise stimulates thirst via the osmoreceptors, or it may be retained by the kidney by action of antidiuretic hormone (ADH). Both mechanisms may operate simultaneously, if necessary, to restore sodium concentration. Water will be drawn from the cells themselves if necessary to restore sodium concentration.

If sodium level decreases, osmoreceptors stimulate the release of aldosterone, which causes the kidneys to retain sodium until concentration is restored. Therefore, a simple decrease in ingested sodium will not produce a measurable saline (sodium in solution) deficit, unless renal sodium-conserving mechanisms are altered. Actual saline depletion usually occurs only when sodium-containing fluids are lost from the body or into a body space.

Ordinarily, these gains and losses of sodium ion and volume are transient, and the volume-regulatory mechanisms operate to restore volume to normal levels. However, in situations where sodium-regulating mechanisms are disturbed, volume problems will occur.

Scribner (1969) categorizes these problems of sodium balance as *saline excess* and *saline depletion*. Body mechanisms work to restore concentration of salt in solution; thus, the volume of *saline* changes, but not the concentration of sodium. Changes in sodium ion concentration are termed problems of water balance; they will be discussed later.

Situations which result in saline volume increase include intrasystem disease, such as chronic renal failure, which decreases normal renal excretion of sodium. Saline losses from the fluid system itself, as in hemorrhage, drainage of hollow organs, vomiting, and burns, also cause volume problems.

Saline Excess When an excess of saline cannot be eliminated, it will remain in the extracellular compartment, eventually collecting in the interstitial space as edema. Both intravascular and interstitial volume will increase with saline excess. However, increasing hydrostatic pressure will ultimately force much of the fluid into the interstitial space. Considerable saline may accumulate before edema is visible. Consequently, rapid weight gain is the most reliable physical indicator of volume increase. One-half kilogram (about 1 lb) gain in twenty-four hours is considered equal to 1 liter of saline. The serum sodium level is normal, as would be expected.

Saline excess is a problem to the patient if the excess volume overburdens the pumping capacity of his heart and leads to pulmonary edema, or creates peripheral edema severe enough to interfere with cellular nutrition by mechanically pushing cells away from their capillaries. Edema is discussed more extensively under "Problems Related to Both Circulatory and Fluid-Electrolyte Status," further on in this chapter.

Saline Depletion Saline depletion occurs through actual loss of body fluid containing sodium: in vomitus, diarrhea, blood, sweat, or urine. As noted earlier, a decreased intake of sodium will not result in saline depletion unless kidney disease prevents normal conservation of sodium. Saline depletion is often called *dehydration*. However, the term dehydration literally means "loss of water." Most problems which are called dehydration are really combined loss of sodium and water, i.e., saline. Literal dehydration may occur; it is discussed further on, under "Water Deficit."

Saline depletion becomes a problem to the patient-client when the loss is severe enough to compromise the vascular volume available for circulation. This situation is called *hypovolemia*—decreased volume. As explained under "Circulatory Status," at the start of this chapter, adequate perfusion of the cells requires an adequate blood pressure. Adequate blood pressure requires sufficient volume for pumping to all parts of the vascular system. In the initial stages of hypovolemia, compensatory constriction of peripheral vessels will maintain blood pressure. With rapid loss of 500 to 1,000 ml, these mechanisms are no longer adequate, and shock may ensue (see "Shock," later in this chapter).

When a patient-client is losing sodium-rich fluid from any source, one aims to detect saline depletion before hypovolemia becomes severe enough to produce shock. Measurement of postural changes in blood pressure and assessment of neck-vein filling are two criteria which are easily used. In addition, the physician may add some laboratory analyses of blood composition.

A drop in blood pressure when the patient changes from lying to sitting or standing position is one of the early signs of hypovolemia. Even though compensatory mechanisms may maintain blood pressure in the supine position, volume is not sufficient to maintain the pressure in the upright position. Scribner (1969) considers a postural systolic drop of 15 mm Hg and a diastolic drop of 10 mm Hg indicative of volume deficit.

Another quick, but not so reliable, indicator of saline depletion is the presence of flat neck veins, or ones which are not normally filled. Ordinarily, if the person lies flat, the neck veins are filled to the jaw level. When blood volume is inadequate, these veins may be filled to a lower level, or they may be flat and fill only when compressed.

The classic signs and symptoms of "dehydration" are not particularly valuable to either the nurse or the physician in early detection of saline depletion. The physical signs—decreased skin turgor (the skin remains in folds when pinched), dry mouth and mucous membranes, and soft eyeballs—occur when hypovolemia is so great that fluid is being drawn from the cells and shock is imminent, if not already present. The subjective symptoms of weakness, dizziness, or fainting may be caused by many conditions other than volume depletion. If these signs and symptoms are present when a nurse first encounters a patient-client whose history is compatible with saline depletion, it is imperative that he see a physician immediately. If, however, a nurse waits for these signs to develop before consulting a physician, he endangers the patient and makes the physician's therapeutic task more difficult.

Water Balance Problems of water balance are caused by alteration in the osmolarity, rather than the volume, of body fluids. Since sodium is the chief regulator of extracellular osmotic activity, changes in the serum sodium level reflect disturbances in water balance. When osmolarity increases or decreases, extracellular fluid is hyperosmolar or hypoosmolar with respect to the cellular fluid. Thus, water will flow into or out of the cells to restore osmolarity. This is a potentially serious situation, for the cells cannot perform their functions when either shrunken or swollen. If cells become too swollen, they burst, or lyse.

The most accurate measure of water balance is the serum osmolarity. Since sodium and its corresponding anion account for almost all the extracellular osmotic activity, the serum sodium level doubled is the easiest guide to extracellular osmolarity, and is accurate enough to guide the physician in therapy (Scribner, 1969, p. 7). Thus, *hyponatremia,* decreased serum sodium concentration, is indicative of water excess. *Hypernatremia,* increased serum sodium level, indicates water depletion. Paradoxically, the serum sodium level is not a good guide to the actual amount of extracellular sodium present, since regulatory mechanisms operate to keep concentration (milliOsmols per liter) constant regardless of amount of sodium. Thus, increases or decreases in sodium concentration reflect disturbances in the *water*-regulating mechanisms. Sometimes both water and sodium regulation are disturbed, and sodium concentration increases or decreases even more than it would have with regulation of aberrant water alone.

Water Excess (Hypoosmolarity) Water excess, also called "water intoxication," occurs when the kidneys cannot excrete water in proportion to intake. It may also occur when parenteral nonelectrolyte solutions, such as dextrose in water, are administered faster than the kidneys can excrete the excess water. Administration of large amounts of tap water in enemas has also been associated with water excess in infants and in the elderly (Gillespie et al., 1959). Retention of water from multiple enemas probably reflects both excess water absorption and decreased renal ability to excrete the excess.

Water excess becomes a problem when intracellular fluid excess is great enough to interfere with cellular function. Cells of the nervous system are particularly susceptible to adverse effects from swelling.

There are symptoms associated with water excess. However, they are not always present and are not so reliable a guide for the physician as the serum sodium level. The signs and symptoms are related to intracellular edema of the brain and include mental confusion, progressing to muscle twitching, vomiting, delirium, convulsions, unconsciousness, and death.

Water Deficit (Hyperosmolarity) Water loss may occur in profound perspiration (perspiration consists of greater amounts of water than of sodium), prolonged diarrhea coupled with low water intake, and metabolic disorders, such as diabetes insipidus, in which renal reabsorption of water is altered. Water deficit may also occur in people who do not have free access to water or who cannot respond to thirst, e.g., those who are unconscious. High solute intake, in high-protein liquid diets or in boiled skim milk, without concomitant increase in water intake may result in total water depletion.

As serum sodium level rises, water is drawn from both interstitial and intracellular compartments in an attempt to restore vascular osmolarity. Hypernatremia, increased specific gravity of urine, and thirst are signs of water deficit. Thirst is the prime regulator of water balance, and the increased specific gravity of urine reflects the renal decrease in water output with normal output of solute.

Medical management of water deficit involves oral and parenteral administration of fluid until serum sodium is within the normal range, or until thirst abates. Alleviation of thirst is not the best criteria, for thirst may persist even when serum sodium reaches rather low levels (Scribner, 1969). Water excess is usually managed by simply restricting fluid until osmolarity approaches normal.

Too rapid correction of water imbalance may create problems which are probably related to the effect of these rapid shifts on nerve and muscle cells. These cells appear to set up new equilibriums with the increased or decreased osmolarity. These alterations require some time to shift back to normal. This implies that the nurse and physician caring for people in water imbalance must be watchful for signs that correction is too rapid. These signs and symptoms, which are related to nerve and muscle malfunction, include increasing mental confusion, nausea and vomiting, muscle twitching, and convulsions.

Concentration of Electrolytes

Body fluid, as noted earlier, is a solution of water and numerous chemical substances. Most of the substances are electrolytes, i.e., ions, or charged particles whose chemical bonds have been broken or which have been dissociated from their molecules. The composition of interstitial fluid and that of the plasma portion of the blood are essentially the same. The most common cation is sodium. In contrast, the most common cation in intracellular fluid is potassium. Since the cell membrane is freely permeable to both sodium and potassium and since diffusion ought to equalize their concentration on both sides of the cell membrane, there is evidently a mechanism which actively keeps potassium in and sodium out of the cell.

The difference in concentration of potassium and sodium appears to be essential in the initiation and propagation of electrical activity in nerve and muscle cells. The high concentration of potassium inside the cell and its low concentration outside create a concentration gradient which promotes diffusion of potassium out of the cell. Ordinarily, this would be matched by an equivalent inward diffusion of sodium ions to maintain a negative charge on the membrane. However, because of the active transport mechanism, the cell membrane is not so permeable to sodium as to potassium, and thus keeps the sodium out. The negative intracellular ions are actively kept within the cell. Thus, the movement of potassium out of the cell positively charges the membrane; there are slightly more positive charges outside than inside. This is called the resting membrane potential. When the membrane is excited, its permeability to sodium rapidly increases; more positive sodium ions move into the cell than remain outside; and the charge on the membrane reverses. This ionic movement, in turn, excites the adjacent membrane of the nerve or muscle fiber, and the electrical current is propagated, or moved. Calcium ion (Ca^{++}) affects the permeability of the cell membrane to sodium; too high an extracellular concentration decreases permeability and thus delays or prevents propagation in the excited membrane. Calcium concentration which is too low increases permeability to sodium and prevents return of the membrane to the resting state. Tetany, or a continued muscle contraction, may result from this prolonged excitation (Guyton, 1971, pp. 52–65).

Abnormally high or low concentration of sodium, potassium, or calcium in the extracellular fluid often causes symptoms of neuromuscular irritability or weakness. This is understandable in light of the effects of electrolyte concentrations on nerve and muscle function.

Thus, we can see that the concentration of dissolved substances in the fluid determines not only the volume of each compartment (see "Volume of Fluid," earlier in the chapter) but also the function of the cells themselves. Sodium and potassium are important in establishing and propagating electrical impulses in nerve and muscle cells; calcium affects the permeability of the cell membrane to sodium, and magnesium acts as a catalyst for intracellular enzymatic reactions, such as those in carbohydrate metabolism. Magnesium may also be a factor, together with potassium, in establishing the concentration gradient which creates membrane potential.

Expressions of Concentration   Concentration of the solute is expressed in terms of chemical activity, osmotic activity, and hydrogen-ion activity.

Chemical Activity   The milliequivalent (mEq) is the unit of measurement of chemical combining ability. Most of the solute in the body consists of charged ions, the electrolytes. An equivalent weight refers to the number of cations available to combine with anions. The milliequivalent is 1/1,000 of an equivalent weight and is used because the quantities of electrolytes in the body are so small in terms of their gram weights. Concentration is expressed in milliequivalents per liter of solution (mEq/L). One milliequivalent refers to one cation or anion of a substance which is available to combine with one cation or anion of another substance. It is related to the actual weight of the ion, but is a better measure of the actual chemical activity than the older expression of milligrams (weight)

per 100 ml. Analogously, to know the total weight of men and women at a dance tells us nothing about how many dancing partners there are. However, to know the number of men and the number of women immediately tells us the potential dancing pairs.

Osmotic Activity   Osmotic activity is expressed in milliOsmols per liter of solution (mOsm/L). As we noted earlier, osmotic force is a function of the concentration of the solution. This includes uncharged as well as charged particles, molecules as well as ions.

Osmolarity is the term used to express the number of osmotically active particles per liter of solution. The prefixes iso-, hyper-, and hypo-indicate whether a solution has approximately the same osmolarity as extracellular fluid (about 300 mOsm per liter) or a greater or lesser degree. Relative osmolarity is of importance in connection with the many medications and solutions used for intravenous and topical therapy. *Tonicity* is another term used in discussing relative osmotic concentrations of solutions and extracellular fluid. However, tonicity is often expressed in percentage of solute in solution, e.g., 0.9 percent saline (normal saline), 5 percent dextrose in water (D_5W). Thus, one has to memorize which solutions are isotonic, hypertonic, and hypotonic. Intravenous solutions are traditionally labeled in percentage terms; therefore, the nurse needs to be aware of which solutions are isotonic. However, manufacturers are currently indicating osmolarity on the labels as well.

Hydrogen-ion Activity   Hydrogen-ion (H^+) concentration is expressed by the pH of the solution. The pH is the reciprocal of the logarithm of the number of hydrogen ions per liter. The number is so small that using the actual concentration would involve cumbersome decimal fractions; e.g., the concentration of normal vascular fluid is 0.00000000735 mEq per liter or pH 7.35. Because the pH is a logarithmic number, very small changes in its value reflect rather large changes in the actual concentration of hydrogen ion. The plasma or serum pH is more easily measured clinically than the interstitial pH, and is thus the standard referent for extracellular fluid pH. The pHs of other body fluids (urine, cerebrospinal fluid, gastric secretions) are quite different from that of the blood.

Potassium Concentration

While potassium-ion concentration is quite low in the extracellular fluid, it is the chief cation found inside the cells. As discussed earlier, potassium has a critical function in the regulation of resting membrane potential in nerve and muscle cells. Therefore, increases or decreases in the extracellular concentration of potassium are reflected in disordered nerve and muscular function.

The relationship of the body potassium capacity—the amount of ion which the body can actually hold—to the amount of potassium actually in the body is the determinant of potassium balance (Scribner, 1969). If capacity exceeds actual amount, potassium deficit results. Conversely, potassium excess reflects total amount of ion which exceeds capacity. It is difficult, however, to measure the total body potassium, since most of it is inside the muscle cells. Fortunately, the serum, or extracellular, potassium level reflects changes in the relationship between potassium capacity and total amount. Normal serum potassium values vary with the laboratory doing the determination; however, the normal range is approximately 3.5 to 5.0 mEq per liter. An increase above the upper limit represents an increase in total potassium over the body's capacity. The excess potassium circulates in the extracellular fluid, since there is no room for it in the cells. Values below the lower limit reflect a potassium capacity greater than the total amount of the ion, i.e., a potassium deficit.

Changes in hydrogen-ion concentration will exert their own effect upon potassium capacity of cells and thus upon serum potassium levels.

The mechanism of this effect will be discussed with hydrogen-ion imbalance later in this chapter. These effects must be taken into account by the physician when interpreting the meaning of potassium levels and in planning therapy.[4]

Because potassium is so important in normal neuromuscular and cardiac function, signs and symptoms of imbalance occur primarily in these systems. These signs and symptoms are less reliable indicators of imbalance than is the serum potassium level, corrected for hydrogen-ion effect. The presence of the signs and symptoms outlined below in a person whose history suggests possible potassium imbalance indicates the need to consult a physician and have serum potassium level determined.

Electrocardiographic changes are often seen with either excess or deficit; cardiac arrest may occur with either extreme excess or deficit. Arrhythmias, which may be palpable as pulse irregularities, may occur with potassium depletion.

Potassium Depletion Potassium depletion is most apt to occur with large losses of potassium-rich fluid (e.g., gastrointestinal fluid in diarrhea or vomiting, or in diuretic therapy, which promotes renal loss of sodium and potassium as well as water). Depletion may also occur when intravenous fluids which do not include maintenance levels of potassium are given for several days to a person who has no oral intake. So many foods contain potassium that it is almost impossible to become potassium-depleted by inadequate diet alone.

The symptoms of potassium depletion—apathy, weakness, paresthesias (unusual sensations)—do not occur until serum potassium is quite low, and are so vague that a patient-client may not contact a physician until the deficit is serious. Consequently, a nurse in contact with a

---

[4] Pocket tools called *nomograms* are available to aid in correcting serum potassium levels for hydrogen-ion changes.

person who has been vomiting or a person who is taking diuretics should suspect possible potassium depletion when the person has "vague complaints."

Potassium Excess Potassium excess is rarely seen except in people with acute renal failure, or in those whose chronic renal failure requires frequent hemodialysis (removal of wastes via an "artificial kidney"). The care of these people is complex and usually not a part of beginning practice.[5] However, a transient and potentially dangerous hyperkalemia may occur if intravenous solutions containing potassium are infused too rapidly. A sudden, high serum potassium level can precipitate cardiac arrest. For this reason, most authorities recommend adding no more than 40 mEq to a liter of solution to prevent fatal concentration even if the whole bottle were to run in rapidly.

Hydrogen-ion Concentration

The pH is the principal expression of the relative acidity or alkalinity of the body fluids—the acid-base balance. Recall that a chemical solution with a pH 7.0 is neutral; acids have a pH less than 7.0; bases, or alkalis, have a pH greater than 7.0. However, since normal plasma pH is 7.4, abnormally high or low values reflect fluid which is *relatively* more acid or more alkaline than normal. Since the upper and lower pH limits compatible with life are generally accepted as 7.0 and 7.8, it is obvious that literal acidemia (acid blood) is fatal. Some body fluids, such as urine and gastric secretions, are acid in the true chemical sense. In this discussion, we will deal only with the hydrogen-ion concentration of the cellular and extracellular fluids, not with that of body secretions and excretions.

The enzyme systems which help cells to perform their specific functions have evolved to

operate within a slightly alkaline environment, pH 7.4. When this environment changes, cells do not function optimally. If the hydrogen-ion concentration increases, pH falls and the environment is more acid; if the ion concentration falls, pH rises and the fluid environs are more alkaline.

Under most circumstances, the body effectively compensates for transient, small changes in hydrogen-ion concentration by two major mechanisms: (1) buffering, or chemically absorbing or releasing hydrogen ion, and (2) eliminating or retaining hydrogen ion as such by the kidneys.

Buffering Buffers are chemical substances which combine with or release free hydrogen ion to maintain a specific hydrogen ion/bicarbonate ratio. The major buffering system is the bicarbonate system (HCO_3^-). Other buffer systems include hemoglobin, protein, and bone.

The bicarbonate system, like all true chemical buffers, continually carries out chemical reactions within the extracellular fluid. The equation for this reaction is as follows:

$$H^+ + HCO_3^- \rightleftharpoons H_2CO_3 \rightleftharpoons H_2O + CO_2$$

Hydrogen ion Bicarbonate Carbonic acid Water Carbon dioxide

Because the reaction is reversible, the bicarbonate (HCO_3^-) or carbonic acid (H_2CO_3) will take up or liberate hydrogen ion as is necessary. Carbonic acid is a weak acid, which means that it is not completely ionized in solution. Consequently, formation of carbonic acid temporarily removes some free hydrogen ion from the solution. If free hydrogen ion decreases, the reaction shifts to the left and more carbonic acid dissociates to free additional hydrogen ion. Remember that buffering reactions simply shift the hydrogen ion about to restore pH. If more hydrogen ion is present than can be buffered, it must be removed indirectly via the kidneys.

A second kind of buffering system is not a chemical buffer at all. Intracellular buffering is the process by which intracellular ionic shifts temporarily add or remove hydrogen ion from

---

[5] See Beland (1970) and Kintzel (1971) for information related to care of such patients.

the extracellular fluid. Actual chemical buffering may occur within the cells. To maintain electrochemical neutrality, a hydrogen ion which is entering or leaving a cell must either take an anion (negatively charged ion) with it or exchange places with another cation. Both these events appear to happen: when extracellular hydrogen-ion concentration rises, hydrogen and small amounts of chloride ion diffuse into the cells, and sodium and potassium ions move out. The reverse is true if extracellular hydrogen ion decreases. Although larger absolute amounts of sodium than potassium shift, the relative increase or decrease of extracellular potassium is greater. Thus, the concentration gradient of potassium necessary for neuromuscular function may be affected by the buffering of hydrogen ion, as well as by absolute increases or decreases in body potassium content. This is why the physician must correct serum potassium values for hydrogen-ion concentration when he tries to estimate potassium excess or deficit.

Elimination or Retention of Hydrogen Ion Buffering is a temporary measure in restoring normal pH. Maintenance or restoration of hydrogen-ion concentration requires some elimination or retention of hydrogen ion. The lungs and kidneys play the major roles in this mecha-

nism. Figure 15-7 shows how these systems interact with the bicarbonate buffer system.

When carbonic acid dehydrates to form carbon dioxide and water, excess carbon dioxide is expired from the lungs, accompanied by some water. Thus some potential hydrogen donor (CO_2) is removed and decreases the potential carbonic acid for a time. The rest of the hydrogen ion is temporarily inactivated in the water remaining in the body. Recall that increase in the serum partial pressure of carbon dioxide (P_{CO_2}) is the normal stimulus for breathing. Therefore, if the buffering system produces more carbon dioxide, the respiratory drive will increase, respiratory rate will increase, and more carbon dioxide and water will leave the body. This mechanism, involving transport to the lungs, operates in about ten to thirty minutes.

Free hydrogen ion must be excreted for day-to-day maintenance of concentration. This excretion occurs via the kidneys. The acid end products of cellular metabolism contain large quantities of hydrogen ion. Excessive amounts would build up if the kidneys could not eliminate free nydrogen ion. If vomiting or other loss of acid secretions depletes hydrogen ion, cellular metabolism cannot keep up with the needs, nor can the weak dissociation of carbonic acid. However, the kidneys can retain as well as

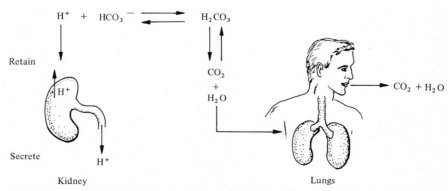

Figure 15-7 Removal of hydrogen ion from the body. Hydrogen ion may be retained or secreted from the kidneys. A small amount of potential hydrogen ion donor (CO_2) may be expired through the lungs.

excrete hydrogen ion to restore balance. Unfortunately, the renal mechanism reacts more slowly than either the buffering or the respiratory mechanisms. This is a problem only when disease creates sufficient imbalance to overwhelm the buffering and respiratory mechanisms.

Disorders of hydrogen-ion concentration are caused by a great variety of metabolic, circulatory, and respiratory disorders. In general, physicians attempt to treat the underlying causes, rather than directly correcting the increase or decrease in pH, which is merely one sign of the disease. In extreme situations, the hydrogen-ion imbalance must be directly attacked so that the patient can live long enough to permit treatment of his basic disease. The care of people with acid-base imbalances and the support of the medical therapy are rather complex and not usually undertaken by beginning nurses. However, many serious alterations in hydrogen-ion concentration can be prevented if the person is brought to medical attention, or if his disease is kept under control. Such preventive activities are well within the scope of beginning practice. Consequently, the terminology and situations which can lead to hydrogen-ion imbalance will be briefly presented here.

Disorders of hydrogen-ion concentration are broadly termed *acidosis* (pH less than 7.4) and *alkalosis* (pH greater than 7.4). These terms, however, tell the physician nothing about the cause of the altered pH. The adjectives "respiratory" or "metabolic" prefacing acidosis or alkalosis indicate not only the state of the pH but also the basic mechanism which is altered.

Respiratory Acidosis and Alkalosis Respiratory acidosis and alkalosis occur because carbon dioxide is either retained or expired abnormally. Any situation which results in *hypoventilation* (decrease in expired carbon dioxide) will create carbon dioxide retention. This will shift the bicarbonate buffer reaction (see "Buffering," above) to the left, release free hydrogen ion, and

produce acidosis. Disorders which impair alveolar gaseous exchange (such as emphysema), decrease lung expansion, or decrease respiratory stimulation may lead to hypoventilation and respiratory acidosis. People who are immobilized or who have painful surgical incisions may breathe shallowly and thus hypoventilate. Nursing care which makes a point of encouraging regular deep breathing can prevent hypoventilation in such instances.

Hyperventilation (increase in carbon dioxide expiration) can cause respiratory alkalosis secondary to the decrease in serum carbon dioxide. This decrease shifts the bicarbonate reaction to the right and removes a potential hydrogen ion donor via the lung. Rapid breathing in itself is not hyperventilation unless it results in a measurably decreased serum carbon dioxide level. Anxiety, pain, and fear are common causes of hyperventilation. Consequently, calm support of a person experiencing these situations can help prevent hyperventilation. Further information about nursing care of people with respiratory problems is found in Part 3, Chapter 16.

Metabolic Acidosis and Alkalosis Metabolic acidosis may occur when the cellular production of organic acid is excessive, as in uncontrolled diabetes or in hypoxia. Excess organic acid is also produced in the metabolism of high doses of such drugs as aspirin. A third cause of metabolic acidosis is renal disease which impairs excretion of metabolically produced acid. Excessive loss of bicarbonate, as in gastrointestinal fluid or diarrhea, creates a relative increase in hydrogen-ion concentration by altering the bicarbonate/carbonic acid ratio.[6]

Metabolic alkalosis can occur when gastric hydrochloric acid is lost, either through vomiting or gastric suction, or when potassium chloride is lost. Potassium loss can lead to alkalosis, because

---

[6] pH is a function of the bicarbonate/carbonic acid ratio. Normal HCO_3^-/H_2CO_3 ratio is 20:1. Thus, changes in concentration of either will result in hydrogen-ion concentration imbalance.

hydrogen moves into the cells to replace the lost potassium ion. Excessive ingestion of bicarbonate in a person with limited renal ability to excrete it can also produce metabolic alkalosis. This sometimes is seen in elderly people who take baking soda (sodium bicarbonate) for "heartburn."

NURSING MANAGEMENT IN FLUID-ELECTROLYTE PROBLEMS

Nurses and physicians share a great many responsibilities in the management of problems related to fluid and electrolyte balance. The physician has primary responsibility in the diagnosis and therapy of actual imbalance, both acute and chronic. Both physician and nurse share responsibility in helping patient-clients to maintain balance. Nurses play a primary role in alleviating or preventing discomfort associated with imbalances or therapeutic management.

Maintaining Normal Fluid and Electrolyte Balance

Most people have no trouble maintaining their fluid balance despite wide variations in intake or output. Even in "ordinary" illnesses such as diarrhea, the regulatory mechanisms of the body keep body fluids within functional volume and concentration ranges. There are, however, groups of people who are more apt to develop problems for which their bodies cannot compensate. These are the people for whom nurses and physicians are responsible, either through advice or actual intervention.

People at risk include those whose regulatory mechanisms cannot adjust to normal environmental or nutritional changes; e.g., those with chronic renal disease. Another group includes people whose regulatory mechanisms do not adjust readily to imbalance caused by illness. The very young (infants) and the very old have such relatively inflexible regulatory mechanisms. For example, infants with diarrhea will rapidly develop saline deficit if fluid intake does not match saline loss. A final group at risk are those who have limited access to fluid. These people are unable to regulate balance by drinking, even though their compensatory mechanisms are normal. This group might include people who have physical handicaps, depressed consciousness, or diminished food and fluid supply.

Nurses and physicians assist people in maintaining fluid balance by helping the person learn to meet his own needs or by actually providing the food and fluid necessary to maintain balance.

Assisting the Person to Meet His Own Needs

Facilitating learning is the appropriate intervention for people who are coping with chronic illness at home, people who are temporarily ill and at home, or hospitalized people who are physically able to use the food and fluid provided them.

As emphasized in Part 3, Chapter 9, facilitating learning is not simply providing information. The nurse-teacher must give information at a level understood and accepted by the learner, provide opportunity to practice behavior which is complex (such as learning a restricted diet), and evaluate with the learner the extent to which he has learned. Responsibility for learning about fluid needs is often shared with the client by several health workers. For example, a person with chronic renal disease may need to adopt a diet greatly restricted in sodium. This is because his mechanism for excreting sodium is impaired. Normal dietary intake thus increases total body sodium; water is retained to restore sodium concentration; and edema, which threatens to overload circulation if mobilized, results. The physician prescribes the diet; he may instruct the patient-client himself or ask a dietitian or a nurse to do so. In turn, the physician, hospital dietitian, or nurse may request that a community health nurse help the client adapt the diet to his home situation and assist in evaluating the efficacy of the diet.

The community nurse may help the client develop menus and find seasoning substitutes, thus providing an opportunity for the client to practice using the diet. In addition, this nurse may evaluate the client's learning by asking him to outline a week's menus or specify foods to be avoided. A record of daily weights and physical examination for edema provide objective evidence of fluid retention or loss.

Direct Assistance

Many people in hospitals or other institutions can meet their fluid needs with little or no help. As long as they have ready access to food and fluid, their own appetite and thirst serve them as well as if they were at home. Others may need direct supervision or help to meet their own needs. For example, people who are severely depressed often feel little motivation to eat and drink. Even though such a person is physically capable of meeting his own needs, he may not be emotionally capable of doing so independently. Therefore, the simple fact that a person is depressed should alert a nurse to assess the client's ability to meet his own fluid needs. If the person is not able to do so, the nurse or family must assume this responsibility temporarily.

Similarly, a person who is physically incapacitated (e.g., weak, paralyzed, or in a restraining therapeutic situation) may be unable to get his own food and fluid. He may be thirsty but hesitate to "bother" anyone. If his level of consciousness is depressed, he may not respond to thirst and may give no clues to the nursing personnel that he needs increased fluids. Professional personnel have particular responsibility to be alert to the fluid needs of such people. There are several reports of severe water depletion (hypernatremia reflecting increased solute concentration) in unconscious patients given high-protein tube feeding (Gault et al., 1968). The high solute load in the liquid diet increases serum osmolarity, but the patient is unable to complain of thirst if sufficient water is not added to compensate for the solute load.

Data for Assessment of the Need for Assistance How does the nurse decide which patient-clients need direct help with their fluid needs, at home or in institutions? The information in the preceding review of fluid and electrolyte balance should guide choice of data needed to assess fluid status. First, what the person actually eats and drinks must be recorded. Table 15-1 shows average amounts of fluid intake and output. The average person ingests about 2,700 to 2,800 ml per day, including about 750 ml which is in food (preformed water). Therefore, if the food intake increases or decreases, free (liquid) fluid should increase or decrease accordingly. The 500-ml output which is called obligatory (i.e., not changed much by internal volume changes) represents the minimal essential intake. However, this allows no margin for volume compensation for such circumstances as temperature change (increased perspiration loss), increased activity (increased respiratory loss), or solute dilution (ingestion of highly salted foods). Consequently, normal people require an intake considerably above the minimum. There are wide variations in normal intake. In a study of the intakes of medical students, medical technologists, and hospitalized patients, the amounts drunk ranged from 600 to 6,000 ml per day. The mean intake for the patients was 2,800 ml and that for the technicians and students between 2,000 and 2,400 ml (Holmes, 1964). Therefore, some knowledge of a client's usual intake is important in determining whether the recorded intake is low, usual, or high with reference to his normal patterns.

People who are ill are generally encouraged to maintain an oral intake between 2,000 and 3,000 ml, including preformed fluid. There is nothing magic about these figures; they simply represent an application of average fluid intakes to people in situations where their fluid requirements may be somewhat raised by the increased metabolic activity associated with illness. People who are apt to develop renal stones or those who have urinary infections may require even more in order to keep the urine dilute and freely flowing.

Actual measurement of output (quantity of urine, number of stools, amount of perspiration) is often unnecessary in determining whether the client needs direct assistance. Inspection of urine and stool gives clues to the person's fluid balance. The presence of small amounts of concentrated urine and hard stools suggests that water is being conserved by the body; large amounts of dilute urine usually indicate elimination of excess water. If these observations are not congruent with recorded intake—e.g., if urine is dilute but intake is low, or urine is concentrated and intake is high—actual measurements should be made.

If the client is being treated for disorders of fluid balance, the physician may wish to gather data about output from all sources—urine, feces, drainage from body cavities, perspiration, and respiration. This type of data can be gathered rather precisely in specialized metabolic research units. For the most part, however, measurement of urine and drainages, counting of stools, and estimation of perspiration are used to give a rough estimate of total output.

Many nurses assume that only a physician can order "intake and output" measurements. This is not so. These measurements are simply one assessment tool which any health professional may use to gain information about the patient-client's needs. Physicians frequently ask that nursing personnel record intake and output to help gather data for the medical diagnosis and therapy. This does not mean, however, that nurses cannot independently gather these data to assess the ability of people at risk to meet their own fluid needs.

The client, his family, and nursing personnel may all be involved in recording the intake on whatever form the health agency uses. If the person is at home, the family may be instructed to measure the amount of fluid held in their glasses, cups, and bowls, and record the amounts taken on a sheet of paper. The patient-client's willingness to assume recording of this intake, and his mental and emotional ability to do so, will determine whether he can help gather these data. The amount of fluid in foods is usually estimated, on the basis of an average of 750 to 1,000 ml in three normal meals. If more exact measures are necessary, hospital dietitians or metabolic research kitchens can calculate the preformed fluid more accurately. Bear in mind that the estimate of fluid intake and output from these recordings is just that, an *estimate*. These records are notoriously inaccurate for a variety of reasons. Nursing personnel in hospitals forget to record on them; output is discarded before amounts are recorded; the patient forgets to record on the form (although he is apt to be more accurate than nursing personnel); and estimates of food consumed or partial amounts of fluid are inaccurate. This means that a pattern of low or imbalanced intake and output should be checked against other data, such as weight and laboratory analysis, the patient's general condition, his usual fluid patterns, and his perception of his intake, before any conclusions are drawn as to the adequacy of his intake.

A second measure of fluid balance is the pattern of weight gain and loss. As stated earlier, a gain or loss of more than 0.5 kg (1.1 lb) in twenty-four hours indicates gain or loss of fluid. Slower gains and losses probably reflect caloric intake.

A final set of observations which the nurse may use to assess the need of people for help in maintaining fluid and electrolyte balance consists of the signs and symptoms of imbalance. These are discussed last, for they are relatively unreliable guides to fluid status. The valuable signs, such as weight gain and loss, postural changes in blood pressure, and thirst, have been discussed previously. Many of the "classic" symptoms are vague and can be caused by many pathological situations. In addition, they usually appear when the imbalance is rather far advanced. Certainly, if a nurse encounters these previously unrecognized signs and symptoms in a patient-client in the community or in the hospital, he should see that the person consults a physician soon. The appearance of these symptoms in a patient under treatment for a fluid and electrolyte imbalance indicates that therapy is not effective and that a physician must be contacted.

Rather than memorizing a long list of similar symptoms and matching them to specific volume and concentration disorders, the nurse should learn the general groups of symptoms, be alert for them in patients at risk to develop imbalances, and seek medical assistance when they are evident.[7] The important point is to note whether a *change has occurred* in the patient's status in the following general categories:

1 Mentation—increasing or decreasing level of consciousness, from lethargy to excitement
2 Muscle tone—flaccidity, twitching, convulsions
3 Tissue turgor—swelling, dryness of mucous membranes, loss of turgor
4 Respiratory rate and depth—shallow to deep and rapid

Diagnosis of the Need for Assistance Once data have been gathered about fluid status, the nurse must decide if the client needs help in

[7] In general, signs and symptoms of electrolyte imbalance reflect neuromuscular malfunction. Apathy, lethargy, and finally coma are one group of symptoms related to the central nervous system effects of volume depletion, potassium deficit, acidosis, and alkalosis. Increasing irritability, muscle twitching, and convulsions are often signs of excessive neuromuscular stimulation due to decreased serum magnesium and calcium. Muscle flaccidity and weakness may characterize potassium depletion and calcium excess. Tissue swelling (edema) is evident in saline excess, tissue dryness in advanced saline depletion.

meeting his own fluid needs. Figure 15-8 shows several alternative paths which the nurse may take regarding problems of oral intake.

If the data indicate that a person with increased risk of developing imbalances is adequately meeting his own needs, no further action is indicated beyond periodic reassessment. Adequate fluid balance would be indicated by a balance between intake and output, intake consistent with his usual patterns and sufficient to meet his current metabolic needs, no unusual weight gains or losses, and absence of signs and symptoms of imbalance.

When a person's physical status and record of intake suggest inadequate fluid ingestion but there are no signs of definite imbalance, he should be offered additional fluids and foods high in water. If his oral intake still does not improve, or if definite signs of volume depletion are evident, a physician should be consulted. In some situations, such as clinics operated by nurse practitioners, the nurse may obtain laboratory analysis of volume and electrolyte status. In most circumstances, the physician will obtain such laboratory work at his discretion. Similarly, evidence of excessive fluid intake (edema, rapid weight gain) calls for consultation with a physician. Once definite abnormalities have been established, it becomes the physician's prerogative to begin therapy.

Management of the Patient's Problems Associated with Therapy of Fluid and Electrolyte Disorders

While the physician has primary responsibility for treating fluid-electrolyte imbalances, the nurse implements much of the therapy. For example, he encourages or restricts intake of oral fluids, monitors administration of intravenous fluids, administers or supervises administration of drugs such as electrolyte supplements or diuretics, and may supervise dietary management. In addition, the nurse's observations contribute data regarding the exact problem and the

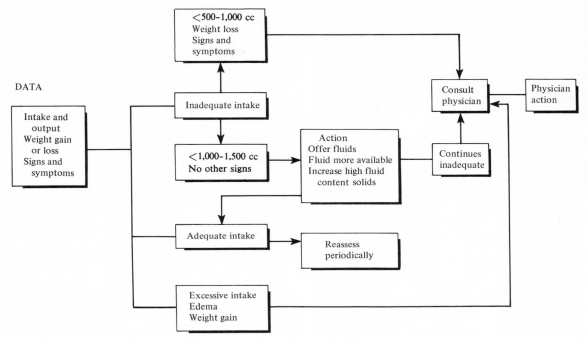

Figure 15-8 Alternative uses of data regarding fluid-intake status. See text for discussion of this diagram.

effect of therapy. Finally, the nurse has primary responsibility in maintaining the patient-client's comfort in problems associated with therapy, such as thirst, immobility imposed by intravenous therapy, and discomfort posed by edema.

Restricting and Increasing Oral Fluid Intake

One of the least complex methods of managing fluid imbalance is to decrease or increase the amount of oral fluid taken. This is commonly called *restricting* and *forcing fluids*. To "force fluids" does not mean literally to subdue the patient and make him drink. It means to increase oral fluid to a specified amount; e.g., 2,500 ml, 3,000 ml, etc. Similarly, fluid intake may be restricted to a specified daily amount—400 ml, 1,000 ml. Fluids are increased for people whose daily intake falls below 1,000 to 1,500 ml, those

who will probably not take sufficient fluids without help, and those who may develop urinary tract stones or infection without a high fluid intake. Fluids are restricted in people who cannot excrete normal amounts of fluid and in those who have a water excess.

Whenever specific fluid goals are to be met, measurement of amounts taken is essential. Estimate your own daily fluid intake and then actually measure it one day. The error inherent in estimations will probably be apparent.

Measurement of all sources of fluid is also important, particularly when fluids must be restricted. Liquids such as water, juice, and milk would be considered fluid by everyone. However, how many consider that gelatin, ice cream, and Junket are also liquids, even though they are semisolid when cold? As noted before, all foods contain some liquid, and this must be taken into account when fluids are severely restricted.

The timing of fluid intake affects the success of both increased and restricted fluid regimens. People whose intake of fluids is restricted and who consume their whole allotment in a few hours may become unbearably thirsty. Those who must consume extra fluids and attempt to do so at one time may feel so full that they refuse to take any more. Spacing of fluids must be based on the person's previous patterns of fluid intake, as well as on the amount to be taken. If the person prefers to drink with his meals, then mealtime is the time to provide a substantial portion of the allotment, or to give extra fluid. Many people do not drink during the night; but if it is the patient-client's habit to do so, some portion of the daily allotment should be reserved for this period.

When a client is regulating his own increased or decreased fluid intake, the nurse may teach him how to measure liquids and to space the daily allotment. If the nursing staff must regulate the fluid intake for a patient, nursing directives must be clear and specific. Specific allotments are made for each working period, including allowances for fluids with meals and with medications. The patient's fluid preferences are also noted.

Even though a patient-client may be unable to regulate his fluid regimen by himself, he can usually help with it. His understanding and cooperation are essential if the regimen is to succeed. Explanations of the reasons for the alteration provide a starting point in gaining his cooperation. A second step may be to have him help devise the plan for types of fluids and spacing. Short-term goals may help him pass the time. For example, a person who must drink extra fluid might be asked to drink a glass of juice before the end of a short television program or a pitcher of water before the afternoon nursing staff comes on duty. Time may pass slowly for a person who has to restrict fluids; therefore, he may benefit from trying to read a certain amount of a book between afternoon fluids and dinner, playing a game with a group of adults or children, or using other diversions. Keeping one's own intake record may provide incentive for people who must increase their intake. Such activity probably only increases the sense of deprivation for people with restricted intake.

Thirst

Thirst is probably the most troublesome sensation for patients whose fluids are restricted. Not only is thirst physically unpleasant, but it is associated symbolically with want, deprivation, and death. Thirst constantly reminds the patient that he cannot have the fluids which most people take for granted. Thirst may become a physical and emotional obsession with some who have severely limited intake. People who have been shipwrecked or lost in the desert and have survived long periods of water deprivation often report their complete obsession with obtaining a drink. Their dreams were full of drinking, streams, and lakes (Wolf, 1958). Because water is so essential to life, giving a man a drink is a symbol of caring and of love. An understanding of the symbolic as well as the physical nature of thirst may help a nurse better understand the patient who begs for water, even though he supposedly "understands" the medical reasons for the restriction.

Thirst is basically a protective sensation. When serum osmolarity is too high, osmoreceptors stimulate the mechanism which produces thirst. The person or animal then drinks sufficient amounts to restore the balance. Many factors in addition to altered osmolarity appear to influence the sensations of thirst and of satiety (sufficiency). The exact mechanisms by which these factors operate is not well understood.

Seeing a favorite beverage or a picture of it may produce the sensation of thirst; this is a learned or conditioned stimulus. Emotional stress, such as fear or anxiety, can produce thirst. An increase in serum osmolarity accompanies such stress in animals (Deaux and Kakolewski, 1970). Mouth breathing, administration of nasal oxygen, or abstinence from food and fluid produce an observably dry mouth. These factors are also associated with the sensation of thirst, even if the person's fluid balance is not altered. Very sweet or salty foods or fluids may create an immediate thirst. Since insufficient time has elapsed for these substances to affect serum osmolarity, this thirst possibly reflects stimulation of osmoreceptors in the mouth (Holmes, 1964).

A number of measures to relieve thirst are suggested in the nursing literature. Unfortunately, few are based on sound physiologic or psychologic principles, and there are few reports of systematic evaluation as to the real efficacy of these measures in groups of thirsty people. Some of the more theoretically sound measures include giving frequent oral care to combat local dryness, spacing liquids in relation to solid intake, providing the illusion of volume, and providing diversion.

Oral Measures Since dryness of the mouth creates the sensation of thirst, it is logical that thirst may decrease if the mucous membranes are moistened. If osmolarity or volume is altered, the relief will be temporary. This will also be true if the cause of dryness, such as mouth breathing or administration of nasal oxygen, persists. Nevertheless, frequent oral care will produce some temporary comfort.

Sham drinking, or holding water in the mouth and then spitting it out, is the simplest oral measure. It provides relief for only about fifteen minutes, and thus must be repeated often (Fenton, 1969).

Sucking hard candy or chewing gum is often recommended for local stimulation of saliva and relief of thirst. It is true that these activities will stimulate the flow of saliva, even in severe water depletion (Holmes, 1964). Absence of salivary action can lead to a condition called *parotitis,* i.e., inflammation of the parotid glands, or *stomatitis,* i.e., inflammation of the mucous membrane and oral structures. Gum chewing may be indicated to prevent such inflammation. However, my personal and clinical experience indicates that gum and hard candy aggravate, rather than alleviate, thirst. The high sugar content creates a hyperosmolar solution in the mouth which draws fluid to the mucous membrane. This temporarily moistens the mouth but probably leaves the membranes ultimately even drier.

Oral hygiene is important in everyone to prevent tooth decay and gum disease. It is doubly important for the person whose fluids are restricted, because oral care prevents accumulation of dried secretions with resultant injury to gums and mucous membranes.

When salivary secretions are decreased or absent and no external moisture is supplied, mucous secretions become thick and accumulate on teeth and mucous membranes. This debris often becomes brown and foul-smelling. Removal of the debris is difficult and often is accompanied by bleeding.

Oral hygiene is frequently mentioned as a measure useful in decreasing thirst; it is probably effective for a short time because of the application of moisture. The few studies done to determine the relative efficacy of various agents used in oral care focus on the cleansing attributes and on objective measures of oral moistness. Reports of subjective appraisal of relief from sensations of thirst from various oral hygiene measures have not been published. Hypertonic oral solutions do cause increased drinking and thirst in both man and animals. Isotonic saline solutions also create thirst, an unexpected finding which is not as yet explained (Holmes, 1964).

Individual nurses and nursing textbooks often emphasize the excellence of one or another oral hygiene agent, such as lemon juice with glycerol, hydrogen peroxide, or aromatic mouthwash. However, the few studies reported have all shown that the agent used makes little difference in the cleansing achieved (Ginsberg, 1961, 1964; Passos and Brand, 1966; Van Drimmelen and Rollins, 1969). Indeed, one of the most commonly used solutions, equal parts of lemon juice and glycerol, is actually drying to the mouth (Van Drimmelen and Rollins) and may promote chemical decalcification of the teeth (Wiley, 1969). The drying properties of lemon juice and glycerol do not affect mechanical cleansing but may promote increased thirst. It is my clinical impression that this is exactly what happens.

Oral care which is effective in cleansing includes toothbrushing or swabbing, and cleaning of the mucous membranes and tongue. If the patient-client is able to do this himself, toothbrushing and rinsing of the mouth are usually sufficient. If he is very ill or physically incapacitated, soft gauze or cotton swabs are often used to cleanse oral tissues. The rating scale of Passos

and Brand for assessing the condition of the mouth is reproduced in Table 15-2 as a general guide to evaluation of the mouth before and after oral care.

DeWalt and Haines (1969) carefully observed physical changes in the oral structures during a five-hour period of mouth breathing and oxygen administration. Secretions were constantly removed by mechanical suctioning. The subject described her sensations of extreme dryness, numbness, and burning. These sensations occurred within the first hour. They were decreased after toothbrushing and swabbing with lemon juice and glycerol. Objectively the mouth was more moist, but the subjective relief lasted only fifteen to thirty minutes.

Spacing Fluids in Relation to Solid Foods The neural regulation of food intake

Table 15-2   Assessment of Condition of the Mouth and Oral Structures

Category	Numerical and descriptive ratings*		
	1	2	3
Saliva	Cavity moist	Scanty, with or without debris	Viscid or ropy, with or without debris
Tongue	Wet or moist, coating absent to small amount of coating	Dry, slight or moderate coating	Dry or moist, with abundant coating
Palates	Wet or moist, debris absent to small amount, soft	Dry, with or without small amount of soft debris	Dry or moist, moderate to large amount of soft or hard debris
Membranes, gums	Wet or moist, debris absent to small amount, soft	Dry, with or without small amount of soft debris; tend to bleed	Dry or moist, moderate to large amount of soft or hard debris, bleed easily
Teeth	Edentulous; debris absent to small amount	Moderate amount of debris	Almost covered with debris
Odor	Sweetish or absent	Trace to moderately unpleasant	Strongly unpleasant
Lips	Smooth and soft, moist to dry	Rough, dry, small or moderate amount of crusting or cracking, tend to bleed	Dry, large amount of crusting or cracking, bleed easily
Nares	Clean, unobstructed, or small amount of soft secretions	Partially obstructed by secretions, with or without nasal tubes	Very dirty, secretions obstruct airway

*This scale defines characteristics of good to poor oral condition. Rating 1 is most desirable, 3 is least desirable.
Source: From Joyce Passos and Lucy Brand, Effects of Agents Used for Oral Hygiene, *Nursing Research,* **15**:199, (1966).

and that of water intake appear to be tied together. The areas in the hypothalamus which affect eating and drinking are separate from each other but in close proximity. Gastric distension will decrease thirst as well as hunger (Morgane and Jacobs, 1969). These facts suggest that methods to alleviate thirst must take into account what food is eaten, when the food is eaten, and when the fluids are consumed.

As Fenton (1969) points out in her review of factors involved in thirst, encouraging the patient to eat will help alleviate thirst for one to two hours by simply distending the stomach. Therefore, if a client is severely restricted in fluid intake, it might be wise to omit fluid altogether from meals and supply a portion of it one to two hours later. If the meal is exceptionally dry, a person accustomed to drinking with his meals may not accept this remedy.

Providing the Illusion of Volume A feeling of deprivation increases the perception of thirst in most people. Therefore, any measure which gives the illusion of greater-than-actual volume of fluid may help decrease this feeling of deprivation. Holmes (1964) suggests the use of large glasses which have a small capacity, such as false-bottomed tumblers. A glass of ice chips is another means to provide the illusion of greater volume. A container of chipped ice will melt to about one-half that volume of water. Thus, a 240-ml glass full of ice would provide 120 ml water. In addition, the coldness of ice seems to relieve many people better than water at room temperature. Popsicles are also effective for the same reasons. Even though they are sweet, the high water content, the cold, and the prolonged sucking seem to help satisfy the oral needs associated with thirst. Obviously, the exact fluid content of either ice or popsicles must be determined by melting a standard measure and then posting this figure where all nursing personnel can find it. The water content of a glass of ice varies a great deal, depending upon whether the ice is in cubes or chipped, and upon how loosely it is packed into the container.

Many people gulp a container of fluid in one swallow. Such people will be very thirsty when fluids are restricted. They may feel less deprived if they can learn to take small mouthfuls at a time.

Diversion Diversion is extremely valuable for the adult or child who is not too ill. The more one thinks about any physical discomfort, the more uncomfortable he becomes. The exact diversion will depend upon the person's level of development and interests. It must be sufficiently interesting to keep him from thinking about how thirsty he is. Television is often not a good diversion for very thirsty patients; it is amazing how many advertisements involve drinking, streams, and the ocean!

Firm Limits Most adults and many older children who must limit fluids will be able to do so, despite their discomfort from thirst and their feeling of deprivation. However, small children and adults who do not accept the medical need for restriction or who have regressed to impulse behavior may need to have external limits imposed on their access to fluid.

Providing only the allowed fluid in small amounts is the first step. However, if the patient-client is able to get about the hospital or home, he has access to drinking fountains, water faucets, and other people's bedside fluids. Patient-clients who feel desperately thirsty have been known to drink the water from their flower arrangements, or bath water, and even their urine. When even small excesses are harmful, as in people in renal failure, strong controls may have to be imposed. These may include such actions as removing the handles from faucets and staying with the patient while he bathes. This is not pleasant for anyone but is best handled with an attitude of, "You are important to us, and we won't let you hurt yourself," rather than with a punitive approach.

Intravenous Therapy

Medical management or prevention of fluid and electrolyte imbalance frequently includes intravenous (IV) therapy. A needle, or flexible plastic catheter, is secured in a vein. Most often, the venous route is used to deliver fluid and electrolyte solutions to restore or maintain volume, osmolarity, and electroneutrality; blood or blood products to restore volume; red blood cells or clotting factors; or specific medications.

The degree to which beginning practitioners are responsible for regulating their patients' intravenous equipment varies. However, when any patient-client is receiving an intravenous infusion, the nurse caring for him is responsible for his comfort, for the patency of the equipment, and for the detection of any untoward (unwanted) effects.

Comfort   From the patient's point of view, comfort or discomfort is of primary importance with intravenous therapy. Many people fear needles and become apprehensive at the sight of the needle or catheter to be used for therapy. Coupled with this fear is the common assumption that one must be seriously ill to require an intravenous infusion. The pain of inserting the needle or catheter into the vein is real, although momentary. If the needle and tubing are well secured, there is rarely any further pain from the equipment itself. However, some medications, such as potassium, cause pain if administered in sufficiently high concentration. Diluting the concentration or slowing the rate is usually sufficient to prevent this pain.

Another cause of pain during infusion (administration of intravenous solution) is thrombophlebitis. Irritation of the vein by the needle or catheter, or by irritating solutions, may cause a local inflammation of the vein. The inflammatory reaction releases substances which promote local blood clotting (thrombus formation). If the inflammation is severe enough, the vein may thrombose for some distance distal to the infusion site. Pain, warmth, and redness along the vein characterize thrombophlebitis. The infusion must be discontinued at that site to prevent serious problems.

Any intravenous equipment may cause thrombophlebitis, but the incidence is greatest with plastic catheters and increases with the length of time they remain in the vein (Cheney and Lincoln, 1964). In light of this, the site for plastic catheters is usually changed every twenty-four to seventy-two hours in long-term therapy. In addition, some physicians add small amounts of steroids to each bottle to decrease the inflammatory reaction to the catheter. Sodium bicarbonate solutions which make the pH of intravenous solution more nearly that of the blood are also sometimes added to decrease irritation by the solution (Pederson, 1970).

Intravenous therapy imposes some immobility on the patient for the duration of the infusion. When needles are used, the patient's activity is significantly related to the frequency of infiltration (leakage of fluid into subcutaneous tissues) and consequent need to discontinue the infusion. The greater the activity, the greater the number of infiltrations (Link, 1967; Sylvester and Bruno, 1966). Consequently, people receiving short-term infusions with needles must remain relatively quiet to avoid dislodging the needle. If therapy must continue for twenty-four hours or more, many clinicians use plastic catheters, which allow much greater mobility but carry their own hazard of thrombophlebitis.

The anxiety of patients who think intravenous infusions imply serious illness may create exaggerated perceptions of the discomforts involved in intravenous therapy. Apparently exaggerated concern over the functioning of the equipment or discomfort from the infusion may be a clue to a patient's fear that his condition may be more serious than anyone has told him. The nurse can help him express this fear by saying something like, "Many people thinking having an IV means they are terribly ill; I wonder if you feel that way." After hearing the person's concern, the nurse can then help him put it in perspective with the actual purposes of the infusion.

Patency of the System   Maintaining the integrity of the intravenous system means more than simply making sure the fluid is still dripping. It involves precautions to keep the needle in the vein, to keep the tubing free, and to keep the rate of flow adequate for the infusion purpose.

Infiltration of the subcutaneous tissues by the intravenous fluid occurs if the needle or, more rarely, the catheter pierces the wall of the vein. This leakage of fluid into the tissues creates a localized edema. The increased tissue pressure secondary to the swelling may eventually stop the flow of fluid. The fluid can be absorbed subcutaneously, but the rate of absorption is variable and erratic. If irritating drugs are contained in the fluid, the site of infiltration may be painful. Some drugs, such as *l*-norepinephrine (Levophed) and antimetabolites (nitrogen mustard), can cause extensive death of the infiltrated tissue.

Pain, swelling, pallor, and coldness along the needle site are indicative of infiltration. Marked slowing of the rate of infusion suggests infiltration, if it is not obviously associated with kinked tubing or contraction of the muscle around the vein. Nurses commonly assume that blood flow into the tubing when the bottle is lowered below the vein (backflow) indicates that infiltration has not occurred. However, blood can return even with infiltration if the needle has pierced the vein but is still partially within it. In addition, a needle which has not infiltrated may be so close to the size of the lumen of the vein as to prevent backflow. For these reasons, Plumer states that checking for backflow is an unreliable method of determining if infiltration exists. She defines only

two criteria: swelling about the needle, and continued infusion when a tourniquet is placed above the needle (1970, p. 62). The infusion must be discontinued and started in another vein when infiltration occurs.

The *rate of flow* is basically determined by the physician's prescription for fluids; e.g., 1,000 ml to run for eight hours; 3,000 ml to run for twenty-four hours. The nurse then calculates the approximate number of milliliters per hour and the approximate length of time it should take to infuse each bottle of solution. Each manufacturer of intravenous equipment has a standard drip meter which is calibrated to deliver a specific number of drops per milliliter. Thus, it is an easy matter to calculate the number of drops per minute needed to deliver a given number of milliliters per hour.[8] Unfortunately, different brands of equipment provide different standards, usually from 10 to 15 drops per milliliter. In addition, companies provide very small drip meters which are used for very slow infusions or for children. These usually deliver 60 drops per milliliter. Consequently, it is important that the nurse be aware of the calibration of the equipment used in his agency.

A number of nursing personnel may be involved in regulating the rate of an infusion. Therefore, each bottle should have a strip of tape or similar label which indicates the rate of flow and approximate level of fluid which should remain at any given time. Thus, each person does not have to calculate for himself whether the infusion is proceeding on schedule.

The rate will not remain as initially set for several reasons. Rate is a function of the pressure of the fluid in the bottle and the resistance it meets from the pressure in the vein. As the fluid level in the bottle decreases, hydrostatic pressure exerted by the fluid also decreases, and the rate slows. Therefore, the rate will need to be ad-

---

[8] $\dfrac{\text{ml / hr}}{60}$ = ml / min × drops / ml = drops / min.

·justed as the bottle empties. Movements of the patient which kink or compress the tubing will also alter the rate mechanically, as will his muscular movements which increase pressure on the vein itself. Consequently, the infusion cannot be left with the assumption that it will continue at the same rate as initially set. Frequent checking and adjustment of rate are necessary.

All too often nurses become so concerned about giving infusions "on schedule" that they adjust the rate to the schedule, not to the needs of the patient. Too rapid administration of fluid to "catch up" may be dangerous. Sudden infusion of large amounts of fluid, particularly saline solution, can overload the circulation and lead to pulmonary edema. Circulatory overload is particularly a danger in adults whose cardiac and renal mechanisms cannot adjust quickly enough. Adults with renal disease and cardiac failure are such persons. Children are also at increased risk of circulatory overload, because their vascular compartments are not large enough to handle sudden large amounts of fluid. Sudden increase in blood pressure, rapid pulse, and dyspnea coincident with a sudden rapid infusion are indications of circulatory overload.

Overrapid infusion is a common accident. The regulating clamp may slip on the tubing, or a curious child or confused adult may accidentally open the clamp wide. Whenever a patient's circulatory status is such that he would not be able to adjust to a sudden, large infusion, precautions must be taken to prevent such accidents. The best precaution is to use bottles which contain no more fluid than the patient could tolerate if all the contents were to flow in within a few minutes. This may be accomplished by using small bottles (100 to 250 ml) or pediatric drip sets which can deliver only small quantities at any one time.

Sudden infusion of high concentrations of potassium poses a danger to any patient-client, for high serum levels of potassium can cause cardiac arrest. Except in extreme hypokalemia, most authorities recommend infusion of no more than 15 to 30 mEq per hour. In most circumstances, no more than 40 mEq potassium should be in a liter of solution to prevent the danger of cardiac arrest, even if the whole liter were suddenly infused.

Untoward Effects   Infiltration and circulatory overload, as discussed above, are certainly unwanted or untoward effects of intravenous therapy. Others include infection and embolism. Nurses and physicians alike are responsible for preventing these effects insofar as possible.

Infection   Infection may be a localized infection of the vein at the site of needle or catheter entry, a generalized bacteremia (bacteria throughout the bloodstream), or septicemia (toxic infection throughout the bloodstream). Local infection is painful to the patient, precludes further use of that vein in long-term therapy, and may give rise to thromboembolism—blood clots which detach from the vein wall and lodge in the lung or, more rarely, in coronary or cerebral vessels. Bacteremia may range in severity from a transient fever to a fatal, widespread septicemia.

Introduction of bacteria into the blood is a possibility whenever intravenous equipment is used. If these bacteria are able to multiply and overwhelm the person's bacteriologic defenses, *septicemia* (infection in the blood) will result. Carelessness in handling open ends of intravenous equipment results in hundreds of incidents of contamination each day. Amazingly, few of these incidents result in actual infection of the patient. This is because the body defense against microorganisms of most people is effective. When systemic infections occur, only careful epidemiologic investigation will determine whether the source is careless handling of equipment or contamination of the solution or tubing by the manufacturer. A recent rash of intravenously induced septicemias was initially thought to be the result of physician-nurse error (Duma et al., 1971). Similar outbreaks throughout the

United States led investigators to discover that the design and composition of the bottle cap of one manufacturer allowed organisms to enter the system after it was sterilized. The organisms did not enter the solution itself until the screw cap was removed ("How the Septicemia Trail . . . ," 1971).

Embolism An embolus is a migrating particle in the bloodstream which is large enough to block circulation at some point. Very small emboli are not stopped until they reach the tiny capillaries; larger emboli may occlude major vessels. Emboli may be composed of blood clots, fat, amniotic fluid, bacteria, and air. Any substance in the bloodstream which does not dissolve or compress sufficiently to pass freely through the circulation may act as an embolus.

Two types of embolism may be associated with intravenous therapy—thromboembolism (blood clots) and air embolism. Both arise in the venous system and are therefore most apt to pass through the chambers of the heart, into the pulmonary circulation, and lodge in the lungs, causing pulmonary embolism. Embolism is a problem to the patient only if the size or number of emboli is such as to interfere with perfusion of the alveoli. Embolism associated with intravenous infusions, particularly air embolism, is rare.

Thromboembolism As discussed earlier, inflammation of the vein at the site of the needle or catheter entry may cause clots which adhere to the vein wall. Clots which are loosely adherent may break free and become emboli. Embolism of thrombi is more apt to occur when veins in the legs are used for intravenous therapy. For this reason, infusions are rarely given in leg veins.

Rather frequently a small clot will form over the tip of the needle or catheter when the infusion has inadvertently slowed or stopped for a period of time. Most hospitals have policies which forbid nurses to apply positive pressure to flush this clot free and thereby allow the infusion to flow again. However, physicians commonly do this, as do practicing nurses. Students of

nursing see this practice and are left wondering if it is or is not safe.

A clot which can be flushed from the needle with a small amount of pressure (i.e., pressure from 2 ml fluid) is so tiny as to represent almost no danger to the patient. It will indeed lodge in tiny pulmonary capillaries, for the lung functions, to some extent, as a sieve to remove such particles from the circulation. Natural mechanisms in the lung tissue act to resolve these small clots within a period varying from hours to a few days (Hume et al., 1970). One or a few such small clots do not endanger the person's ventilation, however.

Some people have an opening between the atria of the heart which is too small to give rise to symptoms but is potentially large enough for a small venous clot to pass through. This is called an *intra-atrial shunt*. In such a case, the clot might be able to pass directly to the coronary arterial or cerebral arterial circulation, provided preexisting lung disease has raised right atrial pressure (Hume, 1970, p. 202). This situation represents a somewhat greater potential danger than pulmonary embolism from a needle clot. However, Friedburg's review (1966) of coronary embolism does not mention any arising from intravenous therapy. I have reviewed the literature extensively and have found no reports of paradoxical arterial embolism associated with intravenous therapy per se.[9]

Since it appears that the actual danger to the patient from this practice is small, irrigating a plugged venous needle ought to be a matter of judgment and accountability, rather than an absolute right or wrong. The decision to irrigate or not to irrigate should be made on the basis of the patient's cardiac and pulmonary status, need

---

[9] There are reports of cerebral embolism associated with the flushing of *arterial* cannulas with amounts of fluid sufficient to force clots to the cerebral circulation (Gaan et al., 1969; Lowenstein et al., 1971).

At this time, novice nurses are not involved in maintaining the patency of arterial cannulas. Nurses who have such responsibilities are referred to the recommendations of Lowenstein et al. (1971).

for intravenous fluids, availability of other veins, and risk of thromboemboli from other sites.

Air Embolism Air can, in large quantities, act as an embolus, because it does not dissolve rapidly enough to allow blood to flow by and through it. The nitrogen content of air accounts for the slow solubility. Large amounts of air accumulate in the left ventricle and interfere with the pumping action of the heart. This can be heard as a characteristic "mill-wheel" sound. The air and blood form a froth which blocks the pulmonary artery (venous pulmonary circulation) when ejected from the heart. Thus, venous blood cannot be oxygenated, and the person may die. If the embolus crosses to the arterial circulation in the heart (via an intra-atrial shunt), death may occur from blockage of the major coronary arteries.

Air in large-enough quantities to cause embolism is most apt to enter the body from veins which have a negative pressure (e.g., the head and neck veins when a person is upright) or when it is forced in under positive pressure. Air embolism most often occurs during surgery of the brain, head, and neck and during pressure pumping of transfusions. The use of plastic containers for blood has almost eliminated the occurrence of air embolism during transfusions under pressure. The plastic bag collapses as blood is infused, and there is no air which can be accidentally pumped into the bloodstream after the blood is gone.[10]

There is always a potential for air embolism with standard intravenous infusion; however, the quantities of air necessary make this an extremely rare occurrence. The minimum lethal quantity in man has not been established experimentally for obvious reasons. It varies somewhat in animals but appears to be between 5.0 and 7.5 cc per kg, or over 350 cc for a 150-lb man (Friedburg, 1966). Considerably less air is fatal if

it crosses to the arterial circulation via a defect in the heart. Even in this rare situation, animal experiments indicate an equivalent of 37.5 cc for a fatal dose for a 150-lb man (Moore and Braselton, 1940). One pathologist suggests that only 10 to 15 cc may be lethal in a severely ill patient (Simpson, 1942). He bases his estimate on conjecture rather than on any objective criteria, but it has unfortunately given rise to some misleading figures in the nursing literature (Metheny and Snively, 1967; Plumer, 1970).

As mentioned before, sufficient air to form a fatal air embolus can enter a vein under negative pressure. Such a potential situation exists when the subclavian or jugular veins are used to insert lines to monitor central venous pressure. There have been several reports of fatal or serious air emboli associated with loose connections or unclamping of portions of these tubes open to the air (Flanagan et al., 1969). Beginning practitioners rarely care for patients with central venous pressure-monitoring equipment, but nurses are apt to do so when working in more advanced situations.

The danger of air embolism from an intravenous line in arm veins is almost nonexistent. Air frequently gets into the tubing, particularly when an infusion bottle runs dry before it is changed. Fluid in the tubing will stop at a level equivalent to the opposing hydrostatic pressure of the vein. Therefore, unless the patient has a decidedly negative venous pressure, the air cannot flow into the vein. Once the new bottle has been attached to the tubing, the air which remains in the tubing should be expelled. Inserting a needle just proximal to the entry point will allow most of the air in the tubing to escape. If the patient has a positive venous pressure at that vein, the tubing can be disconnected to allow the air to be expelled by the force of flow of the solution.

Even though the objective danger from the introduction of small amounts of intravenous air into a vein other than a neck vein is very small,

---

[10] Yeakel (1968) notes that changing the administration set during a plastic bag transfusion under pressure can allow air to enter the bag and lead to fatal air embolism.

the patient may be frightened to see air in the tubing. Nearly everyone has been exposed to murder mysteries in which the malevolent doctor kills someone by injecting 1 cc air into a vein. Consequently, most laymen are alarmed to see air going into *their* veins. For this reason alone, nurses should attempt to remove all air from the tubing. In addition, the patient's expressed or apparent fears about air in the tubing should be explored with him, and he should be accurately told that the amount in the tubing is not sufficient to harm anyone. The entire tubing could hold only about 5 cc air.

PROBLEMS RELATED TO BOTH CIRCULATORY AND FLUID-ELECTROLYTE STATUS

Disorders which may be of primarily cardiac, renal, or fluid origin ultimately affect both circulatory and fluid status. Shock and edema are two such conditions. They are not diseases, but are pathologic states which result from a number of different causes. Regardless of cause, each poses general problems to the patient, and it is these problems upon which we will focus. The physician seeks to determine and correct the underlying disease, and nurses assist in these therapeutic measures. At the same time, the nurse has primary responsibility to support the patient while he is enduring the physical and psychological discomforts.

Edema

Edema is a general term for excess interstitial fluid, whatever the cause. The foot swelling of the person with heart failure, that of the person with chronic renal failure, and that of nearly anyone who has been sitting a long time on a hot day are examples of edema from various causes.

Interstitial swelling occurs when fluid from the vascular compartment flows into the interstitial space faster than it returns, creating a positive interstitial pressure. Net movement is into the interstitial space. In most tissues, the cells are rather loosely held together by a negative interstitial pressure. Once interstitial pressure becomes positive, fluid can accumulate rapidly and cause visible tissue swelling. Guyton (1971) likens this to the rapid expansion of a balloon, once the initial resistance is overcome. Intracellular swelling (excess fluid within the cells themselves) occurs when excess water is in the extracellular compartment; water moves into the cell in response to the greater osmolarity of the cell interior.

Physiological Alterations Basic to Edema   Alterations in osmotic equilibrium and capillary pressure are basic to all types of edema. The disturbances which generally cause interstitial edema include (1) fluid retention by the kidneys with normal water intake, (2) increase in capillary hydrostatic pressure secondary to impaired venous return, (3) decrease in vascular oncotic pressure secondary to a decrease in circulating protein, and (4) impaired lymphatic drainage. Thus alterations in intake and output of fluid and osmotically active substances, and mechanical impairment of circulation are contributory causes of edema.

Saline Retention   Primary sodium and water retention is most commonly seen in renal disease, which impairs renal excretion of sodium, and in heart failure. The exact mechanisms by which the circulatory alterations of a failing heart impair sodium excretion are not well established. However, it is agreed that sodium is retained, and along with it sufficient water to maintain osmotic balance. This excess saline elevates capillary pressure and thus mechanically moves some fluid into the interstitial space.

In heart failure, a large volume of retained saline may be sufficient to overwhelm the heart's ability to pump the blood volume presented to it. When the ventricle cannot pump out all the blood which comes in, some "backs up" in the venous circulation and leads to venous congestion. If the primary congestion is in the pulmonary circulation, the resulting edema is serious indeed. Since pulmonary edema interferes with the oxygenation of blood, the patient may literally drown. Edema resulting from impaired venous return to the right ventricle tends to accumulate in the dependent, or lower, portions of the body.

Increased Capillary Hydrostatic Pressure Localized impairment of venous return may occur when stockings, girdles, or body position cut off venous flow from the legs. The resulting increase in venous, and thus in capillary, hydrostatic pressure below that point results in movement of fluid out of the veins into the interstitial space. Weakness, atrophy, and paralysis of muscles may also impair venous return by inactivating the pumping effect which aids upward venous flow. Blood pools, thus increasing pressure on the capillaries, and edema occurs in these dependent areas.

Impairment of blood flow through an organ such as the liver creates a local increase in hydrostatic pressure and consequent edema. Ascites, or accumulation of fluid in the abdomen, is an example of this.

Decreased Vascular Oncotic Pressure A decrease in circulating plasma proteins and a loss of plasma proteins both decrease oncotic pressure. The plasma proteins raise vascular osmolarity slightly above that of the interstitial fluid, thereby contributing to the net flow of fluid into the vessels. Any loss of protein decreases this oncotic effect and encourages a net fluid flow out of the vascular space. Generalized edema results when the total plasma proteins decrease, as in malnutrition, or when proteins are lost via the kidneys, as in nephrosis.

An increased capillary permeability will allow protein molecules to leave the vascular space, thus decreasing oncotic pressure. The ankle and foot swelling which many people experience on a hot day is due to the increased capillary permeability due to heat. Injured cells may release substances which increase capillary permeability. The resulting edema is usually localized; e.g., the swelling around a sprained ankle or a bee sting.

Impaired Lymphatic Drainage Accumulation of protein in the interstitial fluid is the last major cause of edema. Blockage of the lymphatic system is the primary cause of such accumulation. The lymphatic system removes the small number of proteins which slip through the capillary membrane. If these are not removed, accumulation of protein increases osmotic pressure of the interstitial space and draws water into the compartment.

Surgical removal of lymph glands in cancer therapy may cause at least temporary local lymphatic blockage and subsequent edema. In the tropics, infestation of the lymphatic vessels by the larvae of certain parasites causes severe lymphatic obstruction, commonly called *elephantiasis*. The edema of weak or paralyzed limbs may be partially due to impaired lymphatic return, for the muscles aid lymphatic as well as venous flow.

Problems Posed by Edema Edema is a problem to the patient to the extent that it creates discomfort, tissue damage, or danger to vital functions through circulatory overload or compression of cells.

Discomfort Discomfort from edema may be localized; e.g., tightness of rings or shoes. The discomfort may range from a simple sensation of tightness to actual pain, if swelling is such that the skin is stretched or breaks. Generalized edema may be accompanied by a sensation of heaviness, which may reflect the weight gain accompanying it. Pulmonary edema, in addition to endangering a vital function, produces a great deal of discomfort because of the accompanying dyspnea (difficult breathing). Many people with heart failure cannot sleep lying down because of the increase in dyspnea in this position.

The discomfort from localized edema may be partially relieved by elevating the edematous limb or limbs. If the legs are affected, an elastic stocking will aid venous return. Elevation of limbs may be contraindicated, however, in severe generalized edema because of the possibility of overloading the heart with the mobilized edema fluid. Pooling of some of the fluid in the legs may be uncomfortable but may be sparing the heart. The decision to elevate the legs in generalized edema depends upon the person's cardiac status, the severity of the edema, and the patient's discomfort. The decision is best made in consultation with the physician and more experienced nurse practitioners.

Tissue Damage People with edema are liable to tissue damage, because cells are pushed further from the capillaries and the nutrients therein. Where the body rubs against sheets, open, raw areas are more easily produced on skin covering edematous areas than on nonedematous spots. Pressure sores will develop more easily in edematous areas. Because the sacrum and heels are more apt to develop dependent edema in a bedfast person, a nurse should routinely inspect and protect these areas. Patients who have generalized edema should be given high priority for use of mechanical devices to prevent pressure sores. See Part 3, Chapter 18, for further discussion of pressure sores.

Danger to Vital Functions The most serious problem edema poses is that in which organ and cellular function is impaired. Because the skull offers no room for expansion, edema of the brain compresses cells and blood vessels until they cannot function. Pulmonary edema impairs and prevents ventilation; ascites may compress the diaphragm and interfere with breathing; edema with burns depletes the vascular volume. Management of these serious effects is essentially a medical responsibility, with nursing assistance. However, nurses have a responsibility to help prevent edema which is severe enough to compromise organ function. Records of the patient-

client's daily weight, intake, and output, and observations of presence and extent of swelling, vital signs, and level of consciousness are all means of collecting data regarding the extent and severity of edema.

Shock

The management of a person in severe shock is complex and requires a great deal of medical and nursing skill. Consequently, beginning practitioners are rarely involved in such care. However, many patients and clients with whom such students deal could develop shock. Prevention of shock and recognition of early stages are important nursing responsibilities. Therefore, the beginning nurse needs to have some knowledge of the types and mechanisms of shock, the people at risk of developing shock, and the characteristic signs and symptoms. More detailed readings are given in the bibliography at the end of this chapter.

Basic Mechanisms *Shock* is a general term for a clinical state in which tissue perfusion is inadequate because of an acute circulatory impairment. Cells which are not perfused cannot do their job in living tissues. When inadequate perfusion is widespread throughout the body, clinical shock exists.

Clinically, shock is usually evidenced by hypotension, decreased urine output, pale and clammy skin, and mental changes ranging from apprehension to stupor and loss of consciousness. The lay public uses the term shock to mean almost any kind of physical or emotional blow, regardless of whether any circulatory problem is involved. For health workers, shock refers to a clinical state resulting from acute circulatory insufficiency.

Most commonly, people think of shock in terms of hemorrhage—loss of large amounts of blood. Hemorrhagic shock is one kind of *hypovolemic* shock: circulatory deficit resulting from decreased circulating volume. Anyone who has lost or is losing blood or fluid volume is at risk of hypovolemic shock. Blood loss may be visible: from a nosebleed, surgical wound, in bloody diarrhea, or from the vagina after childbirth. Bleeding may be internal: into the abdomen after trauma or surgery, into an arm or leg after a fracture, or into the throat after a tonsillectomy.

Volume loss need not be due to loss of blood. Severe vomiting, diarrhea, even perspiration can deplete blood volume if the fluid is not replaced. This is particularly true in infants, whose blood volume is so small to begin with.

Shock may also be *cardiogenic,* caused by inadequate output from the heart. Total fluid volume is relatively unchanged. Cardiogenic shock may be caused by sudden cardiac failure in a myocardial infarction, or by compression of the heart by blood in the chest cavity.

Another form of shock is *neurogenic:* failure of the sympathetic nervous impulses which constrict peripheral blood vessels and thus maintain blood pressure. Blood pools in the dilated veins and is essentially lost to the central circulation. Spinal anesthesia or injury to the spinal cord can cause neurogenic shock by interfering with transmission of neural impulses. Endotoxic, or *septic,* shock is also caused by pooling of peripheral blood. However, the defect is apparently in the action of toxins on vessels themselves, rather than in neural regulation of vasoconstriction (Weil and Shubin, 1967, p. 160). People with severe infections are candidates for septic shock.

Although the circulatory dynamics which initiate each type of shock differ, the end result is the same: effective circulating blood volume decreases, and capillary perfusion of the cells is diminished. If adequate volume or cardiac output is not restored, compensatory mechanisms cannot maintain central blood pressure and cardiac output; small capillaries dilate, and the vascular space expands; blood stagnates in these capillary beds; circulating volume is reduced even further; insufficient oxygen reaches the cells; anaerobic (without oxygen) metabolism occurs; organic acid end products build up and produce metabolic acidosis; and the person dies.

A fairly large volume (as much as 1,500 to 1,700 ml) of fluid may be lost before blood pressure begins to fall. This is often termed a stage of *compensated shock:* peripheral vessels constrict (increase resistance) to compensate for the lower stroke volume and thus maintain blood pressure. When these mechanisms no longer maintain blood pressure, shock is overt or uncompensated.

In all shock, prevention of the potentially fatal tissue acidosis depends upon treating and reversing the underlying cause in order to restore adequate circulating volume. In hypovolemic shock, the lost volume, plus whatever is needed to compensate for vascular expansion, must be given intravenously. Peripheral vasoconstriction must be restored in neurogenic shock; vasoconstrictor drugs are usually used for this. The basic infection is treated vigorously in septic shock to prevent further bacterial toxins from maintaining vasodilatation. Cardiac output must be augmented or supported in cardiogenic shock. No really successful methods have been devised for this, and the mortality from cardiogenic shock is quite high (Haddy, 1970).

Nursing Management Nursing management generally consists of recognition of signs of impending and compensated shock states, assistance with therapy of overt shock, and assistance with emergency treatment of sudden severe shock. Implicit in assisting with therapy are the monitoring of vital signs and of urine output, observations of physical and mental changes indicative of a worsening state, and emotional support of a frightened person or family.

The responsibilities of a beginning nurse lie primarily in preventing and recognizing impending or compensated shock states in a person at risk. On rare occasions, the beginning nurse may be involved in emergency treatment of sudden shock. Ongoing responsibility for nursing care of a person in shock should not be undertaken by the beginner without adequate and close supervision.

Signs and Symptoms of Shock No one sign or symptom is exclusively diagnostic of shock. The patient's clinical status must be evaluated in the light of his history of potential shock state and the constellation of signs present.

Hypotension is almost always present in shock but may occur unrelated to it. However, decreased blood pressure, coupled with tachycardia; pale, clammy skin; and apprehension are likely to indicate shock.

Because of peripheral vasoconstriction, hypotension will not be evident during the stage of compensated shock. A volume of as much as 1,500 to 1,700 ml may be lost before any change in blood pressure occurs. Absolute blood pressure readings are of little value. However, a steadily decreasing trend and a narrowing pulse pressure suggest that decompensation is imminent. Scribner et al. (1969) feel that inability to maintain postural adjustments in blood pressure will occur before overt shock is present in volume depletion. They consider a systolic drop of 15 mm Hg and/or a diastolic drop of 10 mm Hg significant. Assessment of postural change is definitely contraindicated in people liable to neurogenic or septic shock—a sudden change in position may precipitate hypotension and shock, since the ability to constrict peripheral vessels in response to change may be completely lacking in these people.

A decrease in urine output is a relatively early sign of decreased blood volume through the kidneys. When circulation is impaired, blood is shunted to the heart, lungs, and brain in preference to the other organs. If the patient has an indwelling catheter, a decrease in hourly urine output will be evident. Urine flow less than 20 ml per hour is generally considered indicative of shock in clinical situations compatible with that diagnosis. Obviously, the nurse needs to make

certain that mechanical obstruction of tubing or catheter is not the cause of the decreased output.

The patient's subjective symptoms are also important as indications of early shock. Increasing restlessness, agitation, and anxiety frequently accompany early states and probably reflect mild hypoxia. Thirst is a frequent symptom with hypovolemic shock. When a patient who might develop shock (e.g., one who has just had an operation or has just delivered a baby) suddenly becomes restless and apprehensive and complains of thirst, the alert nurse will check for overt blood loss and will summon the physician regardless of whether vital signs have changed. Increased drowsiness and loss of orientation and consciousness, coupled with other signs of shock, indicate a rapidly worsening state.

When a nurse feels that a patient is in compensated or early shock, he should summon a physician and be prepared to assist with therapy. In addition, he or someone he delegates should remain with the patient, both to observe him and to provide emotional support. The apprehension characteristic of impending shock is certainly increased when people are scurrying about without any explanation to the patient as to what is going on.

Emergency Management Shock creates an emergency situation when sudden vascular collapse occurs or when unrecognized early shock decompensates. Both conditions are characterized by sudden drop in blood pressure, prostration, and sometimes loss of consciousness. A physician should be summoned as quickly as possible, and emergency equipment brought to the bedside. Most important is intravenous equipment. Regardless of the cause of shock, an infusion will be needed, either to restore volume or to infuse vasoconstrictive drugs in neurogenic shock. Adequate ventilation is equally important, for hypoxia from airway obstruction will compound circulatory hypoxia. Consequently, endotracheal tubes and equipment for oxygen administration should be available. An adequately stocked emergency cart will have all the drugs and equipment needed for the emergency treatment of shock.

Until recently, nurses have been taught to place a patient in shock in the head-down, or Trendelenburg, position. The rationale was that the effect of gravity would increase venous return to the heart, thereby increasing cardiac output. Research with both animals and human beings, however, shows that this position does not increase cardiac output or cerebral blood flow. In fact, it may decrease cardiac output and carotid flow in human beings (Guntheroth et al., 1964; Taylor and Weil, 1967). In addition, the abdominal viscera fall against the diaphragm and increase the work of breathing. Thus, despite even some recent nursing recommendations of Trendelenburg position, the evidence from shock research units contraindicates its use as an emergency measure.

Simeone (1966) recommends a 45° elevation of the legs in order to aid circulating volume temporarily. This is more apt to be of value when blood has pooled in the legs than when large volumes are lost from the body. This modified Trendelenburg position has not been shown to be harmful and may be of some help. The horizontal position is preferable for long-term management of shock (Weil and Shubin, 1967, p. 339).

Summary of Common Problems, with Approaches

Problem	Approach
Saline depletion (extracellular volume depletion)	Provide added salt and water for people losing saline via normal routes (sweat, urine) to prevent hypovolemia
	Note abnormal saline losses (vomiting, diarrhea, wound drainage)
	Assist physician in therapy of saline depletion
Hypovolemic shock	Attempt to prevent by noting signs early:
	a Amounts of saline loss
	b Postural hypotension
	c State of neck-vein filling
	d Trends in vital signs
Saline excess	Prevention:
	Carefully monitor intravenous therapy
	Note rapid weight gain
	Teach about low-sodium diets
Edema	Elevate limbs
Localized	Use elastic stockings
	Prevent prolonged pressure on veins
Generalized	Prevent prolonged pressure on skin
	Use discretion in elevating limbs depending on cardiac status
	Observe for signs of pulmonary edema, cerebral edema
Thirst	Provide frequent oral hygiene
	Encourage sham drinking
	Space fluid intake in relation to solid intake
	Encourage sucking of frozen fluid
	Provide diversion
Discomfort from intravenous therapy	Alleviate fears
	Secure needle or cannula firmly
	Observe for phlebitis
	Maintain mobility of limbs not involved
	Maintain desired rate of flow

REFERENCES

Books

Circulatory Status

Beland, Irene, "Clinical Nursing: Pathophysiological and Psychosocial Approaches," 2d ed., The Macmillan Company, New York, 1970.

Friedberg, Charles, "Diseases of the Heart," 3d ed., W. B. Saunders Company, Philadelphia, 1966.

Jones, Mary, "Accuracy of Pulse Rates Counted for Fifteen, Thirty, and Sixty Seconds by Graduate Nurses and Basic Nursing Students," Unpublished Master's Thesis, University of Washington Library, Health Sciences Division, Seattle, 1967.

Kirkendall, W. M., et al., "Recommendations for Human Blood Pressure Determination by Sphygmomanometers," American Heart Association, 1967.

Moidel, Harriet, et al., "Nursing Care of the Patient with Medical-Surgical Disorders," McGraw-Hill Book Company, New York, 1971.

General Fluid and Electrolyte Status

Guyton, W., "A Textbook of Medical Physiology," 5th ed., W. B. Saunders Company, St. Louis, 1971.

Kintzel, Kay (ed.), "Advanced Concepts in Clinical Nursing," J. B. Lippincott Company, New York, 1971.

Scribner, B. H. (ed.), "A Teaching Syllabus for the Course on Fluid and Electrolyte Balance," 7th rev., University of Washington School of Medicine, Seattle, 1969.

Thirst

Holmes, J. H., Thirst and Fluid Intake Problems in Clinical Medicine, in M. J. Wagner (ed.), "First International Symposium on Thirst in the Regulation of Body Water, 1963," The Macmillan Company, New York, 1964.

Wolf, A. V., "Thirst: Physiology of the Urge to Drink and Problems of Water Lack," Charles C Thomas, Publisher, Springfield, Ill., 1958.

Intravenous Therapy

Hume, M., S. Sevitt, and D. P. Thomas, "Venous Thrombosis and Pulmonary Embolism," Harvard University Press, Cambridge, Mass., 1970.

Link, Marlene, "A Study to Investigate the Incidence of Infiltration and Possible Relationships of Selected Factors in Continuous Intravenous Infusions," Unpublished Master's Thesis, University of Washington Library, Health Sciences Division, Seattle, 1967.

Metheney, N., and W. Snively, "Nurses' Handbook of Fluid and Electrolyte Balance," J. B. Lippincott Company, Philadelphia, 1967, p. 138.

Plumer, Ada L., "Principles and Practice of Intravenous Therapy," Little, Brown and Company, Boston, 1970.

Shock

Hardaway, R. M., et al., "Clinical Management of Shock," Charles C Thomas, Publisher, Springfield, Ill., 1968.

Shoemaker, William, "Shock," Charles C Thomas, Publisher, Springfield, Ill., 1967.

Weil, Max, and Herbert Shubin (eds.), "Diagnosis and Treatment of Shock," The William & Wilkins Company, Baltimore, 1967.

Periodicals

General Fluid and Electrolyte Status

Gault, M. H., et al.: Hypernatremia, Azotemia, and Dehydration Due to High-protein Tube Feeding, *Annals of Internal Medicine,* **68**:790 (1968).

Gillespie, J. B., G. A. Miller, and J. Schloreth: Water Intoxication Following Enemas for Roentgenographic Preparation, *American Journal of Roentgenography,* **82**:1059 (1959).

LeGros Clark, F.: Food Habits as a Practical Nutrition Problem, *World Review of Nutrition and Dietetics,* **9**:56–84 (1968).

Thirst

Deaux, E., and J. W. Kakolewski: Emotionally Induced Increase in Effective Osmotic Pressure and Subsequent Thirst, *Science,* **169**:1226–1228 (Sept. 18, 1970).

Fenton, M.: What to Do about Thirst, *American Journal of Nursing,* **69**:1014–1017 (1969).

Morgane, P. T., and H. L. Jacobs: Hunger and Satiety, *World Review of Nutrition and Dietetics,* **10**:120 (1969).

Oral Care

DeWalt, E. M., and A. K. Haines: The Effects of Specified Stressors on Healthy Oral Mucosa, *Nursing Research,* **18**:22–27 (1969).

Ginsberg, M.: A Study of Oral Hygiene Nursing Care, *American Journal of Nursing,* **61**:67–69 (1961).

——— and A. E. Yoder: The Effectiveness of Some Traditional Methods in Oral Hygiene Nursing Care, *Journal of Periodontia,* **35**:513–518 (1964).

Passos, J., and L. Brand: Effects of Agents Used for Oral Hygiene, *Nursing Research,* **15**:196–202 (1966).

Van Drimmelen, S., and H. Rollins: Evaluation of a Commonly Used Oral Hygiene Agent, *Nursing Research,* **18**:327–332 (1969).

Wiley, S.: Why Glycerol and Lemon Juice? *American Journal of Nursing,* **69**:342–344 (1969).

Intravenous Therapy

Cheney, F. W., and J. R. Lincoln: Phlebitis from Plastic Intravenous Catheters, *Anesthesiology,* **25**:650–652 (1964).

Duma, R., J. Warner, and H. Dalton: Septicemia from Intravenous Infusion, *New England Journal of Medicine,* **284**:257–259 (Feb. 4, 1971).

Flanagan, J. P., et al.: Air Embolus—A Lethal Complication of Subclavian Venipuncture, *New England Journal of Medicine,* **281**:488–489 (Aug. 28, 1969). Letters reporting additional cases: **281**:966 (Oct. 23, 1969); **281**:1425 (Dec. 8, 1969).

Gaan, D., et al.: Cerebral Damage from Declotting Scribner Shunts, *Lancet,* **2**:77–79 (July 12, 1969).

How the Septicemia Trail Led to the IV Bottle Cap, *Hospital Practice,* **6**:35–45, 151–154 (August, 1971).

Lowenstein, E., J. W. Little, and H. H. Lo: Preventing Cerebral Embolization from Flushing Radial Artery Cannulas, *New England Journal of Medicine,* **285**:1414–1415 (Dec. 16, 1971).

Moore, R. M., and C. W. Braselton: Injection of Air and Carbon Dioxide into a Pulmonary Vein, *Archives of Surgery,* **112**:212–218 (August, 1940).

Pederson, B. M.: A Solution for Post-infusion Thrombophlebitis, *American Journal of Nursing,* **70**:325 (1970).

Simpson, K.: Air Accidents during Transfusion, *Lancet,* **242**:679–698 (June 13, 1942).

Sylvester, M., and P. Bruno: Factors Associated with Infiltration during Continuous Intravenous Therapy, *Nursing Research,* **15**:255–258 (1966).

Yeakel, D. E.: Lethal Air Embolism from Plastic Blood Storage Container, *Journal of the American Medical Association,* **204**:267–269 (1968).

Shock

Cohn, J.: Monitoring Techniques in Shock, *American Journal of Cardiology,* **26**:565–569 (1970).

Guntheroth, W. G., F. L. Abel, and G. L. Mullins: The Effect of Trendelenburg's Position on Blood Pressure and Carotid Flow, *Surgery, Gynecology and Obstetrics,* **119**:345–348 (1964).

Haddy, F. J.: Pathophysiology and Treatment of the Shock of Myocardial Infarction, *Annals of Internal Medicine,* **73**:809–827 (1970).

Simeone, F. A.: The Treatment of Shock, *American Journal of Nursing,* **66**:1290–1295 (1966).

Taylor, J., and M. A. Weil: Failure of the Trendelenburg Position to Improve Circulation during Clinical Shock, *Surgery, Gynecology and Obstetrics,* **124**:1005–1010 (1967).

Respiratory Status

Pamela Mitchell
Judith West
Margaret Auld

Data to Be Assessed

Objective	Subjective
Airway patency	History of disease affecting respiratory status
Respiratory rate, depth, character	Sensation of difficult breathing
Effort or lack of effort	Tolerance to activity
Regularity	Environmental influences
Chest expansion	Aids to ventilation:
Breath sounds	Home therapy—IPPB, medications, oxygen, exercises
Mentation	Altered airway—tracheostomy, endotracheal tube
Level of consciousness	Assisted or controlled ventilation
Anxiety, restlessness	Oxygen therapy
Posture, body position	
Cough—secretions	
(presence, pattern, character)	
Laboratory values: Po_2, Pco_2, pH	
Pulmonary function tests	

RESPIRATION: GAS EXCHANGE

Respiration is the most fundamental of life processes. All others either contribute to the movement and exchange of gas by the cells, or are dependent upon adequate respiration of the component cells. For example, brain cells cannot survive more than four to five minutes without oxygen. Muscle cells can function considerably longer but must "pay back" the oxygen "debt."

Some physiologists categorize respiration into two phases: internal and external. Internal, or cellular, respiration is the exchange of oxygen and carbon dioxide between cells and the surrounding capillaries, and the utilization of oxygen by the cells. External respiration consists of the mechanical movement of gases in and out of the pulmonary airways, and the movement of gases into and out of the alveolar capillaries—ventilation and diffusion. The element common to both phases of respiration is the circulating blood.

Thus, respiratory status is determined by the function of three systems: pulmonary (lung and airway), circulatory, and cellular. Comroe (1965) refers to the lungs as the gas exchanger; the airways and alveoli function to bring air into the lungs, provide oxygen, and eliminate carbon dioxide. The circulation then acts as the gas mover, carrying oxygen (both dissolved and combined with hemoglobin) to the cells and carbon dioxide from the cells, and promoting exchange of gases between capillaries and cells. Finally, the cells are the gas users, dependent upon a constant supply of oxygen for biochemical reactions, and a constant elimination of excess carbon dioxide to maintain the pH necessary for the reactions to occur.

Many people erroneously believe that changes in respiratory status indicate only disorders of the lungs or upper airways. Similarly, many beginning nursing students feel that changes in breathing rate and quality are indicative only of pulmonary disease. From the preceding paragraphs we can see that changes in breathing may be caused by any of the three components of respiration. Conversely, one must observe more than just breathing function to assess respiratory status; the state of circulation and partial pressures of dissolved gases and hydrogen-ion concentration in arterial blood also give us clues to respiratory status. In this chapter, we will present the factors affecting oxygenation of cells and removal of carbon dioxide from the cells, manifestations of normal and abnormal function, and nursing management in problems of dysfunction. The focus of beginning nursing practice will be on maintaining function, preventing further dysfunction, and sustaining the person in his dysfunction.

Alterations in Normal Gas Exchange

Alterations in normal gas exchange may lead to *hypoxia*—inadequate cellular oxygen; *hypoxemia*—decreased oxygen tension in the blood; *hypercapnia*—increased carbon dioxide tension in the blood; and *hypocapnia*—decreased carbon dioxide tension in the blood. Factors contributing to the development of these abnormal states include changes or abnormalities in the following: the composition of inspired air, the ability of the pulmonary system to move air uniformly, the ability of the circulatory system to carry oxygen and carbon dioxide, the cellular need for oxygen, and the ability of the cells to use oxygen. The general causes and manifestations of hypoxia, hypoxemia, hypercapnia, and hypocapnia will be discussed in the following section in relation to the function of the three systems involved in respiration. This section is not intended to be a comprehensive review of the physiology of normal and abnormal respiration. The student may wish to review a textbook of normal physiology for such information. In addition, Comroe's *The Physiology of Respiration* (1965) is a highly readable and thorough source.

Hypoxia

Two terms used to describe oxygenation abnormalities are *hypoxemia* and *hypoxia*. Although the two abnormalities are related, the terms are not synonymous. Hypoxemia means a decrease in the partial pressure of oxygen in arterial blood; it is discussed further on. Hypoxia, commonly used to mean tissue hypoxia, refers to inadequate supply of oxygen to tissues. The inadequate oxygen supply may occur either because oxygen delivery is not sufficient for tissue requirements or because utilization of oxygen is blocked at the cellular level.

Cellular need for oxygen will ultimately determine whether the amount inspired and transported is adequate. For example, exercise increases cellular oxygen requirements (metabolic rate) severalfold, depending upon the level of exertion. Similarly, each degree of fever increases the metabolic rate at least 7 percent. Conversely, a decrease in activity decreases the need of active cells for oxygen. Muscular exercise is not the only stimulus to increased metabolic activity; greater than normal demands from any of the organ systems increases the need for oxygen. Problems in respiration result when oxygen delivery is not adequate to meet cellular needs.

A second variable affecting cellular respiration is the ability of the cells to utilize oxygen from the blood. Some poisons, such as cyanide, formaldehyde, arsenic, and some heavy metals, directly inhibit cell use of oxygen or interfere with the enzymes which catalyze oxidative reactions in the cells (Wintrobe et al., 1970).

Oxygen delivery is a function of both cardiac output and the amount of oxygen carried per unit of blood. This is expressed in the following equation:

Cardiac output, as discussed in Chapter 15, is the product of heart rate and stroke volume. Oxygen content of the blood consists primarily of the oxygen bound to hemoglobin (expressed as hemoglobin saturation) and of a small amount of dissolved oxygen (measured by the partial pressure of oxygen—Po_2). Thus conditions which affect the circulating blood volume, the amount of dissolved oxygen, and the oxygen-carrying capacity of the blood can all result in hypoxia. Shock, high altitude, and anemia are examples of such situations.

Hypoxia may be local, as when blood flow is cut off to a part of the body or to an organ, or systemic (throughout the body). An example of systemic hypoxia is that which results from decreased cardiac output in hemorrhagic shock, or that which results from severe ventilatory defects. Certain signs (e.g., increased pulse rate, cyanosis, restlessness, apprehension, and unconsciousness) are seen in hypoxia but are not reliably specific to it. Some of these signs may also be present in hypercapnia or nonhypoxic states. A decreased Po_2 value in conjunction with some of the above signs is indicative of hypoxia.

Hypoxemia

As stated previously, hypoxemia is defined as a decrease in the partial pressure (also called tension) of oxygen in the arterial blood. (Normal arterial Po_2 is 90 to 100 mm Hg.) There are four major causes of hypoxemia: (1) decrease in environmental (ambient) oxygen concentration, (2) alveolar hypoventilation, (3) shunting of blood (blood which passes from the right side to the left side of the heart without being exposed to oxygen), and (4) ventilation-perfusion abnormalities. Impairment of gas diffusion (so-called

$$O_2 \text{ delivery} = (\text{cardiac output}) \times (O_2 \text{ content})$$
$$\phantom{O_2 \text{ delivery} = } (\text{rate} \times \text{stroke volume}) \quad (\text{dissolved } O_2 + \text{hemoglobin-bound } O_2)$$

"alveolar-capillary block") was once considered a cause of hypoxemia. However, recent evidence has shown that oxygen is so highly soluble in tissues that an impossibly thick membrane would be needed to interfere sufficiently with diffusion (Pontoppidan, 1970).

Decrease in Ambient Oxygen Concentration Decreases in ambient oxygen are generally encountered only at very high altitudes or when air is breathed in a closed system. Such a situation occurs during administration of anesthesia if oxygen breathed is not replaced or if it is replaced with another gas.

The partial pressure of ambient oxygen is one factor which determines how much oxygen diffuses into the blood. Movement of gas molecules in the air at sea level creates a pressure of 760 mm Hg. Each gas composing the air mixture exerts a part of this pressure, or a *partial pressure.* Because oxygen comprises 20.93 percent of air, it exerts a partial pressure of 20.93 × 760 mm Hg, or 159.1 mm Hg in dry air. If atmospheric pressure is reduced, e.g., at altitude, the partial pressure of oxygen will be 20.93 percent of that decreased atmospheric pressure, so that the concentration of oxygen will be reduced.

Alveolar Hypoventilation Ultimately the air moved in and out of the lungs must reach the alveoli in order to diffuse into the blood and be used by the cells. Movement of gas in and out of the lungs is called *ventilation.* When the minute ventilation (amount of air moved into the lungs per minute) is decreased, the carbon dioxide which has diffused from the blood to the alveolus tends to remain in the alveolus. This causes an increase in the carbon dioxide tension in the alveolus, which impairs the release of carbon dioxide from the blood to the alveolus. Thus the partial pressure of carbon dioxide in the blood rises (hypercapnia) and, by displacement, the oxygen tension drops (hypoxemia). Alveolar hypoventilation, then, is defined as hypercapnia secondary to reduced movement of alveolar gas.

In addition, the person will have hypoxemia unless he is breathing an oxygen-enriched mixture. Hypoventilation may be suspected in a person who breathes shallowly, but is not confirmed unless laboratory evidence of hypercapnia is present. Situations in which hypoventilation may occur include bed rest, weakness of respiratory muscles, postoperative pain which results in conscious inhibition of deep breathing, and narcotic sedation. Nursing measures to prevent hypoventilation are discussed later in this chapter.

Shunting A shunt is defined as the passage of blood from the right side to the left side of the heart without being oxygenated. The end result of a shunt is a mixture of oxygenated and unoxygenated blood, or hypoxemia. Shunts may occur within the heart itself (e.g., in congenital structural abnormalities) or in the lungs. Anatomic anastomoses of pulmonary arterial to venous circulation will result in shunting of blood back to the heart without contact with alveoli. A shuntlike effect has the same physiological result as an anatomic shunt. This effect occurs when a pulmonary capillary perfuses (flows by) nonventilated alveoli and thus receives no oxygen. Those situations which result in nonventilated alveoli include pneumonia, in which alveoli are filled with inflammatory products, and atelectasis, in which alveoli are collapsed. Atelectasis is clinically detectable only when a large number of alveoli in one area of the lung are collapsed or not ventilated; collapse of a few alveoli is referred to as microatelectasis. The concepts of alveolar hypoventilation and of shunting are important in the care of immobilized and postoperative patients and will be discussed under "Nursing Management," further on in this chapter.

Ventilation-Perfusion Abnormalities Although the lungs are often depicted schematically as two balloons filled with air, they are actually composed of several million little "balloons"—the alveoli. Because of the large number of ventilatory structures, the ventilation throughout the lung is not uniform. For example, in the upright person, the base of each lung receives more air than does the apex. In general, areas of greater ventilation receive greater perfusion and areas of lesser ventilation receive less perfusion. Thus, ventilation and perfusion tend to be matched throughout the lung.

Gas exchange within the lungs depends not only upon ventilation of air and perfusion of blood per se, but also on the matching of these two processes throughout the lungs. Hypoxemia will result when there are substantial areas in which the ventilation is reduced relative to the perfusion. In each alveolus ventilation must replenish the amount of oxygen taken up by the perfusing pulmonary capillary and must remove the amount of carbon dioxide released from the capillary. If the ventilation to one area of the lung becomes decreased without a change in the perfusion to that area, then the rate of oxygen replenishment and the rate of carbon dioxide removal are reduced. Consequently, in these alveoli the oxygen tension will fall and the carbon dioxide tension will rise to new levels, and the blood leaving this area will have a reduced Po_2 and an increased Pco_2. Such blood will mix with blood from other areas of the lung.

Because of the nature of carbon dioxide transport, increased ventilation in one area of the lung can compensate for decreased ventilation in another part, and thus result in a normal arterial Pco_2. However, because of the characteristics of oxygen-hemoglobin dissociation, the increased ventilation in one area will compensate only partially for the decreased ventilation in another; hence some degree of arterial hypoxemia will result. (A shunt might be considered the extreme of a ventilation-perfusion abnormality: i.e., in a shunt there is no ventilation of a perfused area.)

In addition to causing hypoxemia, imbalance of ventilation to perfusion results in inefficient overall ventilation. This is because some areas have to be overventilated to compensate for those which are poorly ventilated. This inefficiency is apt to result in breathlessness.

The mechanisms by which ventilation-perfusion abnormalities result in hypoxemia are more complex than warrants discussion here. However, it is important that nurses be aware of such abnormalities, as they constitute perhaps the most common cause of hypoxemia and are an important cause of breathlessness. Many chronic conditions, such as heart failure, asthma, and chronic obstructive pulmonary disease, have ventilation-perfusion abnormalities as a prominent feature. When a physician has diagnosed such an abnormality as the cause of hypoxemia, he attempts to increase ventilation to the portion of the lung involved.

Hypoxemia in Relation to Oxygen Content Although hypoxemia reflects abnormal pulmonary gas exchange, it does not necessarily mean that the oxygen content of the blood is reduced sufficiently to produce tissue hypoxia. As shown in the equation regarding oxygen delivery, dissolved oxygen, or Po_2, is only a part of the oxygen content of the blood. The majority of the oxygen is carried via the hemoglobin (the portion of the red blood cell which has an affinity, or attraction, for oxygen). The percentage of oxygen to hemoglobin in relation to the total capacity is called *percent saturation* or simply saturation. Hemoglobin is normally 97 to 98 percent saturated with oxygen.

Partial pressure of oxygen is one of the factors (along with pH and temperature of the blood) which determine the association or dissociation of oxygen with hemoglobin (saturation). The relation between partial pressure of oxygen and hemoglobin saturation is not linear. The hemoglobin-oxygen dissociation curve is shown in Fig. 16-1. At the top, or flat part, of the curve, hemoglobin is saturated in the 90 percent and greater range and continues to be so until Po_2 has dropped to below 60 mm Hg, a 40 mm Hg drop in oxygen tension. Even at a Po_2 of 45 mm

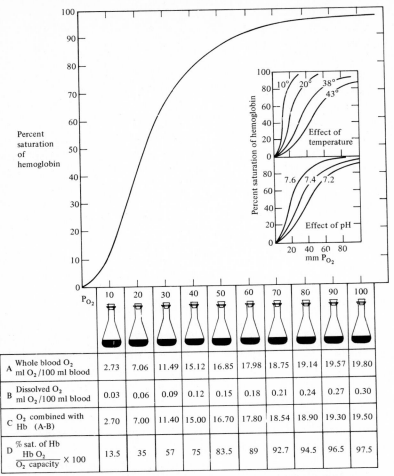

Figure 16-1 Hemoglobin-oxygen dissociation curves. The large graph shows a single dissociation curve, applicable when the pH of the blood is 7.40 and the temperature 38°C. The curve shifts to the right or left when temperature, pH, or Pco_2 is changed, as shown in the small graphs. Note the large drop which must occur in Po_2 before the percent saturation (line D) drops significantly. Note also the extremely small amount of oxygen which the dissolved oxygen (line B) contributes to the total blood oxygen content (line A). *(Reproduced from Julius H. Comroe, "The Physiology of Respiration: An Introductory Text," Year Book Medical Publishers, Inc., Chicago, 1965. By permission of the publishers.)*

	Po_2	10	20	30	40	50	60	70	80	90	100
A	Whole blood O_2 ml O_2/100 ml blood	2.73	7.06	11.49	15.12	16.85	17.98	18.75	19.14	19.57	19.80
B	Dissolved O_2 ml O_2/100 ml blood	0.03	0.06	0.09	0.12	0.15	0.18	0.21	0.24	0.27	0.30
C	O_2 combined with Hb (A-B)	2.70	7.00	11.40	15.00	16.70	17.80	18.54	18.90	19.30	19.50
D	% sat. of Hb $\dfrac{Hb\ O_2}{O_2\ capacity} \times 100$	13.5	35	57	75	83.5	89	92.7	94.5	96.5	97.5

Hg (less than half the normal value), hemoglobin is about 80 percent saturated with oxygen. This saturation would be sufficient for resting cell oxygen needs, provided a normal amount of hemoglobin is circulating. Once Po_2 drops below 45 to 50 mm Hg, the percent saturation of hemoglobin changes markedly with each decrease in oxygen tension. Knowledge of the effect of oxygen tension on hemoglobin saturation is important to nurses in understanding that the Po_2 value alone does not provide sufficient information to determine if hypoxia is necessarily present with hypoxemia.

Conversely, hypoxia may occur without hypoxemia. The total amount of oxygen carried by hemoglobin depends upon the number of red blood cells as well as the percent saturation of each hemoglobin molecule. When red blood cells are not available in sufficient quantity (as in anemia) or when the hemoglobin preferentially combines with a substance other than oxygen (as in carbon monoxide poisoning), blood will contain lesser amounts of oxygen even in the presence of normal gas exchange and a normal arterial oxygen tension. If the deficit is severe enough, an inadequate amount of oxygen will be delivered to the cells and tissue hypoxia will result.

Hypercapnia

Hypercapnia, or hypercarbia, is the elevation of carbon dioxide tension in the arterial blood (P_{CO_2}). The normal value for arterial P_{CO_2} is 40 ± 2 mm Hg. Carbon dioxide is produced by the metabolic activity of cells, and must be eliminated to maintain normal pH (hydrogen-ion concentration). Since carbon dioxide hydrates to form carbonic acid, which dissociates into free hydrogen ion and bicarbonate, it must be eliminated or buffered to prevent dangerous alterations in plasma pH. The alveoli serve to eliminate carbon dioxide through expiration. (An expanded discussion of the role of carbon dioxide in regulation of hydrogen-ion concentration is given in Chapter 15.) Hypercapnia occurs when ventilation is inadequate for the amount of carbon dioxide produced by the body. There are no truly reliable signs of hypercapnia except arterial P_{CO_2} determinations. Certain signs may accompany the state, but they are not specific enough for definitive diagnosis. These signs include headache, dyspnea, increased pulse rate and blood pressure, irritability, difficulty in concentrating, and unconsciousness. Such signs are related to the effects of altered pH on cells and do not occur when hypercapnia develops slowly, as in chronic pulmonary obstructive disease. In such instances, renal compensatory mechanisms have had time to adjust and maintain blood pH near normal.

Hypocapnia

Hypocapnia, or hypocarbia, is a decreased carbon dioxide tension in the arterial blood. Such a decrease affects the hydrogen-ion concentration by removing free hydrogen ion and thus raising pH. Hypocapnia is caused by hyperventilation—an increase above normal in the amount of air exhaled per unit of time. This elevated minute ventilation initially "blows off" carbon dioxide, decreasing the concentration of carbon dioxide in the alveoli and thus in the blood. If the hyperventilation is sustained, a new steady state is reached, in which the arterial carbon dioxide tension is less than normal. Anxiety, fever, hypoxia, and metabolic acidosis are among the situations causing hyperventilation. Although increased rate of breathing may be associated with hyperventilation, it is not synonymous with it. Hypocapnia is thus the only reliable criterion for hyperventilation. The concomitant alkalosis (rise in pH) leads to several rather nonspecific signs, such as irritability, numbness, muscle cramps, headache, dizziness, and cardiac arrhythmias.

ASSESSMENT OF RESPIRATORY STATUS

It should be apparent from the preceding discussion that one needs to evaluate far more than the pattern of breathing when determining respiratory state or respiratory adequacy. For the purposes of this discussion, assessment data will be divided into three groups: objective data, subjective data, and laboratory data. We shall look first at normal findings, then at some manifestations of dysfunction, and finally at nursing help to maintain function and to assist during dysfunction.

Certain groups of people are at increased risk of respiratory difficulty and should have their respiratory status observed more closely than that of others. This group includes people who have acute cardiac problems, those in shock, those with acute pulmonary disease or decompensation of chronic disease, those with increased intracranial pressure, and anyone who begins to have difficulty in breathing.

Rate, Rhythm, and Character of Respirations

The number of breaths per minute (respiratory rate) is the most common, most easily measured, and probably least valuable observation regarding respiratory status. Like the other common vital signs discussed in Chapter 15, respiratory rate is at best a partial estimate of ventilation. Rate in itself tells us nothing about the volume inspired in each breath; however, minute ventilation—the product of rate and tidal volume—is a better indicator of air movement and, thus, of ventilatory ability. Currently, tidal volume can be measured at the bedside, but it is measured only for selected patients or in respiratory-care units. Nurses will become more and more involved in such clinical measurement in situations in which estimation of ventilatory ability is needed. At present, most nurses will continue to record only respiratory rate and to observe changes in the depth of respiration. Such observation should be made with the knowledge that it provides only the roughest of clues to volume inspired. Similarly observations about the character of breathing—rhythm and apparent ease or difficulty of respiration—are also only rough indicators of abnormal function.

Regulation of Respiratory Rate and Depth Somewhere along the continuum between rapid, shallow breathing and slow, deep breathing, normal frequencies have evolved for the various species. In the human being, approximately 15 breaths per minute at 500 cc oxygen per breath provide necessary ventilation with the least work (Fenn, 1960). Deeper respirations expand volume so that the work required for each breath rises. Respiratory rate and depth may be altered by several voluntary and involuntary processes, including physiological regulatory mechanisms and the effects of posture and movement.

Physiological Regulation of Rate Physiological mechanisms operate to maintain normal carbon dioxide tension, normal hydrogen-ion concentration (pH), and adequate supplies of oxygen in the blood. Although it might seem logical that alterations in the arterial oxygen tension (Po_2) would be the primary trigger for changes in respiration, physiological research has demonstrated that the regulatory mechanisms are more responsive to changes in carbon dioxide tension (Pco_2) and hydrogen-ion concentration than to oxygen tension.

The respiratory center in the pons and medulla is directly sensitive to the carbon dioxide tension and the resultant effect on hydrogen-ion concentration. An increased Pco_2 and hydrogen-ion concentration (decreased pH) stimulates deeper and faster breathing, which in turn increases alveolar ventilation. Conversely, a decreased Pco_2 or hydrogen-ion concentration (increased pH) may lead to slower respiration.

The interdependence of these two factors is apparent if you recall from Chapter 15 that an increase in the level of carbon dioxide, under appropriate conditions, can shift the plasma bicarbonate reaction to form carbonic acid (H_2CO_3); the weak acid then dissociates to form free hydrogen ion.[1] It is to the body's advantage to "blow off" the excess carbon dioxide and thus eliminate a potential hydrogen-ion donor. Increased rate and depth of respiration accomplish this. Conversely, if insufficient carbon dioxide is present in the plasma, less hydrogen ion will be formed; carbon dioxide tension falls, pH rises (remember that pH reflects the reciprocal of the hydrogen-ion concentration); the respiratory center is inhibited; respiratory rate decreases; less carbon dioxide is eliminated; and the balance is restored.

In normal people the periodic deep sighing during sleep occurs because of this mechanism. In conditions which produce a state of altered

$$^1 CO_2 + H_2O \underset{\text{carbonic}}{\rightleftharpoons} H_2CO_3 \rightleftharpoons H^+ + HCO_3^-$$
$$\text{anhydrase}$$

consciousness, decreased respiratory depth may lead to a buildup of carbon dioxide levels in the blood. If the respiratory center in the brain is depressed pharmacologically by drugs, or mechanically by increased intracranial pressure, the center may not be so sensitive to increasing carbon dioxide or hydrogen-ion concentrations.

A secondary determinant of respiratory rate is the *hypoxic drive*. A markedly decreased oxygen supply in the blood flowing to chemoreceptors in the aortic and carotid bodies stimulates an increase in the rate of breathing. Because the chemoreceptors depend upon a certain amount of oxygen per unit of time, they can be triggered either by a decrease in oxygen content with normal blood flow, or by a slow blood flow with normal content. The receptors take more oxygen from any milliliter of blood if the total delivered in one minute is decreased. Chemoreceptors are also sensitive to carbon dioxide tension and hydrogen-ion concentration, but these are less potent stimuli here than they are at the respiratory center in the brain.

With normal blood flow, P_{O_2} must decrease to about 50 mm Hg to stimulate the chemoreceptors. If blood flow is one-half to one-fourth normal (as in hemorrhage or other causes of severe shock), the receptors fire with a P_{O_2} near normal (Comroe, 1965, p. 47).

Thus, in most instances, it is the *drive to eliminate carbon dioxide* that sets the rate of respiration. Only when systemic or ambient oxygen is in short supply does the *hypoxic drive* regulated by the chemoreceptors operate. This is an important concept in the care of persons with chronic obstructive pulmonary disease. Such persons cannot effectively eliminate carbon dioxide; they thus live with prolonged elevation of P_{CO_2}. The respiratory center is no longer stimulated by this level of carbon dioxide, and breathing is stimulated only by hypoxia at the chemoreceptors. Consequently, if high concentrations of oxygen are administered to such persons, e.g., when they are in acute respiratory distress, the hypoxic drive is abolished and the person may stop breathing. Emergency administration of oxygen to persons whose respiratory disease status is unknown is obviously unwise.

Effect of Movement and Posture on Rate and Ventilation Excitation of joint and muscle proprioceptors during exercise increases pulmonary ventilation by stimulating increased rate and depth of breathing. Movement of the limbs causes transmission of impulses from the proprioceptors in the joints to the respiratory center, which can stimulate a severalfold increase in ventilation even if that movement is passive (Guyton, 1971). Therefore, assisting the immobilized person with range-of-motion exercises improves alveolar ventilation, in addition to the local effects on joint mobility (see Chapter 12).

The volume of air which can be inhaled varies with posture. Lying supine reduces vital capacity by approximately 200 to 300 cc, because of compression of the chest and increased intrathoracic blood volume. Both these effects decrease the available space within the thorax for lung expansion (Wade and Gilson, 1951). In normal people, lung elasticity decreases in the supine position and mechanical resistance to air flow increases; both changes require increased muscular work to maintain ventilation (Attinger, 1956). Moreover, the ventilation-perfusion relationship is adversely altered in the supine position. Simply turning to the lateral lying position raises arterial P_{O_2} and apparently improves ventilation-perfusion changes created in the supine position (Clauss et al., 1968).

Terms Describing Rate Deviations from normal or easy breathing *(eupnea)* may be defined by generally accepted terms. These terms should be accompanied by the actual counted rate and other indications of respiratory status, including the patient-client's subjective feeling of difficulty, change in mentation or state of consciousness, and use of accessory muscles of respiration. *Tachypnea* may be used to describe respirations of more than 24 per minute and *bradypnea* for a rate of fewer than 10 respirations per minute.

Cessation of breathing is called *apnea*. The continued absence of respiration is obviously incompatible with life. Mechanical airway occlusion, carbon dioxide narcosis (loss of hypoxic drive), severe head injury affecting the respiratory center in the brain, or intracranial pressure elevations may be sufficient to arrest breathing.

Measuring Respiratory Rate   In hospitals, respiratory rate is one of the "vital signs" checked rather routinely on all patients. Depending upon the institutional routine, these measurements may be taken from one to four times daily. The accuracy of measurement and the need for such determinations in the average hospitalized person have been questioned time and again in recent years. In 1957, Kory surveyed physicians' and hospital records regarding the need for respiratory rate data and the correlation of such data with clinical change in the condition of patients. Such measurement appeared to be indicated or useful in less than 5 percent of the several thousand patients involved. In addition, observers checked the accuracy of respiratory rates recorded by nursing personnel. The nursing staff recorded rates between 18 and 22 per minute, whereas the actual respirations (taken seconds later by trained observers) ranged from 11 to 33 per minute. Nursing personnel recorded only the rate, while notations about the depth and character of breathing were omitted.

Eisman (1970) interviewed 48 registered nurses regarding their practice in counting respirations. Slightly greater than half actually counted the rate; the remainder "estimated" the number. Kory's study and empirical observation suggest that nurses and auxiliary personnel estimate rate on the basis of the prevalent notion that a range of 18 to 20 respirations per minute is normal, rather than on the basis of a range of the 14 to 16 respirations per minute, as documented by physiologists.

The nurses in Eisman's study who both counted and estimated rates made their decision as to which method to use on the basis of the "patient's appearance" (usually difficulty in breath-ing, color change, and vague "looked bad") and the medical diagnosis which suggested increased risk of respiratory problems (e.g., postoperative thoracic surgery, acute head injury). One suspects that these nurses "estimated" some rates because they felt expected to fill in a number on the vital sign sheet, although the patient's status did not indicate any need for this measurement.

In Chapters 15 and 17 we emphasize the need for nurses to decide *when* to measure vital signs in assessing circulatory and temperature status, and to make such decisions on the basis of the patient's status and potential difficulties, rather than on the basis of an institutional routine alone. The same is true with respiratory rate. The physician may well determine the frequency of measurement by his need for data about a patient's rapidly changing status. The nurse may wish to increase the frequency of such data collection if the person's condition worsens. In contrast, stabilization of status may indicate a decreasing need for frequent determination. Routine measurement of circulatory, temperature, and respiratory status for patients who have no pathologic condition which directly affects such status and who are not undergoing therapy that affects it is wasteful of time and money. Kory estimated that upward of $5 million is wasted in such routine. Inflation since 1957 would markedly increase that figure today.

Character of Breathing

Effort Associated with Breathing   Normal respiration appears effortless, and a person is usually not consciously aware of his breathing. A number of pathological or mechanical factors may result in increased and visible muscular effort associated with breathing. This increased effort may be characterized by increased rate and depth of breathing, use of accessory muscles of breathing, and a subjective feeling of breathlessness or difficult or painful breathing, which is called *dyspnea*. Observation of a person's effort or lack of effort in breathing provides some rough clues as to the stability or instability of his respiratory status.

Increased rate and depth of breathing may be the result of a normal response to such factors as exercise, fear, or strong emotion. Such a response may also be triggered when disease alters oxygen requirements, metabolic acid production, or carbon dioxide production. The deep, rapid breathing characteristic of diabetic acidosis is one such example.

The accessory muscles of breathing are used when the major respiratory muscles (the diaphragm and the external intercostals) are weak or paralyzed, or when the effort of the major muscles cannot provide sufficient ventilation to meet the body's oxygen demands. Severe muscular exercise, acute obstruction of the airways, and collapse of a substantial portion of the alveoli (atelectasis) are among the normal and abnormal situations which might provoke use of the accessory muscles. The primary accessory muscles are the scalene, sternomastoid, trapezius, and latissimus dorsi muscles. In severe exercise, use of these muscles is valuable in increasing the volume of inspired air per minute. In acute obstruction of the airways, or severe pulmonary disease, the use of accessory muscles indicates inability to inspire sufficient air; it may not result in adequate ventilation, and may soon exhaust the person.

The unpleasant sensation of breathlessness and difficult breathing is commonly called *dyspnea*. It occurs in some but not all situations which result in increased breathing effort. Frequently an observer can see the dyspneic person's visible efforts at breathing; sometimes, however, the person feels breathless but does not appear to be having labored respirations. Dyspnea is discussed more fully under "Subjective Data," later in this chapter.

The concept of *work of breathing* is related to, but not synonymous with, the energy cost of breathing. Strictly speaking, work is a physical term defined as force × distance or pressure × volume. However, common usage frequently equates work with energy expended. The muscles of breathing must overcome primarily two resistances: (1) the elasticity of the lung tissue, and (2) the resistance to air flow within the airways. In order to measure the work performed by these muscles in ventilating the lungs, one would have to measure the pressure which the muscles exert necessary to move a normal amount of gas. Such a measurement can be made in the laboratory using a tank respiratory (iron lung) to perform the work of the respiratory muscles (Comroe, 1965). However, this is purely an investigative procedure.

The metabolic or energy cost of the work of breathing is the amount of oxygen consumed by the muscles of respiration during breathing. This is an extremely difficult measurement and cannot be made directly. By indirect means, physiologists calculate that the ratio of useful work to energy expended in breathing is rather low and that the energy cost becomes disproportionately greater when minute ventilation (volume moved per minute) increases, as in rapid, deep breathing. Although this increased energy cost of breathing is often assumed to be critical relative to total oxygen requirements in people with acute respiratory insufficiency, recent work suggests that, on the contrary, even greatly increased work of breathing contributes little to overall body oxygen requirements (Pontopiddan et al., 1970).

Clinically, because the work of breathing cannot be measured easily, we can only make some inferences regarding the energy expenditure of people in certain disease categories, or with certain structural or functional alteration. For example, there is some evidence that obese persons and those with chronic obstructive pulmonary disease use more energy when they breathe (Comroe, 1965). We cannot, however, measure the *extent* of the increase in work.

In normal man and in many disease conditions, the respiratory regulatory mechanisms somehow compensate for changes in pulmonary elasticity and resistance so that energy expended remains near normal (Otis, 1964). For example, people with asthma tend to automatically take long, slow breaths, which decreases the effort needed to inspire and expire against the increased airway resistance. If, however, the asthmatic person becomes fearful that he cannot breathe, he may begin rapid, deep breathing or gasping, which increases the energy that he must expend but does not increase the volume of inspired air. In instances such as the one just described and others where regulatory mechanisms cannot maintain efficient ventilation, therapy is aimed toward remedying or arresting the underlying pathologic change—e.g., relieving bronchospasm in asthma, increasing ventilation in postoperative atelectasis, reversing the diabetic acidosis which precipitates hyperventilation, or decreasing anxiety which may also stimulate hyperventilation.

Breathing Sounds Another set of objective data consists of the sounds of breathing, both those heard with the unaided ear and those heard when a stethoscope is placed on the chest. Normal respiration is characterized by quiet inspiratory and expiratory excursions. Abnormal sounds indicate constriction of airways, expansion of deflated airways, consolidation of lung tissue, or the presence of fluid in large airways.

Marked constriction of the airways produces *wheezing,* or whistling sounds, generally on expiration. Severe constriction of the trachea produces on inspiration a harsh, crowing sound called *stridor.* This sound, accompanied by use of the accessory muscles of respiration, indicates a respiratory emergency.

Crackling, rattling, or bubbling sounds are commonly referred to as *rales* or *rhonchi.* Because of the disagreement and confusion as to the usage of these terms, several British physicians have proposed classifying abnormal sounds only as crackling or wheezing (Robertson, 1957; Forgacs, 1969). Wheezing is used as defined above. Crackling sounds include those caused by passing of air through mucus or fluid in the large airways (large-airway sounds are not commonly called rales) or by the equalization of gas pressure when inspiration opens small, deflated airways. This explosive sound in the absence of evident fluid is often called dry rales. However, Forgacs emphasizes that even in fluid-filled lungs (pulmonary edema), crackling sounds in areas other than the large airways are probably caused by the opening of airways compressed by edema fluid, rather than by air flowing through fluid. Crackling or bubbling in fluid-filled large airways (commonly called rhonchi) occurs both during inspiration and expiration and in random sequence, whereas crackling in the small airways occurs only during inspiration (as the airways open) and is repetitively rhythmic.

Consolidation of lung tissue, as in pneumonia, exaggerates normal breath sounds. The consolidated tissue acts to amplify the normal sounds.

Physicians auscultate, or listen to, the chest to gain some clues as to the nature and extent of pulmonary disease. Radiographic examination, pulmonary function testing, and the patient's clinical course are then used to supplement these clues. Nurses can use auscultation to evaluate the effect of medical therapies which they administer. For example, if a person requires nasotracheal suction to raise mucus, the nurse may listen over the affected areas for coarse crackling before and after suctioning to determine if the effect of secretions on airway patency has indeed been corrected. Similarly, if a patient is to assume prescribed postures for the purpose of draining specific lung areas (postural drainage), auscultation of the area before and after treatment will provide some notion as to the efficacy of therapy.

Beginning nurses may have little responsibility in the therapy of persons with acute respiratory disease and thus may not use or learn auscultatory skills. However, they may need to acquire these skills eventually in order to care for such patients.

Mental Status

Because cortical brain cells are so vulnerable to lack of oxygen or buildup of carbon dioxide, inadequate gas exchange is rapidly reflected by subtle changes in mentation. Restlessness, diffuse anxiety, irritability, and apathy are all early signs of cerebral hypoxia and hypercapnia. Consequently, when such types of behavior appear in a person with known respiratory insufficiency or one at risk of difficulty, frequent observation of the state of mentation and graphic recording of the data are essential. Lack of cooperation is a common but poor label for the restlessness, lack of interest, and irritability which are characteristic but subtle early signs of hypoxia. Measurement of arterial blood oxygen and carbon dioxide tensions (blood gases) is the only reliable index of hypercapnia and hypoxemia. However, it is often the nurse who is alerted to the need for laboratory confirmation by subtle behavioral changes in the patient.

Color and Temperature

Skin color is discussed as the last of the objective data because, though it is a traditional source of data regarding respiratory status, it is relatively unreliable. Normal color and temperature of skin, mucous membranes, and nail beds suggest adequate circulation and oxygenation of the peripheral blood. The red or pink tint is imparted from the oxyhemoglobin in the red blood cell. Venous blood is more blue-purple because the hemoglobin is desaturated. Consequently, cyanosis (bluish color) of the skin, mucous membranes, and nail beds strongly indicates that these areas are being perfused by blood with unsaturated hemoglobin.

The absence of cyanosis, however, in no way rules out the presence of hypoxemia, because it is the amount of reduced hemoglobin which determines whether a bluish color is present. In anemic conditions, the total amount of hemoglobin is decreased; thus there is not enough hemoglobin to produce a noticeably blue color when reduced. In carbon monoxide poisoning, a person's color may be cherry red because of the color imparted by the carboxyhemoglobin (the compound formed when carbon monoxide in preference to oxygen combines with hemoglobin. However, the hypoxia is severe, as little oxygen can combine with the hemoglobin. Even when cyanosis is present, it is a relatively insensitive sign and indicates that large quantities of hemoglobin have little oxygen bound to them.

Paleness of the conjunctivas and mucous membranes is suggestive of anemia. Since the pink tint of these membranes is imparted by oxygenated hemoglobin, lack of hemoglobin would lead to a paler color. The mucous membrane of the eye (conjunctiva) is one of the best places to observe for pallor in all races. Again, this physical sign is not so reliable as laboratory determination of the red blood cell count, the hemoglobin, and the hematocrit.

Subjective Data

Subjective data are those which the patient-client supplies himself. Since most lay persons think of respiration in terms of breathing, the client is most apt to describe his perceptions of his breathing abilities and of the events or situations which affect these abilities. Because circulatory status and pulmonary status are so closely related, persons with disorders of the heart, red blood cells, or lungs are all apt to have symptoms (subjective sensations) related to breathing. The physician uses the patient's account of his breathing problems in conjunction with his own observations, laboratory analysis, and radiographic evidence (x-rays) to determine the cause of the breathing problem, to institute appropriate therapy, or to prevent further disability. The nurse uses the subjective and objective data primarily to assist the person to live within his limitations and to prevent respiratory insufficiency. These data will also aid the nurse in understanding and intelligently assisting in the medical therapy of the basic respiratory disorder.

Subjective data consist primarily of the person's recollection of previous or current pulmonary, cardiac, or red blood cell disorders (the history); his impressions of impairment in breathing and in daily activities due to difficult breathing or fatigue; and his impressions of limitations imposed on him by these difficulties.

History of Medical Disorders The patient-client's impressions of his current or previous disease not only serve to corroborate physical findings and to provide the physician with direction in his medical examination, but also provide both physician and nurse with valuable clues as to the person's understanding and perception of any disease which he may have. Such clues are essential to planning teaching in connection with chronic disease, such as congestive heart failure or chronic obstructive pulmonary disease (COPD). Discussion of the manifestations, therapy, and teaching involved in such disorders is not within the intent of this textbook. However, such information may be necessary when a beginning practitioner helps a specific client and may be found in most advanced medical-surgical nursing textbooks.

Impression of Breathing Difficulties The person's own impressions of his difficulties are commonly called symptoms (as differentiated from signs, which are objective data). The dominant symptom, or subjective sensation, associated with respiratory difficulty is called *dyspnea*. Although dyspnea is probably the most common symptom associated with respiratory dysfunction, agreement is not complete as to its definition or the physiological reasons for its occurrence. People state that they feel "breathless," "out of breath," "short of breath," or "unable to get enough air." Health personnel tend to lump all these descriptions into the term "dyspnea"— literally, difficult breathing. Some clinicians restrict application of the term dyspnea to sensations of distressing, uncomfortable, or labored breathing; others include awareness of the need for more air, awareness that ventilation has increased, and awareness of difficult or painful breathing (Rapaport, 1971). Those who feel that dyspnea should be restricted to its literal meaning propose using the term "breathlessness" to include sensations of need for more air, or awareness of increased ventilation. Because we are most interested in the person's evaluation of his own sensation, perhaps this problem is best resolved by simply quoting his statement of difficulty and avoiding the label of dyspnea altogether. The observer may note any increases in effort involved in breathing, and the patient can tell us if he feels that his difficulty is increasing or decreasing.

A number of conditions may result in the sensation of breathlessness or difficult breathing. Among the most common are cardiac failure, respiratory disease in which there is either decreased elasticity of lung tissue or increased airway resistance, pulmonary emboli, severe anemia, and strong anxiety. Common to all situations which result in breathlessness is a disproportion between the need for ventilation and the ability to meet the need. It is not completely clear what physiological mechanisms trigger these sensations in such diverse physical and emotional states. Over the years several theories have been proposed which postulate that dyspnea results when respiratory muscles require more oxygen than is supplied to them (oxygen-cost theory); when the work of breathing is increased; or when inappropriate relationships in the length and tension of respiratory muscles exist. None of the theories accounts for dyspnea in all situations, however. Rapaport (1971) and Snider (1969) review current theories regarding dyspnea.

Limitations Imposed by Breathing Difficulties In addition to the client's own descriptions of his breathing difficulties, we wish to know how these difficulties limit him, what precipitates them, and what helps relieve them. The person in severe respiratory distress will not have the breath to relate such information. Indeed, one look at him will indicate that his ability is limited to the efforts merely to take each breath, and that he may soon be too exhausted to do even that. However, the majority of persons with respiratory difficulties are not in such acute situations, and the information they can provide about their breathing limitations will help the nurse in planning daily activities with them.

Many persons who experience breathlessness or difficult breathing do so only when they are increasing their activity, or exercising (this is commonly called "dyspnea on exertion"). Anyone who is "out of shape" has experienced this type of breathlessness after running hard, playing an active game of tennis, or swimming several laps rapidly. The person with cardiac problems, severe anemia, or pulmonary disease may become breathless after climbing a flight of stairs or simply walking across the room. It is important to have the client describe the exact activities which produce breathlessness: exactly how far he can walk or how many stairs he can climb. Not only does this specific information provide a base line against which to measure improvement or decline in physiological condition, but it helps nurse and patient to plan ways to maintain the patient's independence within physical limitations. For example, a person admitted to a hospital with pulmonary disease which causes severe breathlessness when he walks 50 ft could be assigned either to a room with its own bathroom or to a room adjacent to a common bathroom. Thus he may maintain the independence of using the bathroom and not be forced to use a urinal or bedpan. Similarly, a community health nurse might work with an occupational therapist and social worker to help a woman with cardiac disease redesign her home so that she can do much of her work sitting down. She can thus reduce her energy costs and the breathlessness which is a symptom of the inability of her heart to circulate sufficient oxygen to meet these energy costs. The woman could remain independent in her homemaking role, yet live with limitations imposed by disease.

Finally, the client's impressions of situations which precipitate difficult breathing, and of those measures which remedy the situation provide clues to helping him adjust his activity so that he can maintain as much independence as possible within his limitations. Precipitating events can include walking up stairs, picking up a grandchild, worry (anxiety) over his health and failing abilities. Anxiety about getting enough air occurs frequently when a person is having difficulty in breathing, and may contribute to the breathlessness.

The patient-client with disease which has resulted in frequent episodes of breathlessness has probably found certain positions or ways of breathing which help relieve the sensation. Most of these patients find an upright, slightly forward position the most comfortable. Such a position allows maximum ventilation for the least work. The person who is experiencing sudden, acute breathlessness may not automatically assume a position most favorable to ventilation, and may markedly increase his respiratory work because of both anxiety and the physiological regulatory efforts. In such situations, the nurse may be able to help him decrease some of his wasted effort. Measures to accomplish this are discussed under "Nursing Management," below.

Laboratory Data

Certain laboratory tests and analyses are valuable to the physician in confirming or determining the diagnosis of structural or functional pathologic changes and in following changes in the patient's condition. These include radiological examinations (x-rays), pulmonary function tests, blood gas analyses (Po_2, Pco_2, pH, and HCO_3^- concentration), and hemoglobin analyses. Advanced nurse clinicians are beginning to utilize these data to evaluate the effects of nursing care.

Pulmonary function tests are an integral part of the medical diagnosis and management of persons with respiratory or cardiopulmonary dysfunction. Aspects of pulmonary function which are assessed include lung *volumes* and *capacities* (total lung volume, residual volume, vital capacity, and tidal volume) and measurements of the mechanics of breathing (forced expiratory volume, maximal expiratory and inspiratory flow rates, and the maximum breathing capacity). By providing a diagnostician with objective data, the pulmonary function tests assist the physician in detecting, characterizing, and interpreting the severity of the disease. A good reference for further understanding of the nurse's role in this aspect of pulmonary care is an article by Foley (1971).

NURSING MANAGEMENT

Nurses assist persons with problems in respiration in many ways. They may participate in programs aimed at preventing pulmonary and circulatory disorders (e.g., educational programs about the relationship of smoking to cardiopulmonary disease), in citizen groups attempting to reduce air pollution, or in programs aimed toward prevention of nutritional (iron-deficiency) or genetic (sickle-cell) anemia. Nurses have a more direct role in preventing respiratory insufficiency in the postoperative, immobilized, or unconscious person; in helping persons cope with the limitations imposed by compensated respiratory insufficiency and in helping these same persons avoid further insufficiency; and in

participating in the medical therapy of problems in respiration. We emphasize again that respiratory problems encompass *all* phases of respiration—ventilation, gas exchange, circulation, and cell utilization; therefore nursing help in respiratory insufficiency may be given to persons with a wide variety of circulatory, pulmonary, and cellular disorders, as well as to the "well" population in terms of preventive measures.

Beginning students are most apt to work with patients and clients whose needs are for preventive care or for help in coping with compensated respiratory insufficiency—i.e., living within respiratory limitations. Novice practitioners may be involved in implementing some medical therapies, and may find Beland (1970), Secor (1969), and Shafer et al. (1971) helpful references in understanding and applying specific therapies. The person in sudden or acute respiratory insufficiency is in a life-threatening position and requires expert medical and nursing care. Beginning students should seek help immediately if one of their patients experiences sudden respiratory distress, and should not undertake sole responsibility for care of such persons. The following discussion of nursing management focuses on activities in relation to preventing respiratory problems and helping persons maintain function within their limitations. Specific diseases causing respiratory problems will not be discussed, except to exemplify points. Emergency action in the event of sudden respiratory insufficiency is discussed from the perspective of what any responsible citizen should do in such a situation.

Preventing Problems in Respiration

Environmental Prevention Nurses have a responsibility, as do all health professionals, for education of laymen in the environmental factors which predispose persons to disease affecting respiration. The relationship of smoking to lung cancer, heart disease, and chronic pulmonary disease (bronchitis and emphysema) has become increasingly clear over the years in which it has been studied. There is no question that the relationship of heavy cigarette smoking (involving inhalation of the smoke) and the incidence of lung cancer is very strong; it has led to the Federal requirement in the United States that all packages of cigarettes bear a warning about the danger of smoking to one's health. There is also a strong relationship between smoking and the incidence of heart disease and obstructive pulmonary disease. When such diseases exist, cigarette smoking definitely aggravates their symptoms; cessation of smoking appears to increase the affected person's chances of longevity and improved health (*Smoking and Health,* 1964). In the 1964 Surgeon General's report, women appeared less vulnerable than men to disease related to smoking. However, the increased incidence of heavy smoking in women has been paralleled by a rise in the incidence of smoking-associated disease and changes in respiratory function (Woolf and Suero, 1971). Despite these facts and the wide publicity the Surgeon General's reports and recommendations have received, many millions of people in the United States and throughout the world continue to smoke. Health professionals have an obligation to contribute to and participate in programs which aim at early education about the consequences of smoking, and to set an example for lay persons by not smoking.

Environmental pollution is another factor contributing to and aggravating respiratory problems in many persons. Inhalation of tiny particles of asbestos has been shown to contribute to the incidence of lung cancer many years later (Selikoff et al., 1968). At one time, asbestos miners and their families were the only persons at risk from this hazard; however, with the increased use of sprayed asbestos insulation in public buildings, construction workers and a large part of the population may be exposed when the tiny sprayed particles float to ground level and are inhaled by passersby (Brodeur, 1968, 1971). Concerned scientists are pressing for legislation requiring better safety controls in the use of such materials.

Particulate matter from automobile exhaust and from industrial plants ("smog") are examples of air pollutants with a potential for causing pulmonary and systemic disease in large groups of the population (Carnow et al., 1970). Persons with existing lung disease are particularly affected by air pollution. The rates of illness and death from pulmonary and cardiac disease predictably rise in such situations as the severe air pollution in London prior to strict controls over coal burning, and the long-term high "smog" levels in Los Angeles and some industrial cities.

Nurses, as informed professionals, can join with other concerned citizens in supporting legislation to reduce the pollutants from industry and, more importantly, to support alternative methods of transportation to decrease the massive polluting effect of the automobile.

Preventing Respiratory Problems in the Patient-Client Hypoventilation is one of the most common preventable problems encountered by nurses in hospitals. As discussed earlier, alveolar hypoventilation is defined as hypercapnia secondary to decreased movement of air into and out of alveoli. Hypoxemia may be present when the person breathes room air. For beginning students, postoperative patients comprise the largest single group at risk to develop significant hypoventilation. The nurse's role in preventing hypoventilation may assume major significance in the rate at which the patient-client regains or returns to his preillness or presurgery state. Many factors predispose postoperative patients to problems resulting from hypoventilation. Among these factors are postoperative laryngeal edema from intubation (use of a tube that provides the anesthesiologist free access to the trachea during surgery; tight dressings or a hematoma of the neck following procedures on the neck; and depression of normal periodic deep breathing by general anesthesia, sedatives, and narcotics. Impairment of the muscles of ventilation as a result of the use of muscle relaxants, spinal anesthesia, and surgical measures may also occur. Pain may be a major factor in the hesitancy and reluctance of many postoperative patients to breathe deeply enough to expand the alveoli adequately. Restrictive plaster casts or multiple drainage tubes following surgery may contribute to further restriction of chest movement.

Although we usually see candidates for hypoventilation postoperatively, the nurse should be aware that people who are markedly obese, who have skeletal defects (e.g., kyphosis or scoliosis) or neurological disorders which alter regulation of breathing, or who may be medically restricted to bed (as with a myocardial infarct) are also candidates for this condition. As discussed in Chapter 12, any immobilizing condition is a risk factor for hypoventilation. The assumption of a slouched position, restrictive girdles, belts, or other clothing may also contribute to hypoventilation in a person otherwise predisposed to hypoventilatory problems.

Operative and postoperative factors may lead to the development of small or large areas of alveolar collapse which will cause hypoxemia. Microatelectatic areas of the lung are found in normal lungs, as some of the alveoli collapse normally at the end of expiration and fail to reexpand with normal respirations. Involuntary periodic sighing and deep breathing reverse this process (Bendixin, 1964), preventing hypoxemia. In the anesthetized person, the combination of preoperative medications, assumption of one position for an extended period of time, decrease in sighing or deep breathing (as the respirations may be mechanically controlled or controlled by the anesthesiologist), shallow breathing, constant tidal volume, the anesthetic agent, pain, and location of the incision site may either induce or contribute to the further development

of *microatelectasis* or *atelectasis* (Alexander, 1969). Microatelectatic areas are undetectable upon radiological or physical examination. Breath sounds may be normal, with no fever or tachycardia. Large patchy areas of microatelectasis, however, are directly responsible for *hypoxia*, as they functionally remove the diffusion surface of the lung. As microatelectasis becomes more diffuse, and as more secretions collect in the lungs, bronchioles are obstructed and atelectasis occurs. An increase in shuntlike effect and a reduction in functional residual capacity also occur (Laver et al., 1966). Obstructions may be visible on the radiological examination, as well as detectable through the changed breathing and breath sounds heard with a stethoscope, and the changed temperature and heart rate associated with pulmonary infections.

Preventing detectable atelectasis and hypoxemia is a major responsibility of the nurse who works with postoperative patients and with those patients whose breathing rate and depth have been diminished because of unconsciousness, general anesthetics, sedatives, restrictive casts or frames, spinal cord injuries, or other immobilizing conditions. Nurses have generally assumed that such measures as turning the patient and having him cough and breathe deeply prevent hypoventilation. It has been difficult to support this assumption in clinical studies. Wyness (1972) investigated the effect of frequency of deep breathing, coughing, and turning; she compared the effects of treatment given every hour and every two hours, but her clinical evidence did not unequivocally prove the value of one treatment frequency over the other. Her results suggested only that in the nine patients studied, the vital capacity postoperatively was diminished in all, and that any difference in effect of treatment given hourly and every two hours was clinically insignificant.

Alexander (1969) studied the effectiveness of specific ventilatory measures (deep breathing, coughing, yawning, and mechanical intermittent positive pressure) in promoting lung reexpansion in patients following surgery on the upper part of the abdomen. Again, the study did not identify any one ventilatory measure as being consistently more effective in lung reexpansion (and therefore in the prevention of atelectasis). However, Alexander suggested that the measures utilized appear to have been more effective when the patient was in greater ventilatory distress, as revealed by the Po_2 values and tidal volume. Some investigators believe that the prevention and reduction of atelectasis depend not so much on a specified technique or device as on whatever measures effect an increase in tidal volume (Jones, 1968; Thomas, 1967).

Both mechanical and nonmechanical measures are commonly used in the prevention of hypoventilation and hypoxia. Mechanical means include equipment such as hand-operated resuscitator bags (Ambu), intermittent positive-pressure breathing machines (IPPB), blow bottles, and carbon dioxide–rebreathing apparatus. The mechanical methods were popular and acclaimed for a time as the best method of preventing atelectasis and hypoxemia; they have been demonstrated to be no more effective than simple deep breathing (Ward, 1966). The nonmechanical means are perhaps the nurse's most potent measures for preventing or reducing hypoventilation, hypoxia, and atelectasis. Teaching or assisting the patient to *breathe deeply* (often seen written as "DB") will counteract the effects of decreased or absent spontaneous deep breathing. For deep breathing to be effective, use of the diaphragm should be encouraged so that the lower, lateral, and apical lobes are expanded. To be effective in removing retained secretions, *coughing* requires the inspiration of a volume of air to expand the lung, followed by violent expiration. *Turning* is thought to aid in promoting ventilation to the dependent areas of the lungs and in promoting drainage of the lungs. *Sighing* is a normal physiological process which is usually involuntary. A characteristic sigh in

normal clinical subjects entailed about three times the average tidal volume (Bendixen, 1964).

Yawning is an involuntary process which further expands the chest wall following deep inspiration. The mouth is held open for approximately three seconds. The hyperinflation which results from the deep inspiration is thought to diminish alveolar collapse and prevent further hypoxemia. *Ambulation,* frequently complicated and prevented by postoperative pain, is thought by many to be the ultimate therapy in the prevention of respiratory complications. Spontaneous respirations increase in depth and rate, secretions are mobilized to be coughed up and out of the lungs, and tidal volume is increased (Cassara, 1971). The pain that follows surgery restricts deep breathing, coughing, turning in bed, and walking, and predisposes to reduced clearing of airway secretion, atelectasis, and possibly pneumonia (Donnenfeld, 1971). The administration of narcotics for the relief of pain interferes with periodic deep breathing, restricts voluntary motion, and promotes ileus (decreased or absent peristalsis). Ileus leads to abdominal distension, elevated diaphragm, and a restricted tidal volume, which compound the predisposition to pulmonary complications. The use of continuous-infusion segmental peridural analgesia, early ambulation, and preventive pulmonary therapy is currently being investigated by Pflug et al. (1971). At seventy-two hours after surgery, 7 of the 19 patients in the continuous peridural anesthetic groups and 11 of the 19 patients in the nonperidural anesthetic groups had postoperative atelectasis (a 40 percent reduction). The mean hospital stay for the peridural groups was reduced by three days when compared with the nonperidural groups. Nurses may be involved in further investigation of this treatment; they should be expected to extrapolate from this study that early ambulation makes a difference in postoperative prevention of respiratory complications, and to assist the patient in early ambulation.

Mechanical means of assisting the patient to increase ventilation are available. *IPPB* (intermittent positive-pressure breathing) improves ventilation through forcible distension of the alveoli. The physician must order the use of IPPB, and the patient must be carefully instructed in the proper use of the machine. It is a frightening experience for any patient to have his lungs expanded mechanically; therefore early introduction (preoperatively) should be a part of the overall nursing-care plan for any patient who might be using IPPB postoperatively. Traver (1968) compared IPPB and the use of the *carbon dioxide-rebreathing tube* as methods of encouraging deep breathing and coughing. Her findings demonstrate that both treatments significantly increased the tidal volume of postsurgical patients, although the rebreathing tube was more successful than the IPPB in producing a productive cough. *Blow bottles* are aids both in increasing the inspiratory capacity (deep breathing) and in prolonging the expiratory phase of respiration. The efficacy of resistance breathing depends upon an initial large, sustained deep breath, with prolonged, gradual transfer of fluid from one bottle to another (Colgan, 1970). Blowing up *rubber gloves* and *balloons* also requires the patient to inspire deeply and produce a forceful expiration for an extended period of time. These last two measures seem to constitute the favorite regimen for pediatric patients. The use of mechanical means is not intended to displace the effective nursing measures without machines, for any method which effectively increases the tidal volume will promote respiratory health.

Chest physiotherapy has been thought to aid in diminishing postoperative complications. Bendixin et al. (1965, p. 32) have suggested several chest physiotherapy techniques: conscious relaxation to avoid muscle splinting; use of the normal and accessory muscles of respiration for effective coughing; and postural drainage and manual assistance to coughing to aid in secretion removal. Thoren investigated 392 patients with gallbladder surgery. The relationship between chest physiotherapy and the incidence of atelectasis or pneumonia in these patients is presented below:

Chest physiotherapy	Incidence of atelectasis or pneumonia, %
Before and after surgery	12
After surgery only	27
No chest physiotherapy	42

Using chest physiotherapy made a statistically significant difference in diminishing or preventing atelectasis or pneumonia (Thoren, 1954). Levine (1967) states that no apparatus will function by itself and be successful. The nurse's choice of method to prevent hypoxemia secondary to shuntlike effect depends upon both the patient's abilities and the nurse's understanding of how the measure works. In general, mechanical devices should be reserved for those patients who are not capable of breathing deeply enough or coughing well enough by themselves.

Emergency Measures in Acute Insufficiency Sophistication in cardiopulmonary resuscitative skills is expected of nurses who work in special-care units (intensive care, coronary care, or respiratory care) and in emergency rooms. For those who work less frequently with acute or critically ill patients, and those who are new to nursing, there are a few skills that are useful in dealing with acute insufficiency situations.

Upper-airway obstruction may occur from many causes and may lead to respiratory embarrassment. It is not necessarily due to lung disease (Viswanathan, 1970). Acute respiratory embarrassment is a medical emergency. Actions that the nurse may institute often result in aiding the person with acute respiratory insufficiency and those in whom breathing has stopped. *Gain the assistance* of others; many of these measures are best carried out by two people. Two measures of great importance before any other measures are instituted are *proper positioning* and *clearing of the mouth or pharynx* of secretions or foreign bodies. The patient's nose, mouth, and pharynx should be in midline with the trachea, the mandible should be extended to prevent the tongue from occluding the back of the throat, and the mouth should be inspected for foreign bodies or suctioned for vomitus and secretions. The most effective method of positioning the head to overcome upper-airway obstruction is to elevate the jaw with a finger placed at the angle of each side of the mandible. If these actions do not lead to the immediate reversal of the apneic period, the nurse must *ventilate* the patient. Mouth-to-mouth ventilation for adults and mouth-to-nose-and-mouth of infants and small children may be used if no mechanical apparatus (Ambu or Hope hand-operated resuscitator) is available. The rate of artificial ventilation will need to be adjusted to the patient's age; generally, the younger the patient, the greater number of ventilations necessary per minute. Once the patient-client begins to ventilate voluntarily, if his heart is still beating, he will need to be closely observed for further deterioration and reversal of this condition. If his heart has stopped beating, he has had a *cardiac arrest.* In this instance, *cardiac resuscitation,* in addition to ventilation, is necessary to restore cardiac output. Beginning nursing students may or may not be taught the techniques of cardiopulmonary resuscitation (CPR). The techniques are well presented in medical-surgical nursing textbooks. The student is referred to these to recall or review these techniques.

Maintaining Function: Living within Limitations

One of the most helpful services of nurses in both institutions and the community is to assist persons to maintain their function within the limitations of their respiratory problem. The majority of people with respiratory limitations will probably figure out for themselves how to compensate for their disabilities. However, a number of persons, through lack of knowledge, resources, or imagination, require some help to do this. It is this group which nurses can help most. The only way to determine which patients or clients are in this group is to discuss with them their impressions of their limitations and what they do to work around the limitations, and then to observe them functioning in their normal settings. It is sometimes not possible to observe the client at home, for example, and the nurse may wish to get his family's impressions of his abilities and disabilities. It is important not to use one's own impressions or those of a family as "proof" that the person can or cannot compensate as he says he does, but to use them simply as another set of observations. If discrepancies exist between what the person is observed to do and what he says he can do, one needs to discuss this further with the client and try to find the reason for the discrepancy.

Designing Daily Activity within Ability Many people automatically reduce their activity when they have respiratory insufficiency: they may simply do less; they may take several rest stops but continue to walk to the store; or they may request transfer to a job requiring less physical exertion. These persons are reducing their metabolic (O_2) needs. Bed rest for the person with severe insufficiency does the same thing. Some persons may resist "slowing down" or pacing themselves, and consequently make themselves exhausted and frustrated by their inabilities. In such situations, the nurse may want to work with the person to determine and define what his goals are. If his goal is, for example, to be able to continue taking a daily walk, the nurse could suggest that he can still do this but may have to compromise by resting every block. As described earlier, he may help a client to rearrange his work area so that more work can be done sitting down, or so that fewer steps are necessary between work zones. Or a person might be helped to find a new place to live which has elevators rather than steps. Such activities are shared by several health workers, such as occupational therapists, nurses, and social workers. Frequently, a nurse may be the one to recognize that such a problem exists; he may then enlist the help of other health workers who have specialized resources to effect the change.

In a hospital, where the person is quite dependent upon others to reduce his metabolic needs, the nurse in conjunction with the physician may have to determine how best to reduce such needs. Even if the patient is on bed rest, he may have increased oxygen needs because of such conditions as fever and anxiety. Some of the measures used to prevent the detrimental effects of immobility (Chapter 12) have increased metabolic costs, and their use must be weighed in terms of the person's apparent ability to tolerate the increased energy costs against the beneficial effect of such passive or active exercise. Although one rarely measures the actual oxygen consumption at the bedside, changes in the pulse and respiratory rate and depth in response to activity provide some clues to the patient's ability to tolerate such activity.

Adjusting to Changed Abilities The person with a newly changed respiratory status (e.g., one with emphysema who now becomes breathless in one block instead of two, or the person with chronic bronchitis who can no longer work at his job) has to cope with a change in ability and in image of himself just as much as the person who is being rehabilitated after a stroke or an amputation. Consequently, the suggestions which seem so logical to the nurse may be resisted by the client. In time, he may come to use them as he works through his realization that death is closer (if his disease is chronic and incurable) and that he will get steadily worse. Nurses who are attempting to help people in

situations such as these will need to refer to the literature on rehabilitation, grief, and mourning, as well as that on pulmonary or cardiac disease (see Chapters 9 and 12 for some discussion of these topics).

Actions to Maintain Respiratory Function Certain people with chronic obstructive pulmonary disease (commonly called *bronchitis* and *emphysema*) benefit from a program of drainage of secretions from their lungs, and of breathing exercises to help them maintain function. Nurses, physical therapists, and inhalation therapists often interchange roles in implementing such programs.

People with obstructive lung disease often have thick, tenacious secretions which are difficult to cough up. Such secretions, if retained in the lung, can predispose to lung infection and may occlude or block off airways. An effective means of moving these secretions to the larger airways, where they can then be coughed out, is called *postural drainage*. The large airways in each portion of the lung can be drained by the influence of gravity. The upper lobes will drain with the person in the upright position; the middle lobe and the lower lobes do not drain unless the person assumes a lying or head down position. The head-down position is rather uncomfortable; it may be modified to a lateral position for the person who cannot tolerate it. Rie (1968) and most textbooks of advanced medical-surgical nursing describe the techniques well.

Many observers feel that persons with chronic obstructive disease can benefit from a program of controlled breathing, or training to make the most efficient use of the muscles of respiration. Although there is no good evidence that objective measures of pulmonary function improve, many patients feel subjectively improved after such a program. Further work needs to be done to evaluate both objective and subjective results of breathing exercises and to determine whether limited resources and personnel can be best used in such training programs. Rie describes a number of exercises used to promote relaxation and increase efficient use of muscles of respiration.

Many times nurses are asked to help the person with obstructive disease learn to control his exhalation and thus prevent entrapment of air in the alveoli. During expiration there is a normal tendency for bronchi to collapse because of high positive intrathoracic pressures. This is increased in the pathological changes which occur in emphysema. For this reason persons with chronic obstructive pulmonary disease must learn to force the exhaled air out slowly through a narrowed outlet formed by pursing the lips. This allows pressures in the bronchi to remain higher, thus keeping the bronchi open. Exhalation is prolonged about two times the length of inspiration (Secor, 1969, p. 154). Physiological results of one study indicated decreased respiratory rate and decreased arterial P_{CO_2} in males with chronic obstructive pulmonary disease (COPD) during the ten minutes following pursed-lip breathing. The findings were attributed to more effective alveolar ventilation (Ingram and Schilder, 1967).

Sustaining during Dysfunction

Most of the persons who have respiratory insufficiency have chronic cardiopulmonary disease; thus activities that help them live within their limitations also sustain them in their insufficiency—e.g., prevent the insufficiency from worsening, or prevent decompensation. Frequently, however, particularly in the acute-care hospital, nurses need to help people with respiratory dysfunction to maintain some kind of stable state while their body defense mechanisms are coping with the underlying disease. Such situations occur, for example, in pulmonary infection (pneumonia, lung abscess), postoperatively, or in the person with chronic pulmonary or cardiac disease who is hospitalized for other reasons or

who has undergone surgery. The major ways in which beginning nurses can help such persons are to position them to maximize ventilatory effort, assist them to clear secretions and to cough effectively, and minimize the discomfort associated with the respiratory problems. The expert nursing care necessary for persons in acute and severe insufficiency is more and more being provided in specialized respiratory-care units, similar in intent and nature to coronary-care and intensive-care units.

Use of Body Position   As noted earlier in this chapter, posture has definite effects on ventilation. The sitting, leaning-forward position is the most advantageous for maximum vital capacity with minimal muscular effort, whereas sitting while leaning back restricts expansion of the chest wall. The forward-sitting position is usually the one automatically adopted by persons with breathing difficulties who are strong enough to sit. The nurse can sometimes aid the weak person to maintain this posture by using an over-bed table and pillows to support his head and arms. The least desirable position is the supine, not only because of the lowered vital capacity, but because secretions tend to pool in the airways, increase resistance to air flow, and predispose the person to atelectasis and pneumonia (Cameron, 1972; Erwin, 1966). As mentioned previously, simply turning the supine person to the lateral position improves ventilation-perfusion relationships. When the lateral position must be used for any length of time (as in the unconscious person or one who must be flat), frequent turning is necessary to allow the dependent lung to ventilate more fully and to stimulate movement of secretions in the dependent lung.

Clearing Secretions   We all have mucous secretions in our airways; the tracheobronchial tree is coated with mucus, which is moved by the cilia toward the pharynx, carrying any inhaled particulate matter with it. In nonsmokers free of respiratory tract infection, this ongoing activity maintains airway patency without the need to cough. Normally, irritants which stimulate excess mucus production (allergic reactions, cigarette smoke, dust, infection) will stimulate coughing, which in turn removes the excess mucus and its contents and clears the airways.

Stasis of material within the respiratory tract impedes ventilation and predisposes to infection. As the quantity and viscosity of mucus increase, the cilia can only churn. Repeated bouts of coughing are ineffective in preventing the exudate from blocking low passageways and, eventually, the nonciliated alveoli.

In normal people the cough mechanism is sufficient to clear abnormal secretions from the airways. Cough is an active, forceful expiration and thus requires work. If the cough is nonproductive (i.e., dry), violent, or constant, the person may become exhausted with the effort. If it is nonproductive, attempts are usually made to suppress it, as it serves no useful purpose. Both over-the-counter and prescription drugs are available to suppress cough. The most effective contain codeine and thus require a physician's prescription and sensible use.

If the cough is productive, i.e., if mucus or sputum is produced, it is serving to clear the airways and should be encouraged. However, many people do not cough effectively and tire themselves with shallow, hacking coughing. In such situations, the nurse can help the person to cough deeply and forcefully once or a few times, rather than nonproductively several times. Persons who have had thoracic or abdominal incisions are particularly reluctant to cough forcefully as it is so painful. Supporting the person's incision with a "bear hug" or a cloth support can help stabilize it and make the exercise less painful. Persons who must bring up secretions but are reluctant to cough can be stimulated to do so by external pressure on the trachea, nasotracheal suctioning, or manual vibration of the chest as they exhale. Rie (1968) and Ungvarski (1971) describe the techniques well.

Occasionally, a patient may be unable to cough up his excessive or abnormal secretions. The situations which might contribute to this inability include unconsciousness, muscular weakness or paralysis, pain severe enough to cause voluntary inhibition of coughing, and secretions too viscous to raise unaided. A variety of measures may be used to help such persons. Humidity and liquefying agents are sometimes used in hopes of making secretions less viscous. When increased viscosity is related primarily to fluid depletion, simply increasing fluid intake may help. Tracheal suction may be employed either to stimulate cough in persons unable to cough alone, or to help clear large airways of secretions which the person cannot expel himself. Persons who are unconscious or very weak or who have tracheostomies (temporary openings into the trachea) are among those who need such assistance. The cough-stimulating effect of tracheal suction will aid in raising secretions to the trachea, where the negative pressure of the suction apparatus removes them. There are dangers in removal of secretions by suction, including stimulation of laryngospasm and the inducing of hypoxemia by removing air as well as secretions. Laryngospasm may lead to complete tracheal occlusion. Reduction in arterial Po_2 secondary to removing air plus the stimulation of the vagus nerve associated with tracheal irritation may be sufficient to cause cardiac arrhythmias and cardiac arrest. Thus, it is obvious that tracheal suctioning should not be undertaken by anyone who has not been trained in the technique and the hazards, nor should it be used without definite indication. References regarding techniques of suctioning are given in the additional readings for those readers who may be involved in supervised use of nasotracheal suctioning.

Minimizing Discomfort The final way in which beginning practitioners may help people with respiratory problems is to decrease their discomfort as much as possible. The discomfort associated with dyspnea or severe breathlessness is probably a combination of physical distress over the sensation and fear of suffocating. The nurse can alleviate some of the physical discomfort by assisting the person to a position favoring ventilation if he has not already found this position, and providing supports for his head and arms if he can be sitting. Remaining with the person and telling him that you or someone else will be there until he no longer feels in imminent danger is a simple but important step. Anxiety alone can lead to rapid shallow breathing which is not efficient, requires effort that is disproportionate to the degree of ventilation achieved, and thus results in greater dyspnea.

A less frightening source of discomfort is the dry, bad-tasting, or crusted mouth and mucous membranes so often associated with difficult respiration. Dryness and cracking of mucous membranes occur often in mouth breathing and are aggravated by the drying effect of nasal oxygen and mechanical suctioning of oral secretions. DeWalt and Haines (1969) describe the objective and subjective effects of four hours of mouth breathing, nasal oxygen, and suction in a normal person. The subject's mouth changed from pink to red to pale with blisters; saliva became thick; lips became cracked; the tongue and teeth became coated with debris, felt numb, and burned; and all taste was altered for forty-eight hours. Oral care with lemon juice and glycerol resulted in increased saliva and restoration of moistness to mucous membranes. No particular method of oral care has been demonstrated as superior to any other by either subjective or objective measures (see Chapter 15); the important factor is to provide moisture and to clean teeth and tongue of debris.

Summary of Common Problems, with Approaches

Problem	Approach
Postoperative hypoventilation	Turn, encourage coughing, deep breathing, sighing, and yawning
	Use mechanical devices if unable to get ventilation through other measures
	Position for maximum ventilation
	Control pain by decreasing respiratory drive
	Promote early ambulation
Severe breathlessness (dyspnea)	Support position of choice
	Plan daily activities to reduce need for increased ventilation
	Remain with patient to decrease anxiety, or give him means of summoning help
Discomfort associated with mouth breathing and secretions	Provide oral hygiene as frequently as necessary
Excessive or viscous secretions	Assist patient to cough effectively
	Position patient to mobilize secretions
	Provide adequate hydration and humidity
	Provide mechanical suctioning if patient unable to raise secretions unaided
Sudden, unexpected cessation of breathing	Summon assistance
	Position patient to provide airway (keep tongue from occluding pharynx)
	Remove foreign bodies or secretions from mouth or pharynx manually
	Ventilate (mouth-mouth or mechanical ventilation)
	Provide cardiopulmonary resuscitation if cardiac arrest has occurred

REFERENCES

Books

Bendixin, H. H., et al., "Respiratory Care," The C. V. Mosby Company, St. Louis, 1965.

Comroe, Julius H., "The Physiology of Respiration: An Introductory Text," Year Book Medical Publishers, Inc., Chicago, 1965.

Guyton, Arthur C., "Textbook of Medical Physiology," 5th ed., W. B. Saunders Company, Philadelphia, 1971, pp. 502–503.

Otis, A. B., The Work of Breathing, in W. O. Fenn and A. Rahn (eds.), "Handbook of Physiology," sec. 3, Respiration, vol. I, American Physiological Society, Washington, D.C., 1964, pp. 463–476.

Secor, Jane, "Patient Care in Respiratory Problems," W. B. Saunders Company, Philadelphia, 1969.

"Smoking and Health: Report of the Advisory Committee to the Surgeon General of the Public Health Service," U.S. Department of Health, Education, and Welfare Publication 1103, 1964.

Wintrobe, Maxwell M., et al. (eds.), "Harrison's Principles of Internal Medicine," 6th ed., McGraw-Hill Book Company, New York, 1970, pp. 643–667.

Periodicals

Alexander, Ardyth: "A Study of Nursing Measures for Improved Ventilation Following Surgery," Unpublished Master's Thesis, University of Washington, Seattle, 1969.

Attinger, Ernest O., et al.: The Mechanics of Breathing in Different Body Positions. I. In Normal Subjects, *Journal of Clinical Investigation,* **35**:904–911 (1956).

Bendixin, H. H., Gere Smith, and Jere Mead: Pattern of Ventilation in Young Adults, *Journal of Applied Physiology,* **19**:195–198 (1964).

Brodeur, Paul: A Reporter at Large: The Magic Mineral, *The New Yorker,* **43**:117–165 (Oct. 12, 1968).

———: Department of Amplification, *The New Yorker,* **48**:147–153 (Oct. 15, 1971).

Cameron, John L., and George D. Zuidema: Aspiration Pneumonia, *Journal of the American Medical Association,* **219**:1194–1196 (1972).

Carnow, B. W., et al.: The Role of Air Pollution in Chronic Obstructive Pulmonary Disease, *Journal of The American Medical Association,* **214**:894–899 (1970).

Cassara, Evelyn L.: Chest Physical Therapy, *International Anesthesiology Clinics,* **9**(4):159–171 (1971).

Clauss, Roy H., et al.: Effects of Changing Body Position upon Improved Ventilation-Perfusion Relationships, *Circulation,* **37**:214–217, suppl. II (1968).

Colgan, Frank J., et al.: Resistance Breathing (Blow Bottles) and Sustained Hyperinflation in the Treatment of Atelectasis, *Anesthesiology,* **32**:543–550 (1970).

DeWalt, Evelyn, and Ann K. Haines: The Effects of Specified Stressors on Healthy Oral Mucosa, *Nursing Research,* **18**:22–27 (1969).

Donnenfeld, Robert S.: Atelectasis, *International Anesthesiology Clinics,* **9**(4):103–127 (1971).

Eisman, Roberta: "Criteria Registered Nurses Reportedly Use in Making Decisions Regarding the Observation of Respiratory Behavior of Patients," Unpublished Master's Thesis, University of Washington, Seattle, 1970.

Erwin, W. S., D. Zolov, and H. A. Bickerman: The Effect of Posture on Respiratory Function in Patients with Obstructive Pulmonary Emphysema, *American Review of Respiratory Disease,* **94**:865–871 (1966).

Fenn, Wallace O.: The Mechanism of Breathing, *Scientific American,* **202**:138–148 (1960).

Foley, Mary F.: Pulmonary Function Testing, *American Journal of Nursing,* **71**:1134–1139 (1971).

Forgacs, Paul: Lung Sounds, *British Journal of Diseases of the Chest,* **63**:1–12 (1969).

Ingram, Roland H., Jr., and Donald P. Schilder: Effect of Pursed Lip Expiration on the Pulmonary Press-flow Relationship in Obstructive Lung Disease, *American Review of Respiratory Disease,* **96**:381–388 (1967).

Jones, Frederick L.: Increasing Post-operative Ventilation: A Comparison of Five Methods, *Anesthesiology,* **29**:1212–1214 (1968).

Kory, Ross C.: Routine Measurement of Respiratory Rate: An Expensive Tribute to Tradition, *Journal of the American Medical Association,* **165**:448–450 (Oct. 5, 1957).

Laver, Myron B., and Henrik H. Bendixin: Atelectasis in the Surgical Patient: Recent Conceptual Advances, *Progress in Surgery,* **5**:1–37 (1966).

Levine, Edwin Rayner: Inhalation Therapy—Aerosols and Intermittent Positive Pressure Breathing, *Medical Clinics of North America,* **51**(2):307–321 (1967).

Pflug, A. Eugene, Terence Murphy, and Stephen Bulter: Evaluation of a Method of Post-operative Care Using Bupivacaine (Marcaine) Continuous Infusion Segmental Peridural Analgesia, Early Ambulation and Preventive Pulmonary Therapy, abstract of USPHS grant GM 15991–03, Grant RR–133, University of Washington School of Medicine, Department of Anesthesiology and the Anesthesiology Research Center, Seattle, 1971.

Pontopiddan, H., M. B. Laver, and B. Griffin: Acute Respiratory Failure in the Surgical Patient, *Advances in Surgery,* **4**:163–254 (1970).

Rapaport, Eliot: Dyspnea: Pathophysiology and Differential Diagnosis, *Progress in Cardiovascular Diseases,* **13**:532–545 (1971).

Rie, Marcia Wasenius: Physical Therapy in Nursing Care of Respiratory Disease Patients, *Nursing Clinics of North America,* **3**:463–478 (1968).

Robertson, A. J.: Rales, Rhonchi, and Laenec, *Lancet,* **2**:417 (1957).

Selikoff, Irving J., E. Cuyler Hammond, and Jacob Churg: Asbestos Exposure, Smoking, and Neoplasia, *Journal of the American Medical Association,* **204**:104–112 (Apr. 8, 1968).

Snider, Gordon: Physiologic Causes of Dyspnea, *Advances in Cardiopulmonary Diseases,* **4**:145–160 (1969).

Thomas, P. A., et al.: Incidence of Contralateral Pulmonary Atelectasis after Thoracotomy: An Evaluation of Preventive Aftercare, *Diseases of the Chest,* **51**:282–291 (1967).

Thoren, L.: Post-operative Pulmonary Complications: Observations on Their Prevention by Means of Physiotherapy, *Acta Chirurgie Scandinavia,* **107**:193–205 (1954).

Traver, Gayle A.: Effect of Intermittent Positive Pressure Breathing and Use of Rebreathing Tube upon Tidal Volume and Cough, *Nursing Research,* **17**(2):100–103 (1968).

Ungvarski, Peter: Mechanical Stimulation of Coughing, *American Journal of Nursing,* **71**:2358–2361 (1971).

Viswanathan, R.: Respiratory Failure, *The Indian Journal of Chest Diseases,* **12**:25–31 (1970).

Wade, O. L., and J. C. Gilson: The Effects of Posture on Diaphragmatic Movement and Vital Capacity in Normal Subjects, *Thorax,* **6**:103 (1951).

Ward, Richard J., Fred Danziger, J. J. Bonica, G. D. Allen, and John Bowers: An Evaluation of Post-operative Respiratory Maneuvers, *Surgery, Gynecology and Obstetrics,* **123**:51–54 (1966).

Woolf, Colin, and Jesus Suero: The Respiratory Effects of Regular Cigarette Smoking in Women, *American Review of Respiratory Disease,* **103**:26–37 (1971).

Wyness, Margaret Anne: "An Examination, over Specified Time Period, of the Effect of Deep Breathing, Coughing, and Turning Frequency on the Respiratory Function of Selected Patients with Abdominal Surgery," Unpublished Master's Thesis, University of Washington, Seattle, 1972.

ADDITIONAL READINGS

Beland, Irene, "Clinical Nursing: A Psychophysiological Approach," 2d ed., The Macmillan Company, New York, 1970.

Jaquette, Germaine: To Reduce Hazards of Tracheal Suctioning, *American Journal of Nursing,* **71**:2362–2364 (1971).

Respiratory Tract Aspiration, Programmed Instruction, *American Journal of Nursing,* **66**:2483–2510 (1966).

Shafer, Kathleen, et al., "Medical-Surgical Nursing," 5th ed., The C. V. Mosby Company, St. Louis, 1971.

Body-temperature Status

Margaret E. Auld

Data to Be Assessed

I   Factors affecting body temperature
   A Age
   B Diseases
     1 Neoplasm
     2 Infection
     3 Endocrine disorder
     4 Cardiac dysfunction
     5 Tissue injury
     6 Hypersensitivity
   C Time of day
   D Sex
   E Diet
   F Emotional status
   G Menstrual/ovulation cycle
   H Drugs
   I Absence of sweat glands
   J Environmental factors
     1 Living conditions
     2 Working conditions
     3 Natural weather conditions
       a Temperature
       b Wind-air movement
       c Humidity
     4 Clothing
   K Activity

II Skin
   A Color
   B Temperature
   C Presence or absence of
     1 Mottling
     2 Goose pimples
     3 Perspiration
     4 Shivering
     5 Chills
   D Subjective feeling of warmth, coldness
   E Exposure to weather
     1 Cold
     2 Wind
     3 Wet
     4 Heat

III Body temperature
   A Oral
   B Rectal
   C Skin (axillary)

Body temperature is a measure of the balance of heat production and heat loss of the body. Heat production (by exercise or shivering, unconscious tensing of muscles, diseases, and metabolism of food) and heat loss (by sweating, skin circulation, radiation, convection, vaporization, and conduction) are balanced in health to maintain the narrow range of normal. Heat production and heat loss are diagramed in Fig. 17-1.

The extremely narrow range of human body temperature compatible with life is well known. As a homeotherm, man is capable of maintaining his internal body temperature at a near-constant state. Unless the circumstances of cold or heat are extreme and/or rapid, the body can maintain its temperature balance by adaptation to cold or hot weather. The precision of temperature control is evidenced by the fact that normal body temperature rarely fluctuates more than 1.4°F in its diurnal variation (Selle, 1952). This narrow range is maintained in extremes of climates, increased or decreased cellular activity, skeletal muscle activity, and combustion of ingested food. The maintenance of body heat within a narrow range is essential for proper functioning of enzyme and central nervous sys-

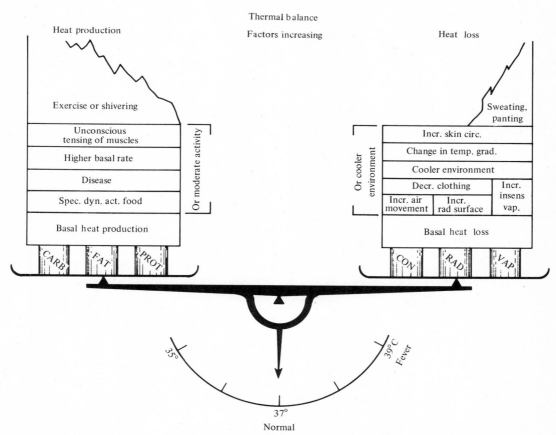

Figure 17-1   Balance between factors increasing heat production and heat loss. *(From Eugene F. DuBois, "Fever and the Regulation of Body Temperature," 1948. Courtesy of Charles C Thomas, Publisher, Springfield, Ill.)*

tems. These systems are temperature-sensitive, and a rise or fall of a few degrees interrupts proper functioning.

Because body temperature is used as one indicator of a person's health status, deviations from the normal range may bring the person to the attention of a health team member. Elevated or depressed body temperature is a nonspecific vital sign, reflective of various disorders. However, no one temperature may be considered "normal," for normal ranges vary among persons. When speaking of body temperature, we usually speak of the interior (core) temperature, rather than skin or tissue temperature. Skin temperature rises and falls with the surrounding temperature. The temperature of a tissue or organ reflects its own heat production, its insulation from the environment, and the flow rate of the blood perfusing it (Cranston, 1966).

Multiple factors affect temperature maintenance and regulation. The external environment (i.e., room temperature, ventilation, amount of clothing), the internal environment (i.e., the amount of adipose tissue, illness, fluid and electrolyte status), sex, age, time of day, emotional status, activity, diet, and drugs are all reputed to affect temperature balance.

Temperature measurement has been possible since Galileo's invention of a temperature-measuring device 400 years ago. Gabriel Fahrenheit altered the basic temperature-measuring device, and, since 1714, we have used a mercurial instrument similar to his. Only since the late nineteenth century has the glass thermometer been widely used. Physicians at first were very possessive of the clinical use of this instrument; currently, it is considered unusual if a person does *not* know how to use a glass thermometer. Since the early 1960s, electronic thermometers have been available for use in hospitals and care facilities. They are thought to be better than glass thermometers in that they register temperature more quickly, accurately, conveniently, and safely (Hagerman, 1971). The accuracy of clinical glass thermometers is disputed (Knapp, 1966).

Body temperature is usually measured in the mouth, rectum, or axilla. Placement sites (Nichols et al., 1966), as well as the angle and depth of insertion (Tate, 1968), seem to affect the recorded measurement. Another major factor in accurate temperature measurement is the length of time of placement in the mouth, rectum, or axilla; this factor is probably related to the blood flow to the orifice or skin.

TEMPERATURE REGULATION IN HEALTH

As stated previously, the body temperature in health exists within an extremely narrow range of normal. DuBois (1948) stated that normal persons may have a recorded temperature anywhere between 36 and 40°C (97 and 104°F). He maintains, however, that under ordinary conditions, rectal temperatures above 37.5°C (99.5°F) should be regarded with suspicion. This narrow range is presented in Fig. 17-2.

The main thermoregulatory mechanism is considered to be in the hypothalamus (Hemingway, 1968; Myers, 1970). Current laboratory work with cats (Myers, 1970) suggests that the mechanism to maintain the temperature in or around 37°C depends upon a constant and inherent balance between sodium and calcium ions within the posterior hypothalamus. Myers hypothesized that the constancy of extracellular ion concentration maintains the firing rate of the neurons in the posterior hypothalamus. Recall that alterations in cation concentration result in movement of anions across the cell membrane. This shift of electrolytes alters the electrical potential of the membrane and thus alters depolarization, or firing. Shifts of sodium or calcium in the extracellular space then might result in hyperthermia or hypothermia. However, animal studies are not necessarily true for human beings. Sodium and calcium serum levels in febrile persons (those with fever) may indeed show a

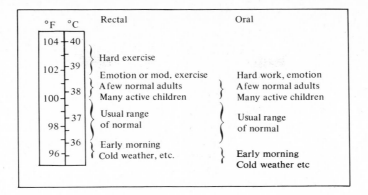

Figure 17-2A An estimate of the ranges in body temperature found in normal persons. *(From Eugene F. DuBois, "Fever and the Regulation of Body Temperature," 1948. Courtesy of Charles C Thomas, Publisher, Springfield, Ill.)*

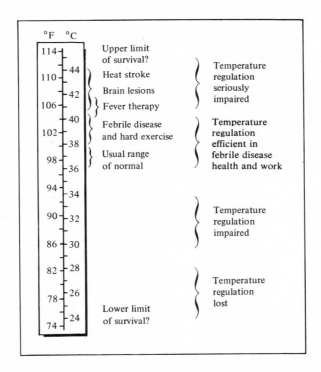

2B Extremes of human body temperature, with an attempt to define the zones of temperature regulation. *(From Eugene F. DuBois, "Fever and the Regulation of Body Temperature," 1948. Courtesy of Charles C Thomas, Publisher, Springfield, Ill.)*

shift. No studies of this apparent phenomenon in human beings are available at this time.

Maintenance of a constant body temperature is a result of a negative feedback system. Simply, the system has receptive, effective, and integrative structures. They sense, alter, and compare sensed temperature to the "set point," and activate motor responses to raise or lower the temperature. Figure 17-3 is a schematic representation of this mechanism. Brengelmann (1965) emphasizes that the "set point" or "reference temperature" does not necessarily represent an existing temperature in the hypothalamus (or

anywhere else in the body); rather it represents the point at which the temperature mechanisms are activated to raise or lower the body temperature. This concept is important in understanding the raising of the "set point" in fever.

Heat Production

Heat production consists of obligatory and adjustable components. Obligatory heat is produced by metabolic activity. Additional heat production is added to our basal metabolic rate (BMR) by activity, exercising, unconscious tens-

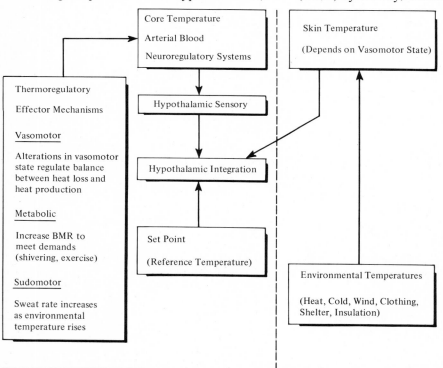

Stabilization of central temperature
through the negative feedback loop

Outside of the negative feedback loop
but contributes to temperature stability

Figure 17-3 Negative feedback regulating temperature basis. A deviation of central temperature from one direction tends to activate opposing mechanisms. Heat gain in the central temperature activates heat loss; a fall in the central temperature activates heat-conservation mechanisms. *(Adapted from George Brengelmann and Arthur C. Brown, Temperature Regulation, in Theodore C. Ruch and Harry D. Patton (eds.), "Physiology and Biophysics," 19th ed., W. B. Saunders Company, Philadelphia, 1965.)*

ing of muscles, hypersensitivity reactions, endocrine disorders, infections, trauma, and emotions. Greatly increasing activity, shivering, or exercise can increase the heat production further. Shivering may increase the nonshivering heat production rate five times (Hemingway, 1968). Shaking chills may cause a 600 percent increase in heat production (Perera, 1941; Selle, 1952). For every degree Fahrenheit above "normal," there is a 7 percent increase in the BMR (Bennett and Petersdorf, 1970).

Thyroxin secretion (from the thyroid gland) and an increased adrenocortical secretion rate in response to cold may also affect heat production. The exact mechanism of both these factors is unknown.

Heat production is lowest during sleep and periods of inactivity, and conversely is highest when skeletal muscles are active. Depending upon the environmental conditions, the great amount of heat produced may be desirable (as in cold weather) or undesirable (as in hot weather). Acclimatization occurs in prolonged exposure to unusual environmental temperatures.

Heat Loss

Heat loss is dependent upon the environmental conditions. Adaptation or lowering of the body temperature may be observed in acclimatization to cold. Man can lose heat by increasing the skin circulation (cutaneous vasodilatation), sweating (which provides rapid evaporative cooling), changing the temperature gradient (use of air conditioning), and increasing air movement (as with fans and removal of clothing). Clothing serves as a trap for warm air.

Four physical principles explain the mechanisms for heat loss: *radiation, conduction, convection,* and *vaporization of water.* These principles do not function independently of one another, and two or more principles may be observed in operation at one time. The relative importance of each varies with environmental conditions.

Selle (1952) reported that at laboratory environmental temperatures of 70 to 80°F, the loss of body heat by radiation constitutes 60 to 65 percent of the total, and loss by evaporation 20 to 30 percent. However, in laboratory conditions of 93 to 95°F, radiation and conduction are no longer the main factors in heat dissipation; evaporation (vaporization) becomes the major heat dissipator.

Radiation Radiation is the transfer of heat from the surface of one object to that of another without physical contact between the two. Radiation or any other form of heat transfer presupposes that a temperature gradient (difference in the temperature) exists between the two objects. However, as one object loses heat and the other gains heat, the temperature gradient tends to disappear. The heat losses are proportional to the surface area.

The body radiates heat to every object relatively near it—window panes, floors, ceilings, pavement, or bodies of water. Radiation may hinder physiologic functioning; i.e., transfer of heat may be disadvantageous to the body. Imagine a lightly clothed person standing on a cement pavement in 25°F weather without any wind; the person loses heat by radiation. To diminish losses to the pavement or air, assumption of a curled-up position would reduce the surface area exposed and, subsequently, the amount of radiation. Other factors to increase heat (shivering, piloerection, and vasoconstriction) would attempt to maintain body temperature at a normal level despite the abnormally large heat loss.

Conduction Conduction is the transfer of thermal energy (heat) from one molecule to another, or from one atom to another. This simple transfer of heat from one molecule or atom to another requires a temperature gradient. It represents only a minute amount of heat loss (Hickey, 1965).

Selle (1952) states that the direction of heat

transfer tends to oppose the body's needs. Falling into a cold sea or sitting nude in a cold metal chair causes the body to lose heat to the sea or chair. Conversely, when the air temperature is greater than or equal to the body temperature, conductive heat loss is prevented, because the temperature gradient is in opposition, preventing heat dissipation. Rather than giving off any heat, the body may gain heat.

Convection Convection is the process whereby transfer of heat from the body occurs as air next to the body is heated, moves away, and is replaced by cool air. This process is always occurring, as warm air rises (because it is less dense) and is replaced by cool air.

We apply the principles of convection when we use fans in treatment to reduce fevers, open doors and windows to create drafts, or fan ourselves in high environmental temperatures. However, much heat is lost to the environmental air when there is a high wind and the skin is exposed, or when the body is inadequately clothed for weather conditions.

Convection aids in conductive heat exchange by continuously maintaining a supply of cool air. Without convection, loss of heat by conduction would be negligible.

Most physicists and physiologists group conduction and convection together when speaking of the human body. These two mechanisms of heat loss are of less importance than is radiation.

Vaporization of Water The fourth physical process by which the body dissipates heat is the vaporization of water (evaporation). The amount of heat loss by vaporization that occurs depends upon several factors: the body's surface area, the respiratory rate, the velocity of air movement, and the vapor pressure of the air (humidity). Vaporization of water is almost continuously occurring as insensible perspiration and through the respiratory passageway. Each gram of water vaporized causes a loss of 0.6 cal

at a temperature of 33°C under physiological conditions.

In hot, humid weather, vaporization of water does not occur—and consequently, we feel hotter. Vaporization from the body cannot occur when the air surrounding it is already saturated. A hot, humid climate, such as that found in New Orleans, Louisiana, is much less comfortable than the climate in Scottsdale, Arizona, where the hot air is usually accompanied by a dry desert climate. Any evaporation of water from the skin, then, in the latter climate is almost instantaneous, and maintenance of physiologically correct temperature at other than basal levels is easier than in a hot, humid environment.

Factors Affecting Temperature Regulation and Maintenance

Multiple factors affect body temperature regulation and maintenance. Some may directly influence the temperature change; others are observations that investigators have noted but have not yet investigated thoroughly.

Felton (1970) studied the *effect of time-cycle change* [from standard time to daylight saving time (DST)] on the blood pressure and temperature of 32 junior and senior nursing students. Her results also provided base-line information regarding circadian temperature cycles. The *time-of-day* temperature rhythm was lowest in the early morning, increased during the day to a high in the early evening, then began to decline. Five days after the change to DST, the temperature rhythm of lows and highs had not adjusted to the new time. Variation in body rhythms could be expected to occur following jet travel across time zones, with hospitalization which may impose an unfamiliar rhythm, or when changing work shifts.

Age is also a factor in heat control and measurement. Nichols (1968) found that children seven to twelve years old required ten minutes for adequate oral temperature measurement, as opposed to adults, who required seven minutes (Nichols et al., 1966). Body-temperature maintenance is markedly poor in the early days of life (Guyton, 1971). Because of an immature heat-regulating system, neonates are unable to regulate their heat production and heat loss within the same narrow limits as the adult organism. Brengelmann states that infants and young children may have a normal temperature as much as a degree higher than that of adults (Brengelmann, 1965).

Increased progesterone secretion at the time of *ovulation* raises body temperature about ½ to 1°. The mechanism by which ovulation raises and maintains the temperature at a higher level is uncertain (Cranston, 1966). In premenopausal women, temperatures taken at the same time each day, in the same orifice, are lower in the first half than in the second half of the menstrual cycle.

Other *sexual differences,* also mainly hormonal, affect body-temperature regulation. Both estrogen and testosterone increase the BMR. Estrogens also cause an increased deposition of fat in the subcutaneous tissue which serves to insulate the female more than the lean, muscular male. Because most body heat is produced in the core of the body, the skin and subcutaneous tissues, particularly the fat, then assist to maintain internal temperatures.

Changes in temperature due to *illness* are well known. The most common manifestation of a disease or illness observed is pyrexia (fever). Not all diseases, however, are accompanied by elevated temperatures. A deficiency of thyroid hormone results in a lower BMR and lower body temperature. Substances such as foreign proteins, the breakdown products of protein, and bacterial by-products can act as pyrogens, which raise the set point of the hypothalamic thermostat. In disease conditions, then, it is the breakdown of body tissue or toxic bacteria that releases pyrogens, causing fever. The exact mechanism by which pyrogens affect the set

point is unknown. We would, therefore, expect alterations of temperature to occur with bacterial or viral illness, following tissue disruption, or after trauma.

Extremes of *emotional* behavior and state may alter the BMR (Cranston, 1966). When the metabolic rate is increased, the body reflects the increased heat production by a rise in temperature. Renbourne (1960), studying boxers' temperatures, found that before championship bouts their temperatures were 0.5°C higher than before practice bouts. The difference could not be accounted for by activity and appeared to be due to their heightened emotional state.

Voluntary factors can greatly affect the maintenance and regulation of temperature. Adjustments in the amount of clothing or the environment are the most obvious of these. Clothing can significantly alter man's response to extremes in weather and environment. During World War II and the Korean War, it became imperative to develop clothing that would protect soldiers from the extreme heat of the Far East and from the extreme cold in mid-Europe. The Army and Navy medical researchers studied the environment, man's reaction to extremes in temperature, and materials which provided optimum protection from heat, cold, and the effects of wind-chill factors. Subsequently, many people, from novice mountaineers to Mt. Everest expeditioners, have applied findings from these military studies to their needs. Ventilating, insulating, and protecting layers of clothing can adequately protect man from cold. Layering of garments is particularly important when the weather is cold and wind speed is high. In cold weather, the wind speed creates a *chill factor.* At any given temperature, the wind, by conduction and convection, causes the body to lose heat as if the still-air temperature was much lower. Thus, the chill factor creates a lower effective temperature than the still-air temperature registered on a thermometer. Figure 17-4 diagrams the wind-chill factor.

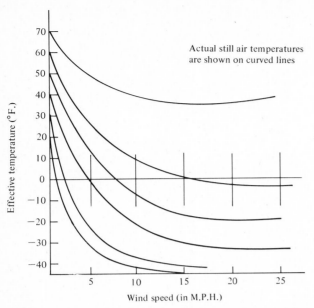

Figure 17-4 Wind chill. To find effective temperature, read vertically from wind speed to actual still-air temperature; then read horizontally to the left-hand scale. At a wind temperature of 10 m.p.h. and a temperature of 50°F, the effective temperature is − 10°F.

Purposeful alterations in environmental conditions are not new to the twentieth century. Early man sought shelter in caves and covered his body with animal skins. The transition from nomadic patterns of living to a more settled existence led to the development of sturdier dwellings and finer controls over individual environment. More recent advancements have made it possible to transform heat energy from sources such as wood, oil, electricity, and solar energy into useful purposes. Air conditioning has made working in hot climates bearable through reduction of the air temperature within a confined space.

"Cold acclimatization," or "cold adaptation," has been extensively studied. As a result of prolonged cold, not great enough to cause freezing, the following adaptive changes are noted to occur: (1) growth of hair; (2) increased thyroid changes with associated metabolic changes; (3) increased ability to tolerate cold without apparent discomfort; and (4) a reduction in visible

shivering (Hemingway and Price, 1968). In animals chronically exposed to cold, metabolic rate can increase without increased muscular activity. This response is thought to be mediated by synergistic activity of the endocrine system and the autonomic nervous system (Brengelmann, 1965).

Adaptation to heat occurs mainly through the acclimatization of the sweat mechanism. There is a difference in adaptation to heat between those who were born in tropical areas and those who are newly exposed to tropical weather. One born and raised in tropical climates secretes almost exactly the amount of sweat that can evaporate from the body; the newly exposed person sweats profusely in droplet form, an ineffective and wasteful mechanism of evaporative cooling. Although much body water and salt are lost at first, the person gradually, over a six-week period, develops a more effective sweat mechanism.

Claims have been made that work production

improves when environmental temperatures are controlled at a level compatible with physiological functioning. We have all experienced lethargy in a "stuffy" hot room, or when cold have been so preoccupied with temperature that our attention span was reduced.

Temperature Measurement

Since the invention and modernization of the thermometer, the nurse has more and more frequently used this "scientific instrument." Temperature determination as a "vital sign" is considered basic to nursing care.

Accurate body-temperature determination will be the result of three main factors: the accuracy of the instrument in use, the accurate placement of the instrument in the body cavity for a minimum time to measure maximally, and accurate reading of the instrument.

Mercurial thermometers (the clinical glass oral or rectal thermometers) operate on the physical principle of expansion of mercury by heat. The manufacturer attempts to standardize the amount and quality of mercury and the calibrations marked on the glass. Nursing researchers routinely standardize their thermometers before instituting their studies (Nichols, 1968; Woodman, 1967). Nichols et al. (1966) calibrated 104 clinical thermometers (52 oral and 52 rectal) to use in her study. She immersed the thermometers in an electronically controlled water bath set at gradually increasing temperatures. After removing those thermometers deviating from the correct reading, she found that at 105.8°F only five oral and three rectal thermometers were accurate. The reader is referred to Nichols's article for a complete summary of the results of her study of mercurial thermometer accuracy. Since inaccuracies in the measurement by the glass thermometer are well known, when a grossly abnormal temperature is obtained it is routine to check the recorded temperature by using another thermometer to obtain an accurate recording.

Electronic thermometers for use in continuous monitoring of temperature were first developed in the early 1960s. They operate on the physical law that heat alters the resistance of a conductor to electrical current. The electric thermometer measures an amount of current running through a resistor (called a thermistor). When heated, its resistance to current rapidly drops, and the increased flow registers on a dial. The dial may be a digital type or a sweep hand.

Hagerman (1971) reviewed information supplied by manufacturers of electronic thermometers. He states that the advantages of electronic thermometers over glass thermometers are speed, accuracy, safety, convenience, and cost. The manufacturers of electronic thermometers claim that temperature reading is almost instantaneous; that the readings are more accurate than those of glass thermometers if the battery is properly charged, if the calibration is correct, and if they are used correctly; and that electronic thermometers are safer because there is less risk of broken glass, mercury ingestion, and cross-infection. They are also more convenient to store and sterilize. The cost is less if calculated in terms of nursing time required to take temperatures with glass thermometers.

Factors Affecting Temperature Recording

Cranston (1966) states that the temperature of the mouth reflects arterial temperature better than rectal temperature. Nurses should be able to obtain an accurate estimate of the core temperature of the body through accurate placement of the instrument in the body cavity (Nichols, 1968; Tate, 1968), accurate interpretation of the instrument, and prevention of extraneous factors that affect the recording.

Since body temperature, like other vital signs, is variable and may reflect minute-to-minute changes in the body, the nurse must be aware that the recorded temperature is a rough estimate of the true temperature of the body at any moment. What we really are looking for are marked or sudden deviations from "normal." When marked or sudden deviations are observed, medical and/or nursing intervention may be initiated.

The nurse is instrumental in determining, on the basis of her knowledge of indications and contraindications, the route by which body temperature is taken. In an institution a physician may order vital signs to be determined at stated intervals; however, the nurse initiates deviations from these orders on the basis of her observations. This may mean that if she observes a patient-client with a chill, she will obtain a temperature recording to compare with the "normal" temperature and be able to supply the physician with objective data. Conversely, if the original order read "VS q4hr" and the patient is to be discharged fully recovered the following day, the nurse makes the decision not to ascertain the vital signs so frequently.

The use of a glass thermometer requires some safety measures. The small amount of mercury used in clinical thermometers, if ingested, will be passed through the gastrointestinal tract without harming the patient-client. The vaporized mercury is, however, toxic, and because of the danger from the toxicity of fumes, the solid mercury should be removed by nursing or hospital safety personnel (*University of Washington Hospital Bulletin,* 1971). Spilled mercury should be vacuumed into a special water vacuum to be disposed of by environmental safety engineers. Disposal of mercury into the sewer or paper-waste containers represents a potential environmental hazard. Hospitals are particularly guilty of poor disposal of mercury (Stilz, 1972). Broken glass represents a safety hazard, whether in the mouth, rectum, or axilla. The nurse must consider several factors before deciding on the route by which a temperature will be taken. These factors include the individual's level of consciousness, his ability to keep his mouth closed, age, ingestion of iced fluids five minutes prior to the time the temperature would be determined, convenience, and maintenance of modesty. (It would not be convenient or protect modesty to obtain

rectal temperatures in a blood bank screening area in full view of others.) Kintzel (1966) was unable to establish that the administration of nasal or tent oxygen significantly altered an oral temperature determination. She suggested, however, that the difference recorded after treatment with O_2 had been initiated was due to a change in site at which the temperature was recorded, and was not a true difference. To prevent this from occurring, her study suggested that, if at all possible, sites of temperature determination should not be changed after another form of therapy is initiated.

Woodman et al.'s (1967) study of normal subjects resulted in two important clinical implications: drinking iced fluids can alter an oral temperature as much as 1.6°F, so that persons who have had iced fluids in their mouths immediately prior to the temperature determination will have a statistically significant error in recorded temperature; and, contrary to instructions in many nursing and medical texts, smoking a cigarette for two minutes immediately prior to temperature determination will not result in a clinically inaccurate oral temperature (although a small temperature change will occur). Forster's study (1970) on the duration of effects of drinking iced water on the oral temperature of 19 males suggests that the oral temperatures stabilized five minutes after ingestion of iced water.

It is axiomatic, then, that a confused, disoriented adult should have his temperature determined by some route other than the oral. The safety of infants and small children needs to be considered before temperature determination is made. Usually their temperatures are measured rectally or in the axilla. If an accurate assessment is made, the temperature recorded should reflect this vital sign correctly.

The nurse needs to use his clinical judgment about when to take temperatures. Because of an order for routine temperature determination, many patient-clients have been awakened in the predawn hours to have their temperatures monitored. Schmidt's study (1958) reported that early-morning temperatures could safely be omitted. A physician in Great Britain studied the time spent by nurses and clerical staff in obtaining and recording temperatures which had been ordered twice daily. Of 13 patients who had elevated temperatures at 6 A.M., 8 had elevated temperatures the previous evening at 6 P.M. Records revealed that medical action was seldom initiated unless the temperature was elevated for several subsequent readings. Therefore, he suggests that omission of an early-morning temperature reading would not delay medical intervention and would allow the patient a longer period of uninterrupted sleep. Sims also suggested that valuable nursing hours could be saved by a single reading around 7 P.M. He felt that this method would effectively screen patients for fever, and would reduce the number of nursing hours spent in obtaining temperatures (Sims, 1965).

Bell (1969) has reported a study in which she surveyed 717 medical and surgical patients to ascertain under what conditions determination of an early-morning temperature provided clinically important information. Only 16 (2.3 percent) of all the patients had an elevated temperature at 7 A.M. that had not been preceded by an elevated temperature at 4 P.M. the previous day. Of these 16 patients, 8 had an inflammatory process or a fever of undetermined origin upon admission. Clearly, nursing judgment would have ascertained that more than once-a-day temperature determination would be essential for these patients.

The circumstances in which Bell states that temperatures should be taken in the early morning are (1) on the operative day; (2) on the first postoperative day; and (3) when a temperature of 99.5°F or over is recorded on the previous evening. Other circumstances in which the nurse exercises clinical judgment to determine whether temperature readings should be made more frequently include critical illness, chilling, diaphoresis, and the use of peritoneal dialysis or hypothermia.

Recommendations for Clinical Temperature Measurement

Placement of the thermometer and length of time it is left in place can enhance accurate determination of oral temperature. With all the confusing instructions about how long to leave thermometers in the mouth, Nichols has the most substantial research evidence regarding length of time in which an accurate reading with a glass thermometer may be obtained. In rooms of 65 to 75°F, the time required for 90 percent of study subjects' thermometers to reach their optimum temperatures was *eight minutes* for men and *nine minutes* for women. In rooms of 76 to 86°F, the optimum placement time is *seven minutes* for all adults (Nichols and Kucha, 1972). On the basis of nursing research, then, the practice of measuring oral temperature with glass thermometers for three to five minutes will result in inaccurate, low measurement. Nichols and Kucha (1972) recommend that *eight minutes* will accurately reflect body temperature in adults, while also making best use of nursing time. The use of any less amount of time will waste nursing personnel time because the recorded temperature will be inaccurate.

Febrile adults (those whose oral temperature had been recorded as at least 100°F) were studied by Nichols et al. in 1969. Again, three to five minutes was insufficient time to obtain an accurate oral measurement. Her study concluded that *six minutes'* placement time would be sufficient to obtain an accurate result in febrile adults.

Oral temperature determination is convenient; it is accurate if the instrument, nurse, and placement are reliable; and it reflects changes in arterial blood temperature rapidly. The length of time necessary to obtain an accurate temperature with a glass thermometer is *six to nine minutes,* contrary to prescribed times in many nursing texts.

Differences in temperatures recorded in the mouth, axilla, and rectum seem to be related to the length of placement time; there do not seem to be any statistically significant real differences in these temperatures (George, 1965; Nichols et al., 1966; Torrance, 1968).

Two minutes has been found to be an adequate length of time to determine rectal temperatures of febrile and nonfebrile adults; the studies of Nichols et al. (1966, 1972) substantiate this clearly. Clinical application based on fact rather than opinion is possible now. Torrance (1968) studied premature infants and the length of time essential to obtain an accurate rectal temperature. At *three minutes,* 95 percent of the 120 premature females and males had registered their greatest temperature recorded.

Prescribed length of time for accurately determining axillary temperature has been ten minutes (Fuerst and Wolff, 1969). This would appear to provide an accurate reading. A study determined that *nine and eleven minutes* are optimum and maximum lengths of time to reflect body temperature adequately (Nichols et al., 1966). Torrance's premature infants required but *four minutes* to register an accurate axillary body temperature (1968).

MANAGEMENT OF COMMON PROBLEMS

Hyperthermic Condition

Fever and Chills Fever is the most widely recognized manifestation of illness. An intact central nervous system is essential for a fever to develop (Cranston, 1966). Fever may be the result of abnormality in the brain itself or of toxic substances or pyrogens which affect the temperature-regulating centers. Elevations in body temperature are common with inflammatory disease; the common factor is tissue injury. Fever is so complicated that physiologists and clinicians describe it as both a friend and a foe (DuBois, 1948; Rodman, 1955).

Simply defined, fever refers to any condition in which the temperature of the body is above the normal range. The absolute rise in temperature is not great, but since man, as a homeotherm, regulates his body temperature within a 6 to 7°C range in health, the increase in temperature is highly significant. Referring to Fig. 17-1, we can see that the upper and lower limits of survival are much different; with medical support, man can survive with an internal temperature below 77°F (Hickey, 1965), but he cannot tolerate temperatures elevated a similar amount. High temperatures can cause irreversible changes in the central nervous system, and can increase the rate of enzymatic and chemical reactions so greatly as to destroy function. In effect, the body "burns up" (a commonly used expression when discussing fevers). Above 41°C the rate of heat production is so great that no amount of physiological regulation can interrupt it. When heat production is so accelerated, the patient-client is in a state of medical emergency. Without aid to diminish his temperature, death will ensue quickly, as high temperatures tend to become higher in cyclic fashion.

A person with a fever regulates his temperature in response to heat, but he has a higher "set point" than the steady-state point of about 37°C. The hypothalamic function is not deranged, but rather responds in a physiologically appropriate manner to the new set point. Cranston's studies (1966) prove that temperature regulation is just as precise during fever as normal. It is the resetting of the central thermostat set point that characterizes fevers.

The onset of a fever is sometimes gradual but may not always be so. A *chill* appears to be the result of the hypothalamic thermostat being rapidly elevated as a response to tissue destruction, pyrogens, or the effects of dehydration. The blood temperature is less than the hypothalamic thermostat, and the autonomic responses normally used to raise body temperature are set into action. Intense vasoconstriction, piloerection, epinephrine secretion, and mass skeletal activity occur. The person rolls up into a ball (reducing radiation), adds blankets, socks, sweaters, and turns up the electric blanket or room temperature. His teeth chatter, and his bed shakes. When the body heat reaches the new set point, these mechanisms stop, and the patient-client feels neither hot nor cold.

When a patient is in a chill, the nurse should determine accurate temperature, maintain the patient's comfort, and, if the client is hospitalized, notify the physician. The physician may wish to obtain a blood sample during a chill, if the chill is thought to be due to pyrogen release into the bloodstream. The identification of a causative organism for the chills and fever may result in more definitive antibiotic therapy.

Fevers not heralded by chills utilize the same mechanism but to a lesser degree. In fevers of unexplained origin (FUO), the nurse should carefully monitor the temperature (Petersdorf and Bennett, 1947; Petersdorf and Beeson, 1961) to help determine characteristic patterns.

Conversely, when the hypothalamus receives stimuli to set the regulating mechanism at a lower or normal level, the person exhibits behavior characteristic of normal heat-loss mecha-

nisms. Profuse sweating occurs, covers and clothing are removed, the skin is hot because of cutaneous vasodilatation, and muscular relaxation is evident. This is frequently called "breaking a fever."

Fevers have long been known to have characteristic patterns. Even before the mechanism was known, physicians were able to predict that their patients were getting well when their fevers "broke." Fevers are classified according to their characteristic rise and fall. They are intermittent (wide fluctuations of high with a return to normal); remittent (a rise each day, followed by a decrease but to a level that is still above normal); and continuous (a high temperature, remaining elevated for several days, with slight fluctuations). Spurious (factitious) fevers characteristically are without such patterns. A typical febrile episode is plotted against time in Fig. 17-5.

In febrile conditions, the goals of nursing care are to assist the patient-client to regain or maintain homeostasis and to provide comfort measures. Removing damp bedding, bathing, changing wet gowns, and arranging the hair so as to

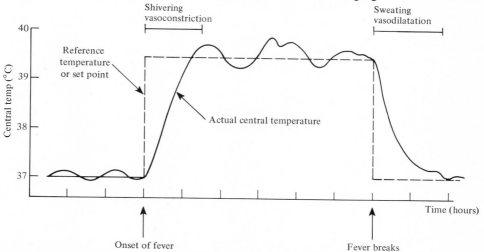

Figure 17-5 Time course of a typical febrile episode. The actual body temperature lags behind the rapid shifts in set point. Note that regulation is maintained during the fever but is less precise, so that temperature fluctuations are generally greater than normal. *(From George Brengelmann and Arthur C. Brown, Temperature Regulation, in Theodore C. Ruch and Harry D. Patton (eds.), "Physiology and Biophysics," 19th ed., W. B. Saunders Company, Philadelphia, 1965. By permission of the publisher.)*

provide more comfort are actions which the nurse can take.

Independently, the nurse can assist the person with chills and fever by adding sources of heat or preventing heat loss. For example, he can offer warmed blankets, reduce physical demands, and remove sources of air movement or drafts, thereby reducing heat loss by conduction and convection. Dependent nursing actions require an understanding of the physiological basis of fever. Some dependent and independent nursing functions are summarized in Table 17-1.

Care of persons with fevers requires that the nurse know how an increased metabolic rate affects other physiological systems and how nursing care can reflect understanding of this knowledge base. Activities of daily living are minimized because of the lack of energy and malaise characteristic of fevers. The nurse should plan to minimize exertion and allow rest periods.

All fevers are accompanied by a 7 percent increase in the metabolic rate per degree Fahrenheit of temperature elevation. Excessive tissue destruction may occur if nutrition is insufficient. If regeneration or repair (as with burns or broken bones) must also occur, additional calories are essential. It has been estimated that 3000 to 5000 calories a day are essential to repair and regenerate burned tissue (Guyton, 1971). Provision, then, of high-calorie, high-protein foods allays tissue destruction by providing a heat source, as well as amino acids essential for tissue repair. However, because febrile patients do not feel like eating, adequate nutrition is not easily provided.

Cellular oxygen consumption is dramatically increased in febrile conditions. Ordinarily, an

Table 17-1 Interdependent and Independent Nursing Functions in Acute Febrile Illnesses (Chills and Fever)

Function	Fever	Chills

Interdependent	1 Administer antipyretics, antibiotics
	2 Rapidly reduce temperature in high fever:
	  a Tepid sponge
	  b Ice-water enemas
	  c Hypothermic blanket
	3 May administer oxygen if temperature and disease warrant it
		1 Notify physician (he may wish to draw blood for examination)

Independent	1 Reduce physical demands, minimize activities of daily living, plan rest periods 2 Increase food and fluids, especially proteins; provide frequent oral care 3 Provide comfort: remove wet clothing; bathe patient to remove wastes on skin 4 Assist patient to lose heat: supply cooling blankets, fans, tepid sponge; remove clothing	1 Add sources of heat: blankets, clothing, heat in room 2 Prevent heat loss; prevent drafts 3 Assist person to position of comfort 4 Monitor vital signs 5 Notify physician if chill occurs

Nurse's goals: (1) Assist the patient-client to regain or maintain homeostasis
          (2) Provide comfort

increase in respiration compensates for this increased oxygen need. Oxygen-consumption measurements in febrile conditions have indicated that there is an increase in oxygen requirement of approximately 7 percent for each degree Fahrenheit (13 percent for each degree Celsius). A patient with a temperature of 106°F (41°C) has an oxygen requirement 50 percent greater than normal (Hopps, 1964). The physician may then wish to administer oxygen, if the clinical need is determined.

Body-water depletion (often called dehydration) frequently accompanies fever, because of an increased need of fluid for metabolic reactions, and because of the loss of water through evaporation during sweating. Electrolyte balance in the bloodstream may be altered. Decreased urinary output is a manifestation of clinical fluid depletion. The nurse can aim to provide fluids of sufficient quantity and caloric requirements. The student is referred to Chapter 15, "Nursing Management in Fluid-Electrolyte Problems."

Many methods of reducing body temperature have been used. *Antipyretics* (such as aspirin) act antagonistically to pyrogens by setting the hypothalamic thermostat at a lower level (Goodman and Gilman, 1970; Strauss, 1964). Antipyretics are ineffective in temperature control when hypoxia or injury to the hypothalamic center is present or when a person suffers heat stroke or neurogenic hyperthermia (Mansfield, 1971).

Bactericidal and *bacteriostatic antibiotics* are used to treat the infection process basic to many fevers. By either destroying or inhibiting the growth of the organism, they give the body's defense mechanisms an opportunity to regroup and assist the body to a homeostatic normal.

A combination of chlorpromazine hydrochloride (Thorazine), promethazine hydrochloride (Phenergan), and meperidine hydrochloride (Demerol) has been used to reduce hyperthermia (Hickey, 1965) and lower temperatures as much as 4°F.

Several physical measures which utilize the principles of radiation, convection, conduction, and evaporation are commonly used to reduce fever. They include hypothermia blankets, removal of clothing, and various types of baths. Lewis (1956) used *hypothermia* (refrigerator) *blankets* on 25 gravely ill hyperthermic patients. He found that use of these blankets was easier and the result more certain in reduction of fevers than use of ice packs, alcohol baths, or aspirin. Thirteen patients recovered fully from temperatures and diseases that normally would have resulted in death. By conduction and convection, body heat is transferred to the cooling blanket.

Removal of clothing in high fevers allows the body to dissipate heat through radiation. Additional heat may be dissipated by *ice-water sponge baths, tepid sponge baths, cold wet sheets, alcohol baths,* and *electric fans.* These mechanisms of heat transfer can significantly alter high temperatures. Controlled nursing studies need to be carried out to determine which method is most successful. Ice-water sponge baths lower temperatures by conduction and evaporation. Such a treatment needs to be continuous until body temperatures drop, to prevent shivering from occurring, which would serve to raise the temperature again. Tepid sponge baths are used to reduce temperature by evaporation. In conjunction with the creation of air movement by fans, this method can be successful. Patients find it more comfortable than cold wet sheets or alcohol sponge baths, and its effect on temperature reduction is acceptable. Cold wet sheets utilize the principles of conduction and evaporation. No studies are available to compare the methods of sponge baths and cold wet sheets. Alcohol sponge baths are based on the rationale that the rapid evaporation of the alcohol from the skin reduces the body temperature. Use of this method, while theoretically sound, is clinically questionable. It is the opinion of the author and several colleagues that the drying effect on the skin could be prevented by use of tepid water, that the shivering frequently produced counteracts the therapy, and that the patients find alcohol sponge baths very uncomfortable. No studies are available at this time which support the superiority of any method.

Heat Stroke Heat stroke occurs as a result of the body's inability to dissipate heat by sweating. This dangerous situation is thus related to the amount of moisture (humidity) in the air. Dry air with some convectional air currents can be tolerated, because of the rapid evaporation of water from the body. Hot climates with a high moisture content do not allow water to evaporate from the skin. Under these conditions, the body's mechanisms for controlling heat dissipation are inadequate, and sweating soon reaches its maximum. Next, the hypothalamus loses its ability to regulate heat, and sweating diminishes. A vicious cycle of heat production and increased body temperature then occurs. Temperatures of 107 to 110°F have been recorded. Such uncontrolled high temperatures may result in brain damage or may be fatal.

Nursing and medical care is directed toward assisting heat dissipation, preventing water and sodium chloride loss, and providing comfort. Heat dissipation is favored by reduction of strenuous physical activity in humid climates, air conditioning, immersion of the body in a tepid bath, or application of ice packs to axilla and groin. Water and sodium losses must be replaced to prevent saline depletion. Actions directed toward heat dissipation and prevention of saline loss will provide comfort. Heat stroke is a medical emergency and needs immediate and constant attention.

Hypothermic Conditions

Hypothermic states are usually prevented by hypothalamic regulation, by increasing the amount and kind of clothing, by increasing skeletal muscle activity, and by preventing exposure. Hypothermia may be either accidentally or artificially induced.

As stated previously, a person can survive with a body temperature markedly lower than normal if supportive medical and nursing care is adequate. All metabolic processes are decreased; oxygen need and combustion and general circulatory rate are slowed. Irregularities in cardiac function are likely to develop at a low temperature level.

Temperature regulation in the hypothalamus is lost when the body temperature is below 85°F. Even at 94°F, the mechanism for temperature maintenance is impaired. Sleepiness and coma reflect the low level of functioning of the nervous system cells.

Accidental Hypothermia Accidental hypothermia is related to low environmental temperatures. Immersion in cold water following a shipwreck may stress the thermostatic mechanisms so greatly as to render them ineffective and cause hypothermia. Cases of accidental hypothermia are also reported following low environmental temperatures and high winds. Elderly people and transients living or traveling in cold environments are usually affected. There is much interest in the cause(s), consequences, and treatment of accidental hypothermia (Cranston, 1966), especially in mountaineering.

Frostbite is the consequence of body exposure to extremely low temperatures. Tissues actually freeze; if they are thawed immediately, damage may be reparable. If the freezing is prolonged, permanent circulatory damage and tissue impairment are so severe that gangrene results. Tissues do not have to be directly exposed (e.g., earlobes and noses) but may be clothed (e.g., fingers and toes). It is of particular importance that wet clothes (gloves and socks) be removed, as the combination of wet and cold causes further heat dissipation.

Purposefully Induced, Artificial Hypothermia Cold can be used therapeutically. It may be generalized or localized, and can be induced internally or externally. Varying degrees of hypothermia can be achieved and for varying periods of time. Hypothermia, achieved by the use of ice packs, can be used to prevent postoperative edema of an extremity; to reduce the amount of bleeding during an operation by reducing the blood flow to an area preoperatively; to reduce the metabolic needs of the central nervous system for delicate neurosurgery; or for open-heart surgery.

Internal methods to reduce body temperature are extracorporeal circulation (heart-lung machine) and use of medications which abolish the heat-production mechanism. Extracorporeal circulation is highly technical, requires constant monitoring, and is usually restricted to use in the operating room for surgical procedures. Medications used are those which have been previously mentioned.

Hypothermia may be externally induced by using commercial electrically controlled hypothermia blankets or ice bags, or by wrapping the patient-client in plastic sheets filled with ice, or by cool baths.

Nursing care is directed towards protection of the integrity of the skin if cold is applied directly to it, and towards making pertinent observations. Use of a thin coat of oil prevents drying of skin, decreases the possibility of frostbite, allows better contact of skin and cooling blankets, and allows more rapid cooling by decreasing insulating air on skin surfaces. Because all body functions are diminished, alertness to changes in other body functions is essential. Irritability of the myocardium observed in hypothermia necessitates close monitoring of the heart rate, rhythm, and regularity. Arrhythmias, ventricular fibrillation, and cardiac arrest all occur as the body temperature falls below 78°F. Renal blood flow diminishes, so that urinary output records must be kept. The respiratory rate also slows during hypothermia, spontaneous respirations usually ceasing at 82°F. Maintenance of respirations by artificial means is then essential (intermittent positive-pressure breathing machines). Prolonged hypothermia requires intensive nursing care (Graves, 1960).

Summary of Common Problems, with Approaches

Problem	Approach	Problem	Approach

Fever and chills	Comfort measures
	  Put on/remove blankets
	  Skin care
	  Dry, clean bed
	  Antipyretics
	Rest
	  Allow rest periods
	  Decrease activity
	Food/fluids: increase to meet
	  metabolic need
	Keep accurate determinations of
	  fluctuations in temperature
	Reduce fevers
	  Antipyretics
	  Cooling blankets
	  Tepid baths
	Assist in treatment of underlying
	  infections: administer
	  antibacterials, antibiotics
		Heat stroke
		
		Hypothermic conditions
			Assist heat dissipation
			  Reduce strenuous activity
			  Air conditioning
			  Tepid-bath immersion
			Comfort measures
			Prevent water and salt losses by
			  adequate intake
			Prevent accidental hypothermia if
			  possible
			Monitor vital signs
			Assess central nervous system
			  functioning
			Assess cardiovascular status
			  (especially for irritability)
			Maintain skin integrity

REFERENCES

Bell, Shirley: Early Morning Temperatures? *American Journal of Nursing,* **69**:764-766 (1969).

Bennett, Ivan, and Robert Petersdorf, "Alterations in Body Temperature," in M. Wintrobe et al. (eds.), "Harrison's Principles of Internal Medicine," 6th ed., McGraw-Hill Book Company, New York, 1970.

Brengelmann, George, and Arthur C. Brown, Temperature Regulation, in Theodore C. Ruch and Harry D. Patton (eds.), "Physiology and Biophysics," 19th ed., W. B. Saunders Company, Philadelphia, 1965, pp. 1050-1059.

Cranston, W. I.: Temperature Regulation, *British Medical Journal,* **2**:69-75 (1966).

DuBois, Eugene F., "Fever and the Regulation of Body Temperature," Charles C Thomas, Publisher, Springfield, Ill., 1948.

Felton, Geraldene: Effect of Time Cycle Change on Blood Pressure and Temperature in Young Women, *Nursing Research,* **19**(1):48-58 (1970).

Forster, Brenda, et al.: Duration of Effects of Drinking Iced Water on Oral Temperature, *Nursing Research,* **19**(2):169-170 (1970).

Fuerst, Elinor V., and LuVerne E. Wolff, "Fundamentals of Nursing," 4th ed., J. B. Lippincott Company, Philadelphia, 1969.

George, Joyce H.: Machines in Perspective: Electronic Monitoring of Vital Signs, *American Journal of Nursing,* **65**:70 (1965).

Goodman, Louis S., and Alfred Gilman, "The Pharmacological Basis of Therapeutics," 4th ed., The Macmillan Company, New York, 1970.

Graves, Nancy: Nursing during Prolonged Hypothermia, *American Journal of Nursing,* **60**:969-970 (1960).

Guyton, Arthur C., "Textbook of Medical Physiology," 5th ed., W. B. Saunders Company, Philadelphia, 1971.

Hagerman, Charles W.: Electric Thermometers—Keeping Your Cool with a Hot Product, *Nursing '71,* **21**:26 (1971).

Hemingway, Allan, and William M. Price: The Autonomic Nervous System and Regulation of Body Temperature, *Anesthesiology,* **29**(4):693-701 (1968).

Hickey, Mary C.: Hypothermia, *American Journal of Nursing,* **65**:116-122 (1965).

Hopps, Howard C., "Principles of Pathology," 2d ed., Appleton-Century-Crofts, Inc., New York, 1964.

Kintzel, Kay Cormen, A Comparative Study of Oral and Rectal Temperatures in Patients Receiving Two Forms of Oxygen Therapy, "ANA Clinical Sessions," New York, Appleton-Century-Crofts, Inc., New York, 1966.

Knapp, Herbert A.: Accuracy of Glass Clinical Thermometers, *American Journal of Surgery,* **112**:139-141 (1966).

Lewis, F. John, et al.: A Technique of Total Body Cooling of the Febrile, Gravely Ill Patient, *Surgery,* **40**:465-470 (1956).

Mansfield, Louise W.: Alterations in Vital Signs and Associated Respiratory Manifestations, in Harriet Coston Moidel et al., "Nursing Care of the Patient with Medical-Surgical Disorders," McGraw-Hill Book Company, New York, 1971.

Myers, R. D., and W. L. Veale: Body Temperature: Possible Ionic Mechanism in the Hypothalamus Controlling the Set Point, *Science,* **70**:95-97 (1970).

Nichols, Glennadee A.: Measurement of Oral Temperature in Children, *Journal of Pediatrics,* **72**:253-256 (1968).

———: Taking Adult Temperatures: Rectal Measurements, *American Journal of Nursing,* **72**:1092-1093 (1972).

——— and Beverly A. K. Gloe: A Replication of Rectal Thermometer Placement Studies, *Nursing Research,* **17**(4):360-361 (1968).

——— and Delores H. Kucha: Taking Adult Temperatures: Oral Measurements, *American Journal of Nursing,* **72**:1091-1093 (1972).

——— and Phyllis J. Verhonick: Time and Temperature, *American Journal of Nursing,* **67**:2304-2306 (1967).

——— and Phyllis J. Verhonick: Placement Times for Oral Thermometers: A Nursing Study Replication, *Nursing Research,* **17**(2):159-161 (1968).

——— et al.: Oral, Axillary, and Rectal Temperature Determinations and Relationships, *Nursing Research,* **15**(4):307-310 (1966).

——— et al.: Taking Oral Temperatures of Febrile Patients, *Nursing Research,* **18**(5):448-450 (1969).

——— et al.: Rectal Thermometer Placement Times for Febrile Adults, *Nursing Research,* **21**(1):76-77 (1972).

Perera, George A.: Clinical and Physiologic Characteristics of Chill, *Archives of Internal Medicine,* **68**:241–260 (1941).

Petersdorf, Robert, and Paul Beeson: Fever of Unexplained Origin: Report of 100 Cases, *Medicine,* **40**:1–30 (1961).

——— and Ivan L. Bennett: Factitious Fever, *Annals of Internal Medicine,* **46**:1039–1061 (1947).

Renbourne, E. T.: Body Temperature and Pulse Rates in Boys and Young Men Prior to Sporting Contests: A Study of Emotional Hyperthermia with a Review of the Literature, *Journal of Psychosomatic Research,* **4**:149–175 (1960).

Rodman, Morton J.: Fever—Friend or Foe? *RN,* **18**:42–45 (1955).

Schmidt, Marie A.: Are All TPR's Necessary? *American Journal of Nursing,* **58**:559 (1958).

Selle, W. A., "Body Temperature: Its Changes with Environment, Disease and Therapy," Charles C Thomas, Publisher, Springfield, Ill., 1952.

Sims, R. S.: Temperature Recording in a Teaching Hospital, *The Lancet,* **1**:535–536 (1965).

Stilz, John, University of Washington Department of Environmental Health and Safety, Personal Communication, Feb. 24, 1972.

Strauss, Walter J.: Fever of Unknown Origin, *Postgraduate Medicine,* **36**:555–559 (1964).

Tate, Gayle V., The Effects of Variation of Angle and Depth of Thermometer Insertion on Rectal Temperature Readings, Unpublished Master's Thesis, Seattle, Washington (1968).

Torrance, Jane T.: Temperature Readings of Premature Infants, *Nursing Research,* **17**(4):312–320 (1968).

University of Washington Hospital Bulletin, Seattle, Fall, 1971.

Woodman, Ellen A., et al.: Sources of Unreliability in Oral Temperatures, *Nursing Research,* **16**(3):276–279 (1967).

ADDITIONAL READINGS

Atkins, Elisha: Elevation of Body Temperature in Disease, *Annals of New York Academy of Science,* **121**:26–30 (1964).

Benzinger, T. H.: The Human Thermostat, *Scientific American,* **204**(1):134–144 (1961).

Cooper, K. E., et al.: Temperature Regulation during Fever in Man, *Clinical Science,* **27**:345–356 (1964).

Knapp, Miland E.: Practical Physical Medicine, Lecture 6, Effects of Heat and Cold, *Postgraduate Medicine,* Part 1:A51–55 (1966); Part 2:A145–150 (1966); Part 3:A123–128 (1966).

Lee, Richard V., and Elisha Atkins: Spurious Fever, *American Journal of Nursing,* **72**:1094–1095 (1972).

Purintun, Lynn R., and Barbara E. Bishop: How Accurate Are Clinical Thermometers? *American Journal of Nursing,* **69**:99–100 (1969).

Walker, Virginia H., and Eugene D. Selmanoff: A Note on the Accuracy of the Temperature, Pulse and Respiratory Procedure, *Nursing Research,* **14**(1):72–76 (1965).

Integumentary Status

Barbara Innes

The integumentary system refers to the skin and its derivatives, the hair and nails. Since it covers the entire body, the integument may be considered the entity which holds inside all the parts of the body. At openings in the body surface, such as the mouth, ear, vagina, and rectum, the skin is continuous with the mucous membrane lining the orifice. The skin, as the largest organ of the body, consists of three layers: the epidermis, the dermis or corium, and the subcutaneous tissue or hypodermis. The *epidermis* is the thin (0.07 to 1.4 mm) outer layer of the skin and is itself made up of from two to four layers. (The outermost of these layers, called the stratum corneum, is actually composed of dead cells which are continually being rubbed or washed away. These

Data to Be Assessed

Skin	Hair
Color	Growth patterns
Turgor	Cleanliness
Elasticity	Shininess
Intactness	Dryness
Character of any lesion	Oiliness
present	Brittleness
Rashes	Presence of lice
Wetness/dryness	Nails
Warmth	Cleanliness
Cleanliness	Shape
Odor	Brittleness
Usual hygiene habits	Condition of
Knowledge base	surrounding tissue
concerning hygiene	Treatment program
needs	ordered for pressure
	sores

lost cells are constantly replaced by cells moving up from the deeper layers.) The middle layer, called the *dermis,* consists of dense connective tissue and contains blood vessels, nerves and nerve receptors, hair follicles, and sweat and oil glands. The *hypodermis,* while thought by some not to be an actual part of the skin itself, is so closely linked with it that it is included in any comprehensive discussion of the integument. This subcutaneous tissue is composed of loose connective tissue and contains fat globules, blood vessels, lymphatic vessels, and nerves. It loosely binds the skin to the underlying structures and provides the springy base for the skin.

The skin is the body's first line of defense. This principle underlies nursing activity related to personal hygiene and to maintaining skin integrity. The skin serves many essential purposes, one of the most important being this protective function. It is rich with nerve receptors which help apprise the body of its external environment through pressure, pain, and temperature sensations. An intact integument is one of the most effective barriers between many of the pathogens in the environment and those parts of the body interior normally free of these organisms. The oils, or *sebum,* secreted by the sebaceous glands help prevent the skin from drying. Excessive drying results in chapping and cracking, thus opening the barrier. The pigment, or *melanin,* of the epidermis helps shield the body from injurious ultraviolet radiation.

Temperature regulation is another major function of the skin. Cutaneous blood vessels and sweat glands respond to temperature changes. In order to reduce the body temperature, the circulatory vessels dilate, bringing an increased blood flow to the exterior, and the sweat glands secrete increased amounts of moisture. This perspiration evaporates from the surface of the skin, thus cooling it. In order to conserve body heat, cutaneous vessels constrict and perspiration decreases.

As mentioned, the skin has secretory abilities and, to a limited extent, some excretory capability. During copious sweating, the skin excretes water, sodium chloride, and nonprotein nitrogen, all of which affect the body's volume and osmotic balance. In advanced renal failure, the skin excretes the urea and salts usually excreted by the kidney; the dried salts produce a white, powdery layer on the skin called "uremic frost." The integument also has a limited capacity for absorption from its surface. This allows some medications, when prepared in a proper vehicle, to produce systemic results following a topical application.

The sebum secreted by the sebaceous glands is an oily substance which has low-grade antibacterial and antifungal properties. At the time of delivery, a newborn's skin is covered with a cheesy material called *vernix caseosa,* which is made of sebum and dead epithelial cells. This protective layer slowly wears off. One of the most important functions of sebum is that it may help maintain the suppleness of the epidermis. The distribution of this oil across the stratum corneum prevents water loss from the tissue. Dry skin actually reflects the loss of water from the skin rather than the lack of skin oil. The percentage of water in the stratum corneum is regulated by internal factors, such as the amount of water in the other tissues, as well as by environmental factors, such as the humidity, temperature, and air movement (Cahn, 1960). Sebum, if allowed to accumulate, may become odoriferous, clog the pores, and cause irritation, especially if it collects in skin folds.

The hair and the nails are accessory structures to the skin. Man's body is almost entirely covered with hair, ranging from very fine and soft to the coarse hair of a man's beard. A newborn baby is often covered by very fine hair, called *lanugo,* which soon disappears and is replaced by more mature hair. The hair's most important function seems to be one of tactile perception. In addition, some feel that in severe burns or lacerations, the epithelium of the hair follicle may have an important role in epidermal regeneration (Crouch, 1965).

The nails protect the susceptible ends of the fingers and toes. They grow from under the proximal nail wall at a rate of approximately 1 mm per week.

ASSESSMENT FACTORS

The skin and its appendages are easily observed; inspection of them may indicate the presence or absence of pathophysiologic changes and their progress.

Skin

Several general categories will guide the nurse to a complete assessment of the skin.

Color The color of a person's skin is produced by a brown pigment called *melanin.* The more melanin present in the layers of the epidermis, the darker the skin. The total lack of this pigment in albinos results in their white color. Sun tanning occurs when exposure to the ultraviolet rays of the sun causes intensification of the melanin.

Assessing color changes in the integument of the darker skinned races may be very difficult. Alterations are best seen in the mucous membranes and sclera. Those used to observing black skin can often note variations in the skin color itself.

Paleness, or *pallor,* of the skin itself is usually the effect of vasoconstriction of the cutaneous blood vessels. This occurs when the body's compensatory mechanisms are striving to conserve body heat or to divert the peripheral blood supply to the vital organs in the central core. This constriction may also be the result of activation of the sympathetic nervous system, which may occur in psychological shock. Anemia is a reduction in the total circulating hemoglobin. The lack of this hemoglobin in the superficial tissues causes a paleness, particularly in the conjunctiva. Mechanical obstruction or constriction of the blood vessel will also result in pallor in the body part usually supplied by the involved vessel.

Any flushing, or reddening of the skin, is also a pertinent observation. It is caused by several different factors. Vasodilatation of the cutaneous blood vessels brings more blood to the surface layer of the skin as the body attempts to lose internal heat. Increased metabolism, such as may be found in febrile states and hyperthyroidism, produces additional body heat which must be dissipated in order to achieve proper body-temperature regulation. An inflammatory response results in the local *hyperemia,* or excessive blood in the part. This may occur as a response to injury, or it may signal that a girdle or brace, for example, is too tight. The intake of alcohol causes vasodilatation. Any of these circumstances brings increased amounts of hemoglobin to the surface of the skin, imparting a redder color. Most people have experienced the kind of flushing resulting from certain emotional states—the blush.

Hypoxia, or the lack of oxygen, in the late stages causes a bluish tinge of the skin called *cyanosis.* The color is the result of excessive amounts of deoxygenated hemoglobin in the cutaneous blood vessels. The degree of cyanosis visible is influenced by the size and number of superficial vessels and is best observed in the earlobes and nail beds and around the mouth (circumoral).

Any bleeding into the superficial tissues causes discoloration of the area. *Ecchymosis* is the medical term for a bruise. When a blood vessel is broken, the blood, which quickly becomes deoxygenated, seeps out into the subcutaneous tissues, turning to a purplish-blue or blue color. As this is reabsorbed, the color changes to yellow and yellow-green. *Petechiae* are round, pinpoint spots of a purplish-red color which result from intradermal or submucosal bleeding. *Purpura* refers to large, merging areas of ecchymosis.

Excessive accumulation of bilirubin in the tissues produces a yellow color and is called *jaundice.* The yellowishness first appears in the sclera but is soon visible all over the body surface. Jaundice occurs when excretion of bilirubin by the liver is impaired, when bilirubin is overproduced, and when there is biliary tract obstruction.

There are many kinds of permanent discoloration of the skin, often called birthmarks. Moles should be observed for changes in their color or size, which may denote a malignant state.

Turgor Tissue *turgor* is defined as the fullness of the tissue; it is related primarily to the amount of fluid surrounding the cells. In late stages of fluid volume depletion, the body fluid is pulled from the peripheral tissues, leaving the skin loose and dry. When the skin is pinched, it does not quickly return to its original shape, as it would with normal tissue turgor, but instead remains in folds or returns slowly to a smooth state. Aged skin has poor turgor, but this is because of loss of subcutaneous fat, rather than fluid imbalance.

With the other extreme of tissue turgor, or edema, an overabundance of fluid in the tissues causes swelling. As edema advances, the skin becomes taut and may become shiny. The swelling obliterates bony prominences in the area and changes the general contour of the part involved.

Elasticity Elastic fibers in the dermis layer allow the skin to retain and regain its usual shape. The skin is stretchable and, under normal conditions, springs back into its original position rather quickly. Sometimes exercises help the process, as with a person who has lost a great deal of weight; if the weight loss has been too rapid, the skin may hang in wrinkles or folds. The elasticity of the skin allows it to stretch and contract repeatedly and without any assistance;

this is seen in the person who is having difficulty with swelling following a sprained ankle.

When the skin is stretched beyond its normal limits, the tissues are damaged, producing a scarlike line called a "stretch mark." This is often seen on obese persons. As demonstrated during pregnancy, the skin over the abdomen has the greatest capacity for distension. However, even so, pregnancy stretches the skin too much, and marks appear on the surface of the abdomen. During pregnancy, these permanent lines are red and called *striae gravidarum;* after delivery, they turn white and are called *lineae albicantes.*

Intactness If the skin is going to fulfill its protective function against microbial invasion, it must be intact, offering no opening to pathogenic organisms. Any traumatic breaks in the skin, such as lacerations, contusions, scratches, and surgical incisions, must be noted. Pressure sores, which will be discussed in depth later, are an important breach in the continuity of the skin. Burns which destroy skin layers open large areas. Environmental conditions, such as wind and sun, as well as frequent hand washing, cause chapping of the skin, which produces minute openings through the barrier. Hangnails may seem rather insignificant, but they constitute another hiatus. Allergies to adhesive tape may cause the skin to be peeled off with the tape.

A common problem in the care of infants and children is diaper rash. This irritation is also found on incontinent persons and persons having poor hygiene habits. It is a painful condition caused by the breakdown of urine and feces into ammonia products, which, when left in contact with the skin, produce a burning effect and proceed to break the integumentary integrity. It is characterized by an inflamed skin surface covering the perineal and buttocks areas and sometimes extending outward, depending on the saturation of the diaper. This irritated skin may have a smooth-appearing surface but more often is blotchy with a sprinkling of redder spots.

Character of Lesions Present   A lesion is any pathological or traumatic discontinuity of the skin; the term is applied to any of those interruptions in intactness mentioned above. Areas around lesions must be observed for signs of local inflammation: swelling, redness *(erythema),* heat, and tenderness. Any drainage from the lesion should be noted and observed as to amount, color, and odor. *Serous* drainage is clear; *serosanguineous* drainage contains both serum and blood. Other colors seen in drainage fluid are white, green, and yellow. Bacteriologic culture is usually made of suspicious drainage products to identify the type of organisms present and the antibiotics to which the organisms are sensitive. In the event of drainage, the skin around the area must be observed closely for signs of irritation.

Rashes   A rash is a temporary eruption on the skin and may be caused by many conditions, such as heat, allergies, disease processes, and emotional states. A *macular* rash is flat with the surface of the skin; a *papular* rash consists of small, solid elevations. Hives are an example of a papular eruption. A rash may be a combination of both macular and papular spots. In addition, a rash may be weeping, with a serous exudate.

Sensation   The skin contains a liberal number of sensory receptors, with some areas more sensitive than others. These receptors permit awareness of certain environmental stimuli, such as heat and cold. They also play an important role in sexual activities. In addition, the skin is capable of pain and of a rather specialized type of discomfort, itching or *pruritus,* which may or may not be found in combination with a rash or other type of lesion. Observations of pruritus should include time of onset, duration, severity, location, activities prior to onset, and results of relief measures tried.

Wetness/Dryness   As discussed earlier, there are, in the epidermis and dermis, sweat glands whose main role is in body-temperature regulation. In response to febrile states, muscular exercise, and increased environmental temperature and humidity, increased amounts of perspiration are secreted onto the surface of the skin, where it can cool the body through evaporation. Excessive perspiration is called *diaphoresis.* Certain emotional states may also produce increased secretion, especially on the forehead, around the mouth, and on the palms and soles.

Continued wetness on the skin, whether from perspiration, urine, or external sources, may lead to *maceration.* Macerated skin becomes softened and wrinkled and liable to trauma. Areas particularly susceptible to this danger are the skin folds, e.g., under pendulous breasts and in the groin. Lying in a wet bed or having continuous wet packs will also produce the same effect. Most people have noticed this wrinkling on their fingers after washing the dinner dishes.

Dryness of the skin may refer to lack of perceptible perspiration, but it is usually evaluated in terms of the oiliness of the skin. The role of the sebaceous glands in maintaining the water content of the skin was described earlier in this chapter. When anything interferes with this oily barrier, such as the lack of sebum production, frequent washing, and the use of soap or alcohol, water is allowed to evaporate from the skin and dryness ensues. Excessive drying results in minute openings through the epidermis, which may allow the entry of microorganisms.

Too much oil production may also be a problem, as will be documented by many teenagers who have struggled with acne. During the adolescent years, and even extending beyond, the sebaceous glands located particularly on the face and back secrete abundant amounts of sebum, which, if allowed to accumulate, plug the duct of the gland, forming a "blackhead." These ducts are then vulnerable to bacterial invasion and infection.

Warmth The warmth of the skin will not only give clues as to the temperature state of the person, but will also suggest the circulatory status of the part. Since the blood itself is warmed in the central core, an adequate supply of blood flowing through the cutaneous vessels will transmit warmth to the surface. With vasoconstriction, the blood flow does not reach the periphery, and thus the skin is cool. The warmth of the skin may be assessed generally over the total surface, or one part may be compared with another. For instance, one of the major observations to be made of a person with a leg in a cast is the warmth of the toes distal to the cast as contrasted with the toes of the other foot. This is done by feeling the parts.

Cleanliness; Odor The cleanliness of a person's skin is often a mirror of his personal hygiene habits. It is easily observed by direct inspection. Odor usually parallels cleanliness. Secretions of the skin contain some waste products, which, as they are decomposed by the surface bacterial flora, produce a characteristic odor. Hairy parts of the body, such as the axillary regions, are particularly susceptible to odor. Unless these secretions are removed, they accumulate, and the odor becomes stronger. Skin odors may also be the result of abnormal body secretions or of substances put on the skin, such as perfumes or medications.

Aging Skin Like most other parts of the body, the skin undergoes physiological changes during the aging process. Probably most visible are the loss of subcutaneous tissue and the loss of skin elasticity, which results in wrinkles and loose, flabby skin folds. The sebaceous glands stop secreting their protective oils, so that the skin becomes dry and flaky. Sweat secretion is greatly reduced. Sometimes the skin becomes so friable that the slightest friction against it will lay back a large layer of skin. These factors contribute to the high vulnerability of the elderly person to pressure-sore formation. The lack of subcutaneous tissue means a greater problem with bony prominences, and the friable skin is more susceptible to traumatic entry.

Special care is often given to aging skin. For example, soap is often left out of the bathing procedure, since it removes whatever protective oils are present, and free use of lotions and creams to replace the oils is encouraged. Baths are often not needed so frequently, since skin secretions are reduced. At the same time, however, the elderly person may need additional assistance with hygiene, especially of the feet and legs because of decreased motor function.

Hair and Nails

The hair is assessed as to cleanliness, dryness or oiliness, brittleness, presence or absence, and growth patterns. Another activity specific to the hair is the inspection for lice. This will be discussed in more detail in the section on personal hygiene, but the presence of lice should be suspected on persons with obviously poor hygiene and when the patient-client is complaining of itching, especially in the hairy areas.

The nails are also inspected for cleanliness and brittleness. In addition, the thickness and shape of the nail should be noted, as well as the condition of the surrounding nail bed.

PERSONAL HYGIENE

Good personal hygiene means different things to different persons. Some of these variations are culturally based, although it must be remembered that not everyone of a culture will necessarily follow all the teachings of that culture. The stereotypical Japanese person is very meticulous about his grooming and appearance and may expect everyone around him to be the same, while a logger living in a mountain logging camp is used to his Saturday night bath and may become very angry if forced into the daily bath routine of a hospital. Family traditions play a big role in the shaping of a person's hygiene habits. Whether or not a daily bath was part of a child's routine will influence the frequency of bathing in his adult years. Peer relationships are also very important, especially during adolescence when the teen-ager needs to be part of the crowd. If all her friends wash their hair every other night, a girl will probably do likewise.

A person's knowledge will also affect his habit patterns. Awareness of the hazards of poor hygiene, both physical and social, may lead toward adequate hygiene, whereas misconceptions may result in unsatisfactory habits. There are people who actually believe that a bath more than once a week, or even once a month, will cause pneumonia. Imagine their anxiety when faced with hospital routine! This knowledge will usually come from formal and informal teaching—from classes, literature and television, health personnel, family, and friends.

In addition to what a person knows about hygiene, several other factors are necessary to maintain his standards of hygiene. The availability of resources is certainly paramount. Such availability may be related to either the person's financial status or his location. To a man on a very limited income, food may be more important than soap. And most camping gear does not include a 6-ft bathtub. How a person feels will also greatly help or hinder his ability to achieve a good hygiene state. If a person is ill or depressed, he may not have enough energy to care how he looks. In these situations, he must depend on others for assistance; if no others are available, these needs will not be met. One of the first signs of improvement may be the patient-client's request for lipstick, a mirror, a shave, or his own pajamas.

Finally, individual need is an important factor in the development of hygiene patterns. Each person has his own particular hygiene problems—heavy perspiration, oily skin, dry hair—

and must build his personal practices on the basis of these needs.

Helping ill persons with their personal hygiene has always been an important function of the nurse. As suggested by the above discussion, this assistance may be facilitated by some assessment before planning this care jointly with the patient-client. Knowledge about his usual hygiene regimen will help toward adaptation of an institutional routine and will present cues as to what kind of health teaching is necessary. Although the professional nurse may not give direct care to each patient who needs help with hygiene, he is responsible for planning how this help shall be given, and for teaching nursing personnel who provide the direct care.

Bathing

Beside the obvious function of removing dirt and dead epithelial cells from the surface of the skin, the bath has several other desirable effects. The friction produced by rubbing with the washcloth and towel stimulates peripheral circulation, increasing nutrition of the cells. Movement during the bathing process provides muscle exercise and allows many of the joints to be put through their range of motion. This movement also increases circulation and improves respiratory function by stimulating deep breathing. These latter effects may be detrimental in the care of a cardiac patient whose heart is being put to rest as much as possible; in this case the exercise phase of bathing may be held to a minimum. Bathing also assists in the removal of transient bacteria on the skin, thus reducing the chance of infection. A detrimental effect is the drying that occurs when soap is left on the skin or the patient-client is not adequately dried.

In addition to the above physiological effects, the bath has a psychological potential. In the American middle-class society, cleanliness and its accompanying lack of distasteful odors have a high value. Most people feel better when they are clean and feel more socially acceptable. A patient-client who has been restless, feverish, or uncomfortable usually feels refreshed after a bath. It may also be sufficiently relaxing that the patient-client falls asleep. A great deal of verbal and nonverbal communication occurs during the bath. Often the nurse can transmit an "I-care-about-you" feeling to the patient-client, and a therapeutic nurse–patient-client relationship ensues. It is a time for verbal interchange, too. Frequently the nurse, especially the beginning nursing student, feels more able to talk with his patient-client when he is doing something with his hands. It is also a time when the patient-client knows he has the nurse's full attention and may feel free to initiate discussion of problems and concerns. And through the casual interchange the nurse and the patient-client get to know each other better.

The bath provides an excellent time for observations by the nurse. The nurse can directly observe all surfaces of the skin, hygiene state, sites of tenderness, range of motion, state of hydration, etc. As the patient-client's abilities progress toward independence, this opportunity diminishes and the nurse will need to plan deliberate direct examination of these areas.

The type of bath given ranges from a complete bed bath, given by the nurse or other personnel, to a tub bath or shower taken completely independently by the patient-client. And within each category there is a wide variety of possibilities, depending on the patient-client's capabilities. Therefore, in a hospital, the nurse must assess these abilities before deciding on the type of bath as well as on how much to allow the patient-client to do for himself. In the home, the nurse may be a consultant to the family about what the patient-client can do for himself and how to adapt care to their particular home.

Sometimes, the physician's orders will determine the type of bath to be used. For instance, if the patient-client is to be kept on bed rest, the possibility of a shower is eliminated. In evaluat-

ing the situation, the nurse must also look at the activities that will be required of the patient-client following the bath. For example, Mrs. S. had abdominal surgery yesterday and, when you go in to meet her this morning, she says that she is feeling pretty good after her pain medication an hour ago. Knowing that she will probably want to feed herself for breakfast and that she must walk out into the hall after her bath, you decide that you will bathe her and allow her to be somewhat passive during that time in order to conserve her energy for the period of ambulation. At other times the nurse will have the patient-client do as much for himself as possible in moving toward rehabilitation.

At times the nurse may decide that the patient-client either does not need or cannot tolerate a complete bath. For instance, if the patient-client has very dry skin, the additional use of soap would increase the dryness. So the nurse decides to omit a complete bath. Sometimes the patient-client is too tired or simply refuses. In these cases, a partial bath is carried out with attention to the face, hands, axillae, perineal area, and back. These are the parts which have priority need for daily care. Any lesions on the skin would also need at least daily care.

When appropriate, most health-care agencies have a written procedure regarding the technique to be used for the different types of baths. After validating the scientific basis of the written procedure, the nurse may use it as a guideline. *Fundamentals of Nursing* (Fuerst and Wolff, 1969) also contains a good discussion of the actual technique. When caring for a patient-client in his home, any of the methodologies can be easily adapted. The main point in any procedure is that it utilize the proper principles of body mechanics, asepsis, and work organization, and provide for the comfort, safety, and individuality of the patient-client.

The cleansing agent used during the bath varies according to the person's needs. Soap is most frequently used, although when the skin is excessively dry, soap should be eliminated, since it further removes the protective oil barrier. Instead, water alone may be used and, in extreme instances, an oil bath may be given. If oil is not used during the bath, lotion should be applied afterwards to replace the skin oils.

Many different kinds of soap are available, but antibacterial soaps are presently the most popular. Fifty percent of the money spent for soap in 1968 purchased this particular type of soap product. Considerable data have been collected which show that these soaps have a residual bacteriostatic effect against gram-positive bacteria when they have been used repeatedly over a period of several days. A study conducted at the U.S. Naval Academy indicated that these soaps can reduce the incidence of superficial skin infections (MacKenzie, 1970). Because of this property, antibacterial soaps have become the soaps routinely used by hospitals on their general units and in nurseries, where they have proved effective in controlling outbreaks of staphylococcal skin infections. When time allows, preoperative skin preparation is done with these soaps; the public uses them to control body odor; and teen-agers use them to avoid the secondary infections of acne.

Hexachlorophene is the active ingredient in these soaps, which, as mentioned, have been used quite freely. In addition, the chemical is used in many cosmetics and deodorants. In the latter part of 1971, the Food and Drug Administration and the Committee of Fetus and Newborn of the American Academy of Pediatrics issued a warning against the use of concentrated hexachlorophene products in the daily bath of newborns. Studies conducted on newborn monkeys showed the development of brain lesions following the accumulation of the chemical in the blood. Newborns bathed daily with the product have also shown high blood levels, but none has demonstrated any toxic symptoms. The FDA felt that the findings were conclusive enough to warrant curtailing the use of concentrated hexachlorophene soaps in nurseries and considering restrictions on use by the general public. Others are concerned about the effect this will have on future staphylococcal epidemics. Research studies are being continued ("Warning Issued against Some Uses of Hexachlorophene," 1972).

Perineal Care

Daily perineal cleansing is particularly important. There are a number of opposing skin surfaces in this area which tend to hold in moisture and secretions. The perineum is an area with a very high potential for bacterial growth. Excretions from the gastrointestinal and urinary systems, as well as from the skin, provide a constant supply of bacteria capable of producing disease if they gain entry into a different site. *Smegma* is a thick, cheesy substance which collects in the perineal area, producing a foul smell and a good medium for bacterial growth. Therefore, the crotch area must be cleaned at least every day in order to avoid excessive bacterial reproduction and an unpleasant odor characteristic of poor hygiene. This becomes even more important when a Foley catheter is present or if the skin or mucous membrane in the area is not intact. The actual technique of perineal care is not very complicated and is described in "Perineal Care of the Incapacitated Patient" (Gibbs, 1969).

In addition to the actual cleansing with soap and water, the use of genital deodorants has become very popular, especially with women. With the increasingly relaxed attitude toward sex, advertising has become more uninhibited, and these products are placed before the public daily with the usual claims of superiority and essentiality. However, there has been an increasing number of reports of vulvar itching or burning and labial swelling. One gynecologist reported treating 30 cases of vulvitis apparently caused by feminine genital sprays ("Should Genital Deodorants Be Used?" 1972).

The major impact of perineal care is psychological. In our culture, the perineal area and its functions have been a very private affair, not to be discussed with others. Therefore the situation may be embarrassing for the nurse and the patient-client alike. This is especially true for the beginning nursing student who has not yet had the opportunity to explore his feelings with his instructor and peers. He often feels that he is the only one having this difficulty. When the patient-client is capable of doing this part of the bath himself, the problem is relatively minor, since the nurse has only to collect the necessary equipment, place it conveniently, position the patient-client properly, and provide adequate privacy. The main obstacle here is how to let the patient-client know what is expected of him, particularly which words to use. Suggestions include, "Now I will leave you to: 'finish your bath,' 'wash your perineal area,' 'crotch,' or 'privates,' or 'wash between your legs.'"

The problem becomes more acute if the nurse is required to do the perineal cleansing himself and is particularly difficult when the patient-client is a young person of the opposite sex. Through experiences and support from those around him, the nurse gains the ability to handle the situation in a matter-of-fact way and to concentrate on the patient-client's feelings, helping him through the situation.

Hair and Nail Care

The routine daily care of the hair consists of daily brushing to distribute the oils along the shaft of the hair and to prevent the accumulative matting and tangling that occur quite rapidly when a person is in bed. Braiding is a comfortable way of handling long hair, but the braids must be undone, brushed thoroughly, and rebraided at least daily. If braiding is too tight, the hair is pulled at the scalp and circulation in the scalp is impaired.

Shampooing and shaving are procedures done as needed or desired by the patient-client. Shaving a man's face is usually done daily, while shampooing the hair and shaving a woman's legs and axillary areas often are put into the category of "nice little extras to do if there is time." However, it is exactly these things that may greatly improve a patient-client's morale and thus improve her physiological progress. Fuerst and Wolff (1969) and DuGas (1972) discuss the procedures involved, as will the procedure books of most health-care agencies.

A problem much too common among people with particularly poor hygiene is that of lice. Although anyone can contact pediculosis, it is distinctly prevalent among people living in crowded, unhygienic conditions. The species infecting the human body are the *Pediculus capitis* (head), *Pediculus corporis* (body), and *Phthirius pubis* (pubic hair). Transmission is by close contact with an infected person. Unless the insects are directly observed first, the main symptom is usually intense itching in the involved area caused by the saliva injected into the skin during feeding and irritation from the excreta deposited. Secondary infection and its accompanying symptoms may occur as the patient-client's scratching further breaks the integrity of the skin. Satisfactory treatment is accomplished with 1 percent gamma benzene hexachloride (Kwell$_{tm}$), which is available in a cream, lotion, and shampoo. One application of the solution is usually enough to achieve the desired results, although repeated treatments are sometimes necessary. Combs, brushes, toilet seats, and other washable items may also be treated with the solution, while clothing and other articles have to be dry-cleaned or otherwise treated (Wexler, 1969).

Nail care involves cleaning and trimming to maintain a safe length and contour, one which will prevent ingrown nails and the resultant infection. Thick, hard nails are better cut after having been soaked in warm water or an oil solution. Because of decreased circulation in the extremities and the danger of ensuing infection, extra caution must be used not to break the skin on the foot of a diabetic patient-client. In fact, some hospitals have a policy restricting this activity to people with special training, such as podiatrists.

Massage

This discussion will deal only with massage of the back. Massage of the extremities, especially the legs, should be done only after checking with the physician or a nurse clinician. This is because of the possibility of dislodging blood clots.

A back massage begins at the base of the buttocks and goes upward, including the trochanters, lumbar and thoracic areas of the back, shoulders, and deltoid regions, and ending with the neck. The nurse must know the fiber directions of the major muscle groups involved: the gluteal group, tensor fasciae latae, external oblique, latissimus dorsi, teres major, deltoid, trapezius, and sternocleidomastoid. Pressure in the longitudinal direction of the muscle fibers aids in venous return.

Physiologically, the desired results of massage are quite similar to those of the bath: increased local circulation and nutrition to the cells and muscle relaxation or stimulation. The sensation of touch is also utilized for its psychological effect. A back rub may be for either relaxation or stimulation, and the end goal will dictate the type of strokes used and the placement of the massage in the schedule of activities. For instance, Mr. J. did not sleep well last night and the nurse would like him to nap this morning. Since the effects of a relaxing back rub would be negated while Mr. J. rolls around during the bed making, the nurse reverses these two activities. When the back massage is completed, Mr. J. can easily slip into a peaceful sleep.

The main component of any nurse's massage technique is that he develop his own habit pattern, one with which he is comfortable. A successful back rub is an art developed through practice.

Before the back rub is begun, the patient-client should be positioned so that he is comfortable and so that the nurse can use proper body mechanics. In the prone position, inversion of the feet augments relaxation of the gluteal muscles. The choice of lubricant used depends on the patient-client's needs. Lotion is the most frequent choice, since it replaces skin surface oils and softens the skin, although powder may also be used if a dry substance is desired. If the patient-client's skin is already oily, alcohol can be utilized for its drying effect. If lotion is used, it should be warmed before the massage.

There are three main types of stroke. *Deep stroking* is a slow, rhythmical movement in which pressure is applied in a generally upward direction. It is usually a long stroke extending from the base of the buttocks to the neck or out to the deltoid regions. It usually begins and ends the back massage and also is used between the other two types. *Kneading* may be defined as a rolling, or lifting, movement which is applied by repeatedly grasping and releasing a muscle with the hands. Each of the superficial muscle groups should be kneaded individually. *Friction* is a deep circular movement in which the skin is made to move in small circles over the underlying tissues. This stroke is used particularly along the vertebrae and around any reddened areas found on the back. However, pressure applied directly over bony prominences will increase local trauma.

The hands should never leave the surface of the skin during the massage; they should be relaxed and should conform to the contour of the area being treated. Fingers should be kept together since individual fingers have very little power and the lack of pressure will cause tickling. When coming to the end of the treatment, signal this to the patient-client by slowing the rhythm and lifting the pressure. The programming of these strokes and skills into an effective technique is the art involved.

The nurse can evaluate the results of the massage by noting muscle relaxation and general flushing of the skin. He may also ask the patient-client how comfortable he is.

PRESSURE SORES

Modern medicine and advances in all realms of health care have increased life expectancies and have greatly improved the chances of surviving diseases and injuries which would have proved fatal some years ago. The result has been a greater incidence of chronic diseases and longer rehabilitative periods. When the life expectancy of an elderly person extended only to the occurrence of his first major illness, there was little problem with geriatric management. This trend has been reversed. These factors have produced several important problems, one of the most paramount being the increased incidence of pressure sores.

The terms "pressure sore," "bedsore," and "decubitus ulcer" are usually used interchangeably to describe the same phenomenon—a phenomenon which is rapidly growing to be a primary health concern as the number of persons at risk increases. Pressure sores are one of the major complications during the care of persons who are chronically ill, are debilitated, or have spinal cord injury. It has been estimated that the average cost of treating a pressure sore is about $5,000, although often the expenditure increases three- to fourfold (Pfaudler, 1968). And these figures do not include the amount of human suffering involved.

Although the physician plays a part in the treatment of pressure sores, the major role in the prevention and management of the pathological process belongs to the nurse. Most of the preventive measures should be done as independent nursing actions, and these same measures should be carried over into the treatment phase, if this is necessary.

Pathogenesis

Pressure sores are areas of cellular necrosis. Cells require adequate supplies of nutrients and removal of metabolic wastes. These functions are accomplished as fluid passes between the capillary and the cell. Any condition which interferes with this exchange between the cell and the blood hinders the proper function of the cell; the ultimate consequence is cell death.

Many factors may predispose a person to pressure-sore development. These will be discussed later as causative and contributory factors. In general, any patient-client whose condition is or has been deteriorating should be considered a high-risk candidate. The majority of patient-clients admitted to a hospital have come because of their declining condition, and Bliss notes that 70 percent of all geriatric patient-clients who develop bedsores do so within two weeks after admission to the hospital. She also states that the pressure sores which develop after admission are often more severe and longer lasting than those present at the time of admission. Whether the deterioration is gradual or sudden seems to make no difference; what matters is that the condition is worsening (Bliss, 1967).

There are specific groups of high-risk patient-clients. Everyone suffers from decreased blood flow to a part each time he sits in one position for any length of time. However, as the ischemia progresses, warning signs of pain, tingling, or numbness occur. As these messages are acted upon, the person either consciously or subconsciously changes position to relieve the ischemia before it causes irreversible damage. Pathological changes in the person's condition may hinder this normal protective mechanism. Persons with decreased sensory input are at a distinct disadvantage in preventing pressure-sore formation, since they lack the normal warning system; the physiological signs just mentioned cannot be so easily perceived by this person—or may not be felt at all. Decreased sensory input occurs in persons with spinal cord lesions or in those suffering from various neurological diseases, such as a stroke. Such persons do not know that they need to change positions.

Another group at risk includes persons who may receive adequate sensory input from the ischemic area, but, because of paralysis or weakness, lack the necessary motor ability to move themselves to a different position. Those persons with a malfunction of both the sensory and motor nervous systems, such as may be caused by medication, anesthesia, and unconsciousness, have a compounded problem. And, in addition to the physiological conditions cited above, psychological disorders, such as may be found in deep depressive states, may reduce the person's ability to react appropriately to the physiological warning signs.

Causative Factors As implied by the name, the principal cause of pressure sores is *pressure.* Bailey asserts that, although the development of pressure sores may be furthered by other intrinsic and extrinsic factors, the actual *cause* is only one thing—pressure. No other causative factor alone will produce a pressure sore, but pressure is capable of doing it without any other help (Bailey, 1967). This pressure narrows or obliterates blood vessels, thereby causing a reduced or completely absent blood flow to the body part normally supplied by the involved vessels.

The problem arises when the amount of pressure exerted on an area is higher than that of the vascular tree supplying the soft tissues. This pressure occurs, for example, when the tissues are squeezed between the external surface and a bone. The blood pressure within a vessel decreases as it moves away from the heart. The pressure in the arteriolar limb is 32 mm Hg, reducing in the midcapillary region to 20 mm Hg, and further decreasing to 12 mm Hg in the venous limb (Leavitt, 1966). Linden et al. (1965) measured the amount of pressure exerted on the

skin areas of persons placed in different positions, and found that the area under the ischial tuberosities, in the sitting position, was exposed to pressures as high as 700 mm Hg. In other positions, many body areas—particularly those covering bony prominences—were subjected to pressures much greater than the blood pressures within the vessels involved (Linden, 1965).

However, since few of us develop pressure sores from sitting, other factors must be involved in addition to the amount of pressure. One such factor is the *duration of the pressure.* High pressures for a short period of time can be tolerated better than low pressures for long periods (Rudd, 1962). The sustained pressure causes more tissue damage, since the cells are without nourishment for an extended time.

Tissues over bony prominences are most apt to develop pressure sores, although necrotic areas do appear in the softer tissues, such as the calf, buttocks, and upper arm. Bony prominences are hard, relatively immovable points which produce a reactive concentrated pressure on the tissue between the skin and bone. As shown with the ischial tuberosities in the sitting position, the pressure may be quite intense. Figure 18-1 shows the major pressure points in unsupported reclining positions. Awareness of these points guides the nurse in his planning of the patient-client's position in bed or a chair.

One would expect that the obese person would be the most susceptible to pressure sores because of the added weight that the body bulk itself places on vulnerable skin surfaces. Actually, the underweight person is just as liable to pressure-sore formation, since the protective subcutaneous tissues, which usually help pad the bony prominences, are not available. Linden found that an underweight 97-lb woman showed slightly higher peak pressures than a 306-lb man. However, the low and medium peak pressures on the man were, of course, spread over a much greater area (Linden, 1965). Therefore, the obese

Supine

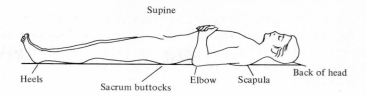

Heels   Sacrum buttocks   Elbow   Scapula   Back of head

Side Lying

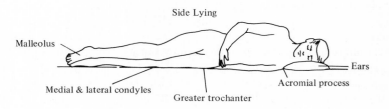

Malleolus

Medial & lateral condyles   Greater trochanter   Acromial process   Ears

Prone

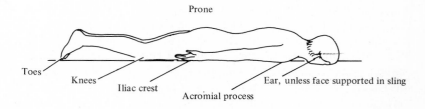

Toes   Knees   Iliac crest   Acromial process   Ear, unless face supported in sling

(plus genitalia — men; breasts — women).

Figure 18-1 Major pressure points in unsupported reclining positions.

and the underweight are equally likely to develop bedsores.

Another factor which results in localized pressure areas is the presence of foreign objects in the bed or chair. Such items as dentures, lipstick cases, bottle caps, buttons, cigarette lighters, pencils, and bobby pins between the bed or chair and the patient-client cause small sites of concentrated high peak pressures on the skin and, if left long enough, can result in skin breakdown in a susceptible patient-client. Wrinkled sheets or clothes can do the same thing.

Shearing force, which occurs when tissue layers move on each other, leads to angulation and stretching of blood vessels passing through the subcutaneous tissue. This constricts the vessels and reduces by various degrees the blood supply to the part involved. One of the most common examples of shearing force occurs in the sacral area. As the head of a patient-client's bed is elevated to 30° or more, the torso tends to slide toward the foot of the bed. The skin remains in a relatively fixed position, since friction anchors it to the bed; the deep fascia is well-attached to the bony structures. However, the deeper portions of the superficial fascia are rather loose and mobile in the sacral region and slide easily on the deeper fascia. This results in the kinking of vessels passing between the superficial and deep fascia layers, particularly the major posterior branches of the lateral sacral and gluteal arteries, and can lead to deep tissue necrosis.

Contributory Factors Although the following factors do not actually *cause* pressure-sore formation, they are definitely contributing factors, increasing the risk of bedsore development and prolonging their duration.

Increased *heat* in an area causes a concomitant increased metabolism. This rise in metabolic rate requires additional nutrient supplies and waste removal. In an area with an already compromised blood supply, this need cannot be met, and cellular necrosis is hastened. The source of heat may be either external or internal (e.g., internal in an inflammatory response).

Maceration reduces the resistance of the skin to other causative and contributory factors. This condition, which occurs when the skin is constantly bathed in moisture, results in softening of the skin layers, making them more susceptible to trauma. Particular areas of danger are those with opposing skin surfaces, such as pendulous breasts.

Friction on the skin removes the protective epithelial layer. It is very common among patient-clients, occurring especially on their heels and elbows as they move themselves around in bed. Moving a patient-client up in bed without a pull sheet causes friction along the length of the back and buttocks. Anything that rubs against the skin, e.g., braces, traction equipment, and clothing, can increase this potential hazard.

Anything that breaks the integrity of the skin, whether it be friction, abrasion, or laceration, opens it to bacterial invasion. This leads to a sequence of events which can predispose an area to breakdown. Inflammatory response increases the heat of the area, the rate of metabolism, and the need for additional nutrients and waste removal; and, at the same time, it is accompanied by swelling and edema, which hinder the exchange process between the capillary and the cell. The larger the number of pathogens that enter the skin, the greater the inflammatory response. Therefore, the status of the bacterial population on the skin surface plays a big part in the development of decubitus ulcers. There is a normal bacterial flora on the skin which naturally grows and reproduces. Hygienic measures are designed to remove periodically excessive accumulations of microorganisms and their environmental dirt. If a susceptible person practices *poor hygiene*, therefore, he increases the chance of this complication during disease or after injury.

Any other factor which interferes with the deliverance of nutrients to a cell brings it closer to death. *Arteriosclerosis* may predispose a person to pressure-sore formation, since it decreases the amount of blood flow in general. As plaque lines the inner walls of the blood vessel, the lumen is constricted, just as it is from external pressure. *Edema* also increases the chances of cellular death. As the distance between the capillary and the cell itself increases, the exchange of nutrients and waste material becomes more difficult. *Anemia* means that the blood is carrying less oxygen and is therefore unable to provide the necessary amounts to the tissue cells.

A person's general state of nutrition is a major component in the formation of pressure sores and the healing process of those already present. General malnutrition means the loss of subcutaneous tissue and muscle. The most important factor concerns proteins, which are essential elements for normal tissue growth and replacement. Illness and injury result in tissue breakdown and loss of proteins from the body. Any condition in which the output of protein exceeds the intake creates a *negative nitrogen balance,* characterized by edema and decreased elasticity, resiliency, and vitality of the skin. In addition, protein intake is necessary for healing. In patient-clients who have large, draining ulcers, the amount of protein lost in the exudate may be as much as 50 gm per day (Schell and Wolcott, 1966). This figure, added to the normal adult daily requirement of 55 to 65 gm, represents a crucial problem, especially when a negative nitrogen balance is accompanied by anorexia.

An *inadequate vitamin C intake* increases capillary fragility. Since this makes the capillary bed more susceptible to trauma and consequent interruption of blood supply to the cells, it is another contributory factor in bedsore development.

Types of Pressure Sores There are generally two differentiations of pressure sore: superficial and deep. Superficial ulcers involve the skin surface and may progress to form shallow craters. They are visible from their onset and usually heal more rapidly than the deeper ones. Deep bedsores may be extensions of superficial ulcers into the subcutaneous and muscle layers, or they may result from shearing force. These lesions are often not visible until they open a tract out onto the skin surface. They are very difficult to heal because of the extensive tissue damage. The ratio of superficial to deep ulcers is about 3:1 (Blinks, 1968). Any combination of these two types may be found. Figure 18-2 shows a superficial ulcer with an underlying deep component.

Another categorization of pressure sores divides them into four major classes: Class I: Primary decubitus ulcer involves epidermal injury, characterized by erythema, edema, pallor, cyanosis, and superficial erosion; it results from localized circulatory collapse in the pressure area. Class II: Secondary ulcers are distinguished by necrosis of the skin and fat which extends to but does not include muscle; they are

also due to localized trauma or irritation. Class III: Terminal pressure sores, with muscle necrosis and bone involvement, occur in the final stages of debilitating illness; they are often numerous and develop rapidly over widespread areas. Class IV: Neutrophic pressure sores develop because of sensation loss and lead to osteomyelitis, septic arthritis, and pathologic fractures (Adams and Bluefarb, 1968).

Development and Healing The first sign of decubitus-ulcer formation is pallor or whiteness of the involved area, the result of lack of blood in the site. This state is extremely transient, since inflammation starts almost immediately, and is rarely seen, although the heel area may remain white for quite a time before breakdown becomes visible.

In the case of a superficial ulcer, the initial pressure-sore indicator usually seen by the nurse is a reddened area (or a warm area in dark-skinned persons). This erythema can ordinarily be connected with pressure over a bony prominence or with foreign objects or wrinkles in the bed or chair. In the early stages, the erythema fades on direct pressure and vascular filling follows release of the pressure. The spot disappears shortly after the pressure is relieved, especially if massage is used to increase circulation to the surrounding area. As development proceeds, the erythema does not fade when pressure is applied and the spot remains for increasing periods of time after the causative pressure is relieved. Progression continues until the superficial skin layers are necrosed, thereby breaking the skin integrity. Figure 18-3 shows a full-thickness superficial skin ulcer. At this point, deterioration of the tissue layers may advance very rapidly because of infection and protein loss.

The first sign of the presence of deep ulcers may be a small opening on the skin, although the nurse may notice a hard lump, purplish discolor-

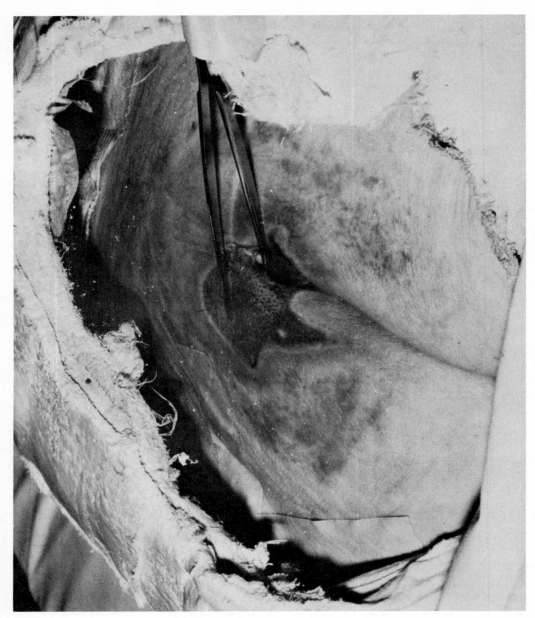

Figure 18-2 Pressure sore with both a superficial and a deep component. Note the plaster cast which originally covered this pressure point. (*Courtesy of University of Washington School of Nursing.*)

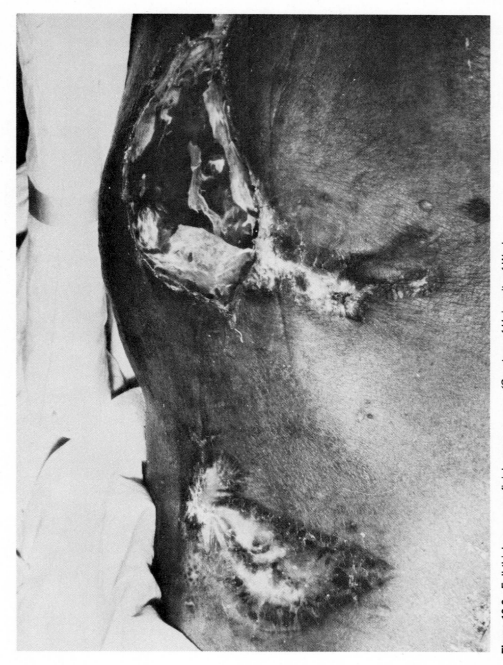

Figure 18-3 Full-thickness superficial pressure sore. *(Courtesy of University of Washington School of Nursing.)*

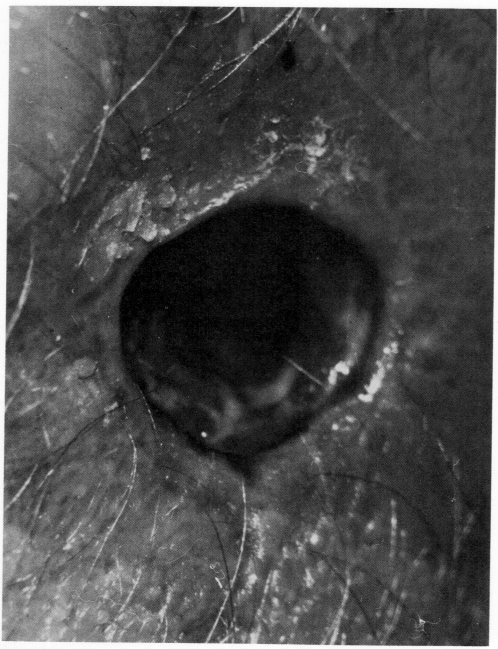

Figure 18-4 Sinus tract leading to deep ulcer. *(Courtesy of University of Washington School of Nursing.)*

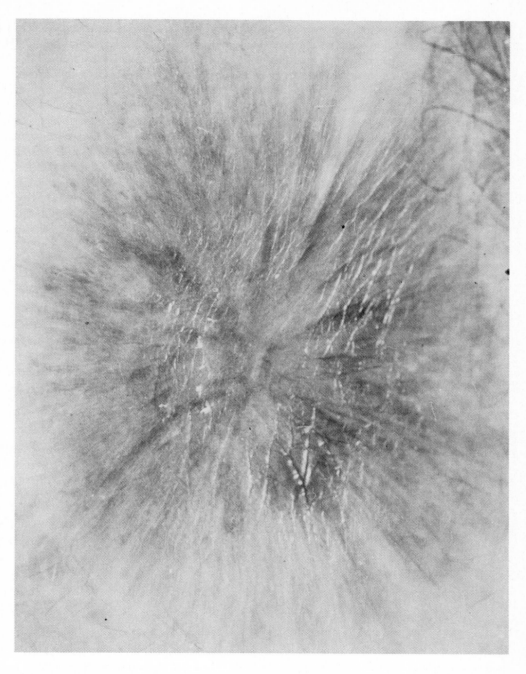

Figure 18-5 Pressure sore which is almost completely healed. *(Courtesy of University of Washington School of Nursing.)*

ation, or tenderness of the skin prior to actual perforation of the skin surface. Figure 18-4 demonstrates a typical sinus tract leading to a deep ulcer. As necrosis occurs in the deep tissues, the products of cellular death (tissue, serous and serosanguineous fluid, and pus), which must find an escape route, force their way out to and through the skin surface. In order to facilitate healing, this tract must be kept open as the ulcer heals from the inside out.

Left unchecked, the tissue necrosis of pressure sores continues its extension to all surrounding structures. The broader the scope of tissue damage, the harder it is to effect healing and the longer the process will take.

Healing by regeneration means the replacement of destroyed cells with cells of a similar type and function. Incisions heal by primary union, but the crater-like wound of a bedsore requires secondary union. Before the surface skin can close over, the cavity must be filled in with granulation tissue. If a pocket remains after the skin occludes the tract, as may happen with a deep ulcer, the area becomes an excellent growth media for anaerobic organisms (e.g., *Clostridia*—"gas gangrene").

Granulation tissue is connective tissue which includes newly formed and forming blood vessels and lymphatic vessels. The formation occurs in response to an inflammatory stimulus. It appears as a soft, somewhat mucinoid, grayish-red tissue which is transparent and slightly granular. It bleeds easily because of the numerous, delicate capillary buds. After the cavity acquires its surface covering of granulation tissue, this tissue continues to proliferate, building up either until the defect is filled in or the opposing margins finally meet. Only then can epithelialization, the final stage of healing, occur. Figure 18-5 shows an ulcerated area that has almost completed its healing process.

Several factors can contribute to poor wound healing: decreased blood supply to the wound; infection which interferes with regeneration directly through the action of bacterial toxins and indirectly because of the altered pH, action of proteolytic enzymes from the leukocytes, edema, etc.; hypoproteinemia which causes local edema and means a lack of the essential amino acids necessary to build new tissue; hypovitaminosis C (collagen cannot be formed without ascorbic acid); and mechanical elements, such as tension on the margins and pressure (Hopps, 1964). Ironically, these are the very factors which contribute to the formation of pressure sores in the first place, which helps explain why these lesions are so difficult to heal.

Prevention

The best way to treat pressure sores is to prevent their formation. Success with this objective would save much money, time, and suffering, both physical and psychological.

Primary responsibility for the prevention of bedsores lies with the nurse. Most of the necessary measures involved are independent nursing actions. The main goals of this nursing care are to (1) prevent sustained pressure, (2) maintain the skin in an intact, healthy condition, and (3) maintain the patient-client in a good nutritional state. One of the main deterrent measures is careful observation; the patient-client, especially if he is paraplegic, is taught to do this himself as soon as possible. Inspection is facilitated by mirrors.

Prevent Sustained Pressure Since the primary causative factor of pressure sores is pressure, the principal preventive measure involves limitation of any prolonged or concentrated pressure. When positioning a patient-client, care must be taken to eliminate intensified pressure over bony prominences. On one or both sides of these projections are indentations in the body contour, such as the waist above the greater trochanter in the side-lying position and above the iliac crests in the prone position. These body hollows result in the high peak pressures over the adjacent bony prominences. Filling in these depressions with pillows, or some other kind of padding, helps distribute the body weight over a greater surface area, thus reducing peak pressures.

Several devices have been made to relieve excessive pressure on the tissues over pressure points. All are based on the goal of equal weight distribution. One of the more successful has been the flotation pad. The underlying principle for this method is Pascal's law, which states that pressure applied to a liquid at any point is transmitted equally in all directions. Therefore, a surface with fluid properties would eliminate unequal pressure points. The silicone gel in the flotation pad is the consistency of human fat and has three important properties. It is a fluid that (1) keeps its shape, (2) is dense enough to support the weight, and (3) is flowable to prevent shearing. This gel is enclosed in a highly elastic membrane which serves only to protect it, not to confine it. The effectiveness was demonstrated in the case of a man with fractures of all four extremities who could not be turned. He was kept in the supine position on a flotation pad for forty days with no signs of pressure breakdown. These pads can fit into the seat of a wheelchair or into a cutout area of a foam mattress cover and are best covered with only a single layer of cloth (Grabenstetter, 1968; Spence, 1967).

Water beds have come into and gone out of vogue periodically over the past years. They are based on Archimedes' principle of displacement, which states that the body loses an amount of weight equal to the amount of fluid displaced. The patient-client is placed on a rubber mattress cover filled with water until the body is floating. This results in the distribution of surface pressure over the entire length of the body. The goal of the water bed, i.e., even weight distribution, has been achieved, but several side effects have prevented its general usage. Persons on complete flotation must be able to tolerate weightlessness; otherwise hallucinations and withdrawal occur.

Proper positioning of the patient-client is impossible, and, because the pelvis tends to lie deeper than the trunk and lower extremities, hip and knee contractures are common. This sinking of the pelvis also causes problems with urine drainage when a Foley catheter is in place. The tubing must be kept full and free of bubbles so that a siphon system is maintained. Many treatment measures are impossible while the patient-client is on a water bed because of its unstable surface. This means that he must be transferred periodically to a flat surface. Skin maceration is also a problem because of the lack of air circulation to the skin surfaces against the bed. A pillow must be placed between the knees to prevent ulcer formation over the medial condyles. Some patient-clients on the water bed have had difficulty with temperature regulation (Pfaudler, 1968; Harwin, 1970).

The University of South Carolina has developed a variation of the water bed, using pumped air as the flotation medium. Because the patient-client tends to float, rather than sink, the problem of hallucinations seems to have been eliminated. In addition to having even weight distribution, the patient-client can turn himself easily with the use of an overhead frame, and the air flow has a drying effect which apparently reduces the amount of drainage. A mild massaging action of the glass spheres in the bed may increase secondary blood flow (Harwin, 1970).

Polyether urethane foam pads are porous and resilient and one of the most easily compressible types of foam obtainable. They are made in various sizes and shapes and are used with positioning to help distribute weight (Line, 1966).

When padding an area to prevent high peak pressures on one site, the nurse must be very careful not to throw the weight onto another area. This has been found to be the result of many cutouts in foam pads. Firm doughnuts do the same thing. When the feet of a person sitting in a wheelchair are supported to take part of the weight, the full pressure is transferred to the ischial tuberosities.

Real and synthetic sheepskins have several functions, one of which is even weight distribution. They also keep the skin surface dry and prevent maceration by the rapid absorption and removal of perspiration. They are resilient, allow circulation of air around the body, and minimize skin abrasions. A new tanning procedure allows easy washing and drying (Brownlowe, 1970). Sheepskin material is made in flat pieces and is also used to line heel and elbow pads, etc.

Prevention of sustained pressure is the other facet under discussion here. The prime intervention is the frequent change of position. Patient-clients in wheelchairs should be taught to lift themselves off the seat about every twenty minutes to avoid ischial ulcerations. For bedridden patient-clients, several methods are available. An alternating-pressure pad is a plastic pad with rows of air-filled cells. A motorized unit causes alternate rows to inflate and deflate, each cycle taking approximately five minutes. This changes the pressure surfaces while the patient-client is lying on it. To be most effective, there must be only one layer of material between the pad and the patient-client, and no pins should be used with the pad.

However, the alternating-pressure pad does not negate the need for position change. Except in total flotation, the conscientious changing of the patient-client's position is the chief way of ensuring that pressure areas will be relieved. The most effective way to do this is to write out a turning schedule and post it in a conspicuous place, as well as noting it in the nursing-care plan. This schedule should take into account the desires and daily activities of the patient-client and the ward activities. For instance, it would not be too convenient to have the patient-client prone during the dinner hour or facing the wall during visiting hours. The traditional time interval between turning is two hours, but the condition and routine of the patient-client must be assessed to find the best time for him. The most important criterion of pressure is the development of reddened areas. The presence of reddened areas that do not disappear immediately when the pressure is relieved is a signal that position must be changed more frequently. Stryker frames and Circolectric beds are also used to accomplish position changes.

Maintain Intact, Healthy Skin   Proper use of the hygiene measures discussed earlier in this chapter is one of the chief means of maintaining healthy, intact skin. This keeps the bacterial flora under control and helps the skin maintain its soft, flexible, intact, clean condition. In addition, any procedure or intervention that reduces the possibility of trauma to the skin layers is desirable. Keeping an incontinent patient-client free of urine and feces accumulation prevents maceration and excoriation in the perineal area. The use of a pull sheet when moving a patient-client reduces the friction between the person and the sheets. Dusting the elbows and heels with talcum powder or cornstarch also reduces the effect of friction. Rubber draw sheets do not allow for the dissipation of moisture and soon are covered with permanent wrinkles. If sheets are placed on the bed with the smooth side of the hem out, the heels will not become irritated as they rub across them. Massage improves local circulation, and exercise increases it generally. Careful assessment of the skin areas around casts and traction and under bandages and binders will pinpoint trouble spots before they become too advanced. The list could go on indefinitely.

Maintain Good Nutrition   A diet chosen from the basic four food groups and containing the proper number of calories for the individual is necessary to maintain the normal day-to-day life of any person. Most illnesses and injuries require an increase in one or more of the dietary constituents. As mentioned before, protein and vitamin C are of particular importance in the prevention of pressure sores. And the weight of the person plays a role in terms of pressure peaks.

As important as the nutritional state is the fluid status. Adequate amounts of fluid intake are necessary to prevent volume depletion, with its resultant dry, cracking skin. Immobilization to any degree is accompanied by an increased need for fluids.

Treatment

If bedsores occur, the treatment measures include continuation of the preventive measures with some alteration and intensification. A pressure sore means that pressure must be removed from the involved area completely. This reduces the number of positions available to the patient-client. The protein intake of the person must be markedly increased; the negative nitrogen balance must be reversed in order for tissue healing to occur. In addition, on the basis of research on the factors in wound healing, some physicians feel that an increased vitamin C intake is beneficial. Then there are some additional actions that can be carried out, most of them in the realm of medical practice, such as use of medications and skin grafting.

However, one area of extreme concern to both the physician and the nurse is that of infection control. The detrimental effects of infection have been discussed; a pressure sore is wide open to this danger. Strict aseptic technique must be used when working with the open wound. There seems to be much controversy as to the best methodology to be followed, with little controlled study as to specific methods. Some observers advocate dressings to prevent contamination from the environment; others feel that the dressings keep any drainage in prolonged contact with the ulcer, providing constant growth media. Some feel that wet dressings may be used to keep an antiseptic solution, such as Burow's or Dakin's solution, next to the lesion; others think that the capillary attraction of the wet material brings too many organisms into the area. Most physicians want the nurse to wash the ulcer periodically with a hexachlorophene soap and then with some other antiseptic solution, such as

Dakin's. Unrestricted use of topical antibiotics is not generally accepted, since the infecting organisms may build up a resistance.

In order to allow normal healing to occur and as a way to reduce the amount of microbial growth, the ulcer crater is frequently debrided, or cleaned of the necrotic tissue. This may be done surgically, or it may be accomplished through the use of proteolytic enzymes, such as Chymar and Elase. Wet-to-dry dressings are a means of mechanical debridement. A dressing soaked in an antiseptic solution is wrung out and placed firmly against the ulcer surface. The dressing is allowed to dry thoroughly and then is pulled off, taking the necrotic tissue with it and leaving a clean bed of granulation tissue.

Another method of infection control concerns the packing of the ulcerated area with granulated sugar after having first cleaned it with hydrogen peroxide. There are several different theories as to why this works. (1) Sugar is the ideal growth medium for the bacteria, so they feed on it rather than on the tissue. (2) The bacteria gorge themselves on the sugar and eventually die. (3) The high concentration of sugar in the tissue alters the pH of that tissue and so influences the toxicity of the invading organisms. (4) The hypertonic solution created brings more serum and nutrients into the tissue, which promotes healing. (5) It stimulates growth of the granulation tissue. (6) It has a possible enzymatic action (Verhonick, 1961).

Local hyperbaric oxygen treatment has been used with some success. Researchers feel that it suppresses bacterial growth and enhances granulation and epithelium formation, although vascularity must be present if the treatments are to be effective. The major action seems to be the absorption of oxygen through the lesion into the ischemic area, which helps relieve the hypoxic state and improve healing (Fischer, 1969).

Heat is also used in an attempt to improve circulation to the area. Heat lamps are used to cause vasodilatation in the site. However, these must be used cautiously, since there is usually a

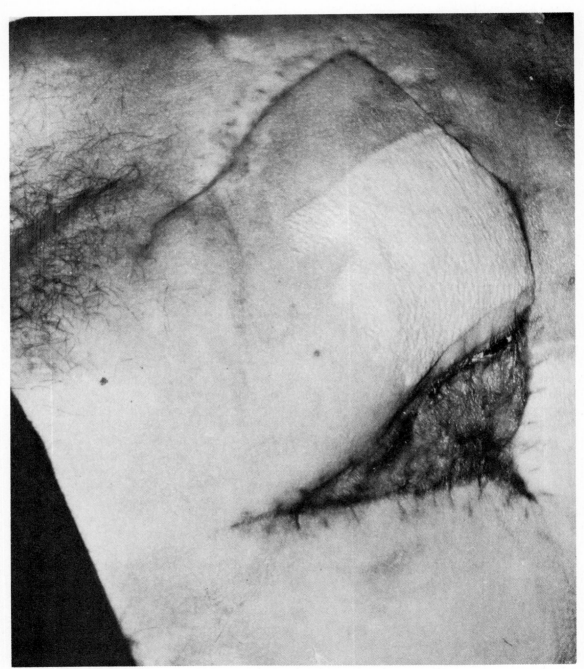

Figure 18-6 Split-thickness skin graft. *(Courtesy of University of Washington School of Nursing.)*

loss of localized sensation and a burn would certainly not help the situation. The heat also helps to dry the lesion.

Frequently the physician must resort to surgical skin grafting in order to get a tissue covering over the ulcer. Figure 18-6 shows a completed full-thickness flap graft.

Other agents, such as Gelfoam, gold leaf, vitamin C paste, and gentian violet, are used by various physicians. In addition, the medical regimen must contain measures to reverse some of the contributory factors, such as anemia and edema.

The whole area of pressure sores is full of controversies, mainly because of a lack of research in the field. Bedsores have been a problem since the beginning of nursing, and today the excellence of nursing care is often evaluated by the absence of pressure sores. However, we know that despite meticulous, expert care, the skin of some patient-clients still breaks down, while that of others, left unattended, does not. Why? What subtle differences make some patient-clients more susceptible than others (Verhonick, 1971)? Research is also needed into the prevention and treatment measures being used now and those that could be used in the future.

Summary of Common Problems, with Approaches

Problem	Approach
Eliminate reddened pressure areas	Relieve pressure, massage around area, observe closely.
Prevent pressure sores	Relieve pressure, change position frequently, pad bony prominences, keep skin dry and clean, provide high-protein diet, increase vitamin C intake, increase fluid intake, massage around area, use aseptic technique, carry out prescribed regimen.
Prevent dry skin	Omit bath, omit soap, apply lotion frequently.
Prevent oily skin	Bathe frequently, apply alcohol.

REFERENCES

Books

Bailey, B. N., "Bedsores," Edward Arnold (Publishers) Ltd., London, 1967.

Crouch, James, "Functional Human Anatomy," Lea & Febiger, Philadelphia, 1965.

DuGas, Beverly, "Kozier-DuGas' Introduction to Patient Care: A Comprehensive Approach to Nursing," 2d ed., W. B. Saunders Company, Philadelphia, 1972.

Fuerst, Elinor, and LuVerne Wolff, "Fundamentals of Nursing," 4th ed., J. B. Lippincott Company, Philadelphia, 1969.

Hopps, Howard, "Principles of Pathology," 2d ed., Appleton-Century-Crofts, Inc., New York, 1964.

Periodicals

Adams, Lawrence, and Samuel Bluefarb: How We Treat Decubitus Ulcers, *Postgraduate Medicine,* **44**:269-271 (1968).

Blinks, F. Allen: Pathogenesis and Treatment of Pressure Sores, *Physiotherapy,* **54**:281-283 (1968).

Bliss, Mary, and Rhoda McLaren: Preventing Pressure Sores in Geriatric Patients, *Nursing Mirror and Midwives Journal,* **123**:434-437ff. (Feb. 10, 1967).

Brownlowe, Miriam: New Washable Woolskins, *American Journal of Nursing,* **70**:2368-2370 (1970).

Cahn, Milton: The Skin from Infancy to Old Age, *American Journal of Nursing,* **60**:993-996 (1960).

Fischer, Boguslav: Topical Hyperbaric Oxygen Treatment of Pressure Sores and Skin Ulcers, *Lancet,* **2**:405-409 (Aug. 23, 1969).

Gibbs, Gertrude: Perineal Care of the Incapacitated Patient, *American Journal of Nursing,* **69**:124-125 (1969).

Grabenstetter, Joan: Synthetic Fat Helps Prevent Pressure Sores, *American Journal of Nursing,* **68**: 1521-1522 (1968).

Harwin, J. Shand, and Thomas Hargest: The Air-fluidized Bed: A New Concept in the Treatment of Decubitus Ulcers, *Nursing Clinics of North America,* **5**:181-187 (1970).

Leavitt, Lewis: Decubitus Ulcers, *Hospital Medicine,* **2**:76-78, 84-85 (November, 1966).

Linden, Olgierd, et al.: Pressure Distribution on the Surface of the Human Body: I. Evaluation in Lying and Sitting Positions Using a "Bed of Springs and Nails," *Archives of Physical Medicine and Rehabilitation,* **46**:378–385 (1965).

Line, Rose: Polyether Urethane Foam: A Nursing Tool in the Prevention and Treatment of Decubitus Ulcers, *Nursing Clinics of North America,* **1**:417–431 (1966).

MacKenzie, Albert: Effectiveness of Antibacterial Soaps in a Healthy Population, *Journal of the American Medical Association,* **211**:973–976 (Feb. 9, 1970).

Pfaudler, Marjorie: Flotation, Displacement and Decubitus Ulcers, *American Journal of Nursing,* **68**: 2351–2355 (1968).

Rudd, T. N.: The Pathogenesis of Decubitus Ulcers, *Journal of the American Geriatric Society,* **10**:48–53 (1962).

Schell, Victor, and Lester Wolcott: The Etiology, Prevention and Management of Decubitus Ulcers, *Missouri Medicine,* **63**:109–112, 119 (1966).

Should Genital Deodorants Be Used? *Consumer Reports,* **37**:39–41 (January, 1972).

Spence, Wayman, et al.: Gel Support for Prevention of Decubitus Ulcers, *Archives of Physical Medicine and Rehabilitation,* **48**:283–288 (1967).

Verhonick, Phyllis: Decubitus Ulcer Care, *American Journal of Nursing,* **61**:68–69 (1961).

———: Clinical Investigations in Nursing, *Nursing Forum,* **10**(1):80–88 (1971).

Warning Issued against Some Uses of Hexachlorophene, *American Journal of Nursing,* **72**:342 (1972).

Wexler, Louis: Gamma Benzene Hexachloride in Treatment of Pediculosis and Scabies, *American Journal of Nursing,* **69**:565–566 (1969).

ADDITIONAL READINGS

Allen, Linda: Facts and Fancies about Cosmetics and Aging Skin, *Nursing Clinics of North America,* **2**:369 (1967).

Carney, Robert: The Aging Skin, *American Journal of Nursing,* **63**:110–112 (1963).

Davis, Bernard: A Patient's View of Backrubs, *American Journal of Nursing,* **47**:112 (1947).

Montagna, William, "The Structure and Function of Skin," 2d ed., Academic Press, Inc., New York, 1962.

Simko, Michael: Foot Welfare, *American Journal of Nursing,* **67**:1895–1897 (1967).

Temple, Kathleen: The Back Rub, *American Journal of Nursing,* **67**:2102–2103 (1967).

Comfort and Sleep Status

**Susanna Lee Garner
and Pamela Mitchell**

Comfort is probably one of our most basic desires and wants. A person who is wet, cold, tired, or in pain tends to focus all or much of his attention on alleviating the discomfort. If he cannot find relief, the discomfort may preoccupy him to the exclusion of all else. Some forms of discomfort may be relatively minor and simply annoying; other forms may be so distressing as to exclude all other concerns.

From the many concepts related to comfort and rest, we have chosen for this chapter the concepts of sleep and of pain. Some of the most common problems facing patient-clients and their nurses involve getting to sleep and gaining relief from pain.

Data to Be Assessed—Sleep

1 Sleep patterns
   a Number of hours each day
   b Usual bedtime and arising time
   c Number of arousals during the night
   d Sleep environment
      (1) Number and type of pillows and covers
      (2) Ventilation
      (3) Amount of light and noise tolerated
      (4) Type of bed
   e Number and length of naps

   f Aids used for sleep
      (1) Bedtime routine
      (2) Beverages
      (3) Warm bath or back rub
      (4) Medications
      (5) Scheduling of activities
   g Personal beliefs about sleep needs
2 Alterations due to health problems
   a Change in usual sleep environment
   b Effect of anxiety

Section A: Comfort and Rest [1]

Most people spend roughly one-quarter to one-third of their lives sleeping. In order to help maximize use of sleep time or to aid with sleep problems, the nurse needs to be knowledgeable about sleep and the many factors that influence it. During the past two decades a great upsurge of interest in and research about all aspects of sleep has resulted in a growing wealth of data, some of which has direct implications for care planning. For example, an awareness of the cyclical nature of sleep and the need for uninterrupted sleep periods will affect the scheduling of activities, treatments, and medications. Some of the current knowledge concerning sleep presented in the following section will provide a scientific basis for problem solving and care planning.

THE NATURE OF SLEEP

Despite its universal occurrence, sleep has yet to be clearly defined. Kleitman, a well-known authority on sleep, briefly defines it as "a periodic temporary cessation or interruption of the waking state. . . ." [2] All descriptions of sleep agree that one necessary criterion of sleep is its reversibility, i.e., a person who is asleep can be aroused. It has also become apparent that although sleep is an interruption of the waking state, this does not imply inactivity. The body is active and functioning during sleep. The difficulty of defining sleep and the nonspecificity of the existing definitions are a reflection of the uncertainty about its true nature.

A recording of the electrical activity in the brain is known as an electroencephalogram (EEG). Such EEG recordings have revealed that sleep in the adult human being is composed of cycles of approximately eighty-five to ninety-five

minutes, although the length may vary between sixty and one hundred and twenty minutes. These cycles are shorter in the neonate (forty-five to sixty minutes) and lengthen as the individual matures. They have been called basic rest-activity cycles (BRAC) or simply sleep cycles (Kleitman, 1969). The average adult has approximately four to six of these cycles per night, with a total of about seven and one-half hours of sleep daily (Webb, 1968). Kleitman (1969) maintains that these basic rest-activity cycles are also operative during wakefulness, thus explaining the occurrence of alternating periods of alertness and drowsiness, such as those which necessitate coffee breaks during the day.

Sleep cycles are composed of two different parts, or phases. The first part of the cycle, which occupies approximately 80 percent of the total sleep time, is called slow-wave or non-rapid-eye-movement (NREM) sleep. This NREM sleep is composed of four stages, known as stages 1 through 4. The second type of sleep, called rapid-eye-movement (REM) sleep, has achieved some notoriety during the past decade because of its relation to dream recall and has probably served as an impetus to the increasing amounts of research being done on sleep. Because it has been studied in many areas and by many different persons, REM sleep has been called by a variety of terms, including desynchronized sleep, dreaming sleep, paradoxical sleep, rhombencephalic sleep, and emergent stage 1 sleep (Berger, 1969, page 19; Kleitman, 1963; Webb, 1968). It is termed rapid-eye-movement sleep because during this period the eyes display clusters of involuntary, jerky movements, as compared with the relatively slow, rolling motions displayed in NREM sleep. The eye movements are binocular and conjugate.

When an adult falls asleep he goes from wakefulness into stage 1 sleep and then proceeds over a period of about twenty to thirty minutes

---

[1] This section was written by Susanna Lee Garner.
[2] Nathaniel Kleitman, "Sleep and Wakefulness," The University of Chicago Press, Chicago, 1963, p. 3.

to progress gradually, in a stepwise manner, through stages 2 and 3, until he reaches stage 4, where he remains for about thirty minutes. At the end of this time the sleeper moves back up through the stages from 4 to 1 or 2 and then moves into a period of REM sleep, where he may remain from ten to thirty minutes. When the REM period is concluded, the individual again progresses from stages 1 or 2 to stages 3 and 4, thus beginning another cycle. If the person is awakened, when he returns to sleep he goes back through the stages in a smooth, stepwise progression and does not resume his cycle at the point he had reached when aroused (Williams, Agnew, and Webb, 1964). The transition into REM sleep is frequently marked by a series of body movements. This description is typical of a sleep cycle in the early part of the night just after sleep commences. As the night continues the character

of the sleep cycle changes so that the length of the NREM sleep periods decreases while the length of the REM periods increases. Therefore, during the first half of the night an individual receives the majority of his stage 3 and 4 sleep, and in the last half of the night he receives the majority of his REM sleep. In fact, the last one to two sleep cycles may not contain any stage 3 or stage 4 sleep (Berger, 1969) (Fig. 19-1).

The progressive change in the character of sleep cycles is also apparent in naps taken during the daytime hours. Naps taken in the morning or recently after awakening from a night's sleep closely resemble in composition sleep cycles which occur during the second half of the night. That is, they have an increased proportion of REM sleep and a decreased amount of NREM sleep. In comparison to morning naps, those taken during the afternoon and evening are

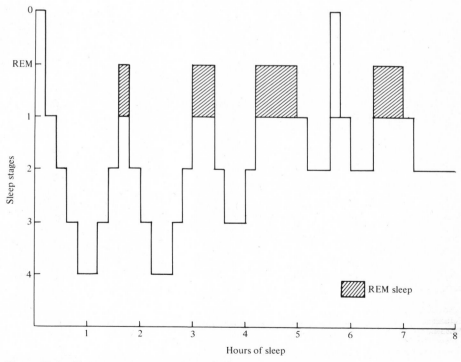

Figure 19-1 Diagrammatic representation of a typical night's sleep.

composed of increasing amounts of NREM sleep (Webb, Agnew, and Sternthal, 1966; Webb, 1969).

The composition of sleep, the pattern of a total night's sleep, and the speed of awakening are all affected by age. As the person ages, REM sleep occupies an increasingly smaller percentage of his total sleep time. Fifty percent of the newborn's total sleep time, 20 to 25 percent of the young adult's, and 13 to 18 percent of the elderly adult's is composed of REM sleep. The length of time a human being spends sleeping also decreases as he approaches maturity, changing from fourteen to sixteen hours per day in the newborn, to twelve and one-half plus or minus two hours at three years of age, and seven to eight hours in the young adult. Man's nocturnal biphasic sleep pattern begins to be established early in life. By the third week the neonate obtains 50 percent of his sleep between 8 A.M. and 8 P.M. The daytime nap in which the child receives the remainder of his sleep usually disappears by the age of five. As a child sleeps less and less during the day, the number of times he awakens during the night also decreases (Webb, 1969). The total sleep time of an elderly person is approximately the same as a young adult's; however, the elderly person awakens more often, stays awake longer, and therefore spends more time in bed to obtain the same amount of sleep. The ability of the organism to attain normal waking function on awakening has been found to be negatively related to age. That is, the younger the person, the longer it takes him to achieve his functional abilities when he awakens from sleep (Feinberg, 1969).

The character of sleep cycles varies greatly between individuals but remains remarkably consistent for any particular person. Webb has identified six factors that influence how long any one person sleeps. These factors include his (1) physiological makeup; (2) temporary changes in his physiological status (disease, addiction); (3) conditioned pattern of sleeping; (4) current stress level; (5) current presence or absence of a task (going to work); and (6) present desires (e.g., deciding to get up early to go skiing) (Webb, 1970).

A variety of other factors affects the composition (amounts of NREM and REM) of a person's sleep. Researchers have found that physical exercise during the day increases the amount of stages 3 and 4 sleep, but if this exercise occurs near bedtime, it disturbs sleep because of physiological activation of the body. Anxiety or a change from one's usual sleep situation may result in the person's taking longer to go to sleep; awakening more often and staying awake longer; having a longer latent period before the first REM period occurs; and having a decreased total amount of REM sleep. As anxiety decreases or the person becomes accustomed to the new sleep situation, these changes in his usual sleep pattern disappear. REM sleep may also be decreased by alcoholic intake before bedtime. Sensory deprivation (see "Sensory-Perceptual Restriction and Overload," Chapter 11) results in both an increase in the length of the first REM period and an increase in the total amount of REM sleep during the night (Baekeland, 1970). Present evidence shows that, following a period of adaptation, sleep obtained during the daytime hours does not vary significantly from that obtained during the night (Webb, 1969). Some common drugs which affect sleep include barbiturates, which reduce the amount of time spent in stage 1 and REM; amphetamines, which reduce the amount of REM time; and some antidepressants, which increase stage 4 (Zung, 1970; Kales and Kales, 1970). When the person stops taking the drug or the effects of the drug wear off, there is a rebound period when the individual spends more than the usual amount of time in the previously deprived stage. For example, when a person stops taking barbiturates (an REM suppressant), he will have an increased amount of REM sleep for several subsequent nights. The withdrawal from REM-suppressant drugs is frequently accompanied by nightmares, insomnia, restlessness, depression, anxiety, and fatigue (Kales and Kales, 1970).

The subjective feeling state of a person in the morning, or whether or not he felt he had a "good" sleep, has been found to depend on the number of times he awakes during the night and on the length of time he slept (Hartmann, 1970). One researcher has found that if people who are making up a sleep loss sleep longer than ten hours, they feel "worn out" on the following day. The conclusion was drawn that there may be a narrow range of optimal sleep time (Globus, 1969).

Several clinical conditions have been demonstrated to have a relation to sleep, especially REM and stage 4 sleep. Patients with coronary artery disease who have attacks of chest pain or angina during the night (nocturnal angina syndrome) usually have these attacks during REM periods. The REM period is also the time when people with duodenal ulcers suffer attacks of epigastric pain caused by an increased output of gastric acid. It has been found that asthmatic patients do not have attacks of dyspnea during stage 4 sleep—indicating that activities such as exercise, which increase stage 4 sleep, may help decrease the incidence of such nocturnal asthmatic attacks. People with untreated hypothyroidism or depression obtain a decreased amount of stage 4 sleep. Successful treatment of their conditions results in an increase of their stage 4 sleep (Kales and Kales, 1970).

PHYSIOLOGICAL CHANGES OCCURRING DURING SLEEP

Physiological changes occur in the body systems during sleep. The systems most visibly affected are the musculoskeletal and autonomic nervous systems. As might be anticipated, REM sleep has a different effect than NREM sleep on these body systems.

During NREM sleep the musculoskeletal system demonstrates a generalized decrease in muscular tone, with postural tone present only in the head and neck. When REM sleep occurs, occasional twitching movements of the face and limbs are apparent and there is a decrease in the postural tone of the head and neck. There is also increased movement in the extraocular muscles of the eye, resembling waking eye movements (Berger, 1969; Snyder, 1967).

With the advent of sleep the autonomic nervous system responds with a decrease in heart and respiratory rate, a fall in systolic blood pressure, and a decrease in body temperature. All these changes are typical of NREM sleep. During REM sleep periods there is a transitory increase in heart and respiratory rate and in the systolic blood pressure, although these rates do not usually reach the waking levels. Other changes which occur in REM sleep include an increase in cerebral blood flow, in the temperature of the brain, and in body oxygen consumption (Berger, 1969; Webb, 1968). Changes in hormonal function and biochemical activity also occur during sleep.

DREAMS

The correlation between dreaming and sleep stages has been a source of great controversy. Some investigators consider that REM sleep is dream sleep; others maintain that dreaming occurs in both REM and NREM sleep. It has been demonstrated that subjects will recall dreams more frequently when awakened from an REM period than when awakened from an NREM period. The exact relation between dreaming and REM sleep, however, has not been established (Berger, 1969). It is quite possible that dreaming and rapid eye movements are both observable manifestations of a more basic physiological or biochemical activity. The ability to recall dreams varies among persons. The content of the dream recall depends on whether a person was awakened from an NREM or an REM period. Thought or dream content from REM periods tends to reflect visible, emotional, movement-oriented activities which are complicated, vivid, and unrealistic. Content from NREM is more realistic and thought-like (Webb, 1968, p. 26).

THE FUNCTION OF SLEEP

Although the exact nature and purpose of sleep are not known at present, sleep experts generally agree that the purpose of NREM is rest and restoration of the body. The body's need is demonstrated by the fact that missed NREM sleep is "made up" and that it is "made up" before missed stage 1-REM sleep. Baekeland and Hartmann (1970) have called NREM sleep *obligatory* sleep and feel that it is necessary for biological health and performance. The need for NREM sleep seems to be quite consistent among subjects studied and in the individual subject (Hartmann, 1970).

The purpose of stage 1-REM sleep is a source of much more controversy. There seems, however, to be a growing body of opinion, theory, and experimental evidence that indicates an interrelationship between stress level, psychological functioning, and the need for stage 1-REM sleep. The fact that recent experiences are often the subject of dreams recalled from stage 1-REM has led Greenberg to postulate that the dream process helps keep the memory "up to date" by integrating recent emotionally meaningful experiences with past experiences and recording how the experience was handled (Greenberg, 1970). Baekeland and Hartmann (1970) called stage 1-REM and stage 2 sleep *facultative* sleep and noted that the need for it seemed to be much more variable than the need for NREM sleep.

SLEEP DEPRIVATION

The fact that sleep is necessary for the normal functioning of the human body is proved by the various psychological changes which occur when a person is deprived of sleep. The types of deprivation which have been most widely studied are total deprivation, stage 1-REM deprivation, and stage 4 deprivation. The last two are examples of stage deprivation.

After approximately four days of total sleep deprivation, healthy people begin to display psychological symptoms such as increasing fatigue, difficulty in concentrating, episodes of disorientation and misperception, feelings of persecution, and general irritability. These changes are most apparent in the early morning hours and least obvious in the afternoon and early evening (Johnson, 1969). Some studies of total deprivation have emphasized the symptoms of delirium, auditory and visual hallucinations, confusion, clouding of consciousness, and progressive disorientation to time, place, and person which occasionally are observed. Since delirium is not found in all people who are sleep-deprived, it is felt that these symptoms probably occur only in susceptible individuals and may not be an inevitable result of total deprivation (Dement, 1960; Johnson, 1969). On recovery nights after total deprivation studies, the percentage of the night's sleep composed of stages 4 and 1-REM is elevated.

Stage 1-REM deprivation is achieved in the laboratory by various means, such as awakening the person every time the EEG recording reveals that he is entering this sleep stage. Because stage 1-REM sleep occurs at the end of a sleep cycle and a person obtains the majority of his stage 1-REM during the last third of the night (Fig. 19-1), stage 1-REM deprivation probably occurs clinically when people are allowed to sleep only for short periods (less than an hour) or when they sleep only a total of three to four hours every twenty-four hours. Some of the behavioral changes which occur with stage 1-REM deprivation include increased appetite, anxiety, irritability, and difficulty in concentrating (Dement et al., 1967). As mentioned earlier under "The Function of Sleep," people who are deprived of stage 1-REM sleep have difficulty in coping with recent stressful experiences. In recovery nights after deprivation, stage 1-REM is made up only after the person has "made up" any missing stage 4 (Greenberg, 1970).

Stage 4 deprivation can be caused in the laboratory in a manner similar to that used in causing stage 1-REM deprivation; it occurs naturally only in chronic alcoholism, depression, and untreated hypothyroidism (Johnson, Burdick, and Smith, 1970; Kales and Kales, 1970).

ASSESSMENT OF SLEEP NEEDS

Knowledge of the nature of sleep, of the factors which affect it, and of the effects of sleep deprivation leads the nurse to the realization that sleep is more than just an incidental event which can be interrupted at will. The human organism requires a definite amount of sleep daily in prolonged periods in order to maintain maximal physiological and psychological functioning.

Awareness of the uniqueness of each patient-client's sleep pattern will guide the nurse's initial assessment. While taking the nursing history, data may be collected on such matters as how long he sleeps, usual bedtime, arising time, the number of arousals during the night, where and in what position he usually sleeps, any bedtime or awakening routines, and whether he habitually uses medication to help him sleep. Additional useful information would be whether and when he naps during the day, the number of blankets and pillows used, the amount of ventilation preferred, the amount of light and noise tolerated, his previous experience(s) with sleeping in different places or in the hospital, and his feelings and beliefs about his sleep needs. If the patient-client has difficulty in communicating,

his family or close friends may be utilized as secondary sources of information. If no data source is available, the patient-client's age may be used as a rough index of his sleep needs.

Once the nurse has collected this information, he can analyze it to determine particular sleep needs of the person and then begin to formulate a care plan to meet these needs.

PLANNING TO MEET SLEEP NEEDS

Each situation or health problem will dictate which of the patient-client's usual routines can be maintained and which cannot. Recognition of usual routines that cannot be followed will allow the nurse to discuss these with the patient-client, to explain the reason for the change, and, if feasible, to plan an alternative with him. At this time, if the patient-client has been hospitalized, the nurse might discuss with him the changes in sleep that occur with anxiety and a change in usual sleeping place (an increased number of awakenings, decreased total sleep time, longer time to fall asleep) and inform him that these changes usually disappear in one to two days.

In addition to following the patient-client's own routine as closely as possible, the nurse can utilize many actions which may relax the patient-client and promote sleep. A good book, a warm bath, a hot drink are helpful to many people. Providing an environment which is conducive to sleep—i.e., one which is quiet, tidy, and dark with suitable ventilation—will decrease disruptions of sleep. In a hospital, the attempt should be made to assign the patient-client to a room with compatible roommates. In the institutional setting, a very common and supremely irritating environmental disturbance is conversation and laughter from staff members in the halls and nursing station. A comfortable bed, freedom from pain, and the knowledge of how to summon help if necessary will contribute to the ability to sleep. Anxiety may be dealt with by allowing the patient-client to express his fears and ask questions, perhaps at the time of a relaxing back rub. If a sleep medication is used, it should be taken so that it begins to act when the patient-client is ready for sleep.

Careful planning and organization will allow the patient-client to sleep better and for longer periods. Treatments, activities, and medications should be scheduled to allow a quiet period to relax prior to bedtime and to avoid awakenings during the night. If arousal is unavoidable, it should be planned so that several things are done at one time and there are as few awakenings as possible. The rationale for routines which require the awakening of patient-clients should be examined to determine whether these routines are logical and should be retained, or whether they are illogical and should be revised or discarded. Why are patient-clients in some settings awakened and washed at 5 A.M.? The nurse can also utilize times when the patient-client awakens himself to make any necessary checks or to do anything required so that he does not have to be reawakened.

A nurse can learn to observe the condition of a sleeping person in a nondisturbing manner so that she can identify changes that may be occurring. For example, she can note increasing restlessness which may indicate pain or shock, or count respirations, noting their quality, and on some patients she may be able to count the pulse. The increasing use of electronic monitors makes some of this information available without touching the patient. Information collected without awakening the patient-client can then be used as a basis for deciding whether he should be disturbed for further assessment or whether he can be left to sleep.

The nurse may observe some of the physiological and behavioral changes which usually occur during sleep to assess whether or not a patient-client is asleep. Lack of purposeful movement and speech are characteristic of sleep. The eyelids of a sleeping person are typically closed or slit. The observable physiological changes are decreased pulse and respiratory rates. Any one of these changes does not indicate that a person is sleeping, but if all are observed the nurse may conclude that the person is probably asleep. The validity of using these physiological changes for deciding that a person is asleep is questionable if he has cardiovascular or respiratory system disease, or if he is dependent on a respirator or a pacemaker (a pacemaker artificially stimulates the heartbeat).

SLEEP DISORDERS

Insomnia

Careful planning of the daily routine may be helpful when a patient-client expresses difficulty in going to sleep and/or remaining asleep, or shows a dependence on drugs. In the initial assessment the exact nature of the problem, its origin, duration, and characteristics, as well as the patient-client's usual daily pattern of activities, should be determined. Then if the person has a sedentary or relatively inactive life style the nurse can help him plan how to increase progressively his exercise and activity during the daytime hours. The evening hours should be occupied with relaxing, uncomplicated, and nonstressful activities. This advice is based on the knowledge that exercise during the day increases stage 4 sleep, but that if it occurs near bedtime it increases wakefulness because of physiological activation. Kales and Kales (1970) advise that the patient-client should try to establish and maintain a regular bedtime; however, he should get into bed only when sleepy and should not stay in bed if he is unable to sleep. These suggestions, in addition to drug therapy, have been found helpful in the treatment of insomnia.

Intensive-care Delirium

Observers in intensive-care situations have described a syndrome known as postcardiotomy or intensive-care delirium, in which the patient-client, after approximately three to five days in the unit, begins to suffer illusions, hallucinations, and sometimes paranoia (Abram, 1966; Heller et al., 1970). The cause of this behavior has not been established, although its pattern closely resembles that displayed by some sleep-deprived people; it commonly disappears after a full night's sleep. In addition to sleep deprivation, sensory deprivation or monotony, age, severity of preoperative illness, duration of surgery, and time spent on the heart-lung machine have all been found to be positively correlated with the appearance of this syndrome (Blachy and Starr, 1964). A collaborative preliminary nursing study found indications that postcardiotomy patients are moderately to severely sleep-deprived during the first week following surgery (Fugate, 1969; Garner, 1969; Hickman, 1969).

Other Sleep Disorders

In addition to insomnia and intensive-care delirium, there are several other sleep-related disorders, including somnambulism or sleepwalking, enuresis or bedwetting, night terrors, and narcolepsy. The incidence of these conditions is relatively low; the interested reader is referred to the literature for further information.

Summary of Common Problems Related to Insomnia, with Approaches

Problem	Approach
Lack of activity	Program of progressively increasing daytime activity
Poor sleep habits	Regular scheduling of day's activities
	Quiet evening activities
	Regular bedtime

Section B: Pain[3]

Pain is one of the most vexing and pervasive of all human problems. Acute and sudden pain may be a warning signal that something is wrong; e.g., the acute abdominal pain associated with appendicitis, or the crushing arm and chest pain which often occurs in myocardial infarction (heart attack). Pain also connotes suffering, intense emotion, sacrifice, and punishment. Indeed, the word is derived from the Greek *poine*, "penalty," and the Latin *poena*, "punishment."

The lay public sees comfort and relief of pain as one of the major functions of nurses (Lysaught, 1970). Beginning nurses usually share this view. Both client and nurse are frustrated and disillusioned when efforts at pain relief do not succeed. Sometimes these efforts fail because they are not based on a sound understanding of the nature of pain, and sometimes because nurse and client expect cessation of pain when only some relief is possible.

The purpose of this section is to present some of the physiological and psychosocial bases of the pain experience in order that practitioners may knowledgeably select measures to help people relieve their pain or, if that is not possible, to cope most easily with it.

THE PAIN EXPERIENCE

Pain can be produced in experimental conditions and in such situations can be measured in terms of threshold and intensity. Moreover, if anxiety can be introduced into the situation, physiological and psychological reactions to experienced pain closely mirror people's responses to pain in the "real" or clinical world. Experimental work with pain has increased our understanding of the neurophysiologic basis for pain and has suggested some avenues of pain management. Sternbach (1968) has written an excellent and highly readable synthesis of experimental work from several disciplines with pain. Readers wishing a more detailed analysis of experimental pain are referred to this work.

[3] This section was written by Pamela Mitchell.

Pain behavior (response to stimulus) has three main components: (1) the neurophysiological transmission of the pain stimulus; (2) the perception and interpretation of the stimulus; and (3) the reaction to the stimulus and to the interpretation of it. A person's response to any single experience with pain is influenced by all preceding experiences, and will influence any subsequent ones. Furthermore, each person's experience with pain is basically a private experience, only some manifestations of which are directly observable.

Neurophysiological Transmission

When an appropriate pain stimulus is present, the sensory nervous system responds in a predictable manner: the stimulus excites sensory neural fibers, which discharge and transmit electrical impulses within the sensory nervous system; the impulses are then interpreted and responded to on a continuum which ranges from "not painful" to "extremely painful."

Notice that even though an appropriate pain stimulus is present, it does not necessarily follow that the neural response to this stimulus will be interpreted by a person as painful. These differences in response to pain stimuli will be discussed later in the chapter.

In order to examine the neurophysiological responses involved in pain, we might look at each component: stimulus, receptor, and peripheral and central pathway.

Stimulus Early investigators of the pain phenomenon felt that the only adequate stimulus for pain is a noxious (harmful) one which causes actual damage to nerve endings. This stimulus, by virtue of altering cellular protein, depolarizes the nerve cell and initiates an action potential along a sensory fiber (Hardy, 1956).

Though there is no doubt that stimuli which produce actual tissue damage do initiate pain behavior, pain also occurs in the absence of apparent physical stimulation, and in some cir-

cumstances, tissue damage can occur without subsequent pain response or perception of pain. There appears to be a neurophysiological basis for these apparent contradictions which can be described if we accept the rather general (and unfortunately circular) notion that an adequate stimulus for pain is a change in physical energy which leads to a pain response (Sternbach, 1968, p. 28). Most of these energy changes involve tissue damage or potential tissue damage by chemical (acid, metabolites), mechanical (cutting, stretching, tearing), thermal (heat, cold), or electrical means. Some body tissues seem to be more sensitive to one kind of energy change. For example, cutting of viscera and hollow organs does not produce a pain response, but stretching (e.g., from gas, an extremely full bladder) does. In the discussion of nerve pathways, we will see how alterations in sensory stimulation other than stimulation of pain fibers, as well as psychological conflict, can also serve as adequate stimuli for the pain experience.

Receptor Undifferentiated free nerve endings appear to be the "pain receptors" both for superficial (skin) stimuli and for the deeper structures and visceral organs. These nerve endings appear to be relatively specific for pain, although in some circumstances, their stimulation can cause other sensations (Sternbach, 1968). Conversely, normal stimulation of other sensory receptors (e.g, those for touch or temperature) can sometimes cause pain (Melzack and Wall, 1965).

Pathways The free nerve endings, whether from superficial or deeper structures, eventually join with two types of sensory nerve fibers— A delta and C. The A delta fibers are small, myelinated ones which presumably transmit rapidly and account for sharp, highly localized sensation. The C fibers are smaller and unmyelinated; they transmit impulses more slowly than A fibers and lead to a diffuse, dull, aching sensation. C fibers are known to mediate touch as well as pain. Sometimes pain sensation is classified as cutaneous (skin and superficial structures), deep (bone, muscle, joint), and visceral (hollow organs). Cutaneous sensation is usually characterized as sharp, bright, acute pain, often followed by an aching dull sensation, whereas deep pain and visceral pain are often experienced as poorly localized, aching, and boring. The differences in quality of "deep" and visceral pain (bone, joint, internal organs) from cutaneous sensation may be partially accounted for by a preponderance of C fibers in the deeper structures.

Those fibers which serve primarily pain sensation join with other sensory fibers from a portion of the body to form a sensory nerve; the nerve, in turn, enters the spinal cord at some dorsal root along its length. The various sensory fibers synapse onto cells in the dorsal horn, in effect split up once again, and ascend the spinal cord in various paths or tracts. Figure 19-2 depicts a simplified representation of these pathways.

Most fibers serving pain cross to the opposite side of the cord at the same level where they enter and ascend to the brain via the lateral spinothalamic tracts. Some fibers ascend directly from the point of entry in the spinal segment via spinothalamic projections other than the opposite lateral one. Some fibers from any one nerve enter the spinal cord several segments above or

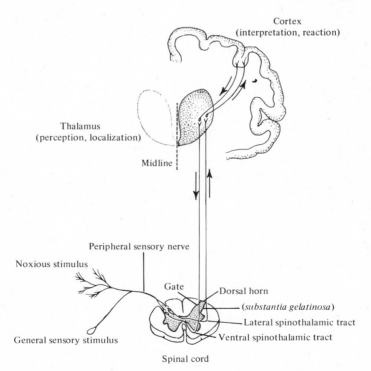

Figure 19-2 Simplified diagram of neural pathway serving pain sensation. Input from both sensory and noxious stimuli reaches the spinal cord via the peripheral sensory nerves. The gate-control theory (Melzack and Wall) proposes that this input is filtered through a gate in the dorsal horn of the spinal cord prior to transmission and perception of the input by the thalamus. From the thalamus, nerve fibers project to the cortex, where the perceived sensation is interpreted and reacted to. The arrows indicate that impulses may travel both up and down these pathways; thus the sensation of pain can be initiated either peripherally or centrally (in the cortex).

below the primary synapses. These multiple and rather confusing articulations are probably one of the reasons why neurosurgical sectioning of specific pain "tracts" often fails to give the expected relief.

Melzack and Wall (1965) propose that within any segment of the spinal cord, certain cells (the *substantia gelatinosa*) function as a "gate" to relay sensory information from all sensory modalities. This gate system essentially filters the information before it reaches the higher perceiving centers in the thalamus. In turn, descending impulses from cortical (central) activity (such as that occurring in anxiety) can influence the sensory input relayed and the central perception of whether it is pain or not.

Specifically, Melzack and Wall theorize that the substantia gelatinosa acts as a gate for sensory input before cells carrying this input synapse with the first cells which transmit impulses to the brain ("T" cells). The gate is always partially open, because of constant, low-level large-fiber activity (general sensory input). Any sudden increase in small-fiber input (specific pain fibers) opens the gate; the T cells fire and activate pain perception in the thalamus. Because the gate opens and shuts on the basis of *relative* increases or decreases in large- and small-fiber activity, an increase in large-fiber activity while pain fibers are firing would tend to close the gate and diminish pain perception. Such large-fiber activity could be generated by rubbing or firm pressure. This would appear to be the basis for the efficacy of counterirritation (hard rubbing or massage) as a measure for pain relief. Similarly, if the gate is partially open from pain firing, any decrease in other sensory input might be expected to increase the experience of pain. As an example, witness the intensified awareness that we have of aches and pains at night.

Finally, if a person has lost many large sensory fibers in a portion of his body (usually from trauma or neurological disease), he also loses the normal gate-closing effect of input over such fibers. Thus, low-level stimulation of small C fibers (which also serve touch and temperature to some degree) could summate over time, and this non-noxious stimulation would be perceived as pain.

According to the gate-control theory, central stimulation (in the brain) as well as peripheral input (outside the central nervous system) can open the gate. Any emotional or cognitive process (anxiety, fear, memory of previous pain experience, sight of a painful source) is transmitted in the brain via electrical activity; this activity can be transmitted downward from the cortex to the thalamus, and opens the gate to peripheral small-fiber input. The neurophysiological sequence by which this occurs and the evidence upon which it is based are rather detailed for presentation here. Interested readers are referred to Melzack and Wall (1965) and to Sternbach (1968, pp. 39-43) for the evidence to support this theory.

Whether one accepts the gate theory of pain or not, it is generally agreed that nerve fibers serving pain transmit impulses to the thalamus, with some projections to the reticular system. The reticular activating system functions to arouse the organism and the thalamus to perceive and localize the painful site.

However, the pain pathways are not quite complete at the thalamic level; even though pain is perceived, it must be interpreted and reacted to in order truly to be a pain experience. Interpretation occurs in the cortex; reaction is moderated via the reflex muscle and autonomic mechanisms in the spinal cord, via the autonomic circuits from the hypothalamus, and via the voluntary skeletal reactions controlled by the cortex.

Interpretation

The experience of people who have had prefrontal lobotomy graphically illustrates that the perception and interpretation-reaction of pain are separate events. Lobotomy is occasionally performed on people with intractable pain; some fibers connecting the thalamus with the frontal lobe are severed. Thereafter the person perceives pain, i.e., he says that he has pain, but shows no emotional or physiological distress over it. He no longer interprets or reacts to the sensation as an unpleasant one.

Although the physical transmission of pain stimuli is reasonably constant among people, interpretation of the meaning of these signals varies considerably. Indeed, it is the variable interpretation of sensory input which makes pain the basically private and personal experience that it is. We can see that a given event might be painful, and we can see some of the person's reaction to that situation, but the actual *experience* is that person's own and is accessible to us only as he describes it.

Interpretation of painful stimuli is a learned process. People learn that we call certain unpleasant feelings "pain" or "hurt"; they also learn which events cause this feeling, or are likely to, and how one reacts to such events. Thus, when signals generated by noxious stimuli reach the cortex of the brain, all these previous learnings are involved in deciding whether these signals do or do not represent pain, and what degree of pain they connote. This learning is influenced by past experience with pain, sociocultural learning about pain, and symbolic meanings attached to pain.

In general, a noxious (harmful) stimulus hurts. Slamming one's finger in the door, being stuck with a diaper pin, and touching a hot stove are all examples of events which hurt. With rare exceptions, every child experiences these painful circumstances from infancy onward. The hurt which occurs soon becomes associated in a child's mind with the words that his parents used at the time—"owee," "hurt," "ouch." Eventually, he learns the abstract word "pain" that encompasses a number of these experiences.

The hurt, or the "owee," is not purely a physical sensation to the child who is much past infancy. Not only does he hear the words which his parents or others ascribe to the event, but he soon perceives their reactions and emotions. Thus, the early experience with pain includes the physical sensation itself, the language others use during and after the event, and the nonverbal behavior which they exhibit.

The language used in conjunction with painful events may assign an abstraction, e.g., pain or hurt, or may describe the sensation and the stimulus event, e.g., burn, sting, pinch. In addition, adults may use words which indicate behavior expected of the child in reaction. For example, when a toddler has touched a hot radiator, the parent may say, or shout, "No—hot." Soon "no" becomes associated with a painful source, and the child may learn to avoid such objects in terms of both the painful experience and the language associated with it. Last, language may indicate value judgments about the hurt. When the baby touches the radiator, his mother may not only shout "No—hot," but also say, "Bad boy, don't touch." When the judgment is frequently coincident with hurt, a child may come to equate his own badness with his hurting and later with pain in general. In the extreme, psychiatrists feel that this association creates in some people a "need" to have pain in order unconsciously to atone for their real or imagined guilt.

The nonverbal behavior of parents and others when a child is hurt is as important in shaping his reactions to pain as is their language. Some parents comfort their children with a minimum of fuss; others "carry on" quite a bit. Children take their cues from these kinds of behavior and react much as their parents do. Similarly, children may react to playground falls as their companions of the moment do. Once a child has had some experience with painful events, he can anticipate hurt if such an event is about to occur again, e.g., when he is about to receive an immunization.

Engel (1958) feels that once one has experienced pain and begun to associate it with certain events and emotional reactions, pain can be experienced without a normally noxious stimulus present. This apparent paradox may be explained as follows:

Anxiety appears to be the primary emotion associated with pain from infancy onward (Szasz, 1957). In the infant, all unpleasant sensations (e.g., hunger, pain, startle) appear to be undifferentiated from anxiety. Eventually, anxiety begins to be separated from other unpleasant sensations and effects. However, anxiety may be associated with pain, depending upon the circumstances in which pain or hurt occurs and, as discussed above, the reaction and language of others. If painful events frequently or consistently occur in conjunction with anxious reactions in others, anxiety will become a strong component of the pain experience and can intensify it.

Similarly, other strong emotions, such as anger and guilt, or even love, may become closely associated with experiences of pain. For example, pain as a result of physical blows may accompany a parent's anger, or a child may be cuddled only after being spanked or beaten. For some people, it appears that these strong emotions may trigger pain in the absence of physically noxious stimuli (Engel, 1958; Kolb, 1962). Since these emotions are physiologically mediated via electrical activity in the cortex, Melzack and Wall's gate theory would suggest that such strong central activity descends the neurological pathway to the gate mechanisms, opens the gate, and allows summated large-fiber (general sensory) input to reach the thalamus and be perceived as pain. Various names have been applied to this type of pain, among them psychogenic pain, central pain, and the pain-prone syndrome.

Engel describes people for whom the psychic portion of the pain experience is dominant as "pain-prone." They experience pain more intensely and frequently than most, seem to suffer more pain than normal persons do when there are demonstrable peripheral lesions, and may suffer without evident noxious stimuli. He attributes this syndrome to developmental experiences in which guilt, anxiety, and gratification of needs were closely tied to pain, as discussed above.

Sociocultural Learning Whether one learns about pain in the more "normal" fashion or in such a way as to contribute to being "pain-prone," sociocultural values, attitudes, and beliefs about pain and how one responds to it are the major factors shaping one's interpretation of pain stimuli.

People who work in hospitals which have clients from several subcultures usually see that patients from different ethnic groups express their experiences quite differently. Zbrowski's classic study (1952) documents the differing expression among Italians, Jews, and Old Americans (U.S.-born, Americanized) and ties these differences to cultural mores defining pain and modes of acceptable expression. The Italian patients interviewed were more verbally expressive of pain and expected their cries to bring sympathy and immediate help. Jewish persons were also openly expressive, but more in concern about getting to the basis of the pain than in immediate symptomatic relief. Last, the Old Americans tended to be stoic, noncomplaining, and expressive only when alone. Even then the expression was apt to be nonverbal or only moaning. Sternbach and Tursky (1965, 1967) have documented physiologically different responses to electric shock among housewives from these same groups. Their findings confirmed Zbrowski's as to ethnic attitudes toward pain and expression, and added that Irish women deliberately suppressed verbal expression of suffering. In addition, they demonstrated significant correlation among pain tolerance, physiological response, and attitudes toward pain in each cultural group. Italians had a lower tolerance to electric shock, and Old Americans adapted most rapidly to it. Those groups who were most expressive of pain showed least tolerance to shock and more autonomic reaction.

If a person changes cultures (e.g., marries a person from another group, becomes a missionary, or moves into another cultural locale), he may find that his own concept of pain and modes of expression are sufficiently different that he either has to change them or be considered deviant. The Italian-American person in a hospital staffed by "Old American" personnel might be in such a position. He may be considered as complaining and a "cry-baby," even though his behavior would be unremarkable in his own group.

These findings are important to nurses and other health workers in understanding and working with culturally derived reactions to painful experiences. However, one must be careful to elicit a person's experience from the person himself, not approach him in terms of an ethnic stereotype.

Symbolic Meaning Both past experiences with pain and one's culture shape the symbols attached to pain. Symbolic meanings of pain include pain as a warning of harm, as a cry for help, as punishment, as suffering, as atonement, or as a means to virtue. In some cases, such symbolism may prompt people to seek pain, e.g., in rites of passage to prove manhood, or in such ancient religious acts as self-flagellation. In other situations, the symbolism or secondary gratifications may prolong the expression and the experience of pain. For example, people who receive solicitude or love only when hurt may experience more pain and unconsciously seek the secondary gratification attached to it. The dictionary definition of pain as punishment, and the derivation of the English word for pain reflect the symbolism of the North American Judeo-Christian-based culture.

An understanding of the symbolic aspects of pain helps one to understand some of the complex reactions which people have to painful situations and experiences, and the complex dynamics of pain which has no apparent physical source.

Reaction to the Pain Sensation

Thus far, we have discussed the first two components of the pain experience—the neurophysiological transmission of stimuli, and the perception and interpretation of the stimuli. The last component is the reaction to pain. Reaction encompasses autonomic and skeletal-muscle reaction, and cortical or psychic activity.

Autonomic Reaction At the reflex level, both autonomic responses and voluntary muscle reaction are activated. When the pain impulse reaches the spinal cord at any level, a reflex arc is initiated. One component signals the sympathetic nervous system to a "fight-flight" response mediated by norepinephrine (Sternbach, 1968, p. 58). The norepinephrine response is characterized by decreased heart rate and cardiac output. Severe pain can produce shock, by decreasing cardiac output sufficiently to depress capillary circulation. Most clinical pain experiences are characterized by varying degrees of anxiety and other general stressors which activate a more general fight-flight response mediated by epinephrine (Adrenalin). Increased heart rate, increased blood pressure, increased oxygen consumption, decreased gastric motility, and peripheral vasoconstriction are characteristic responses to general stress. Activation of both these sympathetic mediators may account for the widely varying pulse and blood pressure response seen in clinical pain.

Skeletal-muscle Reaction Another efferent of the reflex arc stimulates skeletal-muscle activity—one withdraws from external pain sources.

Visceral and deep pain stimulates reflex tightening of muscles over the affected areas. Such tightening, referred to as "guarding," seems to be a protective reflex. However, it may increase the sensation of pain. Labor pain is one such example; tightening of abdominal muscles during a uterine contraction can create the sensation of pain or intensify the sensation which the woman feels.

In addition to reflex muscle activity, there is a great deal of voluntary muscle response. For example, a person may pace the floor, clench his fists, grimace, or toss about restlessly.

Cognitive and Emotional Reaction   The most complex reactions to a pain sensation are those which depend upon our perceptions, thoughts, and feelings about the pain and the painful stimulus. One responds by reflex to a noxious stimulus, with some autonomic and skeletal activity. However, these responses can be augmented or reduced by one's cognitions (thoughts) and feelings.

Zimbardo and others (1966) demonstrated the effect of cognition on pain experience in an ingenious way. Subjects in one group were given a choice as to whether to continue with a series of painful electrical shocks but were given no rationalization for continuing. Members of another group had a choice but were given reasons to continue (e.g., for the benefit of science). Other groups were given no choice. The group with a choice but no reason felt subjectively less pain on the second trial, although the shock was of the same level as in the first. In addition, they had a significantly reduced physiologic response to the second shock. Their responses were quite similar to those of a group who had no choice but whose second shock was of a greatly reduced level. The group with a rationalized choice did not experience less pain on the second trial. This finding might be explained in the following way: in general, people will avoid painful situations; therefore, when a person voluntarily commits himself to a painful experience, his action is not consonant with this pain-avoidance value. According to Festinger's (1957) theory of cognitive dissonance, a person will tend to behave in ways which reduce such dissonance between action and value. In the above experiment a conscious or unconscious reevaluation of the painfulness of the experience is about the only way to reduce this inconsistency. The change in the subjects' response to the second shock cannot be explained as an adaptation to the shock, for other groups which received the same second stimulus intensity did not reduce their subjective and physiological response to it. The attendant physiological response suggests that this redefining was highly effective and probably largely unconscious.

Attention to the pain experience is another aspect of cognition which influences reaction. Nearly everyone has had experiences in which pain disappeared or was unnoticed while he was concentrating on other matters. Kanfer and Goldfoot (1966) used cold to test pain tolerance in several conditions. One group was told only to expect severe pain, another to describe their experience continually, another to set goals by a clock, and the last to view and describe slides. The group which paid the least attention to the pain was that describing slides. This group was considerably more tolerant of the pain than any other group. The next most tolerant group comprised the clock watchers, followed by those expecting pain and the control group (who were given no instructions). The group describing their experience and thus most attentive to it tolerated the pain the shortest period of time.

Anxiety   Anxiety is probably the most significant emotion which occurs in reaction to pain. As discussed earlier, anxiety and pain are initially undifferentiated in the infant. Many aspects of a painful situation create anxiety in later life, such as fear of loss of a hurt body part, fear of loss of affection if the pain is in conjunction with a forbidden activity, and fear of the unknown. In severe and sudden pain one wonders what it means: "Does it mean that I have cancer?" "Does it mean that I will need surgery?" In long-term pain one wonders if it will ever end, or if it will get worse. In intermittent pain, such as labor pain, one wonders if it will get worse, how much worse, and when it will come again. Encompassing all these concerns is a common "Old American" fear that one will not bear up well, will behave disgracefully.

Anxiety, as we have seen before, can precipitate pain and can increase the sensation by increasing and augmenting stimuli to the gate systems. The physiological response to anxiety can produce increasing skeletal-muscle tension, which can increase stimuli over large sensory fibers and thus increase pain when cortical impulses generated by anxiety open the gate. Thus anxiety creates a vicious cycle; pain leads to anxiety which leads to more pain and more anxiety.

MANAGEMENT OF PAIN

How, then, do we help a person who is in pain? How does one choose from the variety of physical, pharmacological, and psychological measures used to relieve pain? Just how much responsibility can a nurse take in choosing means to relieve pain? These are all legitimate questions asked by both beginning and experienced practitioners.

Basic Intervention

Sternbach's model of pain modification is extremely helpful in looking at ways to help people in pain. He reviewed what is known about pain and attempted to integrate all the languages used to describe the experience. Neurologists, psychologists, and psychiatrists all use different ways to describe different aspects of the pain experience. Sternbach concludes that there are two basic ways to modify the physiological and psychological response to a pain stimulus, namely, to (1) alter the sensory input, and (2) alter the degree of anxiety.

Alteration of Sensory Input   The most basic alteration of sensory input is to remove the

noxious stimulus conducted over the pain pathways. There are, however, many vexing circumstances in which the stimulus cannot be removed, as in pain after surgery, or long-term pain associated with malignancy or structural defects. In any of these situations, the experience is such that the person so affected wants help. In some of these situations alteration of general (non-noxious) sensory input can help relieve or decrease the pain experience.

General sensory input includes touch, temperature, sight, hearing, and other modalities. Increasing overall sensory input decreases the pain response; decreasing the input increases the response.

The Kanfer and Goldfoot study cited earlier is an example of increase in cognitive input which decreased the pain response in those whose attention was directed at describing slides. A firm back rub helps many women in labor, by stimulating large sensory fibers for pressure. Blitz and Lowenthal (1966) noted that chronic pain often occurs in people in monotonous, sensorily impoverished environments. They postulate that the decreased sensory input contributes to increased attention to mild pain, increased anxiety, and thus increased pain perception. Some studies of experimental sensory deprivation support the hypothesis that sensory deprivation, particularly visual deprivation, decreases the pain threshold[4] (Vernon and McGill, 1961; Zubek, 1969).

Many of the pharmacologic agents used to modify pain act to alter noxious stimulation. Aspirin apparently alters perception of pain at the thalamus and may act on peripheral fibers as well (Lasagna and Werner, 1966; Goodman and Gilman, 1970). General anesthetics block transmission of input to the cortex, brainstem, and spinal cord; topical anesthetics block transmission of impulses from the periphery.

Behavior modification is another approach to altering sensory input. These techniques are

---

[4] Pain threshold is the point at which pain is first felt; it is not necessarily correlated with pain tolerance.

intended to alter the learned aspects of pain. Recall from the earlier discussion that much of what one interprets as painful and one's modes of reaction to pain are learned phenomena. When a person has pain over a long period of time, others change their responses to that person in terms of his pain, and this pain may become the major focus of interaction. Such a focus may serve to intensify the experience, or may serve to prolong it if the attendant attention is absent except in conjunction with pain.

Fordyce and others (1968) postulate that for some people, particularly some who are "pain-prone," the learned aspects of pain response become dominant over all other responses. They reason that if the reinforcing attention to the pain behavior is withdrawn and given to behavior that is incompatible with pain behavior, the incapacitating behavior will diminish. This is not to say that the person will no longer experience pain, but he will no longer behave as if it is immobilizing him. For example, a person who feels he cannot venture more than a few feet from his chair or bed because of back pain may be ignored whenever he mentions the pain. However, when he does some activity incompatible with his pain behavior, such as attempting to walk a certain distance, or move about unaided, he is given privileges, praise, or whatever has been determined to be a positive reinforcement. Fordyce and his group have had rather remarkable success with this behavior-modification ap-

proach in many people with pain which has been intractable and out of proportion to physical lesions. The principles and methods of such behavior modification are beyond the scope of this book, and should not be undertaken piecemeal by any practitioner. In an appropriate setting, where both the client and trained personnel fully understand the goals of the program, it can be a useful technique.

Alteration of Anxiety The second aspect of pain management is to modify the anxiety generated by the pain. Anxiety and fear are normal reactions to pain; such reactions prepare us, for example, to flee from a fire, to get away from a biting dog, or to fight an attacker. However, a great many painful experiences cannot be fled or fought. Sustained or excessive anxiety in these situations can increase the response to pain and decrease tolerance for it.

There are any number of ways in which nurses and other health workers can help modify the anxiety accompanying pain. The majority of nursing studies reported in the literature use interpersonal approaches which are designed to reduce anxiety, in conjunction with various physical comfort measures. Some of these measures are outlined in Table 19-1.

The goal in modifying anxiety in short-term pain is not to do away with anxiety entirely, for it is a useful part of the reaction. However, one does attempt to reduce anxiety to tolerable

Table 19-1   Summary of some Nursing Measures in the Management of Pain*

Independent measures	Delegated medical therapy
1 Provide physical comfort, e.g., massage, relaxation techniques, repositioning 2 Alter general sensory environment 3 Modify anxiety	1 Pharmacologic agents 2 Placebos 3 Physical measures such as counterirritants, heat, cold, rectal tubes (agency policies determine which measures require physician's order)

*Examples of actions are listed by their category of effect. This table simply represents a summary of actions available; by no means should a nurse attempt to use all the actions in any one category. In many instances actions will be selected from all categories. McCaffery (1972) is suggested as an excellent resource in selecting measures for pain relief.

Mode of action	Examples of action

Modify noxious sensory input	**1** Remove noxious stimulus
	  a Remove splinter
	  b Remove distending gas via rectal tube
	  c Increase circulation; remove constricting bandages, etc.
	  d Cover open nerve endings in burn or open wound
	  e Use bed cradle to keep covers off limbs easily stimulated by touch
	2 Use pharmacologic agents such as aspirin, local anesthetics, narcotics

Modify general sensory input	**1** Stimulate large sensory fibers
	  a Massage
	  b Apply vibration to painful part
	  c Rub with washcloth
	  d Apply ice on burn
	  e Reposition—large-muscle movement
	2 Increase cognitive stimuli
	  a Concentrate on other stimuli, as in "natural" childbirth
	  b Increase social, visual contacts in low-level, long-term pain
	3 Alter responses to pain
	  a Reinforce nonpain behavior
	  b Ignore pain-related verbalizations (these measures should not be used independently of coordinated modification program)
	4 Decrease environmental stimuli: decrease noise and glare in acute pain

Modify anxiety	**1** Decrease the area of the unknown
	  a Provide information
	  b Clarify meaning of experience with patient
	  c Decrease uncertainty about duration, next onset
	  d Discuss pain experience
	    (1) Cue that pain is ending or will end
	    (2) Help patient assimilate experience to decrease anxiety about future similar pain
	2 Discharge anxiety
	  a Listen
	  b Provide for physical activity
	3 Channel energy
	  a Prepare patient for pain whenever possible
	  b Teach patient how to handle pain; relaxation
	  c Indicate help and support available
	  d Help patient exert control in situation
	  e Encourage efforts at control, verbally and nonverbally
	4 Decrease isolation: remain with patient; provide someone to remain with him
	5 Control panic: verbally or physically break into panic behavior until person regains control
	6 Use pharmacologic agents: narcotics, tranquilizers, placebos
	7 Exert "nurse placebo effect" (attitude of confidence in agent or action used)

levels. In long-term pain, anxiety only serves to increase the response; therefore one attempts to decrease it as much as possible.

Health workers can act either to increase or to decrease anxiety. Actions which increase anxiety are often nondeliberate and may include minimizing a client's complaint of pain, expecting that he will bear his pain with minimum complaint, and leaving him alone to wonder what is happening to him. These actions tend to increase the uncertainty about the nature of the pain or the adequacy of one's ability to cope. Actions which help decrease anxiety include decreasing the area of the unknown, discussing fears, channeling anxiety constructively, utilizing the anxiety-decreasing effect of medication, and utilizing the "placebo effect" of the nurse's attitude.

Decreasing the Unknown A major source of anxiety is fear of the unknown: "How long will this last, what does it mean, who will help me?" Therefore, communication which is intended to decrease the area of the unknown can help decrease anxiety and focus it upon specific concerns.

Discussing Fears McCaffery and Moss (1967) point out the importance of discussing pain experiences in order to help the person to (1) mobilize coping abilities, (2) alter his attitudes and anxieties about the source, (3) note cues that the pain is lessening or ending, and (4) assimilate the experience into his learning about coping with pain.

When pain can be anticipated, the physician or nurse can provide information as to what might be expected, the source of the pain, and ways to cope with it. This approach not only decreases the area of the unknown, but helps the person channel the anxiety which he does experience into constructive actions.

When a person is in pain, particularly if it is severe and he is very anxious, a great deal of information will not be perceived by him and the talking may make him more anxious. In such situations, physical presence, touch, and reassurance that someone will be with him and will help him are more appropriate and may decrease his sense of isolation.

Channeling Anxiety A second way either to decrease anxiety or to prevent excessive anxiety is to channel constructively the anxiety that is present—to prepare the client prior to the pain in ways to cope with it, to listen to his expression of fear and anxiety in order to help him discharge it, and to help him exert control in the situation.

Utilizing Anxiety-reducing Effect of Medication Many pharmacologic agents work to decrease anxiety; e.g., narcotics act at least partially upon cortical response, as do tranquilizers. Placebos, i.e., agents which have no actual pharmacological effect but which reduce pain in many people, probably "act" upon the anxiety component of the pain response. When one expects that a pill or injection will bring relief, anxiety lessens and thereby lessens the pain response.

The *placebo effect,* i.e., the druglike effect of inert agents, has generated much study. A number of personality characteristics, such as dependency and low ego strength, have been associated with response to placebos (Walike and Meyer, 1966). However, there appears to be no consistency in such characteristics from study to study, or even in one person from one time to another (Sternbach, 1968). People seem to react to placebos more when under stress, which suggests that reduction of anxiety is a major factor in the responses.

Utilizing "Placebo Effect" of Nurse's Attitude The mental set that a drug will act in a certain way seems to have a great deal to do with the placebo response to any "drug." Therefore, a few investigators have attempted to study the placebo effect of nurses' communication with patients about pain-relieving action.

Billars (1970) used a physical measure, position change, in response to the postoperative pain of 30 patients. No medication was given. In one group, she repositioned the person and said, "I think this will help relieve your pain. . . ." In another group she made the same statement and added that she would return in ten minutes and do something else if the measure did not help. The third group was simply repositioned with no statement of expectation of relief. Only one patient in the group to whom she made no statement of relief actually felt less pain, whereas the majority of persons in the other two groups did feel relief. The investigator expected that those patients to whom she promised to return in ten minutes would have the most relief. However, only 7 out of 10 from that group felt less pain, as opposed to 9 of 10 in the first group. Billars hypothesizes that her statement concerning returning may have led the patients to think the repositioning probably would not work. The differences in subjective assessment of pain reduction among the groups suggests that the nurse's positive attitude about her intervention made the difference.

The following studies were not designed to test the placebo effect of the nurse's statements per se. It seems possible, however, that the nurse's way of discussing the experience with the patient had a general placebo or anxiety-reducing effect. Moss and Meyer (1966) studied the effect of participation by the patient in the choice of action on the relief of pain. The measures were all in the area of repositioning and general comfort; no medications were offered or given. Those patients who participated in choosing the relief measure had significantly less pain than those for whom the nurse chose the action. McBride (1967) and Bochnak (1963) studied the effect of exploring the meaning of a person's pain with him after giving medication. They found that those patients who were allowed to discuss their experience had greater relief from pain than those who were simply given medication.

In another study, when a medication (Darvon—propoxyphene hydrochloride) was administered, the nurse's statements made no significant difference in the reduction-of-pain score, computed from both objective and subjective data (Chambers and Price, 1967). These studies are not comparable, in that different responses to pain were measured (subjective assessment of relief in Billars's study; subjectively and objectively derived scores in the Chambers and Price study). Nor were the groups of patients the same. These contrasts simply suggest that the effect of the nurse's statement may be greatest on the patient's subjective assessment of his experience, or may be greatest when medication is not used. Considerably more work needs to be done in studying the placebo effect of nursing approach.

Assessing the Pain Experience

Although measures of intervention may be classified under two basic modes—alteration of sensory input and alteration of anxiety—the specific actions within each mode are not all equally applicable in any given situation. In order to help a particular patient-client, the nurse must gather as much data as possible about the pain which the person is experiencing, the pathological process possibly operating, and the ways in which the client has attempted to deal with the pain. Using these data, the nurse will be able to select specific approaches which have the greatest probability of success within the scope of nursing practice.

Not all approaches to pain management are directly usable by the nurse; some require a physician's prescription. For example, in most agencies, pharmacologic agents (drugs) and some physical measures (such as heat) must be prescribed by a physician before nurses may administer them. Other measures, such as back rubs, position change, or means to decrease anxiety, are used solely at the nurse's discretion.

The physician is primarily concerned with discovering and removing the cause of pain or, if that is not possible, with finding ways to relieve it. In practice, most physicians concentrate on prescribing drugs or performing surgery aimed at such ends. The nurse is primarily concerned with helping a person find a means to relieve pain and to cope with pain while he experiences it. Thus, a nurse may use prescribed medical therapy, such as narcotics and heat, and may prescribe additional measures such as position change or diversion. Conversely, the nurse may decide that nursing measures alone will be effective. Many medical prescriptions for drugs, to be used both in hospital and at home, prescribe a medication "for pain, PRN," meaning "as needed for pain." Thus the nurse (or the patient if he is at home) must determine when to give medication, when to use other measures, when to use both. Such decisions are made with the help of the same problem-solving process (data collection, analysis, testing of action, and evaluation) described in Part 2. Both nurse and client may use this process to determine what measures might help and actually do help. The following discussion of the data needed to help persons in pain is directed toward the nurse, but it is equally applicable in assisting a client to analyze his pain experience in order to determine when to use medication and when other measures may be equally as effective.

Descriptive Data   In many circumstances the client asks the nurse for help; e.g., he asks for pain medication, or he says, "I hurt." One needs considerably more information about his sensation before providing any help. Such information includes the location of the pain (where), the frequency (when), the duration (how long), his subjective assessment of the intensity (how much), what precipitates the pain, what he does about it, what helps, what does not help, and

what he thinks the pain means. The descriptive data provide one with the person's own perception of the situation and the meanings which he attaches to it. They also provide some clues as to potential help.

Objective Data   At the same time, the nurse can be observing the person's reaction to the pain experience. Skeletal muscle reaction may be noted in such activity as clenching fists, gritting teeth, grimacing, rigid posture, and reflex withdrawal of muscles when the painful area is touched or approached. The absence of such reaction should also be noted. Autonomic reactions may be observed by measuring pulse, blood pressure, and respirations, and by noting presence or absence of perspiration, as well as the state of the pupillary reaction (increased sympathetic activity can lead to dilation of pupils). Finally, verbal reactions and nonverbal behavior may give some clues to the presence or absence of anxiety regarding his experience. Such behavior may range from a relatively calm, matter-of-fact description of a hurt, to complete absorption in the pain experience.

Knowledge of Possible Pain Sources   The last part of the needed data is a knowledge of the pathologic process possibly operating to cause the pain. For example, when muscles have been cut in abdominal surgery, one expects that the person will have some pain afterward; when skin has been burned one also expects pain. However, if the burn is third-degree (i.e., has gone through all the subcutaneous tissue), the nerve endings have been destroyed and one expects pain in those areas to be much less. Consequently, knowledge of the common sources of pain helps the nurse to anticipate which illness situations may be painful to a client. However, absence of a known physical source for pain does not mean that a client "shouldn't" be having his pain. As discussed earlier, anxiety can cause lesser stimuli to be interpreted as pain.

Knowledge regarding pain associated with

various disease processes and treatments can be gained through the literature and through experience in caring for persons in a variety of clinical situations.

Inferences Regarding the Experience Once the nurse has gathered as much data as possible, he makes a judgment about that data; he forms an impression or inference regarding the nature of the patient-client's pain experience and the nature of his reaction. For example, one might ask: Is his reaction primarily physiological? Does there seem to be a large anxiety component? Does it appear out of proportion to a known stimulus? One must be careful at this point to make the inference regarding *what the person is experiencing,* not *how much pain he is having.* Only the person himself, on the basis of his own scale, can quantify how much pain he has. Observers can only attempt to infer the quantity or quality of this private experience. Davitz et al. (1970) found marked differences in the inferences of physical pain and suffering among nurses and persons of lay occupational groups when they were given the same vignettes to rate. The investigators hypothesize that the nurses, by virtue of their constant exposure to pain and suffering, tended to become less sensitive to situations which lay persons considered to be of greater potential distress. It also seems possible that the lay occupational groups looked at the vignettes in terms of what they would feel like if they were in that situation, whereas the nurses may have looked at them in terms of how much pain they thought a person *should have* in this situation.

One does indeed need to know what kind of experience "most people" have in any given situation, e.g., after an appendectomy. If a particular patient-client seems to be experiencing a more severe or more prolonged pain than expected, one begins to search for additional causes for the pain (e.g., an abdominal abscess, signs of peritonitis) or for increased levels of anxiety which may contribute to the reaction.

This is an extremely important step, for if one dismisses the reaction which seems to be out of proportion to what is expected, the patient may either (1) develop a physical complication which is discounted as "crockish," or (2) become increasingly more anxious because no one believes that he is experiencing anything. Since there are so many approaches to reducing sensory input and anxiety, and these are often quite different, one needs to make an accurate inference of the relative strength of the client's reaction in order to choose effective interventions.

Intervening to Relieve Pain

Once a reasonable inference has been made, one begins to propose interventions and test them. Table 19-1 shows several possible actions. In some relatively uncomplicated experiences, simply reducing the input to the nerve endings may be sufficient; with a headache, aspirin may sufficiently relieve pain. Other situations, e.g., a woman in labor, may be more complicated and call both for altering sensory input and for relieving anxiety. For example, a back rub may stimulate large nerve fibers and thus block input from pain fibers; concentration on breathing technique may prevent the person from concentrating on the discomfort; and the presence of a concerned nurse may decrease the woman's fears about being left alone. McCaffery (1972) describes in detail a number of types of nursing intervention, and the reader is referred to her book for more depth in this area.

As the Moss and Meyer (1966) study suggests, collaboration with the patient in choosing the method of relief and in trying it seems to result in greater relief than if the nurse simply acts on his own. This and other nursing studies suggest that in some instances comfort measures alone may be just as effective as medication (Moss and Meyer; Billars, 1970).

Just as the intervention should be planned with the patient-client, the evaluation of its effect cannot be complete without his subjective evaluation. The nurse can observe for any changes in the physiological and skeletal muscle reactions which were noticed during the initial assessment, and for any evidence of a decrease in anxiety. In addition, he must check the patient's perception of relief. No matter what changes there are in physical parameters, if the client does not feel relieved, he is not relieved. Such a situation would suggest that the anxiety factor in the pain experience may be high for that client, and the beginning practitioner may need help from a more experienced nurse in helping such a person.

Many people who are in pain are afraid that they will not be believed, that nurses and physicians will think they are "putting it on." Discussing the experience with the patient-client, consulting with him in planning help and asking his perception of the help received all help a person to know that the professional *is* interested in his impressions of his own pain. People for whom no organic cause of pain can be found are particularly sensitive to anyone's implied judgment that the pain is unreal. One need not dwell on elaborate descriptions of the pain to let such a person know that the nurse appreciates that he (the patient) does have pain, and that the nurse will work with the other health professionals to try and alleviate that experience.

REFERENCES

Books

Comfort and Rest

Berger, Ralph J., The Sleep and Dream Cycle, in A. Kales (ed.), "Sleep Physiology and Pathology," J. B. Lippincott Company, Philadelphia, 1969, pp. 17–32.

———, Physiological Characteristics of Sleep, in A. Kales (ed.), "Sleep Physiology and Pathology," J. B. Lippincott Company, Philadelphia, 1969, pp. 66–79.

Feinberg, Irwin, Effects of Age on Human Sleep Patterns, in A. Kales (ed.), "Sleep Physiology and Pathology," J. B. Lippincott Company, Philadelphia, 1969, pp. 39–52.

Fugate, Nancy, Types of Interruptions of Sleep and Amount of Sleep and Rest Obtained by Selected Post-cardiotomy Patients during the First Eight Post-operative 11:00 PM to 7:00 AM Periods, Unpublished Master's Thesis, University of Washington, Seattle, 1969.

Garner, Susanna, A Study of Sleep Deprivation and Nursing Activities Which Affect Sleep in Post-cardiotomy Patients, Unpublished Master's Thesis, University of Washington, Seattle, 1969.

Hickman, Barbara, Frequency of Interruptions and Amount of Sleep Attained or Potentially Available for Four Open-heart Surgery Patients on the First Eight Post-operative Days, Unpublished Master's Thesis, University of Washington, Seattle, 1969.

Johnson, Laverne C., Psychological and Physiological Changes Following Total Sleep Deprivation, in A. Kales (ed.), "Sleep Physiology and Pathology," J. B. Lippincott Company, Philadelphia, 1969, pp. 206–220.

Kleitman, Nathaniel, Basic Rest-Activity Cycle in Relation to Sleep and Wakefulness, in A. Kales (ed.), "Sleep Physiology and Pathology," J. B. Lippincott Company, Philadelphia, 1969, pp. 33–38.

———, "Sleep and Wakefulness," The University of Chicago Press, Chicago, 1963.

Webb, Wilse, "Sleep: An Experimental Approach," The Macmillan Company, New York, 1968.

———, Twenty-four Hour Sleep Cycling, in A. Kales (ed.), "Sleep Physiology and Pathology," J. B. Lippincott Company, Philadelphia, 1969, pp. 53–65.

Pain

Festinger, Leon, "A Theory of Cognitive Dissonance," Stanford University Press, Palo Alto, Calif., 1957.

Goodman, Louis, and Alfred Gilman (eds.), "The Pharmacologic Basis of Therapeutics," 4th ed., The Macmillan Company, New York, 1970, p. 316.

Lysaught, Jerome, "An Abstract for Action: Report of the National Commission for the Study of Nursing and Nursing Education," McGraw-Hill Book Company, 1970, p. 58.

McCaffery, Margo, "Nursing Management of the Patient with Pain," J. B. Lippincott Company, Philadelphia, 1972.

Sternbach, Richard, "Pain: A Psychophysiological Analysis," Academic Press, Inc., New York, 1968.

Szasz, Thomas, "Pain and Pleasure," Basic Books, Inc., Publishers, New York, 1957.

Zubek, John, "Sensory Deprivation: Fifteen Years of Research," Appleton-Century-Crofts, New York, 1969, p. 252.

Periodicals

Comfort and Rest

Abram, Harry S.: Psychological Problems of Patients after Open-heart Surgery, *Hospital Topics,* **44**:111-113 (1966).

Baekeland, Frederick: Effects of the Day's Events on Sleep, *International Psychiatry Clinics,* **7**:49-58 (1970).

———, and Ernest Hartmann: Sleep Requirements and the Characteristics of Some Sleepers, *International Psychiatry Clinics,* **7**:33-43 (1970).

Blachy, Paul H., and Albert Starr: Post-cardiotomy Delirium, *The American Journal of Psychiatry,* **121**:371-375 (1964).

Dement, William: The Effect of Dream Deprivation, *Science,* **131**:1705-1707 (1960).

———, et al.: Studies on the Effect of REM Deprivation in Humans and Animals, in S. S. Kety, E. V. Evarts, and H. L. Williams (eds.), "Sleep and Altered States of Consciousness," Research Publication, Association for Research in Nervous and Mental Disease, The Williams & Wilkins Company, Baltimore, 1967, vol. 45, pp. 456-486.

Globus, Gordon G.: A Syndrome Associated with Sleeping Late, *Psychosomatic Medicine,* **31**:528-535 (1969).

Greenberg, Ramon: Dreaming and Memory, *International Psychiatry Clinics,* **7**:258-265 (1970).

Hartmann, Ernest: What Sleep Is Good Sleep? *International Psychiatry Clinics,* **7**:59-69 (1970).

Heller, Stanley S., et al.: Psychiatric Complications of Open-heart Surgery, *The New England Journal of Medicine,* **283**:1015-1020 (1970).

Johnson, Laverne C., J. Alan Burdick, and James Smith: Sleep during Alcoholic Intake and Withdrawal in the Chronic Alcoholic, *Archives of General Psychiatry,* **22**:406-418 (1970).

Kales, Anthony, and Joyce Kales: Evaluation, Diagnosis and Treatment of Clinical Conditions Related to Sleep, *Journal of the American Medical Association,* **213**:2229-2235 (1970).

Snyder, Frederick: Autonomic Nervous System Manifestations during Sleep and Dreaming, in S. S. Kety, E. V. Evarts, and H. L. Williams (eds.), "Sleep and Altered States of Consciousness," Research Publication, Association for Research in Nervous and Mental Disease, The Williams & Wilkins Company, Baltimore, 1967, vol. 45, pp. 469-487.

Webb, Wilse: Individual Differences in Sleep Length, *International Psychiatry Clinics,* **7**:44-47 (1970).

———, Harman W. Agnew, and Hyman Sternthal: Sleep during the Early Morning, *Psychonomic Science,* **6**:277-278 (1966).

Williams, Robert L., Harmon W. Agnew, and Wilse W. Webb: Sleep Patterns in Young Adults: An EEG Study, *Electroencephalography and Clinical Neurophysiology,* **17**:376-381 (1964).

Zung, William W. K.: The Pharmacology of Disordered Sleep: A Laboratory Approach, *International Psychiatry Clinics,* **7**:123-146 (1970).

Pain

Billars, Karen: You Have Pain? I Think This Will Help, *American Journal of Nursing,* **70**:2143-2145 (1970).

Blitz, B., and M. Lowenthal: The Role of Sensory Restriction in Problems with Chronic Pain, *Journal of Chronic Disease,* **19**:1119-1125 (1966).

Bochnak, Mary: The Effects of an Automatic and Deliberative Process of Nursing Activity on the Relief of Patients Pain: A Clinical Experiment, Unpublished Master's Thesis, Yale University School of Nursing, New Haven, Conn. Abstracted in *Nursing Research,* **12**:191 (Abstract 77) (1963).

Chambers, Wilda, and Geraldine Price: Influence of Nurse upon Effects of Analgesics Administered, *Nursing Research,* **16**:228-233 (1967).

Davitz, Lois (ed.): Inferences of Physical Pain and Psychological Distress, *Nursing Research,* **19**:338-401 (1970).

Engel, George: Psychogenic Pain, *Medical Clinics of North America,* **42**:1481-1496 (1958).

Fordyce, Wilbert, Roy Fowler, Justus Lehman, and Barbara DeLateur: Some Implications of Learning in Problems of Chronic Pain, *Journal of Chronic Disease,* **21**:179-190 (1968).

Hardy, James: The Nature of Pain, *Journal of Chronic Diseases,* **4**:1-110 (1956).

Kanfer, Frederick, and David Goldfoot: Self-control and Tolerance of Noxious Stimulation, *Psychological Reports,* **18**:79–85 (1966).

Kolb, Lawrence: Symbolic Significance of the Complaint of Pain, *Clinical Neurosurgery,* **8**:248 (1962).

Lasagna, Louis, and Gerhard Werner: Conjoint Clinic on Pain and Analgesia, *Journal of Chronic Disease,* **19**:695–709 (1966).

McBride, Mary A.: Nursing Approach, Pain, and Relief: An Exploratory Experiment, *Nursing Research,* **16**:337–341 (1967).

McCaffery, Margo, and Fay Moss: Nursing Intervention for Bodily Pain, *American Journal of Nursing,* **67**:1224–1227 (1967).

Melzack, Ronald, and Patrick Wall: Pain Mechanisms: A New Theory, *Science,* **150**:971–979 (Nov. 19, 1965).

Moss, Fay, and Burton Meyer: The Effects of Nursing Interaction upon Pain Relief in Patients, *Nursing Research,* **15**:303–306 (1966).

Sternbach, Richard, and B. Tursky: Ethnic Differences among Housewives in Psychophysiological and Skin Potential Responses to Electric Shock, *Psychophysiology,* **1**:241–246 (1965).

Tursky, B., and R. Sternbach: Further Physiological Correlates of Ethnic Differences in Response to Shock, *Psychophysiology,* **4**:67–74 (1967).

Vernon, J., and T. E. McGill: Sensory Deprivation and Pain Thresholds, *Science,* **133**:330–331 (1961).

Walike, Barbara, and Burton Meyer: Relation between Placebo Reactivity and Selected Personality Factors, *Nursing Research,* **15**:119–123 (1966).

Zbrowski, Mark: Cultural Components in Responses to Pain, *Journal of Social Issues,* **8**:16–30 (1952); also in E. G. Jaco (ed.), "Patients, Physicians, and Illness," The Free Press, Glencoe, Ill., 1958.

Zimbardo, P. G., et al.: Control of Pain Motivation by Cognitive Dissonance, *Science,* **151**:217–219 (Jan. 14, 1966).

ADDITIONAL READINGS

Comfort and Rest

Fass, Grace: Sleep, Drugs, and Dreams, *American Journal of Nursing,* **71**:2316–2320 (1971).

Kales, Anthony (ed.), "Sleep Physiology and Pathology," J. B. Lippincott Company, Philadelphia, 1969.

Kety, Seymour S., Edward V. Evarts, and Harold L. Williams (eds.), "Sleep and Altered States of Consciousness," Research Publication, Association for Research in Nervous and Mental Disease, The Williams & Wilkins Company, Baltimore, 1967, vol. 45.

Kleitman, Nathaniel, "Sleep and Wakefulness," The University of Chicago Press, Chicago, 1963.

Long, Barbara: Sleep, *American Journal of Nursing,* **69**:1896–1899 (1969).

Webb, Wilse, "Sleep: An Experimental Approach," The Macmillan Company, New York, 1968.

Williams, Donald H.: Sleep and Disease, *American Journal of Nursing,* **71**:2321–2324 (1971).

Pain

Beecher, Henry: The Powerful Placebo, *Journal of the American Medical Association,* **159**(2):1603–1607 (Dec. 24, 1955).

Berni, Rosemary, Joan Dressler, and Janice Baxter: Reinforcing Behavior, *American Journal of Nursing,* **71**:2180–2183 (1971).

Crowley, Dorothy, "Pain and Its Alleviation," University of California, Los Angeles, 1962.

LeShan, Lawrence: The World of the Patient in Severe Pain of Long Duration, *Journal of Chronic Disease,* **17**:119–126 (1964).

Pain: Parts I and II, *American Journal of Nursing,* **66**:1085–1108; 1345–1368 (1966). (Programmed units: pain assessment and intervention.)

Index

Abilities of patient-clients, identification of, 100-101
Acceptance, 88
Accidents, 179-181
  in the aged, 179
  in children, 179-180
  as health problems, 179, 181
  prevention of, 179-183
Acid-base balance (*see* Fluid-electrolyte homeostasis)
Acidosis:
  metabolic, 340, 341
  respiratory, 340
Adaptation, 7
  to cold (*see* Cold adaptation)
  to heat (*see* Heat adaptation)
  (*See also* Behavior, adaptive, in anxiety)
Adolescent:
  nutritional needs of, 277
  psychosocial development of, 156-157
Adulthood, 157-158
Age:
  effect of: on body temperature, 396-397
    on safety, 179, 181
  relationship of: to sleep patterns, 440
    to urinary incontinence, 300
  sensory stimulation needs, 204-207
  skin characteristics, 415
Agency, social interaction patterns in, 36
Airway obstruction in respiratory distress, 382
  (*See also* Respiration)
Alcohol bath, use of, in fever, 405
Alkalosis:
  metabolic, 340-341
  respiratory, 340

American Nurses' Association:
  definition of nursing functions by, 27
  position paper on nursing education by, 30-31
Anal incontinence, 313-314
Anemia:
  iron deficiency, 276
  pallor, 375, 412
Anger as response to anxiety (fight behavior), 56, 163-165
Anion (*see* Fluid-electrolyte homeostasis)
Anorexia:
  definition of, 289
  related to immobility, 242
Anoxia (*see* Hypoxia)
Anxiety:
  behavioral manifestations of, 15, 159, 164
  causes of, 159
  definition of, 158-159
  effect of, on respiration, 387
  in hypoxia, 359, 365, 375
  levels (continuum), 160-161, 164
  mechanisms to relieve, 161-166
  pain and, 159, 450, 452-453
  in pain response, 452-456
  related to bowel status, 296
  related to hospitalization, 56, 159, 164
  related to sleep, 443
  related to transition from health to illness, 15
  in sensory-perceptual deprivation, 201, 213
  in shock, 359
Apical pulse, 323
Apnea, 371

Appetite, definition of, 282
Arrhythmia, 324-325
Asepsis, 185-186
  techniques used to achieve, 185
  (*See also* Infection, control of)
Assessment, nursing, 76-97
  (*See also* Diagnostic process in nursing)
Atelectasis, 380-381
Atrophy, muscle, 227-230
  prevention of, 230, 260-261
    related to immobility, illustrated, 228, 229
Attitudes, 116-118
  attempts to change, 117-118
  conflicts, 116
  definition of, 116
  toward health, 10-17, 117-118
Auscultation:
  apical pulse, 323
  of chest, 374
Autonomy, 155
Autonomy-authority conflict, 41
Axillary temperature, 402

Back rub (*see* Massage)
Bacteria (*see* Microorganisms)
Basal metabolic rate:
  in immobility, 223, 242
  in temperature maintenance, 394-395
Bathing, 150, 416-418
Bed rest:
  harmful aspects of, 224-244
  therapeutic aspects of, 222-223
  (*See also* Immobility)
Bed sores (*see* Pressure sores)

Behavior:
adaptive, in anxiety, 162
fight, 163–165
flight, 165–166
changes in sensory-perceptual restriction, 201–202, 234
definitions of, 141
individual and group, 35
movements of roles within, 59–60
nonverbal, 55, 86, 91, 151
and nutrition, 276–277
overt, factors in, 51–53
role, 37–38
sociocultural influences on, 42, 144
Bicarbonate:
buffer system, 338–340
carbonic acid/bicarbonate ratio, 340
Bladder, urinary, 297–304
anatomy and physiology of, 297
assessment data, 295
common problems and approaches, 316
cultural considerations in function of, 297–300
(*See also* Urinary diversion; Urinary incontinence; Urinary retention)
Blood:
chemicals, 327–328
clots (thrombi), 239–241, 353–354
gases in, 365
loss of, in shock, 358–359
role of, in respiration, 364, 365
Blood pressure, 322, 325–326
(*See also* Vital signs)
Body temperature (*see* Temperature)
Bowel function, 296–298, 304–315
absorption, 304
assessment data, 295–297
common problems, 316
in immobility, 244–246, 311
motility, 306, 311
reflex activity, illustrated, 305
Bradypnea, 371
Breath sounds, 374–375
Breathlessness, 372–373, 376–377, 386–387
Buffer systems, 338–340

Calcium balance, 335–336
in immobility, 232–233, 242–243
in nerve and muscle function, 335–336
(*See also* Osteoporosis)
California Nurses' Association, definition of nurse's functions by, 31
Carbon dioxide (*see* Respiration)
Cardiac output, 325–326
factors regulating, 325
relationship of, to blood pressure, 325–326
in shock, 358
Cardinal signs (*see* Vital signs)
Cardiogenic shock, 358
Cardiopulmonary resuscitation (CPR), 382–383
as advanced skill, 382
Care plan (*see* Intervention, nursing)
Catheterization, urinary: clinical considerations, 301

Catheterization, urinary: dangers associated with use of, 190, 302, 303
infection from, 190, 302
nursing care, 303
Cation (*see* Fluid-electrolyte homeostasis)
Central nervous system:
in consciousness, 169
in the pain experience, 445–450
in sensory perception, 197–198
in temperature maintenance, 392–394, 402–403
Change, resistance to or facilitation of, 43
Chemoreceptors, role of, in respiration, 370–371
Children:
developmental factors, 65, 155–156, 195, 204–205
hospitalized, 65–66, 207, 226
institutionalized, 204
interpersonal relationships with, 65–67
need for environmental safety, 179
Chill factor, 397
wind chill, illustrated, 398
Chills:
nursing care during, 403
in relation to fever, 403–404
Cigarette smoking, relationship of, to pulmonary disease, 378–379
Circulation:
in edema, 355–356
role of, in respiration, 364, 370
in shock, 357–358
Circulatory status, 321–326
assessment guide, 81, 320
measurement of, 322
Client (*see* Patient-client)
Cold adaptation, 398–399
Collaborative relationship as essential to successful change, 98
Colon (*see* Bowel function)
Colostomy, 164, 172, 314–315
Comfort, 437
and rest status assessment guide, 82
Communication, 38–40, 84
facilitation of, 39, 88, 90–91
models, 39
nonfacilitation of, 91–92
opening, 86
patterns of, 38
Compassion, 63–64, 88
Concept:
basis for diagnosis and intervention, 111–112, 134
definition of, 110, 133
development of, 135–138
identifying properties, 135
information storage system, 133
validation of, 136
Conceptualization:
definition of, 3, 133–134
personal aspects of, 138
in professional practice, 96
steps in development, 135
Conduction as a means of losing body heat, 395–396
Consciousness, level of: alterations in, 169, 222
assessment of, 169–170, 375

Consciousness, level of: awareness of self, 169–171
definition of, 168–169
in fluid-electrolyte imbalance, 344
nursing responsibilities, 171
response, 170
Constipation:
causes of, 244, 310–311
definition of, 311
impaction (*see* Fecal impaction)
preventive measures, 245
related to immobility, 244–246, 310
Consultation, 95–96
Contracture:
illustrated, 231
related to immobility, 230
Convalescence, 19–20
Convection as a means of losing body heat, 396
Cough, 380–381, 386
Crisis:
developmental, 154
illness and, 58–59
situational, 154
Cultural and social systems, 42–43
Culture:
changes in, 43
as factor: in defining health and illness, 4–5, 12–20
in food habits, 280–284
in planning care, 18, 35, 42
in seeking health care, 13–14, 21–22
Cyanosis in hypoxia, 375, 412

Death:
coping with, 146–147
related to value of life, 145
(*See also* Dying)
Deconditioning (*see* Disuse phenomena)
Decubitus ulcer (*see* Pressure sores, contributory factors)
Defecation, 305–307
aids useful in, 306
reflex initiation, 305–306
(*See also* Stool)
Defense mechanisms in anxiety, 161–162
Dehydration (*see* Saline depletion; Water balance)
Denial:
in anxiety, 161, 164
in disability, 265
in dying, 146
Deprivation:
perceptual (*see* Sensory-perceptual restriction)
sensory (*see* Sensory-perceptual restriction)
sleep, 442–443
Dermis, 411
Development, psychosocial: conscience, 155
crisis, 58–59, 154
developmental tasks, 153
effect of illness on, 52, 65
influence of sensory environment, 198, 204–205
support during illness, 50, 65–66

Diagnosis, 74–106
    of behavioral problems, 166–168
    definition of, 47, 69
    diagnostic process compared with
        scientific method, 69–70
    nursing, 75–76
Diagnostic process in nursing:
    assessment tool, functional
        abilities/disabilities, 77–82
    collaboration with client, 97–99, 171
    data: collection of, 74–97
        consultation, 95
        examination and observation, 93–95
        interview, 83–93
        methods, 83
        review of literature, 95–97
        organization of, 100–102
        gaps in, 101–102
    data analysis, 97–103
    inferring problems, 102–103, 166–168
    interpersonal relationships in, 49
    model of, illustrated, 75
    priority of assessment, 96–97
    statement of problem, 102–103
    validation, 91, 98, 168
Diarrhea, 312–313
    causes of, 312
    definition of, 312
    fluid loss in, 312, 333
    losses in, illustrated, 313
    nursing care considerations for, 312–313
    physiological changes with, 312, 333
Diastolic pressure, 325
Diet:
    economics, 281, 290, 292
    group reducing plans, 291
    therapeutic, 289, 291–292
Diffusion, 328–329, 365–366
Disability, adapting to, 265–266
Disinfection, 189
Displacement, 161, 164
Distention, postoperative, 381
    (See also Flatulence)
Disuse phenomena:
    circulatory, 227, 237–241
    cyclical nature, illustrated, 229
    deconditioning, 226
    diagnosis, 248
    elimination, 241, 243–246
    experimental, 225–226
    integumentary, 246–247
    metabolic, 241–243
    musculoskeletal, 227–233
    neurosensory, 233–235
    nursing responsibilities, 248–263
    nutritive, 241–242
    pathological consequences, 227
    respiratory, 235–236
Doctor (see Physician)
Dreams, 441–442
Dying:
    coping with, 146–147
    nurse's reaction to, 146
    stages of, 145
Dyspnea (see Breathlessness)

Eating, 227
    changing eating habits, 282–286

Eating:
    motivation for, 284
    patterns of, 280
Edema, 355–357
    causes of, 239, 355–356
    definition of, 238, 355
    dependent, 355
        related to immobility, 238–239
        as sign of cardiac disease, 356
    in diarrhea, 312
    nursing responsibilities, 239, 357
    pathophysiology, 333, 355–356
    problems associated with, 239, 312, 356
Electrolytes, 326–341
    abnormalities in, 336
        diarrhea, 312
        illustrated, 313
        saline depletion, 333–334
    concentration, 335–337
    osmotic force, 329–330
    pH (see Hydrogen-ion concentration)
    role in function of cells, 326–327,
        335–336
    units of measurement, 336
    volume regulation, 330–331
    (See also Fluid-electrolyte homeostasis)
Elimination:
    assessment guide, 80, 295
    normal patterns, 296–297
        interference with, 314
    sociological considerations, 150, 296
    special problems (see Anal incontinence;
        Urinary incontinence)
    (See also Bladder function; Bowel
        function)
Embolus, 353–355
    air, 354–355
    related to immobility, 227, 239–241
    thromboembolism, 353–354
Emotion:
    in client-nurse relationships, 63–64, 173
    in diarrhea, 312
    in elevated body temperature, 397
    in pain experiences, 450
    (See also Anxiety; Interpersonal
        relationships)
Empathy, 63–64, 88
Enema, 306–307
    hazards associated with, 307
    kinds of, 306
    purpose of, 306
Environment:
    assessment guide, 78
    as factor: in illness, 7–10, 191–192
        in respiratory disease, 378–379
    nurses' role in, 178, 205–211, 378–379
    pathogen control, 183–191
    safety, 178, 179
    sensory, 196
    (See also Sensory-perceptual deprivation)
Epidemiologist, nurse as, 186
Epidemiology in infection control, 185,
    186, 190
Epidermis, 410
Esteem, need for, 53, 56, 143
Evaluation:
    of learned material, 174, 286
    of nursing care, 121–122

Evaporation in body temperature
    regulation, 396
Examination and observation in diagnostic
    process, 93–95
Exercise:
    contraindications for, 261
    effect of, on oxygen requirements, 365
    isometric, 230, 233, 260–261
    isotonic, 233, 260
    range of joint motion, 251, 258–260
    tolerance, related to immobility, 227–228

Fact, definition of, 110
Family:
    effect of illness upon, 152–153
    functions of, 151
    variations in roles, 152
Fecal impaction, 311–312
    definition of, 245, 311
    in immobility, 311
Feminist movement, effect of, on nursing,
    29
Fever(s):
    characteristic patterns of, 403
    and chills, management of, 402–405, 407
    effect of, on basal metabolic rate, 395
    hypothalamic regulation, 402
    metabolic use, 404
    nursing care for, 402–404
    of unknown origin (FUO), 403
    (See also Hyperthermia)
Fibrosis, joint: prevention of, 230, 251,
    258–259
    related to immobility, 230
Filtration, 330
Flatulence, 308–310
    distention, 310
    factors associated with, 309
    normal production of gases, 308–309
    nursing care measures, 310
    postoperative, 310, 381
    relief of symptoms, 310
Flotation pads, 431
Fluid-electrolyte homeostasis, 326–341
    assessment guide, 80–81, 320
    electrolyte concentration, 329, 335–336
    factors regulating fluid movement,
        321–322, 330–335
    high-risk patients, 341
    measurement, 336–337
    (See also Electrolytes)
Fluid volume, 327, 330–335
    in adults, illustrated, 328
    causes of gains and loss in, 332
        illustrated, 331
    in children, illustrated, 328
    depletion of, 333–334
        saline, 332, 333
        water, 332
    losses in, 330
    sodium as regulator, 332–334
Fluoridation as a means of decreasing
    dental caries, 287
Folk medicine, 4, 24–25
Food:
    daily food guide, 273
    eating patterns, 272, 280

Food:
  feeding, 288
  physical factors in intake, 279, 286-287,
      290
  regional and ethnic patterns, 281
  regulation of intake, 278-280
  religious influences, 280, 281
  social and economic factors, 280-282,
      290
  substitutions in diets, 284
Food and Agriculture Organization (FAO),
    resources for nutritional composition
    of indigenous foods, 272
Food and Drug Administration, 273, 418
Food and Nutrition Board, National
    Academy of Sciences, 272
Food habits:
  as affected by social, cultural, and
      environmental factors, 282-286, 288
  changing, 282, 284
  in relation to being fed, 288
Frostbite, 406

Generativity vs. self-absorption, adult
    developmental task, 158
Grief:
  as part of dying, 147
  as part of rehabilitation, 265-266
Guilt during psychosocial development,
    155

Hair, 411, 415
Hallucinations:
  dealing with, 214-215
  in sensory-perceptual restriction, 202,
      214
Handwashing, importance of, to diminish
    spread of pathogens, 186
Health:·
  concept of, 3-4
  definition, of, 5, 6, 10
    affected by sociocultural differences,
        12-20, 149
  and illness, 6, 8-11
  and wellness, 4-5, 9-10
Health care:
  delivery, 21-22
  goals of, 22
  and mobility, 221
  and nursing, 25
  recipients of, 26-27
  scientific models, 4-10, 24
  sociocultural factors as determinants of
      the sick role, 21-22, 149
Health status, 7-8
Health team, 29-32
Heart as example of concept, 134-135
Heat adaptation, 398
Heat stroke, 406
Helplessness as response to anxiety (flight
    behavior), 165
Hemoglobin, saturation, 367-368
Hemorrhage as cause of hypovolemia,
    357-358
Hexachlorophene, 418
  use of: contraindications to, 418
    in preventing skin infection, 418

Homeostasis, 7, 198
  fluid-electrolyte (*see* Fluid-electrolyte
      homeostasis)
Hopelessness, 165
Hospitalization:
  anxiety in, 56, 159-160
  of children, 65
  and limitation on mobility, 223
  and nosocomial infections, 184
  orienting patient to, 57
Hunger:
  factors affecting, 278-280
  stimulus to, 282
Hydrogen-ion concentration, 336-341
  disorders of, 340-341
Hygiene, personal, 415-421
  bathing, 416-418
  hair and nails, 415, 419-420
  handwashing, 186
  influence of values, 416
  maintenance of values, 416
  perineal cleansing, 246, 418-419
  providing for, 417
  role of, in development of pressure
      sores, 424
Hyperbaric oxygen, use of, in pressure sore
    treatment, 433
Hypercapnia (hypercarbia), 364, 369
Hyperemia in pressure sore development,
    246, 425
Hypernatremia, 334, 335
Hyperosmolarity, 334
Hyperthermia, 402-406
Hypocapnia (hypocarbia), 364, 369
Hypodermis, 410
Hyponatremia, 334
Hypoosmolarity, 334
Hypotension, postural, 358
  related to immobility, 237-238
  as sign of compensated shock, 358
Hypothermia, 406-407
  and bradycardia, 324
Hypoventilation, alveolar, 366, 379-382
  approaches to, 387
  definition of, 366
  factors contributing to, 379-380
  pathophysiology, 366
  post-operative, 379
  ventilatory aids, 380-381
Hypovolemia, 333-334
  (*See also* Fluid volume, depletion of;
      Shock)
Hypovolemic shock, 357-358
Hypoxemia, 365-369
  causes of, 365-367, 380
  definition of, 364, 365
Hypoxia, 365
  definition of, 364, 365
  factors contributing to, 365, 368-369
Hypoxic drive, 371

Identity vs. self-diffusion, adolescent
    development task, 156-157
Ileostomy, 314-315
Illness:
  changes in temperature, 397
  children's response to hospitalization, as
      factor in, 65-67

Illness:
  classification of, 5-10
  concept of, 4-10
  data gathering, 18
  definition of, 11-14
    affected by sociocultural differences, 4,
        13-14
  ecological systems theory, 7-10
  experience, 10
  multiple-causation theory, 6-7
  nature of, 21
  nonscientific causes of, 4, 5
  patient experience, 13, 16-18
  perception of, 4, 17-18
  scientific orientation, 4-5
  and sick-role enactment, 16, 20-22
  single-agent theory of, 5-6
  social processes in, 14-15, 20-22, 152
  stages of, 15-19
  symbolic and real loss, 17-18
  transition from health, 15
  transition to wellness, 19-20
  variations in response to, 16-19
  verification of, 17
Immobility:
  concept of, 224
  consequences of, 224
  effects of, 200, 203, 222, 224
  extent of, 224, 248
  nursing management, 247-263, 371
  pathological consequences of:
    contractures, 230
    fracture, 233
    hypoventilation, 380
    loss of muscle tone, 227
    nerve damage, 233
    pneumonia, 236
    pulmonary embolism, 237
    renal stones, 243
    thrombosis, 239-241
    urinary retention, 243
  physiological consequences of (*see*
      Disuse phenomena)
  therapeutic use of, 222-223
  (*See also* Mobility)
Incontinence:
  anal, 313-314
  bladder, 300
  stress, 300
Independence:
  development of autonomy, 155
  development of initiative, 155
  as related to need for achievement, 148
Industry vs. inferiority, developmental task,
    156
Infarct:
  myocardial, 222
  pulmonary, 227
Infection:
  association with nutritional deficiency,
      275
  chain of, 184-185
  control of: antibiotic development,
      183-184
    by epidemiologist, 185, 186
    historical perspective of, 183
    microbial control, 184, 185
    nurses' role in, 185, 190
    resistant strains of pathogens, 184

Infection:
in pressure sores, 433
Infusion, intravenous, 350-355
microbial dangers of, 190
Inhalation therapy:
microbial dangers of, 190
postoperative, 382
Initiative vs. guilt, childhood development task, 155
Insomnia (see Sleep, disorders of)
Integrity vs. despair, late-adult development task, 158
Integument, 410-436
assessment guide, 82
Interaction, 38-40, 51
communication patterns, 38
Intercellular fluid (interstitial), 327
Interpersonal relationship, 49-51
movement in, 59-65
skills useful in, 53-57
tools of self, 49, 55-57
Interstitial fluid, 327
Intervention, nursing, 107-129
basis of, 112
collaboration with patient-client, 97-99, 113
compatibility with client's beliefs and attitude, 113, 115-118
concept selection, 112, 135-138
coordination of activities, 120-121
evaluation of, 112, 119, 121-122, 174
examples of, 107
feasibility of solution, 118-119
goals and objectives of: conflict in, 113-114
defining, 112-119, 174
implementation, 119-121
interpersonal relationships in, 49-50
model, illustrated, 109
modification, 122
objectives, statement of, 113
problems: defining, 108
priority setting, 114-115, 119
process, 108
recording, 122-128
referral, 120
selection of action, 108, 111, 115
sociological factors affecting, 116-118
solutions, 115
use of theoretical base, 108, 115-116
Interview, 83-93
assessment, 85-86
atmosphere favorable to communication, 86
evaluation, 93, 104-106
intentions of nurse, table, 84
maintaining momentum, 85
purpose of, 83-85
roles assumed in, 84-85
setting for, 92-93
structure of, 89-90
techniques: for facilitating communication, 85-88, 90-91
for inhibiting communication, 91-92
termination, 93
Intimacy vs. isolation, adult developmental task, 157
Intracellular fluid, 327
Intravascular fluid, 327

Intravenous therapy, 350-355
complications, 190, 352-355
embolism, 353
hyperalimentation, 242
infection, 190, 352
infiltration, 350, 351
nursing responsibilities, 350-352
patient discomfort, 350
septicemia, 352-353
thrombophlebitis, 350
IPPB (intermittent positive-pressure breathing), 382
Isolation:
for infection control, 191
definition of, 186-187
rationale for selection, 188
setting, 188
types of, 187
social, 191, 199, 207
(See also Sensory-perceptual restriction)
Isometric exercises:
contraindications to, 261
in prevention of muscle atrophy, 230, 260
in prevention of osteoporosis, 233
Isotonic exercises in mobility, 233, 260

Joint mobility:
exercises to maintain, 251, 258-261
loss of, 230
passive exercises for, 251

Kidney, relationship of, to hydrogen-ion concentration, 339

Lanugo, 411
Laxatives, 307
Leadership, 30-31, 41-42
Learning:
in anxiety continuum, 160-161
in changing food habits, 285-286
concept of, 171-172
and malnutrition, 276
meaningful, 171
as part of coping with health problems, 171-172
planning for, 171-175
Lesions, skin, 414
Level of consciousness:
alterations, causes of, 169
assessment of, 169-170
definition of, 169
Life, value placed on, 145
Love, need for, 143

Maceration, 424
Magnesium in fluid-electrolyte homeostasis, 336
Malnutrition:
associated with poverty, 273, 276
effect of: on behavior, 276-277
on health, 274
on mental and physical growth, 275-276

Maslow's hierarchy of human needs, 52-53, 142-144
Massage, 420-421
back, 420
contraindications in extremities, 420
in pressure sore prevention, 432
strokes for, 420
Medical asepsis, 185
Medical record (see Problem-oriented record)
Medical therapy:
differing focus from nursing intervention, 28
in fluid-electrolyte disturbances, 340, 341
in immobility, 222, 248
in pain, 454
table, 458
in shock, 359-360
in thrombophlebitis, 241
Melanin, 411, 412
Mental and emotional status assessment guide, 78, 140
Metabolism:
basal, 223, 242
body heat and, 395
exercise and, 365
fever and, 365
oxygen use and, 373
Microorganisms:
knowledge of, in infection control, 183-184
major types of, in hospital infection, 184
pathogenic, 183
resident, 186
transfer of, 183, 189
transient, 186
Micturition, 297-299
normal innervation, illustrated, 298
process of emptying bladder, 297
reflexes associated with, 297, 299
(See also Urine)
Mistrust (see Trust, development of, in infancy)
Mobility:
factors altering, 221-224
safety factors, 180
(See also Immobility)
Model:
of communication in social systems, 39
of health care, 24-25
the nurse as, of healthy interpersonal relationships, 55
Monotony, perceptual (see Sensory-perceptual restriction)
Motor status assessment guide, 79, 220
Mucus:
function of, 385
removal of, 386

Nails, care of, 419-420
National Commission for the Study of Nursing and Nursing Education, 31
Needs, basic human: definitions of, 52-53, 142
development of, 142-144
effect of, on behavior, 142, 158
hierarchy (Maslow), 52-53, 114, 142
in nurse-client relationship, 52-53, 114

Neurogenic shock, 358
Nitrogen balance as related to immobility, 242
Norms, 35-36
 health, 12-14, 99-100
 implicit and explicit, 35-36
 influence on behavior, 35
 professional, 99
 social and cultural factors, 35-36, 42-43, 99-100
Nosocomial infection (hospital-acquired), 184
Nurse(s):
 associate degree, 31
 in baccalaureate programs, 31
 clinical specialist, 29
 education of, 30-31, 99
 functions of, 29, 30
 licensed vocational, 30
 practitioners, 29
 "Primex," 29
 professional, 30, 31
 registered, 30
 relationship of, with children, 65-67
 role of, in promoting and facilitating change in health care systems, 29, 43
 self-insight of, 57-58
 status and prestige of, 40-41
 technical, 31
Nurses' notes (see Problem-oriented record)
Nursing, 27-32
 career ladders, 32
 focus and goals of nursing care, 27-29
  definition of focus, 28
 and health care models, 25-26
 historical development of, 28-29
 process of (see Diagnostic process in nursing; Intervention, nursing)
 role of, 25-27, 29, 37-38
  collaborative: with client, 97-99, 116
   on health team, 29-30, 120
  independent, 28-29
  modern, evolution of, 29
 team, 29-32
Nursing action (see Intervention, nursing)
Nursing assessment (see Diagnostic process in nursing)
Nursing care planning:
 perception of the illness experience, 17-19
 (See also Intervention, nursing)
Nursing diagnosis (see Diagnosis)
Nursing orders, 120
Nursing process (see Diagnostic process in nursing; Intervention, nursing)
Nursing team, 29-32
Nutrition:
 adequate, definition of, 273
 assessment guide, 80, 270
 cultural and individual variations, 270-272, 280-282
 deviations from good nutritional status, 273-275
 effect of, on physical and mental growth, 275-276
 factors in nutritional status, 277
 guides to assessment of groups, 272-273, 287-288

Nutrition:
 minimum daily requirements, 273
 nursing management and, 287-293
 optimum, 292
 poverty and, 281
 and pressure sores, 424, 432-433
 recommended dietary allowances, 272, 273
 in relation to health and disease, 275
  illustrated, 271
Nutrition Survey, National, 276
Nutritional deficiency diseases, 273, 275, 276, 312

Obesity:
 in association with weight loss and control, 290
 definition of, 289
 and pressure sores, 422-423
 scientific experiments and, 290
 treatment, 290
Objectives:
 in learning, 174
 in nursing care planning, 112-114
Observation in diagnostic process, 83, 93-95
Oral hygiene, 347-348, 387
 evaluation of, 348
 with thirst, 347-348
Organization, social, and role behavior, 37-38
Osmolarity, 329, 336
 (See also Fluid-electrolyte homeostasis)
Osmosis, 329-330
Osteoporosis as related to immobility, 230, 232
Overhydration (see Water balance)
Overload, sensory (see Sensory-perceptual overload)
Overnutrition, 274-275
 (See also Obesity)
Ovulation as a factor in temperature variation, 397
Oxygen (see Respiration)
Oxygenation (see Respiration)

Pain, 445-460
 anxiety in, 448, 450, 452-456
 assessment of, 457-459
 behavior, 446, 449
 "gate-control" theory, 448
 intervention, 459-460
  table, 454-455
 learned aspects, 449
 management, nursing, 453-457
 nervous transmission, 446-448
 "pain-prone" behavior, 450, 454
 reaction to, 446, 449, 451-453
 relation to hypoventilation, 380, 381
 sociocultural factors, 449-451
 symbolism in, 451
Panic as level of anxiety, 160
Parenteral fluids (see Intravenous therapy)
Partial pressure:
 of carbon dioxide, 369
 of oxygen, 365
Pathogen (see Microorganism)

Patient, connotations of the word, 26
Patient-client:
 characteristics of relationship of, with nurse, 58-59
 self-concept of, 57
 usage defined, 26-27
Perineal cleansing, 418-419
Perspiration, 414
pH (see Hydrogen-ion concentration)
Physician:
 focus of care by, 27, 28
  compared with nursing focus, illustrated, 28
 as health team member, 27, 28, 30
 status of, 40
Placebo effect, 456-457
Play as a tool for child assessment, 66-67
Politics, role of, in the concept of authority, 42
Position of bed patient:
 prone, illustrated, 256, 257
 side lying, illustrated, 254, 255
 supine, illustrated, 252, 253
 Trendelenburg, contraindication for shock, 360
 use of, to prevent complications of immobility, 248-251
Posture, use of, in preventing disuse phenomena, 248-251
Potassium, role of, in electrical activity, 335
Potassium concentration, intracellular, 335, 337
Potassium depletion, 337-338
Potassium excess, 338
Power, role of, in the concept of authority, 42
Pressure:
 and circulatory stasis, 239, 241
 and ischemia, 422, 425
 as primary cause of pressure sores, 249, 422
Pressure sores, 421-435
 categorization of, 425
 causative factors, 422-424
 contributory factors, illustrated, 247, 424-425
 definition of, 246
 development and healing, 425-430
 in high-risk patients, 421-422
 immobility, related to, 246-247
 pathogenesis, 421-422
 prevention of, 430-433
 signs of, 246, 425
 treatment for, 433-435
 types of, 425
 water beds, 431
Principle, definition of, 110
Problem-oriented record, 122-129
 advantages of, 128-129
 characteristics of, 123-128
 rationale of, 122
Problem-solving as application of scientific method, 70
 (See also Diagnostic process in nursing; Intervention, nursing)
Professional relationship, 51, 58-59
Prognosis in nursing care, 113
Projection, 161

Proteins:
    deficiencies, 273-274, 312
    in fluid homeostasis, 329
    loss in immobility, 242
    in nutrition, 274, 276
Psychogenic pain, 460
Psychosocial status:
    assessment data, 77, 140
    influence of: on client-nurse relationship,
        141
        on definitions of health and illness, 13,
            141, 149
        on learning, 174
        on nutrition, 280-282
        on outcome of nursing care plan,
            116-118
        on pain experience, 448-450
    as related to immobility, 226-227
Pulmonary function tests, 377-378
    use of, in medical diagnosis of
        pulmonary disease, 378
Pulmonary therapy:
    aids useful in, 381-382
    mechanical assistance, 382
    postural drainage, 382
Pulse:
    determining rate of, 323, 324
    points for palpation, illustrated, 323
Pulse deficit, 324
Pulse pressure, 325

Radiation as means of losing body heat,
    395
Rales, 374
Range-of-motion exercises, illustrated,
    258-259
    (See also Joint mobility)
Rashes, skin, 414
Rationalization, 162
Record, medical (see Problem-oriented
    record)
Reference group as factor in defining
    illness, 15, 19
Regression:
    in anxiety, 162, 165
    in illness, 59, 65, 162, 166
Rehabilitation, 264-266
    nurse's role in, 266
    as a process, 265
    team in, 264
Relationship:
    with children, 65-67
    movements within, 59-62
    nurse-client, 58-63
    professional, 51, 56-57
    tasks within, 58-59
    termination of, 64-65
Religion and health care, 150-151
Repression, 162
Respiration, 364-369
    carbon dioxide, role of, in respiratory
        rate, 370-371
    character and effort of breathing,
        372-374
    disease, 377-379
        history of, 376
        living with limitations, 377, 383

Respiration:
    external, 364
    hypoxic drive, 371
    internal (cellular), 364
    laboratory tests, 377-378
    limitations on activity by disease,
        373-374, 383
    mental changes with increased CO_2 and
        decreased O_2, 375
    metabolism associated with, 373, 383
    nursing care of patients with respiratory
        dysfunction, 374, 378-387
    physiological changes, 370-371, 375
    posture and movement effect on, 371,
        374, 385
    rate, 370, 372-374
        regulation, 370-371
    terminology used to describe, 371
    shunting, 366, 380
    (See also Hypercapnia; Hypocapnia;
        Hypoxemia; Hypoxia)
Respiratory assessment guide, 81-82, 363
Respiratory rate, 372-373
Respiratory status, 369-378
    (See also Respiration)
Restraints, mechanical: precautions for,
    182
    use of, for safety, 182
Resuscitation, cardiopulmonary (CPR),
    382-383
Review of literature:
    in diagnosis, 95-96
    as method of validating, planning, and
        evaluating intervention, 108-112
Rhonchi, 374
Role:
    assumed by health professionals, 37-38
    authority, 40, 41
    behavior, 37-38
    clarifying and changing, 62-63
    complementary, 38
    conflicts in perception, 61
    deliberative establishment, 58, 61
    gaps in health-care delivery, 38
    of interviewee, 88-89
    of interviewer, 84-88
    mothering, 62-63
    of nurse, 27-29, 37, 57-60
        conflict in, 37-38, 62-63
    overlapping of health services, 37
    of patient-client, 61-62
    sick, 15-16, 153
    stereotyping, 60-62

Safety:
    in home, 180
    in hospital, 180-181
    needs for, 142
    (See also Accidents)
Safety hazards, potential, 179
    use of restraints, 182
Saline depletion, 312
Satiety, 278, 282
Science:
    nursing as applied science, 70
    scientific approach to medicine, 4, 24-26

Scientific method:
    comparison between scientist and
        practitioner's use, 72-73
    definition of, 69
    difficulty in use, 71-73
    use of, in nursing, 71
Scientist, 70
Sebum, 411
Self:
    altered by disease, 165, 173, 264-265
    awareness of, as part of consciousness,
        169
    fulfillment of, 143
    perception of, 173
Self-concept, 55-57
    development of, 55
    personal, 55-56, 165
    professional, 56-57
Sensation:
    perception, 195, 197-198
    sensoristasis, 198-199, 211
    sensory modalities, 196-197
    sensory status, 195
Sensitivity in client-nurse relationship,
    59-60
Sensory assessment guide, 78, 194
Sensory-perceptual deprivation (see
    Sensory-perceptual restriction)
Sensory-perceptual overload:
    clinical, 209, 212, 214
        management, 207, 214, 217
        patients, risk of, 192, 209, 212, 213,
            215
    definition of, 200
    differentiation from sensory-perceptual
        restriction, 200, 214
    effects of, 192, 200, 207, 215
    experimental, 198-200
Sensory-perceptual restriction:
    clinical: acute syndrome, 191, 203,
        214-215
        chronic syndrome, 204, 215-216
        management, 205-207, 213-217
        patients, risk of, 191, 209-213
        prevention of, 207, 211-212
    definitions of, 191, 199-200
    developmental effects of, 198, 204-205,
        211-212
    effects of, 199-202
    experimental, 198-202
    as factor in safety, 181
    related to immobility, 200, 234-235
    structuring environment to prevent, 191,
        205-207
    tolerance for, 202, 212-213
Sensory stimulation, 198
Septic shock, 358
Septicemia, 352
Sex:
    discrimination and social status
        differences, 40
    as factor in temperature regulation, 397
Sexuality as part of adult development,
    157-158
Shearing force as causative factor in
    pressure sores, 423-424
Sheepskin (see Pressure sores, prevention
    of)

Shock, 357–360
  classification of, 357–358
  diagnosis, 358, 359
  management, 358–360
  mechanism, 359
Shunting (see Respiration)
Sick role, 16, 153
Sighing, role of, in reducing CO_2 levels, 381
Skin:
  aging, 415
  assessment of, 412–415
  breakdown, 415
  functions of, 411
Sleep, 438–445
  assessment of need for, 443
  character of, 440
  cycles, 438–440
    factors affecting, 440–441
    phases (NREM, REM), 438
  deprivation, 442–443
  disorders, 444–445
  and dreams, 441–442
  function of, 438, 442
  physiological changes during, 441
Smegma, 418
Soap, effects of, on skin, 417–418
Sodium, 332–335
  hypernatremia, 334
  hyponatremia, 335
Sodium balance, 332
Sodium regulation, 332–335
Sponge bath, use of, in fever, 405–406
Status, 40–41
  achieved, 40
  ascribed, 40
  nursing, 40
  patient-client, 41
  and prestige, 40
  social, 40
Sterilization, 189
Stones, renal, related to immobility, 242–243
Stool:
  changes in food or medication affecting, 241, 308
  characteristics of, 307–308
  composition of, 307
    abnormal, 308
    normal, 308
    odor, 308
  (See also Defecation)
Stress, psychosocial, 158, 166–167
  (See also Anxiety)
Sublimation, 162
Suppression, 162
Surgical asepsis, 185
System behavior, 34–37
  components of, 36–37
  cultural, 35
  social, 35
Systems, 34–44
Systolic pressure, 325
  in hypovolemia, 333

Tachypnea, 371
Teaching (see Learning, planning for)
Team (see Health team; Nursing team)

Teeth (see Oral hygiene)
Temperature, 390–409
  assessment guide, 82, 390
  disturbances in maintenance of, 402–407
  effect of shivering, 395
  environmental control, 391, 397–398
  environmental effects, 391
  factors affecting, 396–399
  loss of heat, 391, 395
    adaptive mechanisms, 395
    environmental alterations, 395
    physical principles, 395–396
  maintenance and regulation factors, 391–394, 402–404, 411
  measurement, 392
    recommended time, 401–402
  negative feedback concept, 394
  production of heat, 391, 394–395
    diurnal variations, 396
  role of hypothalamus, 402
  (See also Hyperthermia; Hypothermia)
Temperature recording, 392, 399–402
  accuracy, 399
  clinical studies, 399–401
  determination of route, 399–400
  placement, accurate, as factor, 402
Theories of illness, 5–10
  ecological systems, 7–10
  multiple-causation, 6–7
  single-agent, 5–6
Theory, definition of, 110
Thermometer, 399–400
Thirst:
  associated with fluid restriction, 331, 346, 349
  as a learned or conditioned stimulus, 331, 346–347
  measures to relieve, 347, 350
  physiology, 346
  preventive nursing care, 347–350
Time:
  of day, effect of, on temperature rhythm, 396
  value of, 148–149
Time cycle change, effect of, on body temperature, 396
Trendelenburg position, contraindication for, in shock, 360
Trust:
  in client-nurse relationship, 63
  development of, in infancy, 154
Turgor, skin, 413

Undernutrition, 274
Understanding, 87–88
Urinary diversion, 302–304
Urinary incontinence, 300
Urinary retention, 301–302
  causes of, 243–244, 301
  characteristic signs of, 301
  with overflow, 244
  as related to immobility, 244
Urine:
  abnormal route of excretion, 302–304
  appearance and characteristics of, 299–300
    abnormal, 299
    normal, 299–300

Urine:
  changes in: with drug administration, 241, 299
    in immobility, 242
  formation and storage, 299
  volume excreted, 299

Valsalva maneuver, danger of, 261
Values:
  of freedom, 41
  influence of social class values on behavior, 35, 148–149
  in planning nursing care, 116
Vaporization of water in body temperature regulation, 396
Ventilation:
  abnormalities, 366–367
  alteration with postural changes, 367
  alveolar function, 366, 369
  alveolar hypoventilation, 366
  post-operative complications, 379–380
  (See also Respiration)
Vital signs, 322–326
  blood pressure, 325–326
    changes in saline depletion, 333, 359
    diastolic, 325
    measurement, 325
    mechanism of maintaining, 325
    systolic, 325
  discrimination in routine use of, 326
  pulse, 322–325
    abnormalities, 323
    accuracy, 323
    alterations: in rate, 323
      in rhythm, 324–325
    bradycardia, 324
    deficit, 323
    as indicator of activity tolerance, 324
    tachycardia, 324
    use of, in nursing care, 324
  respiratory rate, 372–378
    as poor single indicator of respiratory status, 372
    (See also Respiration)
  as rough estimate of function, 325
  temperature, 392, 399–402
Volume depletion (see Fluid volume)
Volume excess (see Fluid volume)
Vomiting:
  in electrolyte imbalance, 337, 340
  in volume depletion, 333

Water balance, 334–335
  disturbances in, 333, 334
Water beds, 431
Well role, 13–14
  resumption of, after illness, 19–20
Wellness, 6–7, 9–10
World Health Organization, definition of health by, 6
Wound healing as related to pressure sores, 429–430, 433

Yawning as aid to prevent atelectasis, 380